From the most trusted sou...
he only CPT® codebook wi...
CPT coding rules and guidelines developed
by the CPT Editorial Panel.

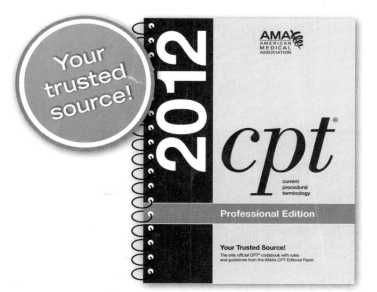

Correctly interpreting and reporting medical procedures and services begins with *CPT® 2012 Professional Edition*. Straight from the American Medical Association (AMA), this is the only CPT® codebook with the official CPT coding rules and guidelines developed by the CPT Editorial Panel. Covers hundreds of code, guideline, and text changes.

Available October 2011, spiralbound, 8 ½" x 11", 760 pages

Item #: EP888812 ISBN: 978-1-60359-568-1

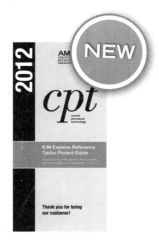

Purchase direct from the AMA and receive a FREE *2012 E/M Express Reference Tables Pocket Guide.** This quick reference guide provides a side-by-side comparison of E/M codes in a CPT section.

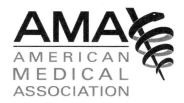

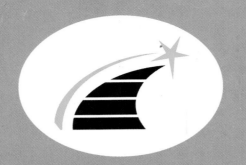
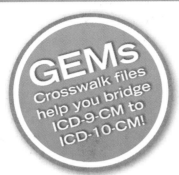
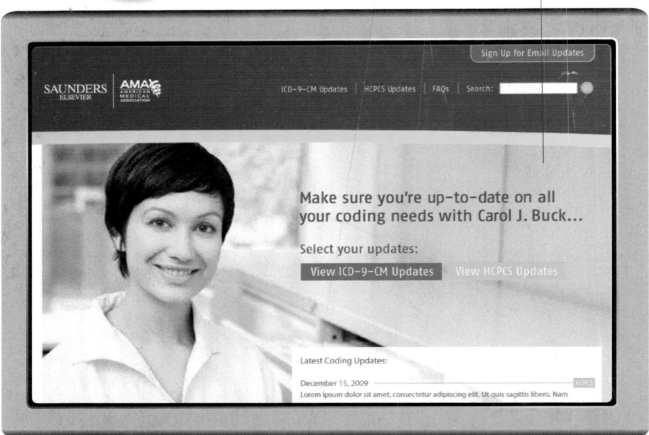

2012
HCPCS Level II

PROFESSIONAL EDITION

INCLUDES NETTER'S ANATOMY ART

2012
HCPCS Level II

Carol J. Buck
MS, CPC, CPC-H, CCS-P

Former Program Director; Medical Secretary Programs
Northwest Technical College; East Grand Forks, Minnesota

ELSEVIER

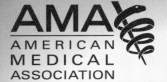

AMA
AMERICAN
MEDICAL
ASSOCIATION

3251 Riverport Lane
St. Louis, Missouri 63043

2012 HCPCS LEVEL II PROFESSIONAL EDITION   ISBN: 978-1-4557-0770-6

Notices

Knowledge and best practice in this field are constantly changing. As new research and experience broaden our understanding, changes in research methods, professional practices, or medical treatment may become necessary.

Practitioners and researchers must always rely on their own experience and knowledge in evaluating and using any information, methods, compounds, or experiments described herein. In using such information or methods they should be mindful of their own safety and the safety of others, including parties for whom they have a professional responsibility.

With respect to any drug or pharmaceutical products identified, readers are advised to check the most current information provided (i) on procedures featured or (ii) by the manufacturer of each product to be administered, to verify the recommended dose or formula, the method and duration of administration, and contraindications. It is the responsibility of practitioners, relying on their own experience and knowledge of their patients, to make diagnoses, to determine dosages and the best treatment for each individual patient, and to take all appropriate safety precautions.

To the fullest extent of the law, neither the Publisher nor the authors, contributors, or editors, assume any liability for any injury and/or damage to persons or property as a matter of products liability, negligence or otherwise, or from any use or operation of any methods, products, instructions, or ideas contained in the material herein.

ISBN: 978-1-4557-0770-6

Publisher: Jeanne Olson
Senior Developmental Editor: Jenna Johnson
Publishing Services Manager: Pat Joiner-Myers
Senior Designer: Amy Buxton

Printed in the United States of America

Last digit is the print number: 9 8 7 6 5 4 3 2 1

TECHNICAL COLLABORATORS

Jacqueline Klitz Grass, MA, CPC
Coding Specialist
Grand Forks, North Dakota

Nancy Maguire, ACS, CRT, PCS, FCS, HCS-D, APC, AFC
Physician Consultant for Auditing and Education
University City, Texas

CONTENTS

Updates will be posted on http://codingupdates.com when available.

Check the Centers for Medicare and Medicaid Services (http://www.cms.gov/Manuals/IOM/list.asp) website and http://codingupdates.com for IOMs.

Notice: 2012 DMEPOS updates were unavailable at the time of printing. Check http://codingupdates.com for updates in December. Also available online are the 2012 PQRI Measures List and Specifications Manual.

GUIDE TO USING THE 2012 HCPCS LEVEL II CODES

Medical coding has long been a part of the health care profession. Through the years medical coding systems have become more complex and extensive. Today, medical coding is an intricate and immense process that is present in every health care setting. The increased use of electronic submissions for health care services only increases the need for coders who understand the coding process.

2012 HCPCS Level II was developed to help meet the needs of today's coder.

All material adheres to the latest government versions available at the time of printing.

Annotated

Throughout this text, revisions and additions are indicated by the following symbols:

◄ **New:** Additions to the previous edition are indicated by the color triangle.

← **Revised:** Revisions within the line or code from the previous edition are indicated by the color arrow.

✔ **Reinstated** indicates a code that was previously deleted and has now been reactivated.

✖ deleted words have been removed from this year's edition.

HCPCS Symbols

✪ **Special coverage instructions** apply to these codes. Usually these special coverage instructions are included in the Internet Only Manuals (IOM) select references at http:codingupdates.com.

◆ **Not covered or valid by Medicare** is indicated by the diamond. Usually the reason for the exclusion is included in the Internet Only Manuals (IOM) select references at http:codingupdates.com.

✳ **Carrier discretion** is an indication that you must contact the individual third-party payers to find out the coverage available for codes identified by this symbol.

NDC Drugs approved for Medicare Part B are listed as NDC (National Drug Code). All other FDA-approved drugs are listed as Other.

A2-Z3 **ASC Payment Indicators** identify the 2012 Final OPPS payment for the code. A list of Payment Indicators is listed in the front material of this text.

A-Y **ASC Status Indicators** identify the 2012 Final OPPS status assigned to the code. A list of Status Indicators is listed in the front material of this text.

Coding Clinic Indicates the American Hospital Association *Coding Clinic for HCPCS* references by year, quarter, and page number.

⚀ DMEPOS identifies durable medical equipment, prosthetics, orthotics, and supplies that may be eligible for payment from CMS

♀ Indicates a code for female only

♂ Indicates a code for male only

A Indicates a code with an indication of age

PQRS Indicates a code included in the 2011 PQRS Quality Measure Specifications Manual.

Qp Indicates there is a maximum allowable number of units of service, per day, per patient for physician/provider services (*see* Appendix A, Medically Unlikely Edits)

Qh Indicates there is a maximum allowable number of units of service, per day, per patient in the outpatient hospital setting (*see* Appendix B, Medically Unlikely Edits)

Red, green, and blue typeface terms are terms added by the publisher and do not appear in the official code set.

SYMBOLS AND CONVENTIONS

HCPCS Symbols

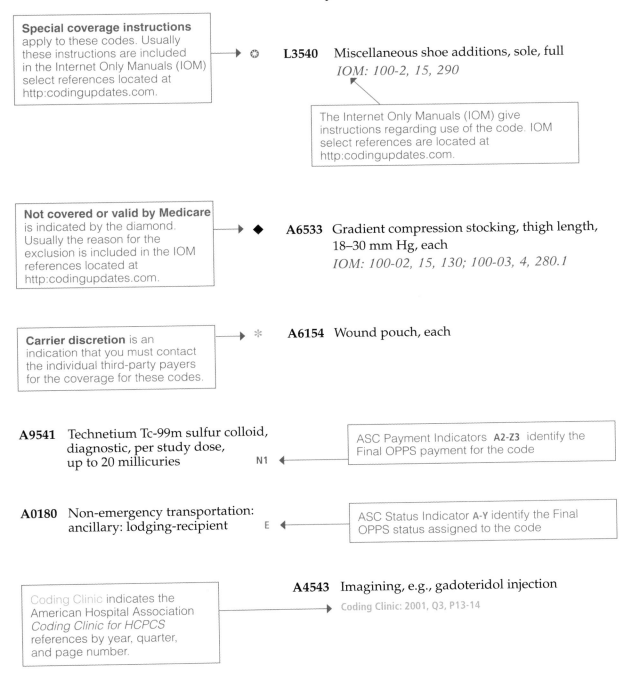

Special coverage instructions apply to these codes. Usually these instructions are included in the Internet Only Manuals (IOM) select references located at http:codingupdates.com.

⊗ **L3540** Miscellaneous shoe additions, sole, full
IOM: 100-2, 15, 290

The Internet Only Manuals (IOM) give instructions regarding use of the code. IOM select references are located at http:codingupdates.com.

Not covered or valid by Medicare is indicated by the diamond. Usually the reason for the exclusion is included in the IOM references located at http:codingupdates.com.

◆ **A6533** Gradient compression stocking, thigh length, 18–30 mm Hg, each
IOM: 100-02, 15, 130; 100-03, 4, 280.1

Carrier discretion is an indication that you must contact the individual third-party payers for the coverage for these codes.

✳ **A6154** Wound pouch, each

A9541 Technetium Tc-99m sulfur colloid, diagnostic, per study dose, up to 20 millicuries   N1

ASC Payment Indicators **A2-Z3** identify the Final OPPS payment for the code

A0180 Non-emergency transportation: ancillary: lodging-recipient   E

ASC Status Indicator **A-Y** identify the Final OPPS status assigned to the code

A4543 Imagining, e.g., gadoteridol injection

Coding Clinic indicates the American Hospital Association *Coding Clinic for HCPCS* references by year, quarter, and page number.

Coding Clinic: 2001, Q3, P13-14

Codes shown are for illustration purposes only and may not be current codes.

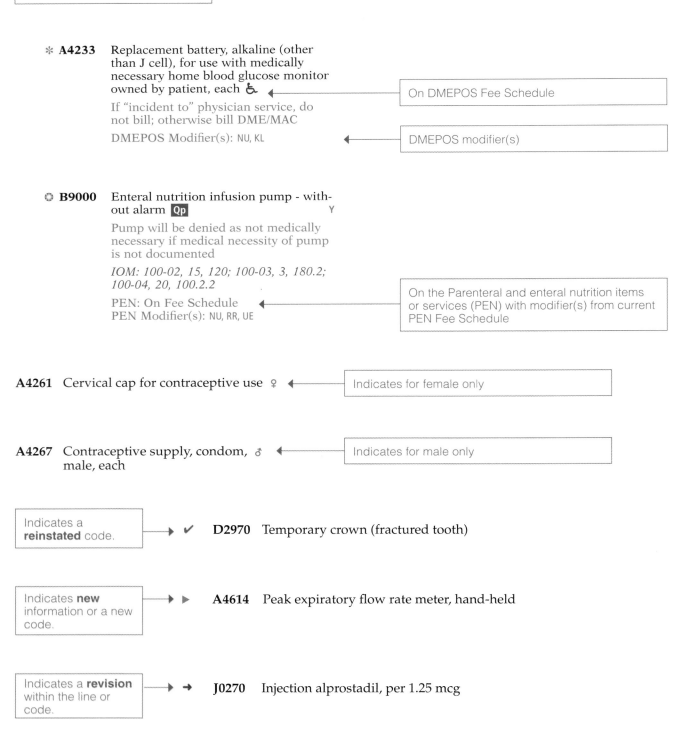

DMEPOS symbol identifies durable medical equipment, prosthetics, orthotics, and supplies that may be eligible for payment from CMS

E2210 Wheelchair accessory, bearings, any type, replacement only, each ♿

※ **A4233** Replacement battery, alkaline (other than J cell), for use with medically necessary home blood glucose monitor owned by patient, each ♿

If "incident to" physician service, do not bill; otherwise bill DME/MAC

DMEPOS Modifier(s): NU, KL

On DMEPOS Fee Schedule

DMEPOS modifier(s)

◐ **B9000** Enteral nutrition infusion pump - without alarm Qp   Y

Pump will be denied as not medically necessary if medical necessity of pump is not documented

IOM: 100-02, 15, 120; 100-03, 3, 180.2; 100-04, 20, 100.2.2

PEN: On Fee Schedule
PEN Modifier(s): NU, RR, UE

On the Parenteral and enteral nutrition items or services (PEN) with modifier(s) from current PEN Fee Schedule

A4261 Cervical cap for contraceptive use ♀

Indicates for female only

A4267 Contraceptive supply, condom, ♂ male, each

Indicates for male only

Indicates a **reinstated** code.

✔ **D2970** Temporary crown (fractured tooth)

Indicates **new** information or a new code.

▶ **A4614** Peak expiratory flow rate meter, hand-held

Indicates a **revision** within the line or code.

➔ **J0270** Injection alprostadil, per 1.25 mcg

Codes shown are for illustration purposes only and may not be current codes.

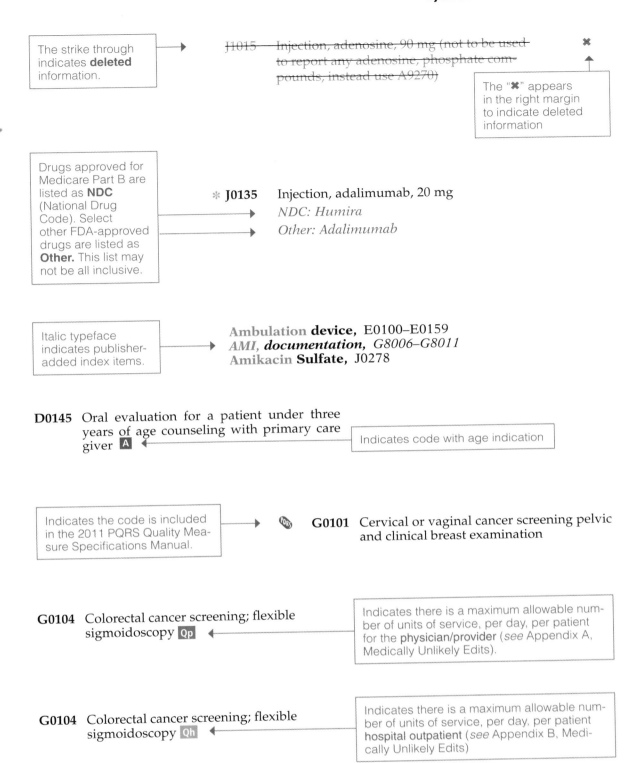

The strike through indicates **deleted** information.

J1015   Injection, adenosine, 90 mg (not to be used to report any adenosine, phosphate compounds, instead use A9270)

The "✖" appears in the right margin to indicate deleted information

Drugs approved for Medicare Part B are listed as **NDC** (National Drug Code). Select other FDA-approved drugs are listed as **Other.** This list may not be all inclusive.

✳ **J0135**   Injection, adalimumab, 20 mg
NDC: Humira
Other: Adalimumab

Italic typeface indicates publisher-added index items.

Ambulation device, E0100–E0159
*AMI, **documentation,** G8006–G8011*
Amikacin Sulfate, J0278

D0145   Oral evaluation for a patient under three years of age counseling with primary care giver **A**

Indicates code with age indication

Indicates the code is included in the 2011 PQRS Quality Measure Specifications Manual.

G0101   Cervical or vaginal cancer screening pelvic and clinical breast examination

G0104   Colorectal cancer screening; flexible sigmoidoscopy **Qp**

Indicates there is a maximum allowable number of units of service, per day, per patient for the **physician/provider** (*see* Appendix A, Medically Unlikely Edits).

G0104   Colorectal cancer screening; flexible sigmoidoscopy **Qh**

Indicates there is a maximum allowable number of units of service, per day, per patient **hospital outpatient** (*see* Appendix B, Medically Unlikely Edits)

Codes shown are for illustration purposes only and may not be current codes.

2012 HCPCS UPDATES

2012 HCPCS New/Revised/Deleted Codes and Modifiers

HCPCS quarterly updates are posted on the companion website (http://www.codingupdates.com) when available.

NEW CODES/MODIFIERS

AY	E0988	G0448	G8653	G8706	G8745	G8783	G8821	G8858	G8895	J2358	L6715
AZ	E1831	G0449	G8654	G8707	G8746	G8784	G8822	G8859	G8896	J2426	L6880
CS	E2358	G0450	G8655	G8708	G8747	G8785	G8823	G8860	G8897	J2507	L8693
DA	E2359	G0451	G8656	G8709	G8748	G8786	G8824	G8861	G8898	J3095	Q0162
GU	E2622	G0908	G8657	G8710	G8749	G8787	G8825	G8862	G8899	J3262	Q0478
GX	E2623	G0909	G8658	G8711	G8750	G8788	G8826	G8863	G8900	J3357	Q0479
NB	E2624	G0910	G8659	G8712	G8751	G8789	G8827	G8864	G8901	J3385	Q2026
PD	E2625	G0911	G8660	G8713	G8752	G8790	G8828	G8865	G8902	J7131	Q2027
PT	E2626	G0912	G8661	G8714	G8753	G8791	G8829	G8866	G8903	J7180	Q2035
A4566	E2627	G0913	G8662	G8715	G8754	G8792	G8830	G8867	G8904	J7183	Q2036
A5056	E2628	G0914	G8663	G8716	G8755	G8793	G8831	G8868	G8905	J7196	Q2037
A5057	E2629	G0915	G8664	G8717	G8756	G8794	G8832	G8869	G8906	J7309	Q2038
A7020	E2630	G0916	G8665	G8718	G8757	G8795	G8833	G8870	G9147	J7312	Q2039
A9272	E2631	G0917	G8666	G8720	G8758	G8796	G8834	G8871	G9156	J7326	Q2043
A9273	E2632	G0918	G8667	G8721	G8759	G8797	G8835	G8872	J0131	J7335	Q4117
A9584	E2633	G0919	G8668	G8722	G8760	G8798	G8836	G8873	J0171	J7665	Q4118
A9585	G0157	G0920	G8669	G8723	G8761	G8799	G8837	G8874	J0221	J7686	Q4119
C1749	G0158	G0921	G8670	G8724	G8762	G8800	G8838	G8875	J0257	J8561	Q4120
C1830	G0159	G0922	G8671	G8725	G8763	G8801	G8839	G8876	J0490	J8562	Q4121
C1840	G0160	G8629	G8672	G8726	G8764	G8802	G8840	G8877	J0558	J9043	Q4122
C1886	G0161	G8630	G8673	G8727	G8765	G8803	G8841	G8878	J0561	J9179	Q4123
C8931	G0162	G8631	G8674	G8728	G8767	G8805	G8842	G8879	J0588	J9228	Q4124
C8932	G0163	G8632	G8682	G8730	G8768	G8806	G8843	G8880	J0597	J9302	Q4125
C8933	G0164	G8633	G8683	G8731	G8769	G8807	G8844	G8881	J0638	J9307	Q4126
C8934	G0428	G8634	G8685	G8732	G8770	G8808	G8845	G8882	J0712	J9315	Q4127
C8935	G0429	G8635	G8694	G8733	G8771	G8809	G8846	G8883	J0775	J9351	Q4128
C8936	G0434	G8642	G8695	G8734	G8772	G8810	G8847	G8884	J0840	K0741	Q4129
C9275	G0436	G8643	G8696	G8735	G8773	G8811	G8848	G8885	J0897	K0742	Q4130
C9279	G0437	G8644	G8697	G8736	G8774	G8812	G8849	G8886	J1290	K0743	Q5010
C9285	G0438	G8645	G8698	G8737	G8775	G8813	G8850	G8887	J1557	K0744	S0119
C9286	G0439	G8646	G8699	G8738	G8776	G8814	G8851	G8888	J1559	K0745	S0148
C9287	G0442	G8647	G8700	G8739	G8777	G8815	G8852	G8889	J1599	K0746	S0169
C9366	G0443	G8648	G8701	G8740	G8778	G8816	G8853	G8890	J1725	L3674	S3722
C9367	G0444	G8649	G8702	G8741	G8779	G8817	G8854	G8891	J1786	L4631	S8130
C9732	G0445	G8650	G8703	G8742	G8780	G8818	G8855	G8892	J1826	L5312	S8131
C9800	G0446	G8651	G8704	G8743	G8781	G8819	G8856	G8893	J2265	L5961	T1505
E0446	G0447	G8652	G8705	G8744	G8782	G8820	G8857	G8894			

REVISED CODES/MODIFIERS

Change in Short Description
GA
RA
RB
V5
V6
V7
A4399
A5112
A6011
A6248
A6260
A6261
A6262
A7013
B4034
B4035
B4036

E0637
E0638
E0641
E0642
E0691
G0151
G0152
G0153
G0154
G0406
G0407
G0408
G0425
G0426
G0427
G0431
G0432
G0433
G0435

G8427
G8428
G8431
G8432
G8433
G8447
G8448
G8482
G8509
G8510
G8511
G8539
G8542
G8553
G8573
G8574
G8575
G8576
G8577

G8578
G8580
G8583
G8586
G8605
G8608
G8611
G8614
G8617
G8620
G8623
G8626
J0129
J0220
J0256
J0598
J1561
J9060
L2005

L3671
L3677
L6000
L6010
L6020
L7368
Q0499
Q4101
Q4102
Q4103
Q4104
Q4105
Q4106
Q4107
Q4108
Q4110
Q4111
Q4112
Q4113

Q4115
Q4116
S9900

Change in Administration
SC
A6530
A6533
A6534
A6535
A6536
A6537
A6538
A6539
A6540
A6541
A6544
A6545

A6549
E0765
E0978
E1161
G0306
G0307
G0339
G0340
K0730

Change in Short Description
J9208
K0669
K0899

Miscellaneous Change
A4619

DELETED CODES/MODIFIERS

C9255
C9256
C9258
C9259
C9260
C9261
C9262
C9263
C9264
C9265
C9266
C9267
C9268
C9269
C9270
C9271
C9272
C9273
C9274
C9276
C9277
C9278
C9280
C9281
C9282
C9283
C9284
C9365
C9406
C9729
C9730
C9731
C9801
C9802
E0220
E0230
E0238
E0571

G0430
G0440
G0441
G8006
G8007
G8008
G8009
G8010
G8011
G8012
G8013
G8014
G8015
G8016
G8017
G8018
G8019
G8020
G8021
G8022
G8023
G8024
G8025
G8026
G8027
G8028
G8029
G8030
G8031
G8032
G8033
G8034
G8035
G8036
G8037
G8038
G8039

G8040
G8041
G8051
G8052
G8053
G8054
G8055
G8056
G8057
G8058
G8059
G8060
G8061
G8062
G8075
G8076
G8077
G8078
G8079
G8080
G8081
G8082
G8085
G8093
G8094
G8099
G8100
G8103
G8104
G8106
G8107
G8108
G8109
G8110
G8111
G8112
G8113

G8114
G8115
G8116
G8117
G8129
G8130
G8131
G8152
G8153
G8154
G8155
G8156
G8157
G8159
G8162
G8164
G8165
G8166
G8167
G8170
G8171
G8172
G8182
G8183
G8184
G8185
G8186
G8193
G8196
G8200
G8204
G8209
G8214
G8217
G8219
G8220
G8221

G8223
G8226
G8231
G8234
G8238
G8240
G8243
G8246
G8248
G8251
G8254
G8257
G8260
G8263
G8266
G8268
G8271
G8274
G8276
G8279
G8282
G8285
G8289
G8293
G8296
G8298
G8299
G8302
G8303
G8304
G8305
G8306
G8307
G8308
G8310
G8314
G8318

G8322
G8326
G8330
G8334
G8338
G8341
G8345
G8351
G8354
G8357
G8360
G8362
G8365
G8367
G8370
G8371
G8372
G8373
G8374
G8375
G8376
G8377
G8378
G8379
G8380
G8381
G8382
G8383
G8384
G8385
G8386
G8387
G8388
G8389
G8390
G8391
G8402

G8403
G8407
G8408
G8409
G8423
G8424
G8425
G8426
G8429
G8434
G8435
G8436
G8437
G8438
G8439
G8440
G8441
G8443
G8445
G8446
G8449
G8453
G8454
G8455
G8456
G8457
G8466
G8467
G8479
G8480
G8481
G8488
G8507
G8508
G8518
G8519
G8520

G8534
G8537
G8538
G8636
G8637
G8638
G8639
G8640
G8641
G8675
G8676
G8677
G8678
G8679
G8680
G8681
G8684
G8686
G8687
G8688
G8689
G8690
G8691
G8692
G8693
G9041
G9042
G9043
G9044
J0128
J0170
J0559
J0560
J0570
J0580
J0704
J0970

J1390
J1470
J1480
J1490
J1500
J1510
J1520
J1530
J1540
J1550
J1785
J1825
J2321
J2322
J7130
J7184
J9062
J9080
J9090
J9091
J9092
J9093
J9094
J9095
J9096
J9097
J9110
J9140
J9290
J9291
J9350
J9375
J9380
K0734
K0735
K0736
K0737

L1500
L1510
L1520
L3672
L3673
L3964
L3965
L3966
L3968
L3969
L3970
L3972
L3974
L4380
L5311
L7266
L7272
L7274
L7500
Q0179
Q1003
Q2025
Q2040
Q2041
Q2042
Q2044
Q4109
S0146
S0161
S0181
S0196
S0625
S2270
S2344
S3628
S3905
S9075

A2-Z3 ASC Payment Indicators

Final ASC Payment Indicators for CY 2012	
Payment Indicator	**Payment Indicator Definition**
A2	Surgical procedure on ASC list in CY 2007; payment based on OPPS relative payment weight.
D5	Deleted/discontinued code; no payment made.
F4	Corneal tissue acquisition, hepatitis B vaccine; paid at reasonable cost.
G2	Non office-based surgical procedure added in CY 2008 or later; payment based on OPPS relative payment weight.
H2	Brachytherapy source paid separately when provided integral to a surgical procedure on ASC list; payment OPPS rate.
J7	OPPS pass-through device paid separately when provided integral to a surgical procedure on ASC list; payment contractor-priced.
J8	Device-intensive procedure; paid at adjusted rate.
K2	Drugs and biologicals paid separately when provided integral to a surgical procedure on ASC list; payment based on OPPS rate.
K7	Unclassified drugs and biologicals; payment contractor-priced.
L1	Influenza vaccine; pneumococcal vaccine. Packaged item/service; no separate payment made.
L6	New Technology Intraocular Lens (NTIOL); special payment.
M5	Quality measurement code used for reporting purposes only; no payment made.
N1	Packaged service/item; no separate payment made.
P2	Office-based surgical procedure added to ASC list in CY 2008 or later with MPFS nonfacility PE RVUs; payment based on OPPS relative payment weight.
P3	Office-based surgical procedure added to ASC list in CY 2008 or later with MPFS nonfacility PE RVUs; payment based on MPFS nonfacility PE RVUs.
R2	Office-based surgical procedure added to ASC list in CY 2008 or later without MPFS nonfacility PE RVUs; payment based on OPPS relative payment weight.
Z2	Radiology service paid separately when provided integral to a surgical procedure on ASC list; payment based on OPPS relative payment weight.
Z3	Radiology service paid separately when provided integral to a surgical procedure on ASC list; payment based on MPFS nonfacility PE RVUs.

CMS-1525-FC, Final Changes to the ASC Payment System and CY 2012 Payment Rates, http://www.cms.gov/ASCPayment/ASCRN/list.asp#TopOfPage

A-Y ASC Status Indicators

	Final OPPS Payment Status Indicators for CY 2012	
Indicator	**Item/Code/Service**	**OPPS Payment Status**
A	Services furnished to a hospital outpatient that are paid under a fee schedule or payment system other than OPPS, for example:	Not paid under OPPS. Paid by fiscal intermediaries/MACs under a fee schedule or payment system other than OPPS. Services are subject to deductible or coinsurance unless indicated otherwise.
	• Ambulance Services	
	• Clinical Diagnostic Laboratory Services	Not subject to deductible or coinsurance.
	• Non-Implantable Prosthetic and Orthotic Devices	
	• EPO for ESRD Patients	
	• Physical, Occupational, and Speech Therapy	
	• Routine Dialysis Services for ESRD Patients Provided in a Certified Dialysis Unit of a Hospital	
	• Diagnostic Mammography	
	• Screening Mammography	Not subject to deductible or coinsurance.
B	Codes that are not recognized by OPPS when submitted on an outpatient hospital Part B bill type (12x and 13x)	Not paid under OPPS. • May be paid by fiscal intermediaries/MACs when submitted on a different bill type, for example, 75x (CORF), but not paid under OPPS. • An alternate code that is recognized by OPPS when submitted on an outpatient hospital Part B bill type (12x and 13x) may be available.
C	Inpatient Procedures	Not paid under OPPS. Admit patient. Bill as inpatient.
D	Discontinued Codes	Not paid under OPPS or any other Medicare payment system.
E	Items, Codes, and Services:	Not paid by Medicare when submitted on outpatient claims (any outpatient bill type).
	• That are not covered by any Medicare outpatient benefit based on statutory exclusion.	
	• That are not covered by any Medicare outpatient benefit for reasons other than statutory exclusion.	
	• That are not recognized by Medicare for outpatient claims alternate code for the same item or service may be available.	
	• For which separate payment is not provided on outpatient claims.	
F	Corneal Tissue Acquisition; Certain CRNA Services and Hepatitis B Vaccines	Not paid under OPPS. Paid at reasonable cost.
G	Pass-Through Drugs and Biologicals	Paid under OPPS; separate APC payment.
H	Pass-Through Device Categories	Separate cost-based pass-through payment; not subject to copayment.
K	Nonpass-Through Drugs and Nonimplantable Biologicals, including Therapeutic Radiopharmaceuticals	Paid under OPPS: separate APC payment.
L	Influenza Vaccine; Pneumococcal Pneumonia Vaccine	Not paid under OPPS. Paid at reasonable cost; not subject to deductible or coinsurance.
M	Items and Services Not Billable to the Fiscal Intermediary/MAC	Not paid under OPPS.
N	Items and Services Packaged into APC Rates	Paid under OPPS; payment is packaged into payment for other services. Therefore, there is no separate APC payment.
P	Partial Hospitalization	Paid under OPPS; per diem APC payment.

A-Y ASC Status Indicators—cont'd

Final OPPS Payment Status Indicators for CY 2012		
Indicator	**Item/Code/Service**	**OPPS Payment Status**
Q1	STVX-Packaged Codes	Paid under OPPS; Addendum B displays APC assignments when services are separately payable. (1) Packaged APC payment if billed on the same date of service as a HCPCS code assigned status indicator "S," "T," "V," or "X." (2) In all other circumstances, payment is made through a separate APC payment.
Q2	T-Packaged Codes	Paid under OPPS; Addendum B displays APC assignments when services are separately payable. (1) Packaged APC payment if billed on the same date of service as a HCPCS code assigned status indicator "T." (2) In all other circumstances, payment is made through a separate APC payment.
Q3	Codes That May Be Paid Through a Composite APC	Paid under OPPS; Addendum B displays APC assignments when services are separately payable. Addendum M displays composite APC assignments when codes are paid through a composite APC. (1) Composite APC payment based on OPPS composite-specific payment criteria. Payment is packaged into a single payment for specific combinations of service. (2) In all other circumstances, payment is made through a separate APC payment or packaged into payment for other services.
R	Blood and Blood Products	Paid under OPPS; separate APC payment.
S	Significant Procedure, Not Discounted when Multiple	Paid under OPPS; separate APC payment.
T	Significant Procedure, Multiple Reduction Applies	Paid under OPPS; separate APC payment.
U	Brachytherapy Sources	Paid under OPPS; separate APC payment.
V	Clinic or Emergency Department Visit	Paid under OPPS; separate APC payment.
X	Ancillary Services	Paid under OPPS; separate APC payment.
Y	Non-Implantable Durable Medical Equipment	Not paid under OPPS. All institutional providers other than home health agencies bill to DMERC.

CMS-1525-FC, Final Changes to the ASC Payment System and CY 2012 Payment Rates, http://www.cms.gov/ASCPayment/ASCRN/list.asp#TopOfPage

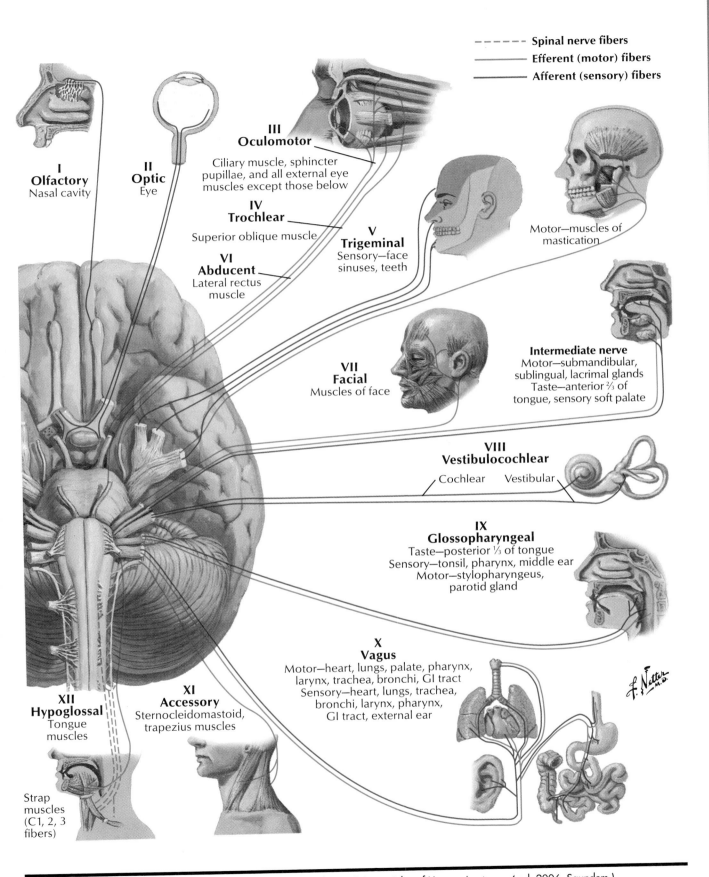

I Olfactory
Nasal cavity

II Optic
Eye

- - - - - Spinal nerve fibers
———— Efferent (motor) fibers
———— Afferent (sensory) fibers

III Oculomotor
Ciliary muscle, sphincter pupillae, and all external eye muscles except those below

IV Trochlear
Superior oblique muscle

VI Abducent
Lateral rectus muscle

V Trigeminal
Sensory—face sinuses, teeth

Motor—muscles of mastication

VII Facial
Muscles of face

Intermediate nerve
Motor—submandibular, sublingual, lacrimal glands
Taste—anterior ⅔ of tongue, sensory soft palate

VIII Vestibulocochlear
Cochlear   Vestibular

IX Glossopharyngeal
Taste—posterior ⅓ of tongue
Sensory—tonsil, pharynx, middle ear
Motor—stylopharyngeus, parotid gland

X Vagus
Motor—heart, lungs, palate, pharynx, larynx, trachea, bronchi, GI tract
Sensory—heart, lungs, trachea, bronchi, larynx, pharynx, GI tract, external ear

XII Hypoglossal
Tongue muscles

XI Accessory
Sternocleidomastoid, trapezius muscles

Strap muscles (C1, 2, 3 fibers)

f. Netter m.d.

NETTER ANATOMY PLATE

Plate 118   Cranial Nerves (Motor and Sensory Distribution): Schema. (Netter: Atlas of Human Anatomy, 4 ed, 2006, Saunders.)

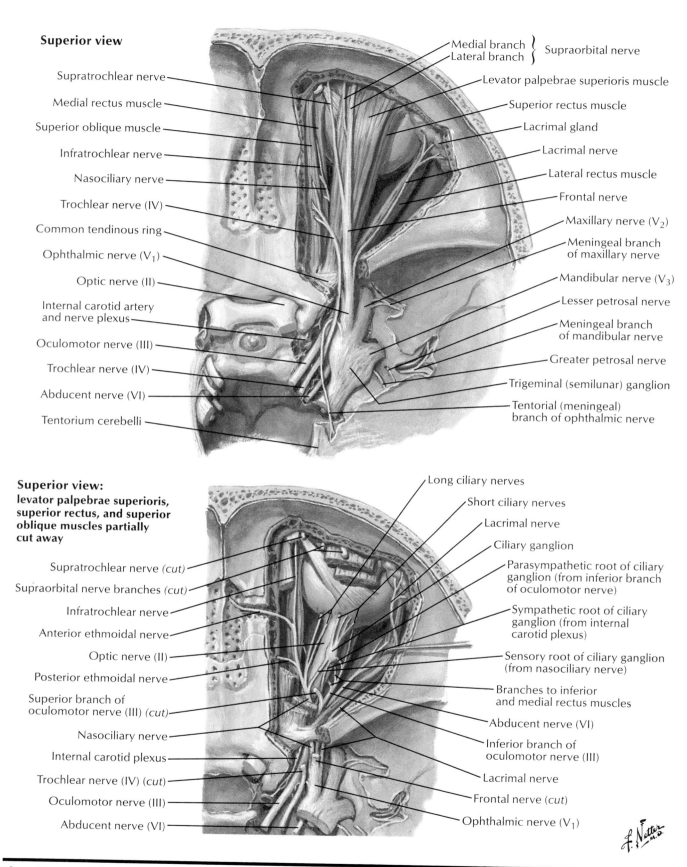

Superior view

Supratrochlear nerve

Medial rectus muscle

Superior oblique muscle

Infratrochlear nerve

Nasociliary nerve

Trochlear nerve (IV)

Common tendinous ring

Ophthalmic nerve (V₁)

Optic nerve (II)

Internal carotid artery and nerve plexus

Oculomotor nerve (III)

Trochlear nerve (IV)

Abducent nerve (VI)

Tentorium cerebelli

Medial branch } Supraorbital nerve
Lateral branch

Levator palpebrae superioris muscle

Superior rectus muscle

Lacrimal gland

Lacrimal nerve

Lateral rectus muscle

Frontal nerve

Maxillary nerve (V₂)

Meningeal branch of maxillary nerve

Mandibular nerve (V₃)

Lesser petrosal nerve

Meningeal branch of mandibular nerve

Greater petrosal nerve

Trigeminal (semilunar) ganglion

Tentorial (meningeal) branch of ophthalmic nerve

Superior view:
levator palpebrae superioris, superior rectus, and superior oblique muscles partially cut away

Supratrochlear nerve *(cut)*

Supraorbital nerve branches *(cut)*

Infratrochlear nerve

Anterior ethmoidal nerve

Optic nerve (II)

Posterior ethmoidal nerve

Superior branch of oculomotor nerve (III) *(cut)*

Nasociliary nerve

Internal carotid plexus

Trochlear nerve (IV) *(cut)*

Oculomotor nerve (III)

Abducent nerve (VI)

Long ciliary nerves

Short ciliary nerves

Lacrimal nerve

Ciliary ganglion

Parasympathetic root of ciliary ganglion (from inferior branch of oculomotor nerve)

Sympathetic root of ciliary ganglion (from internal carotid plexus)

Sensory root of ciliary ganglion (from nasociliary nerve)

Branches to inferior and medial rectus muscles

Abducent nerve (VI)

Inferior branch of oculomotor nerve (III)

Lacrimal nerve

Frontal nerve *(cut)*

Ophthalmic nerve (V₁)

Plate 86 Nerves of Orbit. (Netter: Atlas of Human Anatomy, 4 ed, 2006, Saunders.)

NAP-2

NETTER ANATOMY PLATE

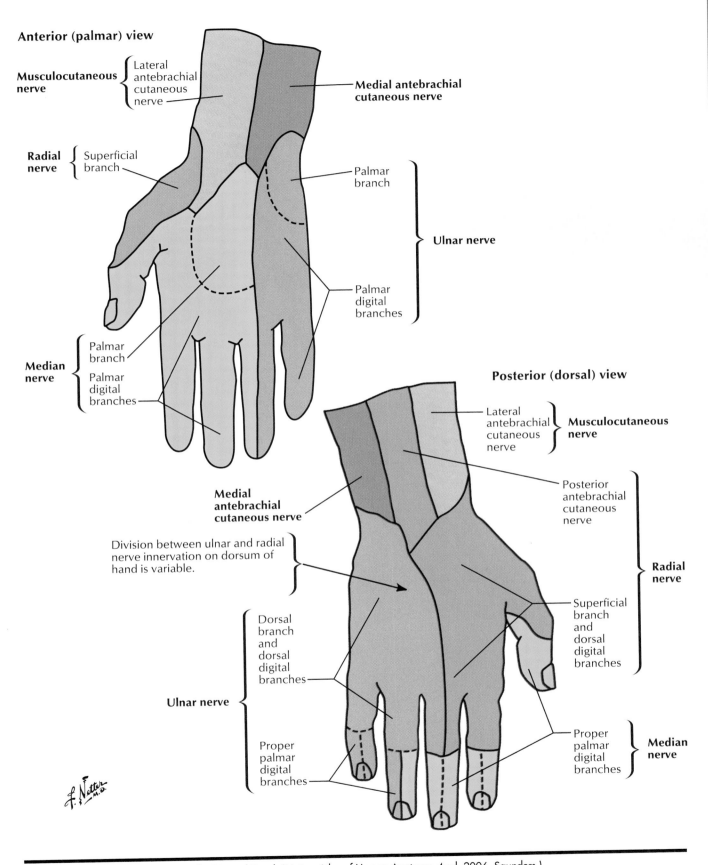

Anterior (palmar) view

Musculocutaneous nerve — Lateral antebrachial cutaneous nerve

Medial antebrachial cutaneous nerve

Radial nerve — Superficial branch

Palmar branch
Palmar digital branches
} Ulnar nerve

Median nerve — Palmar branch / Palmar digital branches

Posterior (dorsal) view

Lateral antebrachial cutaneous nerve } Musculocutaneous nerve

Medial antebrachial cutaneous nerve

Posterior antebrachial cutaneous nerve

Division between ulnar and radial nerve innervation on dorsum of hand is variable.

Radial nerve

Superficial branch and dorsal digital branches

Ulnar nerve — Dorsal branch and dorsal digital branches / Proper palmar digital branches

Proper palmar digital branches } Median nerve

NETTER ANATOMY PLATE

Plate 472 Cutaneous Innervation of Wrist and Hand. (Netter: Atlas of Human Anatomy, 4 ed, 2006, Saunders.)

NAP-3

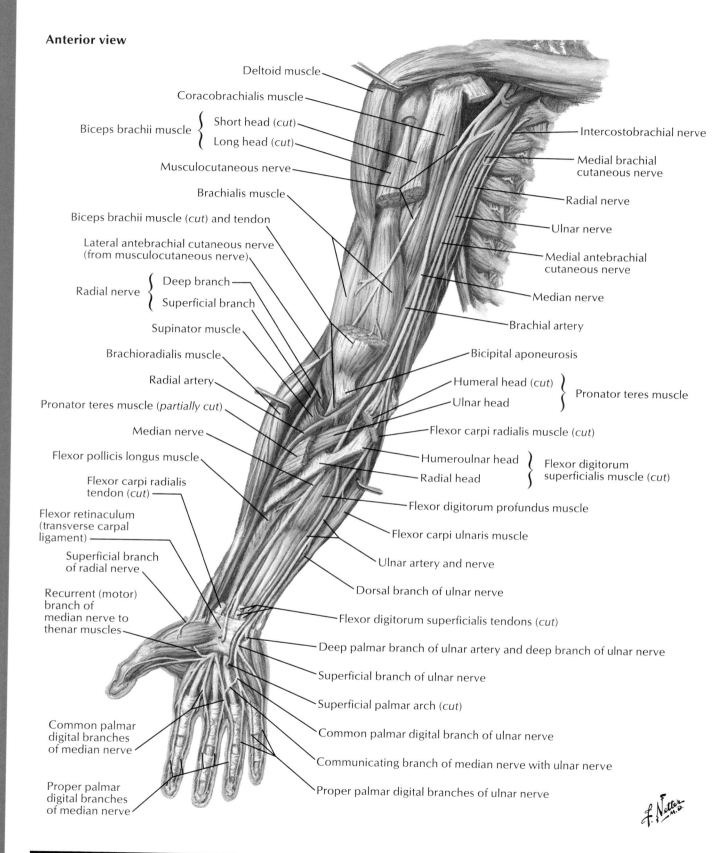

Anterior view

Deltoid muscle

Coracobrachialis muscle

Biceps brachii muscle { Short head (cut)

Long head (cut)

Musculocutaneous nerve

Brachialis muscle

Biceps brachii muscle (cut) and tendon

Lateral antebrachial cutaneous nerve (from musculocutaneous nerve)

Radial nerve { Deep branch

Superficial branch

Supinator muscle

Brachioradialis muscle

Radial artery

Pronator teres muscle (partially cut)

Median nerve

Flexor pollicis longus muscle

Flexor carpi radialis tendon (cut)

Flexor retinaculum (transverse carpal ligament)

Superficial branch of radial nerve

Recurrent (motor) branch of median nerve to thenar muscles

Common palmar digital branches of median nerve

Proper palmar digital branches of median nerve

Intercostobrachial nerve

Medial brachial cutaneous nerve

Radial nerve

Ulnar nerve

Medial antebrachial cutaneous nerve

Median nerve

Brachial artery

Bicipital aponeurosis

Humeral head (cut) } Pronator teres muscle

Ulnar head

Flexor carpi radialis muscle (cut)

Humeroulnar head } Flexor digitorum superficialis muscle (cut)

Radial head

Flexor digitorum profundus muscle

Flexor carpi ulnaris muscle

Ulnar artery and nerve

Dorsal branch of ulnar nerve

Flexor digitorum superficialis tendons (cut)

Deep palmar branch of ulnar artery and deep branch of ulnar nerve

Superficial branch of ulnar nerve

Superficial palmar arch (cut)

Common palmar digital branch of ulnar nerve

Communicating branch of median nerve with ulnar nerve

Proper palmar digital branches of ulnar nerve

Plate 473 Arteries and Nerves of Upper Limb. (Netter: Atlas of Human Anatomy, 4 ed, 2006, Saunders.)

NAP-4

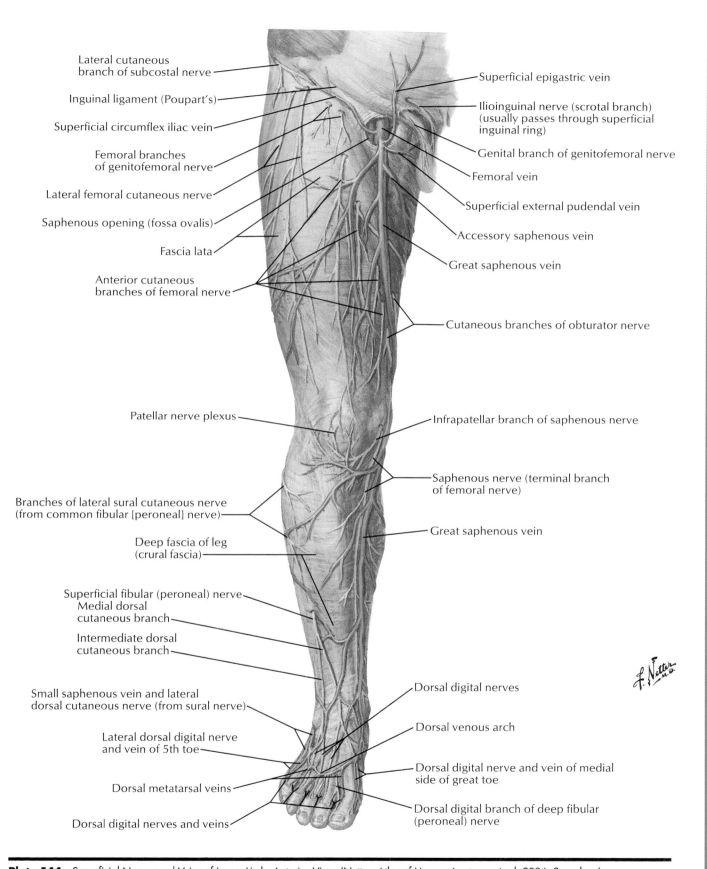

Lateral cutaneous branch of subcostal nerve

Inguinal ligament (Poupart's)

Superficial circumflex iliac vein

Femoral branches of genitofemoral nerve

Lateral femoral cutaneous nerve

Saphenous opening (fossa ovalis)

Fascia lata

Anterior cutaneous branches of femoral nerve

Patellar nerve plexus

Branches of lateral sural cutaneous nerve (from common fibular [peroneal] nerve)

Deep fascia of leg (crural fascia)

Superficial fibular (peroneal) nerve
Medial dorsal cutaneous branch

Intermediate dorsal cutaneous branch

Small saphenous vein and lateral dorsal cutaneous nerve (from sural nerve)

Lateral dorsal digital nerve and vein of 5th toe

Dorsal metatarsal veins

Dorsal digital nerves and veins

Superficial epigastric vein

Ilioinguinal nerve (scrotal branch) (usually passes through superficial inguinal ring)

Genital branch of genitofemoral nerve

Femoral vein

Superficial external pudendal vein

Accessory saphenous vein

Great saphenous vein

Cutaneous branches of obturator nerve

Infrapatellar branch of saphenous nerve

Saphenous nerve (terminal branch of femoral nerve)

Great saphenous vein

Dorsal digital nerves

Dorsal venous arch

Dorsal digital nerve and vein of medial side of great toe

Dorsal digital branch of deep fibular (peroneal) nerve

NETTER ANATOMY PLATE

Plate 544 Superficial Nerves and Veins of Lower Limb: Anterior View. (Netter: Atlas of Human Anatomy, 4 ed, 2006, Saunders.)

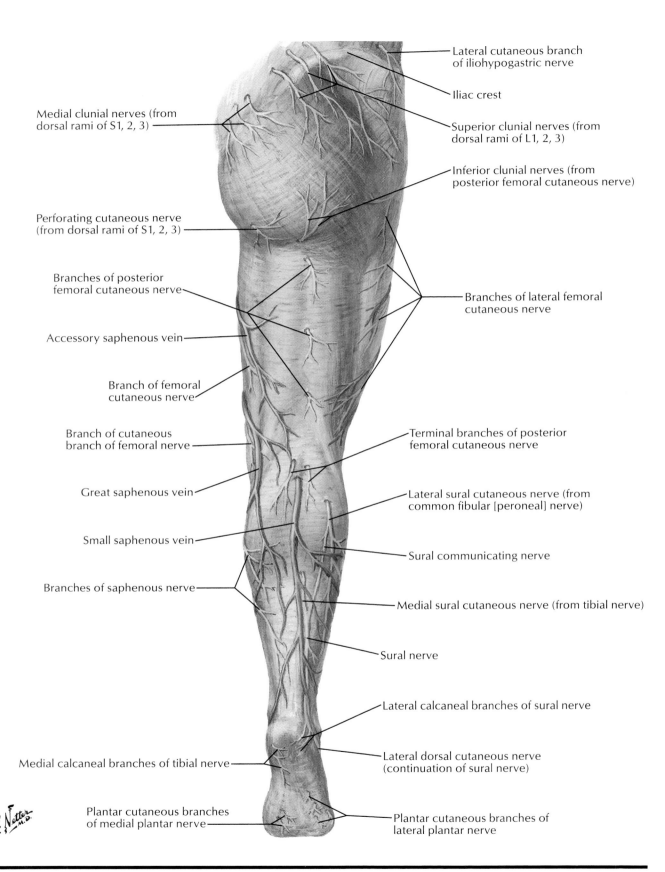

Lateral cutaneous branch
of iliohypogastric nerve

Iliac crest

Superior clunial nerves (from
dorsal rami of L1, 2, 3)

Inferior clunial nerves (from
posterior femoral cutaneous nerve)

Medial clunial nerves (from
dorsal rami of S1, 2, 3)

Perforating cutaneous nerve
(from dorsal rami of S1, 2, 3)

Branches of lateral femoral
cutaneous nerve

Branches of posterior
femoral cutaneous nerve

Accessory saphenous vein

Branch of femoral
cutaneous nerve

Terminal branches of posterior
femoral cutaneous nerve

Branch of cutaneous
branch of femoral nerve

Lateral sural cutaneous nerve (from
common fibular [peroneal] nerve)

Great saphenous vein

Sural communicating nerve

Small saphenous vein

Medial sural cutaneous nerve (from tibial nerve)

Branches of saphenous nerve

Sural nerve

Lateral calcaneal branches of sural nerve

Medial calcaneal branches of tibial nerve

Lateral dorsal cutaneous nerve
(continuation of sural nerve)

Plantar cutaneous branches
of medial plantar nerve

Plantar cutaneous branches of
lateral plantar nerve

Plate 545   Superficial Nerves and Veins of Lower Limb: Posterior View. (Netter: Atlas of Human Anatomy, 4 ed, 2006, Saunders.)

NAP-6

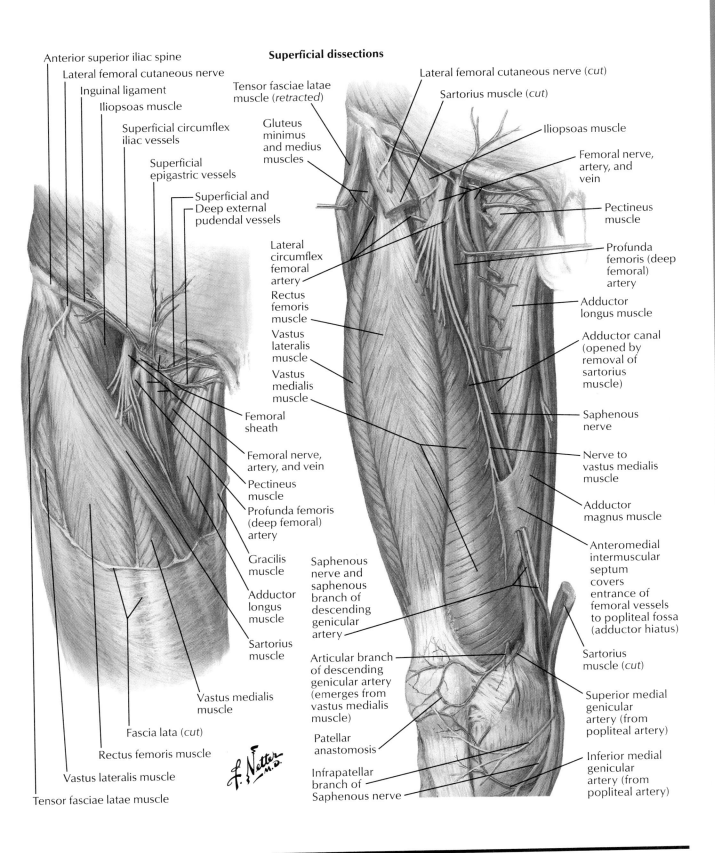

Superficial dissections

Anterior superior iliac spine

Lateral femoral cutaneous nerve

Inguinal ligament

Iliopsoas muscle

Superficial circumflex iliac vessels

Superficial epigastric vessels

Tensor fasciae latae muscle (*retracted*)

Gluteus minimus and medius muscles

Superficial and Deep external pudendal vessels

Lateral circumflex femoral artery

Rectus femoris muscle

Vastus lateralis muscle

Vastus medialis muscle

Femoral sheath

Femoral nerve, artery, and vein

Pectineus muscle

Profunda femoris (deep femoral) artery

Gracilis muscle

Adductor longus muscle

Sartorius muscle

Vastus medialis muscle

Fascia lata (*cut*)

Rectus femoris muscle

Vastus lateralis muscle

Tensor fasciae latae muscle

Lateral femoral cutaneous nerve (*cut*)

Sartorius muscle (*cut*)

Iliopsoas muscle

Femoral nerve, artery, and vein

Pectineus muscle

Profunda femoris (deep femoral) artery

Adductor longus muscle

Adductor canal (opened by removal of sartorius muscle)

Saphenous nerve

Nerve to vastus medialis muscle

Adductor magnus muscle

Anteromedial intermuscular septum covers entrance of femoral vessels to popliteal fossa (adductor hiatus)

Sartorius muscle (*cut*)

Superior medial genicular artery (from popliteal artery)

Inferior medial genicular artery (from popliteal artery)

Saphenous nerve and saphenous branch of descending genicular artery

Articular branch of descending genicular artery (emerges from vastus medialis muscle)

Patellar anastomosis

Infrapatellar branch of Saphenous nerve

f. Netter M.D.

Plate 500 Arteries and Nerves of Thigh: Anterior View. (Netter: Atlas of Human Anatomy, 4 ed, 2006, Saunders.)

Deep dissection

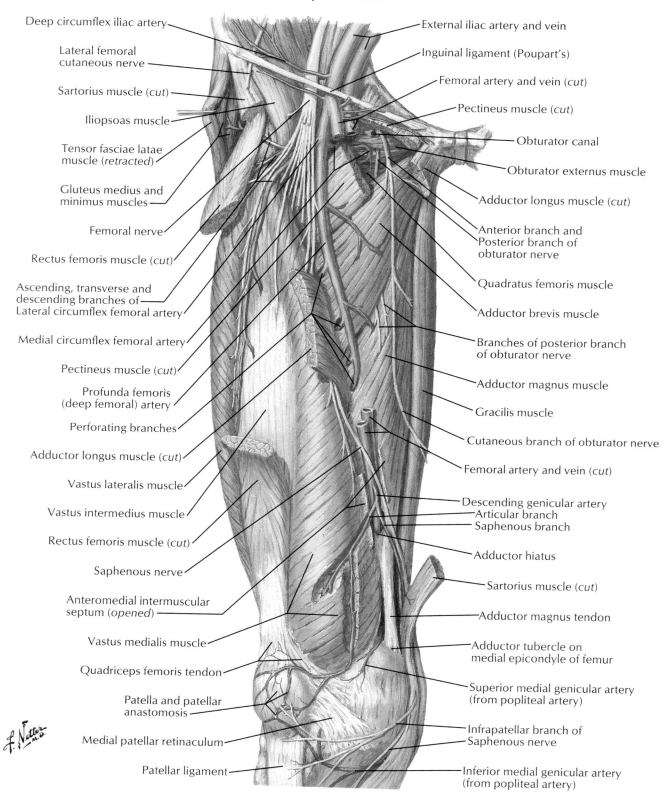

Deep circumflex iliac artery

Lateral femoral cutaneous nerve

Sartorius muscle (*cut*)

Iliopsoas muscle

Tensor fasciae latae muscle (*retracted*)

Gluteus medius and minimus muscles

Femoral nerve

Rectus femoris muscle (*cut*)

Ascending, transverse and descending branches of Lateral circumflex femoral artery

Medial circumflex femoral artery

Pectineus muscle (*cut*)

Profunda femoris (deep femoral) artery

Perforating branches

Adductor longus muscle (*cut*)

Vastus lateralis muscle

Vastus intermedius muscle

Rectus femoris muscle (*cut*)

Saphenous nerve

Anteromedial intermuscular septum (*opened*)

Vastus medialis muscle

Quadriceps femoris tendon

Patella and patellar anastomosis

Medial patellar retinaculum

Patellar ligament

External iliac artery and vein

Inguinal ligament (Poupart's)

Femoral artery and vein (*cut*)

Pectineus muscle (*cut*)

Obturator canal

Obturator externus muscle

Adductor longus muscle (*cut*)

Anterior branch and Posterior branch of obturator nerve

Quadratus femoris muscle

Adductor brevis muscle

Branches of posterior branch of obturator nerve

Adductor magnus muscle

Gracilis muscle

Cutaneous branch of obturator nerve

Femoral artery and vein (*cut*)

Descending genicular artery
Articular branch
Saphenous branch

Adductor hiatus

Sartorius muscle (*cut*)

Adductor magnus tendon

Adductor tubercle on medial epicondyle of femur

Superior medial genicular artery (from popliteal artery)

Infrapatellar branch of Saphenous nerve

Inferior medial genicular artery (from popliteal artery)

Plate 501 Arteries and Nerves of Thigh: Anterior View. (Netter: Atlas of Human Anatomy, 4 ed, 2006, Saunders.)

NAP-8

NETTER ANATOMY PLATE

Deep dissection

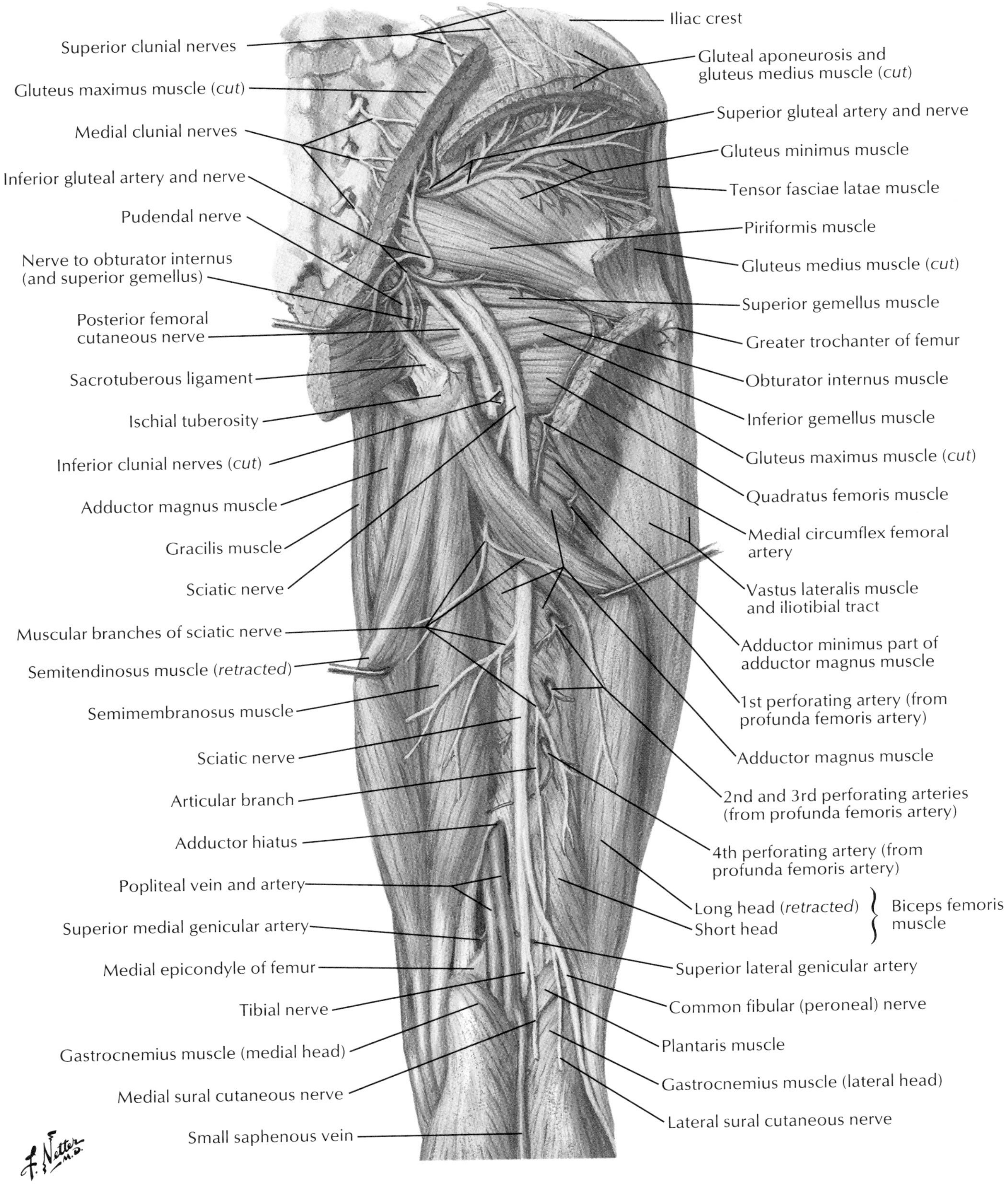

Superior clunial nerves

Gluteus maximus muscle (*cut*)

Medial clunial nerves

Inferior gluteal artery and nerve

Pudendal nerve

Nerve to obturator internus (and superior gemellus)

Posterior femoral cutaneous nerve

Sacrotuberous ligament

Ischial tuberosity

Inferior clunial nerves (*cut*)

Adductor magnus muscle

Gracilis muscle

Sciatic nerve

Muscular branches of sciatic nerve

Semitendinosus muscle (*retracted*)

Semimembranosus muscle

Sciatic nerve

Articular branch

Adductor hiatus

Popliteal vein and artery

Superior medial genicular artery

Medial epicondyle of femur

Tibial nerve

Gastrocnemius muscle (medial head)

Medial sural cutaneous nerve

Small saphenous vein

Iliac crest

Gluteal aponeurosis and gluteus medius muscle (*cut*)

Superior gluteal artery and nerve

Gluteus minimus muscle

Tensor fasciae latae muscle

Piriformis muscle

Gluteus medius muscle (*cut*)

Superior gemellus muscle

Greater trochanter of femur

Obturator internus muscle

Inferior gemellus muscle

Gluteus maximus muscle (*cut*)

Quadratus femoris muscle

Medial circumflex femoral artery

Vastus lateralis muscle and iliotibial tract

Adductor minimus part of adductor magnus muscle

1st perforating artery (from profunda femoris artery)

Adductor magnus muscle

2nd and 3rd perforating arteries (from profunda femoris artery)

4th perforating artery (from profunda femoris artery)

Long head (*retracted*)
Short head
} Biceps femoris muscle

Superior lateral genicular artery

Common fibular (peroneal) nerve

Plantaris muscle

Gastrocnemius muscle (lateral head)

Lateral sural cutaneous nerve

Plate 502 Arteries and Nerves of Thigh: Posterior View. (Netter: Atlas of Human Anatomy, 4 ed, 2006, Saunders.)

NETTER ANATOMY PLATE

Horizontal section

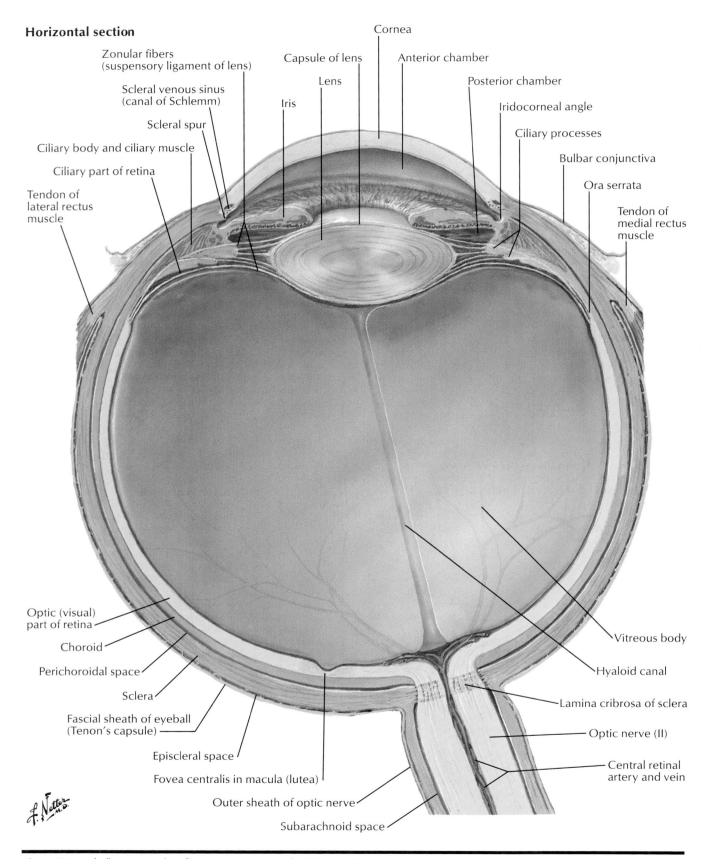

Zonular fibers (suspensory ligament of lens)

Scleral venous sinus (canal of Schlemm)

Scleral spur

Ciliary body and ciliary muscle

Ciliary part of retina

Tendon of lateral rectus muscle

Iris

Capsule of lens

Lens

Cornea

Anterior chamber

Posterior chamber

Iridocorneal angle

Ciliary processes

Bulbar conjunctiva

Ora serrata

Tendon of medial rectus muscle

Optic (visual) part of retina

Choroid

Perichoroidal space

Sclera

Fascial sheath of eyeball (Tenon's capsule)

Episcleral space

Fovea centralis in macula (lutea)

Outer sheath of optic nerve

Subarachnoid space

Vitreous body

Hyaloid canal

Lamina cribrosa of sclera

Optic nerve (II)

Central retinal artery and vein

Plate 87   Eyeball. (Netter: Atlas of Human Anatomy, 4 ed, 2006, Saunders.)

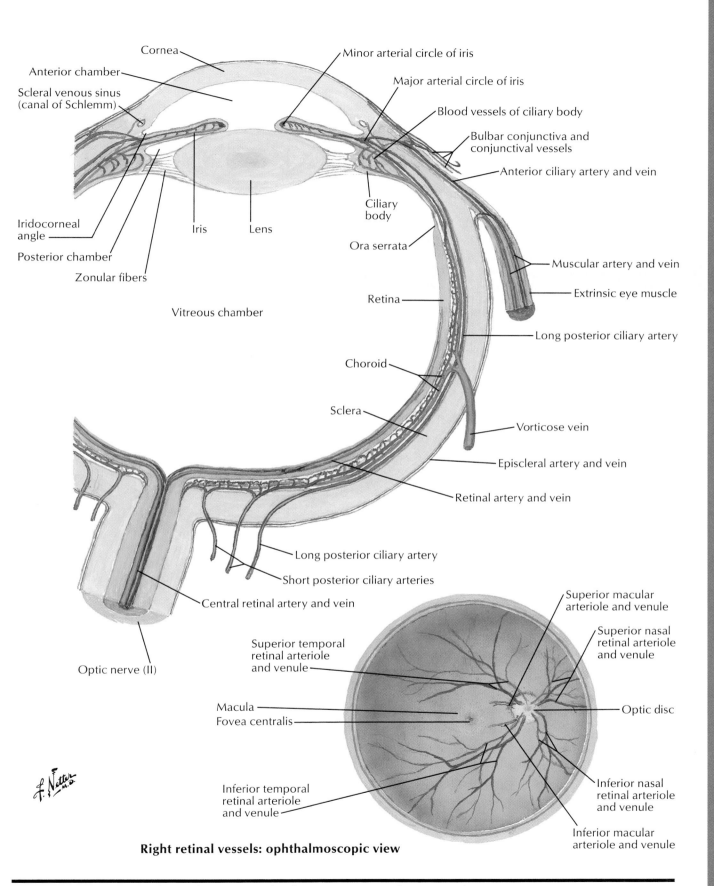

Cornea

Anterior chamber

Scleral venous sinus
(canal of Schlemm)

Minor arterial circle of iris

Major arterial circle of iris

Blood vessels of ciliary body

Bulbar conjunctiva and
conjunctival vessels

Anterior ciliary artery and vein

Iridocorneal
angle

Iris   Lens

Ciliary
body

Ora serrata

Posterior chamber

Zonular fibers

Muscular artery and vein

Extrinsic eye muscle

Retina

Long posterior ciliary artery

Vitreous chamber

Choroid

Sclera

Vorticose vein

Episcleral artery and vein

Retinal artery and vein

Long posterior ciliary artery

Short posterior ciliary arteries

Central retinal artery and vein

Optic nerve (II)

Superior macular
arteriole and venule

Superior nasal
retinal arteriole
and venule

Superior temporal
retinal arteriole
and venule

Optic disc

Macula

Fovea centralis

Inferior temporal
retinal arteriole
and venule

Inferior nasal
retinal arteriole
and venule

Inferior macular
arteriole and venule

Right retinal vessels: ophthalmoscopic view

Plate 90   Intrinsic Arteries and Veins of Eye. (Netter: Atlas of Human Anatomy, 4 ed, 2006, Saunders.)

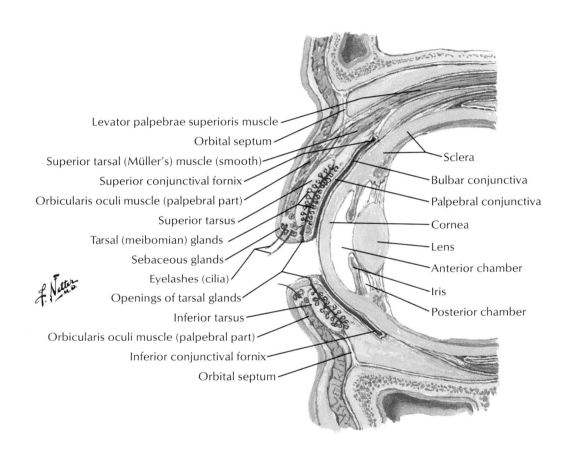

Levator palpebrae superioris muscle
Orbital septum
Superior tarsal (Müller's) muscle (smooth)
Superior conjunctival fornix
Orbicularis oculi muscle (palpebral part)
Superior tarsus
Tarsal (meibomian) glands
Sebaceous glands
Eyelashes (cilia)
Openings of tarsal glands
Inferior tarsus
Orbicularis oculi muscle (palpebral part)
Inferior conjunctival fornix
Orbital septum

Sclera
Bulbar conjunctiva
Palpebral conjunctiva
Cornea
Lens
Anterior chamber
Iris
Posterior chamber

Plate 81, Middle   Eyelid. (Netter: Atlas of Human Anatomy, 4 ed, 2006, Saunders.)

NAP-12

Superior palpebral conjunctiva: tarsal (meibomian) glands shining through

Seen through cornea { Pupil
Iris

Corneoscleral junction (corneal limbus)

Bulbar conjunctiva over sclera

Inferior conjunctival fornix

Inferior palpebral conjunctiva: tarsal glands shining through

Superior lacrimal papilla and punctum

Plica semilunaris

Lacrimal caruncle in lacrimal lake (lacus lacrimalis)

Inferior lacrimal papilla and punctum

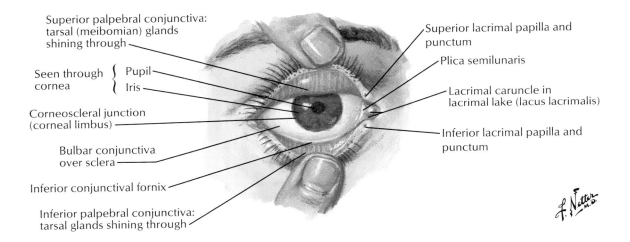

Plate 81, Upper Eyelid. (Netter: Atlas of Human Anatomy, 4 ed, 2006, Saunders.)

NAP-13

NETTER ANATOMY PLATE

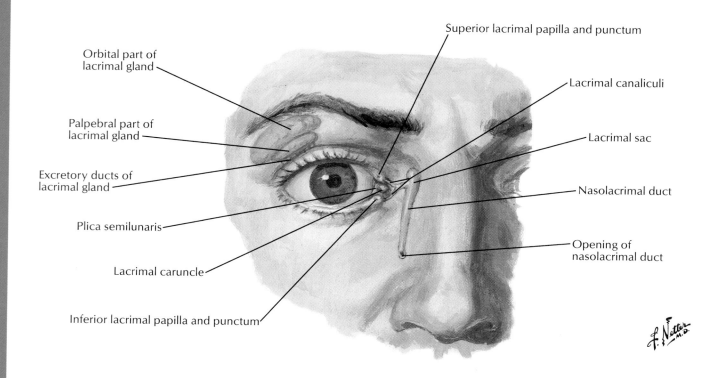

Orbital part of
lacrimal gland

Palpebral part of
lacrimal gland

Excretory ducts of
lacrimal gland

Plica semilunaris

Lacrimal caruncle

Inferior lacrimal papilla and punctum

Superior lacrimal papilla and punctum

Lacrimal canaliculi

Lacrimal sac

Nasolacrimal duct

Opening of
nasolacrimal duct

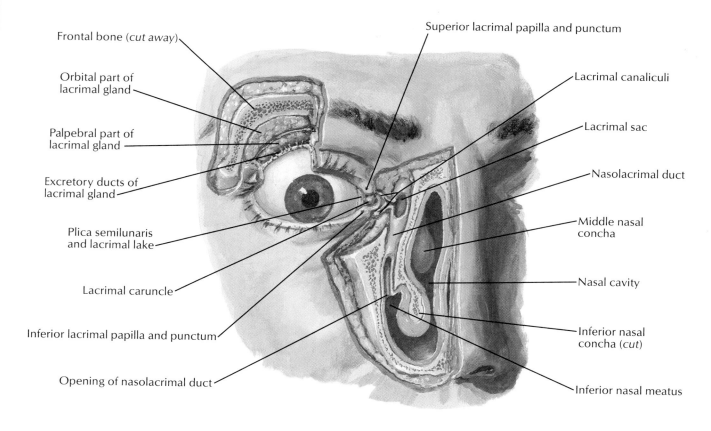

Frontal bone (cut away)

Orbital part of
lacrimal gland

Palpebral part of
lacrimal gland

Excretory ducts of
lacrimal gland

Plica semilunaris
and lacrimal lake

Lacrimal caruncle

Inferior lacrimal papilla and punctum

Opening of nasolacrimal duct

Superior lacrimal papilla and punctum

Lacrimal canaliculi

Lacrimal sac

Nasolacrimal duct

Middle nasal
concha

Nasal cavity

Inferior nasal
concha (cut)

Inferior nasal meatus

Plate 82   Lacrimal Apparatus. (Netter: Atlas of Human Anatomy, 4 ed, 2006, Saunders.)

Frontal section

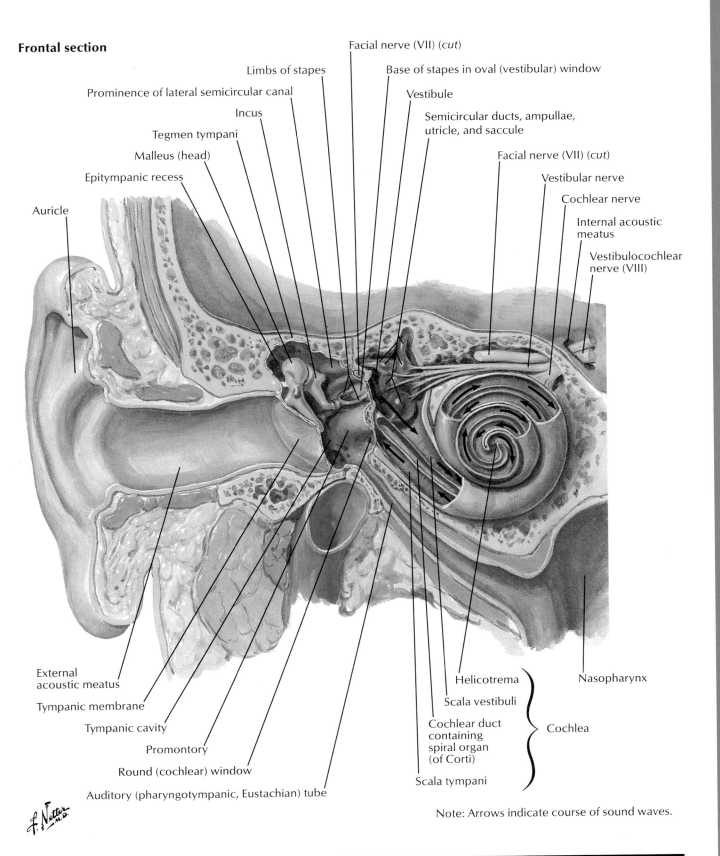

Facial nerve (VII) (*cut*)

Limbs of stapes

Base of stapes in oval (vestibular) window

Prominence of lateral semicircular canal

Vestibule

Incus

Semicircular ducts, ampullae, utricle, and saccule

Tegmen tympani

Malleus (head)

Facial nerve (VII) (*cut*)

Epitympanic recess

Vestibular nerve

Cochlear nerve

Auricle

Internal acoustic meatus

Vestibulocochlear nerve (VIII)

External acoustic meatus

Helicotrema

Nasopharynx

Tympanic membrane

Scala vestibuli

Tympanic cavity

Cochlear duct containing spiral organ (of Corti)

Cochlea

Promontory

Round (cochlear) window

Scala tympani

Auditory (pharyngotympanic, Eustachian) tube

Note: Arrows indicate course of sound waves.

Plate 92 Pathway of Sound Reception. (Netter: Atlas of Human Anatomy, 4 ed, 2006, Saunders.)

NAP-15

Medial wall of tympanic cavity: lateral view

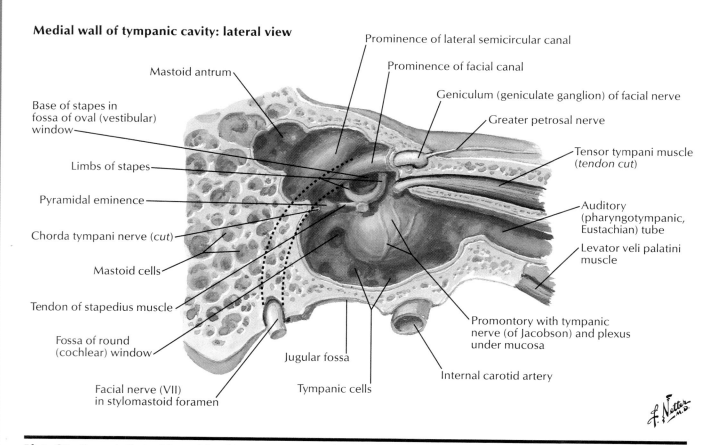

Mastoid antrum

Prominence of lateral semicircular canal

Prominence of facial canal

Geniculum (geniculate ganglion) of facial nerve

Greater petrosal nerve

Base of stapes in fossa of oval (vestibular) window

Limbs of stapes

Pyramidal eminence

Chorda tympani nerve (cut)

Mastoid cells

Tendon of stapedius muscle

Fossa of round (cochlear) window

Facial nerve (VII) in stylomastoid foramen

Jugular fossa

Tympanic cells

Internal carotid artery

Promontory with tympanic nerve (of Jacobson) and plexus under mucosa

Tensor tympani muscle (tendon cut)

Auditory (pharyngotympanic, Eustachian) tube

Levator veli palatini muscle

Plate 94   Tympanic Cavity. (Netter: Atlas of Human Anatomy, 4 ed, 2006, Saunders.)

Otoscopic view of right tympanic membrane

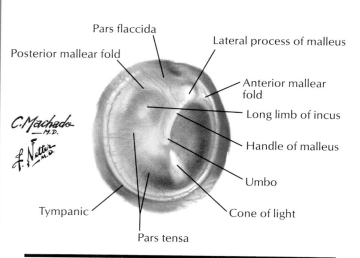

Pars flaccida

Posterior mallear fold

Lateral process of malleus

Anterior mallear fold

Long limb of incus

Handle of malleus

Umbo

Cone of light

Tympanic

Pars tensa

Plate 93   Tympanic Cavity. (Netter: Atlas of Human Anatomy, 4 ed, 2006, Saunders.)

Dissected right bony labyrinth (otic capsule): membranous labyrinth removed

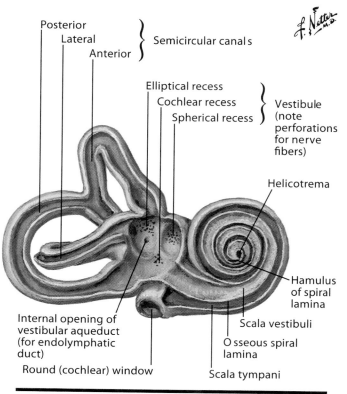

Posterior

Lateral

Anterior

Semicircular canals

Elliptical recess

Cochlear recess

Spherical recess

Vestibule (note perforations for nerve fibers)

Helicotrema

Hamulus of spiral lamina

Scala vestibuli

Osseous spiral lamina

Scala tympani

Internal opening of vestibular aqueduct (for endolymphatic duct)

Round (cochlear) window

Plate 95   Bony Membranous Labyrinth. (Netter: Atlas of Human Anatomy, 4 ed, 2006, Saunders.)

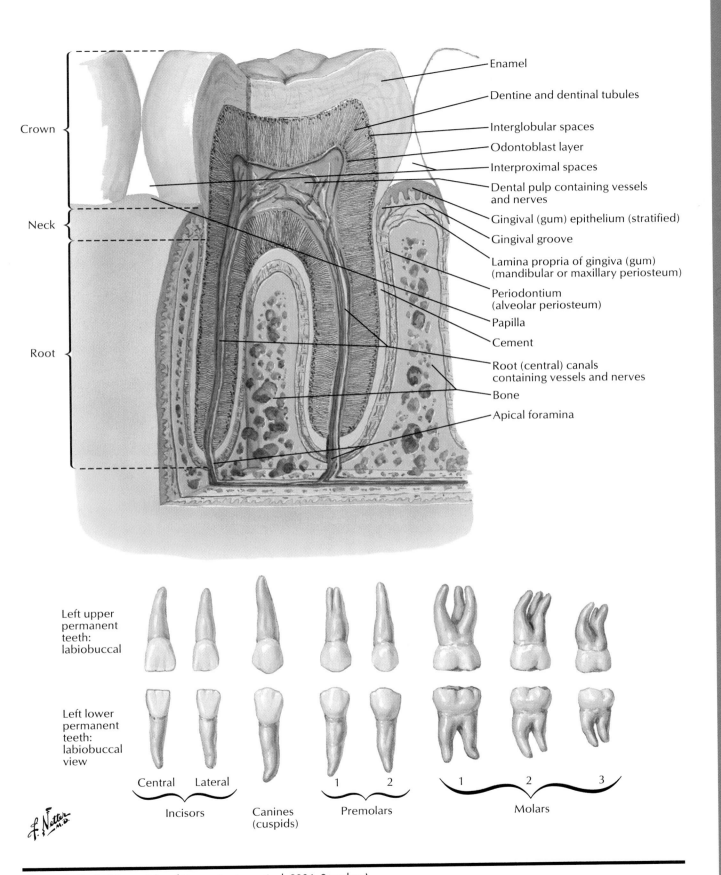

Crown

Neck

Root

Enamel

Dentine and dentinal tubules

Interglobular spaces

Odontoblast layer

Interproximal spaces

Dental pulp containing vessels and nerves

Gingival (gum) epithelium (stratified)

Gingival groove

Lamina propria of gingiva (gum) (mandibular or maxillary periosteum)

Periodontium (alveolar periosteum)

Papilla

Cement

Root (central) canals containing vessels and nerves

Bone

Apical foramina

Left upper permanent teeth: labiobuccal

Left lower permanent teeth: labiobuccal view

Central   Lateral   1   2   1   2   3

Incisors   Canines   Premolars   Molars
                  (cuspids)

Plate 57 Teeth. (Netter: Atlas of Human Anatomy, 4 ed, 2006, Saunders.)

Tongue

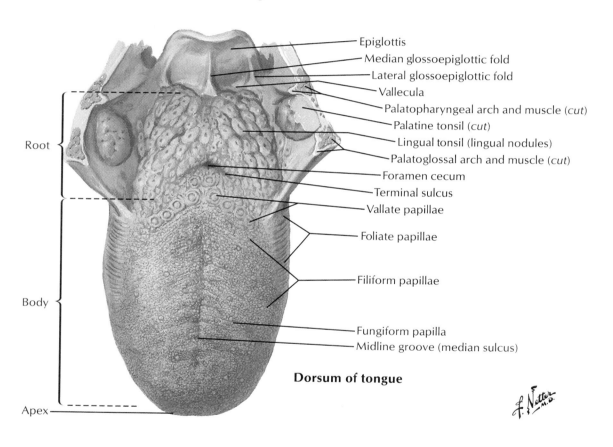

Epiglottis
Median glossoepiglottic fold
Lateral glossoepiglottic fold
Vallecula
Palatopharyngeal arch and muscle (*cut*)
Palatine tonsil (*cut*)
Lingual tonsil (lingual nodules)
Palatoglossal arch and muscle (*cut*)
Foramen cecum
Terminal sulcus
Vallate papillae
Foliate papillae
Filiform papillae
Fungiform papilla
Midline groove (median sulcus)

Root

Body

Apex

Dorsum of tongue

Plate 58 Tongue. (Netter: Atlas of Human Anatomy, 4 ed, 2006, Saunders.)

NAP-18

NETTER ANATOMY PLATE

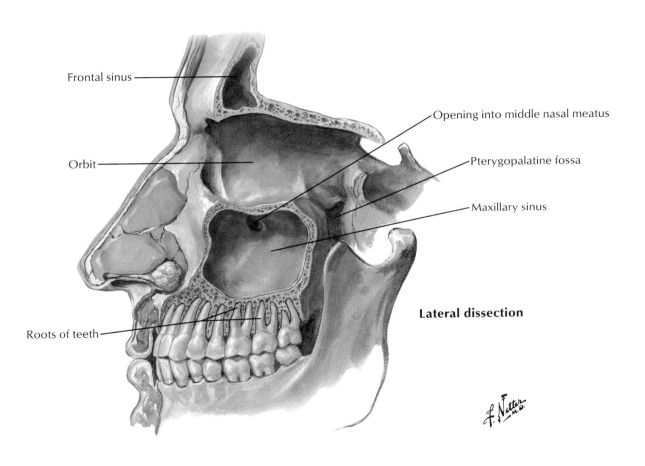

Frontal sinus

Orbit

Roots of teeth

Opening into middle nasal meatus

Pterygopalatine fossa

Maxillary sinus

Lateral dissection

Plate 49 Paranasal Sinuses. (Netter: Atlas of Human Anatomy, 4 ed, 2006, Saunders.)

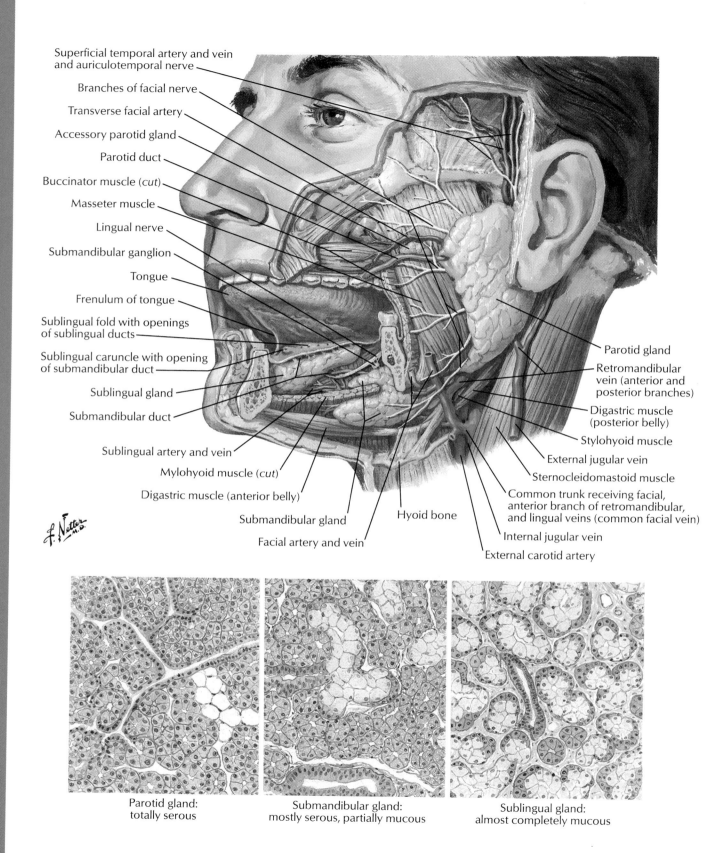

Superficial temporal artery and vein and auriculotemporal nerve

Branches of facial nerve

Transverse facial artery

Accessory parotid gland

Parotid duct

Buccinator muscle (*cut*)

Masseter muscle

Lingual nerve

Submandibular ganglion

Tongue

Frenulum of tongue

Sublingual fold with openings of sublingual ducts

Sublingual caruncle with opening of submandibular duct

Sublingual gland

Submandibular duct

Sublingual artery and vein

Mylohyoid muscle (*cut*)

Digastric muscle (anterior belly)

Submandibular gland

Facial artery and vein

Parotid gland

Retromandibular vein (anterior and posterior branches)

Digastric muscle (posterior belly)

Stylohyoid muscle

External jugular vein

Sternocleidomastoid muscle

Common trunk receiving facial, anterior branch of retromandibular, and lingual veins (common facial vein)

Internal jugular vein

External carotid artery

Hyoid bone

Parotid gland:
totally serous

Submandibular gland:
mostly serous, partially mucous

Sublingual gland:
almost completely mucous

Plate 61   *Salivary Glands. (Netter: Atlas of Human Anatomy, 4 ed, 2006, Saunders.)*

Right coronary artery: left anterior oblique view

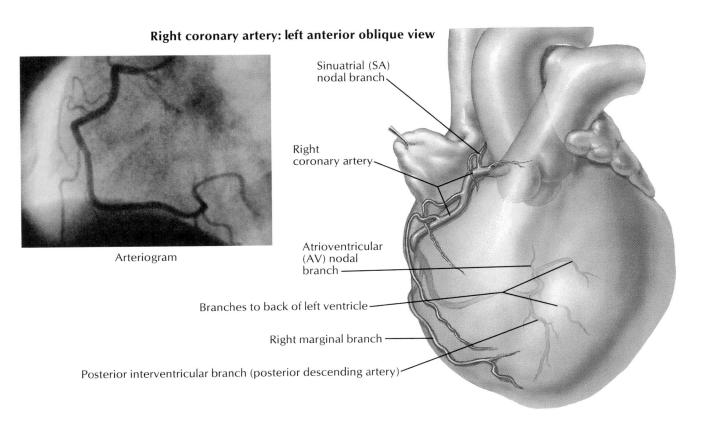

Arteriogram

Sinuatrial (SA) nodal branch

Right coronary artery

Atrioventricular (AV) nodal branch

Branches to back of left ventricle

Right marginal branch

Posterior interventricular branch (posterior descending artery)

Right coronary artery: right anterior oblique view

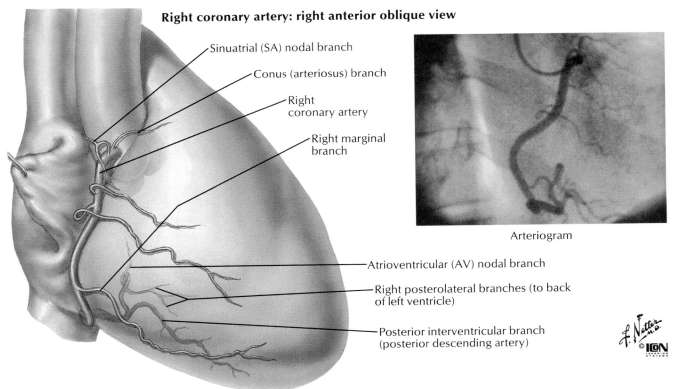

Sinuatrial (SA) nodal branch

Conus (arteriosus) branch

Right coronary artery

Right marginal branch

Arteriogram

Atrioventricular (AV) nodal branch

Right posterolateral branches (to back of left ventricle)

Posterior interventricular branch (posterior descending artery)

Plate 218   Coronary Arteries: Arteriographic Views. (Netter: Atlas of Human Anatomy, 4 ed, 2006, Saunders.)

NAP-21

NETTER ANATOMY PLATE

Left coronary artery: left anterior oblique view

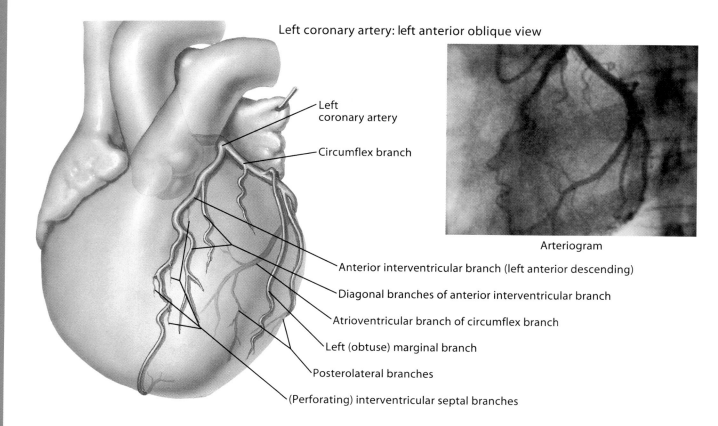

Left coronary artery

Circumflex branch

Arteriogram

Anterior interventricular branch (left anterior descending)

Diagonal branches of anterior interventricular branch

Atrioventricular branch of circumflex branch

Left (obtuse) marginal branch

Posterolateral branches

(Perforating) interventricular septal branches

Left coronary artery: right anterior oblique view

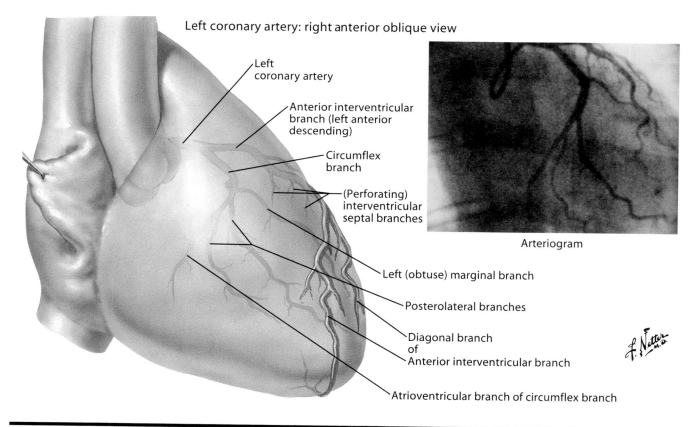

Left coronary artery

Anterior interventricular branch (left anterior descending)

Circumflex branch

(Perforating) interventricular septal branches

Arteriogram

Left (obtuse) marginal branch

Posterolateral branches

Diagonal branch of Anterior interventricular branch

Atrioventricular branch of circumflex branch

f. Netter M.D.

Plate 219   Coronary Arteries: Arteriographic Views. (Netter: Atlas of Human Anatomy, 4 ed, 2006, Saunders.)

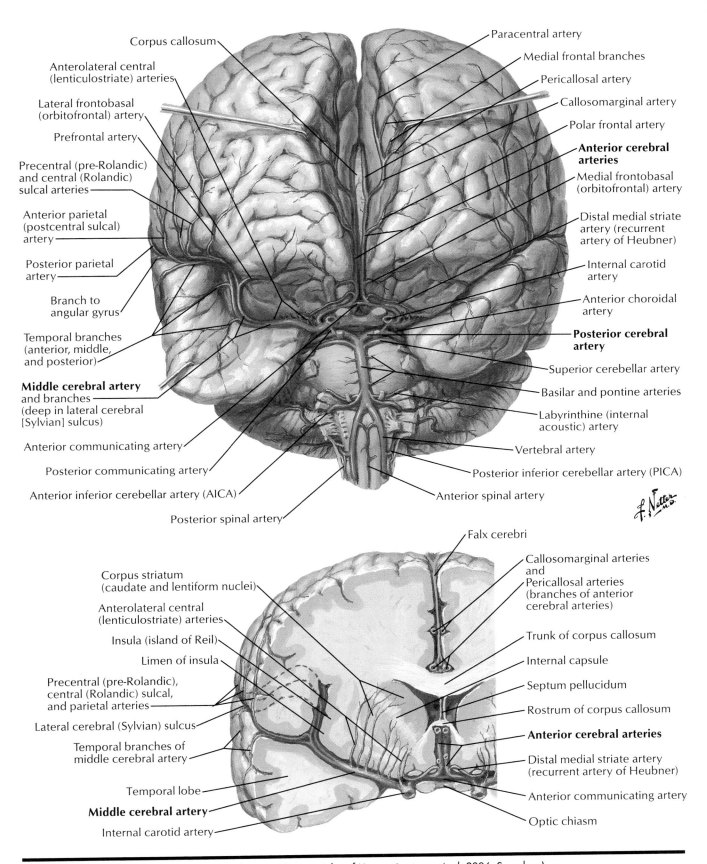

Corpus callosum

Anterolateral central (lenticulostriate) arteries

Lateral frontobasal (orbitofrontal) artery

Prefrontal artery

Precentral (pre-Rolandic) and central (Rolandic) sulcal arteries

Anterior parietal (postcentral sulcal) artery

Posterior parietal artery

Branch to angular gyrus

Temporal branches (anterior, middle, and posterior)

Middle cerebral artery and branches (deep in lateral cerebral [Sylvian] sulcus)

Anterior communicating artery

Posterior communicating artery

Anterior inferior cerebellar artery (AICA)

Posterior spinal artery

Paracentral artery

Medial frontal branches

Pericallosal artery

Callosomarginal artery

Polar frontal artery

Anterior cerebral arteries

Medial frontobasal (orbitofrontal) artery

Distal medial striate artery (recurrent artery of Heubner)

Internal carotid artery

Anterior choroidal artery

Posterior cerebral artery

Superior cerebellar artery

Basilar and pontine arteries

Labyrinthine (internal acoustic) artery

Vertebral artery

Posterior inferior cerebellar artery (PICA)

Anterior spinal artery

Corpus striatum (caudate and lentiform nuclei)

Anterolateral central (lenticulostriate) arteries

Insula (island of Reil)

Limen of insula

Precentral (pre-Rolandic), central (Rolandic) sulcal, and parietal arteries

Lateral cerebral (Sylvian) sulcus

Temporal branches of middle cerebral artery

Temporal lobe

Middle cerebral artery

Internal carotid artery

Falx cerebri

Callosomarginal arteries and Pericallosal arteries (branches of anterior cerebral arteries)

Trunk of corpus callosum

Internal capsule

Septum pellucidum

Rostrum of corpus callosum

Anterior cerebral arteries

Distal medial striate artery (recurrent artery of Heubner)

Anterior communicating artery

Optic chiasm

NETTER ANATOMY PLATE

Plate 141 Arteries of Brain: Frontal View and Section. (Netter: Atlas of Human Anatomy, 4 ed, 2006, Saunders.)

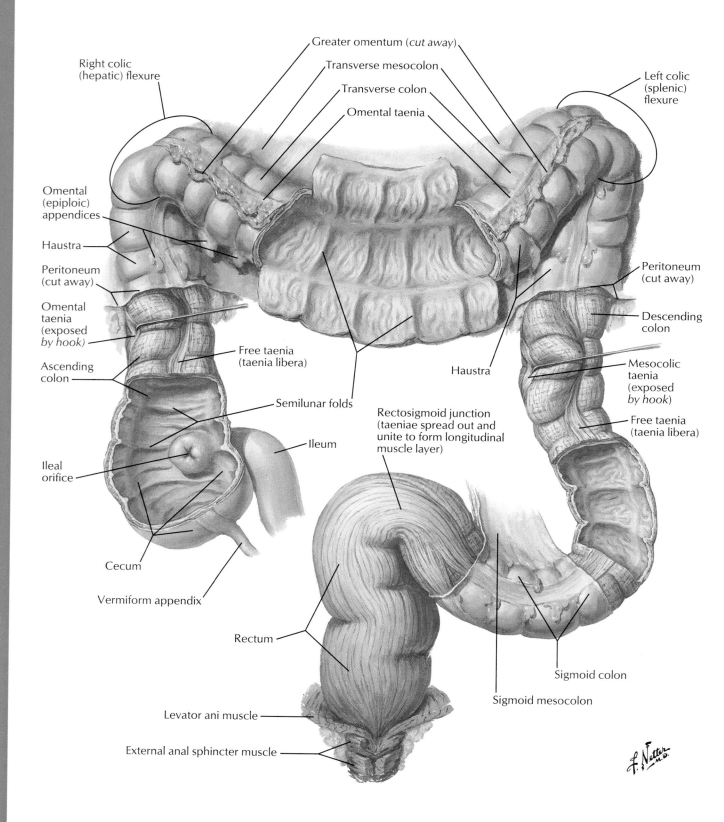

Greater omentum (*cut away*)

Transverse mesocolon

Transverse colon

Omental taenia

Right colic (hepatic) flexure

Left colic (splenic) flexure

Omental (epiploic) appendices

Haustra

Peritoneum (cut away)

Omental taenia (exposed *by hook*)

Ascending colon

Ileal orifice

Cecum

Vermiform appendix

Free taenia (taenia libera)

Semilunar folds

Ileum

Rectum

Levator ani muscle

External anal sphincter muscle

Rectosigmoid junction (taeniae spread out and unite to form longitudinal muscle layer)

Haustra

Peritoneum (cut away)

Descending colon

Mesocolic taenia (exposed *by hook*)

Free taenia (taenia libera)

Sigmoid colon

Sigmoid mesocolon

Plate 284   Mucosa and Musculature of Large Intestine. (Netter: Atlas of Human Anatomy, 4 ed, 2006, Saunders.)

Transverse Section: T3–4 Intervertebral Disc, Manubrium

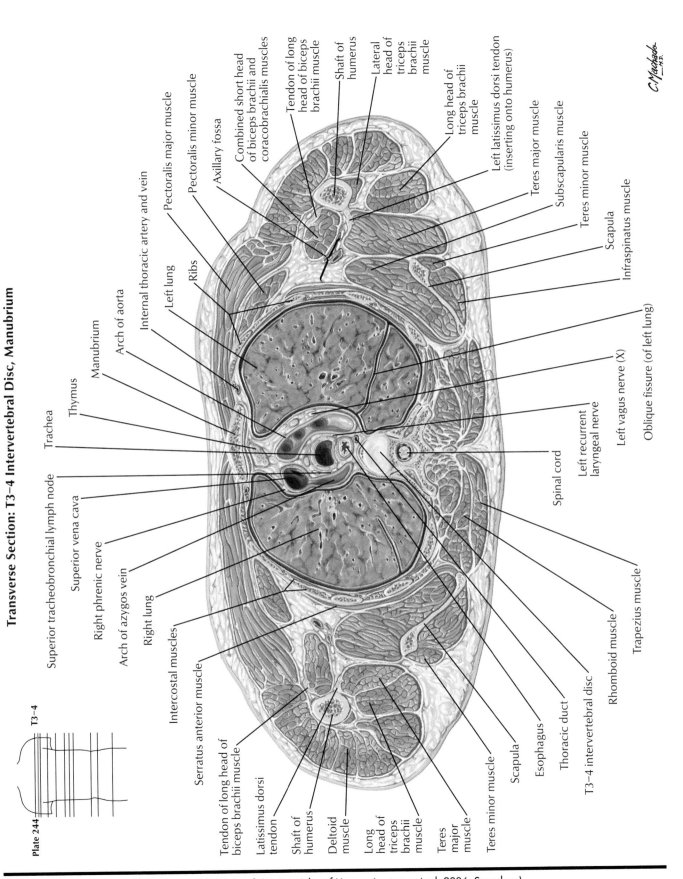

Plate 244 Cross Section of Thorax at T3-4 Disc Level. (Netter: Atlas of Human Anatomy, 4 ed, 2006, Saunders.)

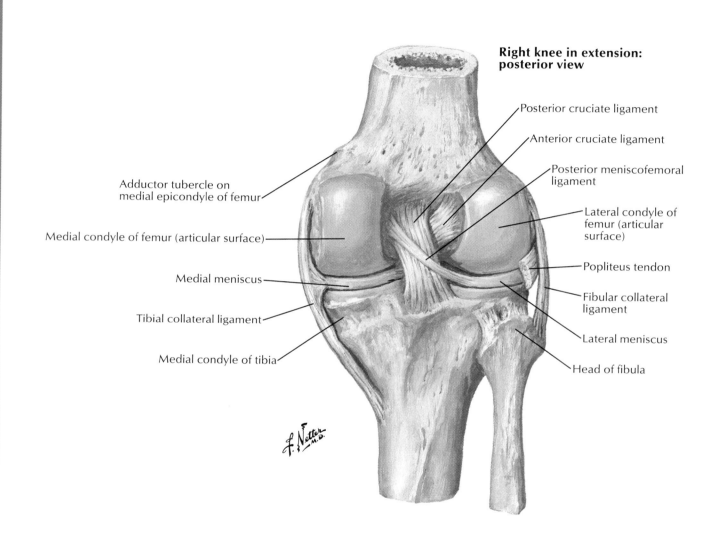

Right knee in extension: posterior view

Posterior cruciate ligament

Anterior cruciate ligament

Posterior meniscofemoral ligament

Adductor tubercle on medial epicondyle of femur

Lateral condyle of femur (articular surface)

Medial condyle of femur (articular surface)

Popliteus tendon

Medial meniscus

Fibular collateral ligament

Tibial collateral ligament

Lateral meniscus

Medial condyle of tibia

Head of fibula

Plate 509   Knee: Cruciate and Collateral Ligaments. (Netter: Atlas of Human Anatomy, 4 ed, 2006, Saunders.)

HCPCS 2012 INDEX

A

Abatacept, J0129
Abciximab, J0130
Abdomen
  dressing holder/binder, A4462
  pad, low profile, L1270
Abduction **control, each,** L2624
Abduction restrainer, A4566
Abduction **rotation bar, foot,** L3140–L3170
AbobotulinumtoxintypeA, J0586
Absorption **dressing,** A6251–A6256
Access, site, occlusive, device, G0269
Access **system,** A4301
Accessories
  ambulation devices, E0153–E0159
  artificial kidney and machine (*see also* ESRD),
    E1510–E1699
  beds, E0271–E0280, E0300–E0326
  wheelchairs, E0950–E1030, E1050–E1298, *E2201–*
    E2295, E2300–E2399, K0001–K0109
ACE/ARB therapy, G8468–G8475
Acetaminophen, J0131◄
Acetazolamide **sodium,** J1120
Acetylcysteine
  inhalation solution, J7604, J7608
  injection, J0132
Activity, therapy, G0176
Acyclovir, J0133
Adalimumab, J0135
Adenosine, J0150, J0152
Adhesive, A4364
  bandage, A6413
  disc or foam pad, A5126
  remover, A4455, A4456
  support, breast prosthesis, A4280
  wound, closure, G0168
Adjunctive, dental, D9110–D9999
Administration, **Part D**
  supply, tositumomab, G3001
  vaccine, hepatitis B, G0010
  vaccine, influenza, G0008
  vaccine, pneumococcal, G0009
Admission, observation, G0379
Administrative, **Miscellaneous and**
  Investigational, A9000–A9999
Adrenalin, J0171
Advanced **life support,** *A0390, A0426, A0427, A0433*
Aerosol
  compressor, ~~E0571,~~ E0572
  compressor filter, K0178–K0179
  mask, K0180
AFO, E1815, E1830, L1900–L1990, L4392, L4396
Agalsidase **beta,** J0180
Aggrastat, J3245
A-hydroCort, J1710
Aide, **home, health,** *G0156, S9122, T1021*

Aide (Continued)
  bath/toilet, E0160–E0162, E0235, E0240–E0249
  services, G0151–G0156, G0179–G0181, S5180,
    S5181, S9122, T1021, T1022
Air **bubble detector, dialysis,** *E1530*
Air **fluidized bed,** E0194
Air **pressure pad/mattress,** E0186, E0197
Air **travel and nonemergency transportation,** A0140
Alarm
  not otherwise classified, A9280
  pressure, dialysis, E1540
Alatrofloxacin **mesylate,** J0200
Albumin, **human,** P9041, P9042
Albuterol
  all formulations, inhalation solution,
    concentrated, J7610, J7611
  all formulations, inhalation solution, unit
    dose, J7609, J7613
  all formulations, inhalation solution, J7620
Alcohol/substance, **assessment,** *G0396, G0397,*
  H0001, H0003, H0049
Alcohol, A4244
Alcohol **wipes,** A4245
Aldesleukin **(IL2),** J9015
Alefacept, J0215
Alemtuzumab, J9010
Alert **device,** A9280
Alginate **dressing,** A6196–A6199
Alglucerase, J0205
Alglucosidase, J0220
Alglucosidase **alfa,** J0221◄
Alphanate, J7186
Alpha-1-proteinase **inhibitor, human,** J0256,
  J0257←
Alprostadil
  injection, J0270
  urethral suppository, J0275
ALS mileage, A0390
Alteplase **recombinant,** J2997
Alternating **pressure mattress/pad,** A4640, E0180,
  E0181, E0277
Alveoloplasty, D7310–D7321
Amalgam **dental restoration,** D2140–D2161
Ambulance, A0021–A0999
  air, A0430, A0431, A0435, A0436
  disposable supplies, A0382–A0398
  oxygen, A0422
Ambulation **device,** E0100–E0159
Amikacin **Sulfate,** J0278
Aminolevulinate, J7309
Aminolevulinic **acid HCl,** J7308
Aminophylline, J0280
Amiodarone **HCl,** J0282
Amitriptyline **HCl,** J1320
Ammonia **N-13,** A9526
Ammonia **test paper,** A4774
Amniotic **membrane,** V2790
Amobarbital, J0300

◄ New   ← Revised   ✔ Reinstated   ~~deleted~~ Deleted

Amphotericin **B,** J0285
  Lipid Complex, J0287–J0289
Ampicillin
  sodium, J0290
  sodium/sulbactam sodium, J0295
Amputee
  adapter, wheelchair, E0959
  prosthesis, L5000–L7510, L7520, L7900,
    L8400–L8465
  stump sock, L8470–L8485
  wheelchair, E1170–E1190, E1200, K0100
Amygdalin, J3570
Anadulafungin, J0348
Analgesia, dental, D9230
Analysis
  saliva, D0418
  semen, G0027
*Angiography, **iliac, artery,** G0278*
  reconstruction, G0288
  renal, artery, G0275
Anistreplase, J0350
Ankle splint, recumbent, K0126–K0130
Ankle-foot orthosis (AFO), L1900–L1990, L2106–
  L2116, L4361, L4392, L4396
Anterior-posterior-lateral orthosis, L0700, L0710
*Antidepressant, **documentation,** G8126–G8128*
Anti-emetic, oral, Q0163–Q0181, J8498, J8597
Anti-hemophilic factor (Factor VIII), J7190–J7192
Anti-inhibitors, per I.U., J7198
*Antimicrobial, **prophylaxis, documentation,** G8201,
  D4281*
Anti-neoplastic drug, NOC, J9999
Antithrombin III, J7197
Antithrombin recombinant, J7196
Antral fistula closure, oral, D7260
Apexification, dental, D3351–D3353
Apicoectomy, D3410–D3426
Apomorphine, J0364
Appliance
  cleaner, A5131
  pneumatic, E0655–E0673
*Application, **heat, cold,** E0200–E0239*
Aprotinin, J0365
Aqueous
  shunt, L8612
  sterile, J7051
*ARB/ACE **therapy,** G8468–G8475*
Arbutamine HCl, J0395
Arch support, L3040–L3100
  Intralesional, J3302
Arformoterol, J7605
Aripiprazole, J0400
Arm, wheelchair, E0973
Arsenic trioxide, J9017
Artificial
  cornea, L8609
  kidney machines and accessories (*see also* Dialysis),
    E1510–E1699

Artificial (*Continued*)
  larynx, L8500
  saliva, A9155
*Arthrography, **injection, sacroiliac, joint,** G0259,
  G0260*
*Arthroscopy, **knee, surgical,** G0289, S2112, S2300*
Asparaginase, J9020
*Aspiration, **bone marrow,** G0364*
*Aspirator, **VABRA,** A4480*
Assessment
  *alcohol/substance, G0396, G0397, H0001, H0003,
    H0049*
  audiologic, V5008–V5020
  cardiac output, M0302
  speech, V5362–V5364
*Attachment, **walker,** E0154–E0159*
Astramorph, J2275
Atropine
  inhalation solution, concentrated, J7635
  inhalation solution, unit dose, J7636
Atropine sulfate, J0461
Audiologic assessment, V5008–V5020
Auditory osseointegrated device,
  L8690–L8693
Auricular prosthesis, D5914, D5927
Aurothioglucose, J2910
Azacitidine, J9025
Azathioprine, J7500, J7501
Azithromycin injection, J0456

B

Back supports, L0621–L0861, L0960
Baclofen, J0475, J0476
Bacterial sensitivity study, P7001
Bag
  drainage, A4357
  enema, A4458
  irrigation supply, A4398
  urinary, A4358, A5112
Basiliximab, J0480
*Bath, **aid,** E0160–E0162, E0235, E0240–E0249*
Bathtub
  chair, E0240
  stool or bench, E0245, E0247–E0248
  transfer rail, E0246
  wall rail, E0241, E0242
Battery, L7360, L7364–L7368
  charger, E1066, L7362, L7366
  replacement for blood glucose monitor,
    A4233–A4234
  replacement for cochlear implant device,
    L8623–L8624
  replacement for TENS, A4630
  ventilator, A4611–A4613
BCG live, intravesical, J9031
Beclomethasone inhalation solution, J7622

◀ New   ← Revised   ✔ Reinstated   ~~deleted~~ Deleted

Bed
   accessories, E0271–E0280, E0300–E0326
   air fluidized, E0194
   cradle, any type, E0280
   drainage bag, bottle, A4357, A5102
   hospital, E0250–E0270, E0300–E0329
   pan, E0275, E0276
   rail, E0305, E0310
   safety enclosure frame/canopy, E0316
Behavioral, **health, treatment services,**
   H0002–H2037
Belimumab, J0490 ◄
Belt
   extremity, E0945
   ostomy, A4367
   pelvic, E0944
   safety, K0031
   wheelchair, E0978, E0979
Bench, **bathtub** (*see also* **Bathtub**)**, E0245**
Bendamustine **HCl,** J9033
Benesch **boot,** L3212–L3214
Benztropine, J0515
Betadine, A4246, A4247
Betamethasone
   acetate and betamethasone sodium phosphate,
      J0702
   inhalation solution, J7624
Bethanechol **chloride,** J0520
Bevacizumab, J9035, Q2024
Bicuspid **(excluding final restoration), D3320**
   retreatment, by report, D3347
   surgery, first root, D3421
Bifocal, **glass or plastic, V2200–V2299**
Bilirubin **(phototherapy) light, E0202**
Binder, A4465
Biofeedback **device, E0746**
Bioimpedance, **electrical, cardiac output,** M0302
Biperiden **lactate,** J0190
Bitewing, D0270–D0274
Bitolterol **mesylate, inhalation solution**
   concentrated, J7628
   unit dose, J7629
Bivalirudin, J0583
Bladder **calculi irrigation solution,** Q2004
Bleomycin **sulfate,** J9040
Blood
   count, G0306, G0307, S3630
   fresh frozen plasma, P9017
   glucose monitor, E0607, E2100, E2101, *S1030,*
      S1031
   glucose test, A4253
   granulocytes, pheresis, P9050
   ketone test, A4252
   leak detector, dialysis, E1560
   leukocyte poor, P9016
   mucoprotein, P2038
   platelets, P9019
   platelets, irradiated, P9032

Blood *(Continued)*
   platelets, leukocytes reduced, P9031
   platelets, leukocytes reduced, irradiated, P9033
   platelets, pheresis, P9034
   platelets, pheresis, irradiated, P9036
   platelets, pheresis, leukocytes reduced,
      P9035
   platelets, pheresis, leukocytes reduced, irradiated,
      P9037
   pressure monitor, A4660, A4663, A4670
   pump, dialysis, E1620
   red blood cells, deglycerolized, P9039
   red blood cells, irradiated, P9038
   red blood cells, leukocytes reduced, P9016
   red blood cells, leukocytes reduced, irradiated,
      P9040
   red blood cells, washed, P9022
   strips, A4253
   supply, P9010 P9022
   testing supplies, A4770
   tubing, A4750, A4755
Blood **collection devices accessory,** A4257, E0620
BMI, G8417–G8422
Body **jacket**
   scoliosis, L1300, L1310
Body **sock,** L0984
Body, mass, index, G8417–G8422
Bond **or adhesive, ostomy skin,** *A4364*
Bone
   density, study, G0130
   marrow, aspiration, G0364
Boot
   pelvic, E0944
   surgical, ambulatory, L3260
Bortezomib, J9041
Brachytherapy **radioelements,** Q3001
Breast **prosthesis,** L8000–L8035, L8600
   adhesive skin support, A4280
Breast **pump**
   accessories, A4281–A4286
   electric, any type, E0603
   heavy duty, hospital grade, E0604
   manual, any type, E0602
Breathing **circuit,** A4618
Bridge
   recement, D6930
   repair, by report, D6980
Brompheniramine **maleate,** J0945
Budesonide **inhalation solution,** J7626, J7627,
      J7633, J7634
Bulking **agent,** L8604
Buprenorphine **hydrochloride,** J0592
Bus, **nonemergency transportation,** A0110
Busulfan, J0594, J8510
Butorphanol **tartrate,** J0595
Bypass, **graft, coronary, artery**
   documentation, G8160–G8163
   surgery, S2205–S2209

◄ New   ← Revised   ✔ Reinstated   ~~deleted~~ Deleted

C

C-1 Esterase Inhibitor, J0597–J0598
Cabazitaxel, J9043◀
Cabergoline, **oral,** J8515
Caffeine **citrate,** J0706
CABG, documentation, G8160–G8163
Cabinet/System, ultraviolet, E0691–E0694
CAD documentation, G8160–G8163
Calcitriol, J0636
Calcitonin-salmon, J0630
Calcitrol, S0169
Calcium
  disodium edetate, J0600
  gluconate, J0610
  glycerophosphate and calcium lactate, J0620
  lactate and calcium glycerophosphate, J0620
  leucovorin, J0640
Calibrator **solution,** A4256
Canakinumab, J0638
Cancer, screening
  cervical or vaginal, G0101
  colorectal, G0104–G0106, G0120–G0122,
    G0328, S3890
  prostate, G0102, G0103
Cane, E0100, E0105
  accessory, A4636, A4637
Canister
  disposable, used with suction pump, A7000
  non-disposable, used with suction pump, A7001
Cannula, **nasal,** A4615
Capecitabine, **oral,** J8520, J8521
Capsaicin **patch,** J7335
Carbon **filter,** A4680
Carboplatin, J9045
Cardia **Event, recorder, implantable,** E0616
Cardiokymography, Q0035
Cardiovascular **services,** M0300–M0301
Carmustine, J9050
Caries **susceptibility test,** D0425
Care, coordinated, G9001–G9011, H1002
Case **management,** T1016, T1017
Care plan, G0162
Caspofungin **acetate,** J0637
Cast
  diagnostic, dental, D0470
  hand restoration, L6900–L6915
  materials, special, A4590
  supplies, A4580, A4590, Q4001–Q4051
  thermoplastic, L2106, L2126
Caster
  front, for power wheelchair, K0099
  wheelchair, E0997, E0998
Catheter, A4300–A4355
  anchoring device, A5200, A4333, A4334
  cap, disposable (dialysis), A4860
  external collection device, A4327–A4330, A4347

Catheter *(Continued)*
  implanted, A7042, A7043
  indwelling, A4338–A4346
  insertion tray, A4354
  intermittent with insertion supplies, A4353
  irrigation supplies, A4355
  male external, A4324, A4325, A4348
  oropharyngeal suction, A4628
  starter set, A4329
  trachea (suction), A4609, A4610, A4624
  transtracheal oxygen, A4608
  vascular, A4300, A4301
Catheterization, **specimen collection,** P9612, P9615
CBC, G0306, G0307
Cefazolin **sodium,** J0690
Cefepime **HCl,** J0692
Cefotaxime **sodium,** J0698
Ceftaroline **fosamil,** J0712◀
Ceftazidime, J0713
Ceftizoxime **sodium,** J0715
Ceftriaxone **sodium,** J0696
Cefuroxime **sodium,** J0697
CellCept, K0412
Cellular **therapy,** M0075
Cement, **ostomy,** A4364
Centrifuge, A4650
Cephalin **Floculation, blood,** P2028
Cephalothin **sodium,** J1890
Cephapirin **sodium,** J0710
Certification, physician, home, health,
  G0179–G0182
Certolizumab **pegol,** J0718
Cerumen, removal, G0268
Cervical
  cancer, screening, G0101
  cytopathology, G0123, G0124, G0141–G0148
  halo, L0810–L0830
  head harness/halter, E0942
  orthosis, L0100–L0200
  traction, E0855, E0856
Cervical **cap contraceptive,** A4261
Cervical-thoracic-lumbar-sacral **orthosis (CTLSO),**
  L0700, L0710
Cetuximab, J9055
Chair
  adjustable, dialysis, E1570
  lift, E0627
  rollabout, E1031
  sitz bath, E0160–E0162
  transport, E1035–E1039
Chelation **therapy,** M0300
Chemical **endarterectomy,** M0300
Chemistry **and toxicology tests,** P2028–P3001
Chemotherapy
  administration, Q0083–Q0085 (hospital reporting
    only)
  drug, oral, not otherwise classified, J8999
  drugs (*see also* drug by name), J9000–J9999

◀ **New**   ← **Revised**   ✔ **Reinstated**   ~~deleted~~ **Deleted**

Chest **shell (cuirass),** E0457
Chest **Wall Oscillation System,** E0483
  hose, replacement, A7026
  vest, replacement, A7025
Chest **wrap,** E0459
Chin **cup, cervical,** L0150
Chloramphenicol **sodium succinate,** J0720
Chlordiazepoxide **HCl,** J1990
Chloromycetin **Sodium Succinate,** J0720
Chloroprocaine **HCl,** J2400
Chloroquine **HCl,** J0390
Chlorothiazide **sodium,** J1205
Chlorpromazine **HCl,** J3230
Choroid, lesion, destruction, G0186
Chorionic **gonadotropin,** J0725
Chromic **phosphate P32 suspension,** A9564
Chromium **CR-51 sodium chromate,** A9553
Cidofovir, J0740
Cilastatin **sodium, imipenem,** J0743
Ciprofloxacin, **for intravenous infusion,** J0744
Cisplatin, J9060
Cladribine, J9065
Clamp
  dialysis, A4910, A4918, A4920
  external urethral, A4356
Cleanser, **wound,** A6260
Cleansing **agent, dialysis equipment,** A4790
Clofarabine, J9027
Clonidine, J0735
Closure, wound, adhesive, tissue, G0168
Clotting **time tube,** A4771
Clubfoot **wedge,** L3380
Cochlear **prosthetic implant,** L8614
  accessories, L8615–L8617
  batteries, L8621–L8624
  replacement, L8619, L8627–L8629
Codeine **phosphate,** J0745
Colchicine, J0760
Cold/Heat, application, E0200–E0240
Colistimethate **sodium,** J0770
Collagen
  meniscus implant procedure, G0428
  skin test, G0025
  urinary tract implant, L8603
  wound dressing, A6020–A6024
Collagenase, **Clostridium Histolyticum,** J0775
Collar, **cervical**
  multiple post, L0180–L0200
  nonadjust (foam), L0120
Collection and preparation, saliva, D0417
Colorectal, screening, cancer, G0104–G0106,
  G0120–G0122, G0328, S3890
Coly-Mycin **M,** J0770
Comfort **items,** A9190
Complete, blood, count, G0306, G0307
Commode, E0160–E0175
  chair, E0170–E0171
  lift, E0625, E0172

Commode *(Continued)*
  pail, E0167
  seat, wheelchair, E0968
Composite **dressing,** A6203–A6205
Compressed **gas system,** E0424–E0480
Compressor
  aerosol, E0572, E0575
  air, E0565
  nebulizer, E0570–E0585
  pneumatic, E0650–E0676
Compression
  bandage, A4460
  burn garment, A6501–A6512
  stockings, A6530–A6549
Compressor, E0565, E0570, ~~E0571~~, E0572,
  E0650–E0652
Conductive gel/paste, A4558
Conductivity **meter, bath, dialysis,** E1550
Conference, team, G0175, G9007, S0220, S0221
Congo **red, blood,** P2029
Contact **layer,** A6206–A6208
Contact **lens,** V2500–V2599
Continent **device,** A5081, A5082, A5083
Continuous **glucose monitoring system**
  receiver, A9278
  sensor, A9276
  transmitter, A9277
Continuous **passive motion exercise device,**
  E0936
Continuous **positive airway pressure (CPAP)**
  device, E0601
  compressor, K0269
Contraceptive
  cervical cap, A4261
  condoms, A4267, A4268
  diaphragm, A4266
  intratubal occlusion device, A4264
  intrauterine, copper, J7300
  intrauterine, levonorgestrel releasing, J7302
  levonorgestrel, implants and supplies, A4260
  patch, J7304
  spermicide, A4269
  supply, A4267–A4269
  vaginal ring, J7303
Contracts, **maintenance, ESRD,** A4890
Contrast **material**
  injection during MRI, A4643
  low osmolar, A4644–A4646
Coordinated, care, G9001–G9011
Corneal **tissue processing,** V2785
Corset, **spinal orthosis,** L0970–L0976
Corticorelin **ovine triflutate,** J0795
Corticotropin, J0800
Corvert, *see* **Ibutilide fumarate**
Cosyntropin, J0833, J0834
Cough **stimulating device,** A7020, E0482
Counseling **for control of dental disease,** D1310,
  D1320

Counseling, **smoking and tobacco cessation,** *G0436, G0437*

Count, **blood,** *G0306, G0307, S3636*

Counterpulsation, **external,** *G0166*

Cover, **wound**
 alginate dressing, A6196–A6198
 foam dressing, A6209–A6214
 hydrogel dressing, A6242–A6248
 non-contact wound warming cover, and accessory, A6000, E0231, E0232
 specialty absorptive dressing, A6251–A6256

CPAP **(continuous positive airway pressure) device,** E0601
 headgear, K0185
 humidifier, A7046
 intermittent assist, E0452

Cradle, **bed,** E0280

Crib, E0300

Cromolyn **sodium, inhalation solution, unit dose,** J7631, J7632

Crotalidae **polyvalent immune fab,** J0840◀

Crowns, D2710–D2810, D2930–D2933, D4249, D6720–D6792

Crutches, E0110–E0118
 accessories, A4635–A4637, K0102

Cryoprecipitate, **each unit,** P9012

CTLSO, L1000–L1120, L0700, L0710

Cuirass, E0457

Culture **sensitivity study,** P7001

Cushion, **wheelchair,** E0977

Cyanocobalamin **Cobalt C057,** A9559

Cycler **dialysis machine,** E1594

Cyclophosphamide, J9070
 oral, J8530

Cyclosporine, J7502, J7515, J7516

Cytarabine, J9100
 liposome, J9098

Cytomegalovirus **immune globulin (human),** J0850

Cytopathology, **cervical or vaginal,** *G0123, G0124, G0141–G0148*

D

Dacarbazine, J9130

Daclizumab, J7513

Dactinomycin, J9120

Dalalone, J1100

Dalteparin **sodium,** J1645

Daptomycin, J0878

Darbepoetin **Alfa,** J0881–J0882

Daunorubicin
 Citrate, J9151
 HCl, J9150

DaunoXome, *see* **Daunorubicin citrate**

Decitabine, J0894

Decubitus **care equipment,** E0180–E0199

Deferoxamine **mesylate,** J0895

Defibrillator, **external,** E0617, K0606
 battery, K0607
 electrode, K0609
 garment, K0608

Degarelix, J9155

Deionizer, **water purification system,** E1615

Delivery/set-up/dispensing, A9901

Denileukin **diftitox,** J9160

Denosumab, J0897◀

Density, **bone, study,** *G0130*

Dental **procedures**
 adjunctive general services, D9000–D9999
 alveoloplasty, D7310–D7320
 analgesia, D9230
 diagnostic, D0100–D0999
 endodontics, D3000–D3999
 evaluations, D0120–D0180
 implant services, D6000–D6199
 implants, D3460, D5925, D6010–D6067, D6075–D6199
 laboratory, D0415–D0999
 maxillofacial, D5900–D5999
 orthodontics, D8000–D8999
 periodontics, D4000–D4999
 preventive, D1000–D1999
 prosthetics, D5911–D5960, D5999
 prosthodontics, fixed, D6200–D6999
 prosthodontics, removable, D5000–D5999
 restorative, D2000–D2999

Dentures, D5110–D5899

Depo-estradiol **cypionate,** J1000

Dermal **filler injection,** *G0429*

Desmopressin **acetate,** J2597

Destruction, **lesion, choroid,** *G0186*

Detector, **blood leak, dialysis,** E1560

Dexamethasone
 acetate, J1094
 inhalation solution, concentrated, J7637
 inhalation solution, unit dose, J7638
 intravitreal implant, J7312
 oral, J8540
 sodium phosphate, J1100

Dextran, J7100

Dextrose
 saline (normal), J7042
 water, J7060, J7070

Dextrostick, A4772

Diabetes
 evaluation, G0245, G0246
 shoes, A5500–A5508
 training, outpatient, G0108, G0109

Diagnostic
 dental services, D0100–D0999
 radiology services, R0070–R0076

Dialysate
 concentrate additives, A4765
 solution, A4728
 testing solution, A4760

◀ New   ← Revised   ✔ Reinstated   ~~deleted~~ Deleted

Dialysis
  air bubble detector, E1530
  bath conductivity, meter, E1550
  chemicals/antiseptics solution, A4674
  disposable cycler set, A4671
  emergency, G0257
  equipment, E1510–E1702
  extension line, A4672–A4673
  filter, A4680
  fluid barrier, E1575
  forceps, A4910
  home, S9335, S9339
  kit, A4820
  pressure alarm, E1540
  shunt, A4740
  supplies, A4650–A4927
  thermometer, A4910
  tourniquet, A4910
  unipuncture control system, E1580
  unscheduled, G0257
  venous pressure clamp, A4918
Dialyzer, A4690
Diaper, T1500, T4521–T4540
  adult incontinence garment, A4520
Diazepam, J3360
Diazoxide, J1730
Dicyclomine HCl, J0500
Diethylstilbestrol diphosphate, J9165
Digoxin, J1160
Digoxin immune fab (ovine), J1162
Dihydroergotamine mesylate, J1110
Dimenhydrinate, J1240
Dimercaprol, J0470
Dimethyl sulfoxide (DMSO), J1212
Diphenhydramine HCl, J1200
Dipyridamole, J1245
Disarticulation
  lower extremities, prosthesis, L5000–L5999
  upper extremities, prosthesis, L6000–L6692
Disease
  status, oncology, G9063–G9139
Disposable supplies, ambulance, A0382, A0384,
  A0392–A0398
Dispensing, fee, pharmacy, G0333, Q0510–Q0514,
  S9430
DME
  miscellaneous, A9900–A9999
DMSO, J1212
Dobutamine HCl, J1250
Docetaxel, J9171
Documentation
  antidepressant, G8126–G8128
  blood pressure, G8476–G8478
  bypass, graft, coronary, artery, documentation,
    G8160–G8163
  CABG, G8160–G8163
  dysphagia, G8232
  dysphagia, screening, G8232, V5364

Documentation (Continued)
  eye, functions, G8315–G8333
  influenza, immunization, G8482–G8484
  osteoporosis, G8401
  pharmacologic therapy for osteoporosis, G8634,
    G8635
  prophylaxis, DVT, G8218
  prophylactic parenteral antibiotic, G8629–G8632
  prophylaxis, thrombosis, deep, vein, G8218
  urinary, incontinence, G8063, G8267
Dolasetron mesylate, J1260
Dome and mouthpiece (for nebulizer), A7016
Dopamine HCl, J1265
Doripenem, J1267
Dornase alpha, inhalation solution, unit dose
  form, J7639
Doxercalciferol, J1270
Doxil, J9001
Doxorubicin HCl, J9000, J9001
Drainage
  bag, A4357, A4358
  board, postural, E0606
  bottle, A5102
Dressing (see also Bandage), A6020–A6406
  alginate, A6196–A6199
  collagen, A6020–A6024
  composite, A6203–A6205
  contact layer, A6206–A6208
  foam, A6209–A6215
  gauze, A6216–A6230, A6402–A6406
  holder/binder, A4462
  hydrocolloid, A6234–A6241
  hydrogel, A6242–A6248
  specialty absorptive, A6251–A6256
  transparent film, A6257–A6259
  tubular, A6457
Droperidol, J1790
  and fentanyl citrate, J1810
Dropper, A4649
Drug screen, G0434
Drugs (see also Table of Drugs)
  administered through a metered dose inhaler,
    J3535
  antiemetic, J8489, J8597, Q0163–Q0181
  chemotherapy, J8500–J9999
  disposable delivery system, 5 ml or less per hour,
    A4306
  disposable delivery system, 50 ml or greater per
    hour, A4305
  immunosuppressive, J7500–J7599
  infusion supplies, A4230–A4232, A4221, A4222
  inhalation solutions, J7608–J7699
  non-prescription, A9150
  not otherwise classified, J3490, J7599, J7699, J7799,
    J8499, J8999, J9999
  oral, NOS, J8499
  prescription, oral, J8499, J8999
Dry pressure pad/mattress, E0179, E0184, E0199

◄ New   ← Revised   ✔ Reinstated   ~~deleted~~ Deleted

Durable **medical equipment (DME),** E0100–E1830,
 K Codes
Duraclon, *see* **Clonidine**
Dyphylline, J1180
Dysphagia, screening, documentation, G8232,
 V5364
Dystrophic, nails, trimming, G0127

E

Ear **mold,** V5264
Ecallantide, J1290
Echocardiography **injectable contrast**
 material, A9700
Eculizumab, J1300
ED, visit, G0380–G0384
Edetate
 calcium disodium, J0600
 disodium, J3520
Eggcrate **dry pressure pad/mattress,** E0184, E0199
Elastic **garments,** A4466
Elbow
 disarticulation, endoskeletal, L6450
 orthosis (EO), E1800, L3700–L3740, L3760
 protector, E0191
Electric, nerve, stimulator, transcutaneous, A4595,
 E0720–E0749
Electrical **work, dialysis equipment,** A4870
Electromagnetic, therapy, G0295, G0329
Electronic medication compliance, T1505
Electrodes, **per pair,** A4556
Elevating **leg rest,** K0195
Elliotts **b solution,** J9175
Emergency department, visit, G0380–G0384
EMG, E0746
Eminase, J0350
Endarterectomy, **chemical,** M0300
Endodontic **procedures,** D3000–D3999
 periapical services, D3410–D3470
 pulp capping, D3110, D3120
 root canal therapy, D3310-D3353
 therapy, D3310–D3330
Endoscope **sheath,** A4270
Endoskeletal **system, addition,** L5848, L5856–
 L5857, L5925, *L5961*
Endodontics, dental, D3000–D3999
Enfuvirtide, J1324
Enoxaparin **sodium,** J1650
Enema, bag, A4458
Enteral
 feeding supply kit (syringe) (pump) (gravity),
  B4034–B4036
 formulae, B4149–B4156
 nutrition infusion pump (with alarm) (without),
  B9000, B9002
 therapy, supplies, B4000–B9999
Epinephrine, J0171

Epirubicin **HCl,** J9178
Epoetin **alpha,** J0885–J0886, Q4081
Epoprostenol, J1325
Equipment
 decubitus, E0181–E0199
 exercise, A9300, E0935, E0936
 orthopedic, E0910–E0948, E1800–E8002
 oxygen, E0424–E0486, E1353–E1406
 pump, E0781, E0784, E0791
 respiratory, E0424–E0601
 safety, E0700, E0705
 traction, E0830–E0900
 transfer, E0705
 trapeze, E0910–E0912, E0940
 whirlpool, E1300, E1310
Ergonovine **maleate,** J1330
Eribulin **mesylate,** J9179◄
Ertapenem **sodium,** J1335
Erythromycin **lactobionate,** J1364
ESRD **(End-Stage Renal Disease;** *see also* **Dialysis)**
 machines and accessories, E1500–E1699
 plumbing, A4870
 supplies, A4651–A4929
Estrogen **conjugated,** J1410
Estrone **(5, Aqueous),** J1435
Ethanolamine **oleate,** J1430
Etidronate **disodium,** J1436
Etonogestrel **implant system,** J7307
Etoposide, J9181
 oral, J8560
Everolimus, J8561◄
Euflexxa, J7323
Evaluation
 conformity, V5020
 contact lens, S0592
 dental, D0120–D0180
 diabetic, G0245, G0246
 footwear, G8410–G8416
 fundus, G8325–G8328
 hearing, S0618, V5008, V5010
 hospice, G0337
 multidisciplinary, H2000
 nursing, T1001
 ocularist, S9150
 performance measurement, S3005
 resident, T2011
 speech, S9152
 team, T1024
 treatment response, G0254
Examination
 gynecological, S0610–S0613
 ophthalmological, S0620, S0621
 oral, D0120–D0160
 pinworm, Q0113
 ringworm, S0605
Exercise
 class, S9451
 equipment, A9300, E0935, E0936

◄ New ← Revised ✔ Reinstated ~~deleted~~ Deleted

External
    ambulatory infusion pump, E0781, E0784
    ambulatory insulin delivery system, A9274
    power, battery components, L7360–L7368
    power, elbow, L7160–L7191
    urinary supplies, A4356-A4359
Extractions (see also Dental procedures), D7110–
    D7130, D7250
Extraoral films, D0250, D0260
Extremity
    belt/harness, E0945
    traction, E0870–E0880
Eye
    case, V2756
    functions, documentation, G8315–G8333
    lens (contact) (spectacle), V2100–V2615
    prosthetic, V2623, V2629
    service (miscellaneous), V2700–V2799

F

Faceplate, ostomy, A4361
Face tent, oxygen, A4619
Factor VIIA coagulation factor, recombinant, J7189
Factor VIII, anti-hemophilic factor, J7185,
    J7190–J7192
Factor IX, J7193, J7194, J7195
Factor XIII, anti-hemophilic factor, J7180 ◀
Family Planning Education, H1010
Fee
    coordinated care, G9001–G9011
    dispensing, pharmacy, G0333, Q0510–Q0514, S9430
Fentanyl citrate, J3010
    and droperidol, J1810
Fern test, Q0114
Ferumoxytol, Q0138, Q0139
Filgrastim (G-CSF), J1440, J1441
Filler, wound
    alginate dressing, A6199
    foam dressing, A6215
    hydrocolloid dressing, A6240, A6241
    hydrogel dressing, A6248
    not elsewhere classified, A6261, A6262
Film, transparent (for dressing), A6257–A6259
Filter
    aerosol compressor, A7014
    dialysis carbon, A4680
    ostomy, A4368
    tracheostoma, A4481
    ultrasonic generator, A7014
Fistula cannulation set, A4730
Flebogamma, J1572
Flowmeter, E0440, E0555, E0580
Floxuridine, J9200
Fluconazole, injection, J1450
Fludarabine phosphate, J8562, J9185
Fluid barrier, dialysis, E1575

Flunisolide inhalation solution, J7641
Fluocinolone, J7311
Fluoride treatment, D1201–D1205
Fluorodeoxyglucose F-18 FDG, A9552
Fluorouracil, J9190
Foam
    dressing, A6209–A6215
    pad adhesive, A5126
Folding walker, E0135, E0143
Foley catheter, A4312–A4316, A4338–A4346
Fomepizole, J1451
Fomivirsen sodium intraocular, J1452
Fondaparinux sodium, J1652
Footdrop splint, L4398
Footplate, E0175, E0970, L3031
Footwear, orthopedic, L3201–L3265
Forearm crutches, E0110, E0111
Formoterol, J7640
    fumarate, J7606
Fosaprepitant, J1453
Foscarnet sodium, J1455
Fosphenytoin, Q2009
Fracture
    bedpan, E0276
    frame, E0920, E0930, E0946–E0948
    orthosis, L2106–L2136, L3980–L3986
    orthotic additions, L2180–L2192, L3995
Fragmin, *see* **Dalteparin sodium**
Frames (spectacles), V2020, V2025
Fulvestrant, J9395
Furosemide, J1940

G

Gadobutrol, A9585 ◀
Gadofosveset trisodium, A9583
Gadoxetate disodium, A9581
Gait trainer, E8000–E8002
Gallium Ga67, A9556
Gallium nitrate, J1457
Galsulfase, J1458
Gammagard liquid, J1569
Gamma globulin, J1460, J1560
Gammaplex, J1557 ◀
Gamunex, J1561 ←
Ganciclovir
    implant, J7310
    sodium, J1570
Garamycin, J1580
Gas system
    compressed, E0424, E0425
    gaseous, E0430, E0431, E0441, E0443
    liquid, E0434–E0440, E0442, E0444
Gatifloxacin, J1590
Gauze (see also Bandage)
    impregnated, A6222–A6233, A6266
    non-impregnated, A6402–A6404

◀ New   ← Revised   ✔ Reinstated   ~~deleted~~ Deleted

Gefitinib, J8565
Gel
    conductive, A4558
    pressure pad, E0185, E0196
Gemcitabine **HCl,** J9201
Gemtuzumab **ozogamicin,** J9300
Generator
    ultrasonic with nebulizer, E0574
Gentamicin **(Sulfate),** J1580
Gingival **procedures,** D4210–D4240
Glasses
    air conduction, V5070
    binaural, V5120–V5150
    bone conduction, V5080
    frames, V2020, V2025
    hearing aid, V5230
Glaucoma
    screening, G0117, G0118
Gloves, A4927
Glucagon **HCl,** J1610
Glucose
    monitor with integrated lancing/blood sample
        collection, E2101
    monitor with integrated voice synthesizer, E2100
    test strips, A4253, A4772
Gluteal **pad,** L2650
Glycopyrrolate, **inhalation solution,**
    concentrated, J7642
Glycopyrrolate, **inhalation solution, unit**
    dose, J7643
Gold
    foil dental restoration, D2410–D2430
    sodium thiomalate, J1600
Gomco **drain bottle,** A4912
Gonadorelin **HCl,** J1620
Goserelin **acetate implant** (*see also* **Implant),** J9202
Grab **bar, trapeze,** E0910, E0940
Gradient, compression stockings, A6530–A6549
Grade-aid, **wheelchair,** E0974
Granisetron **HCl,** J1626
Gravity **traction device,** E0941
Gravlee **jet washer,** A4470
Guaiac, stool, G0394
Guidelines, practice, oncology, G9056–G9062

H

Hair **analysis (excluding arsenic),** P2031
Hallus-Valgus **dynamic splint,** L3100
Hallux **prosthetic implant,** L8642
Haloperidol, J1630
    decanoate, J1631
Halo **procedures,** L0810–L0860
Halter, **cervical head,** E0942
Hand **finger orthosis, prefabricated,** L3923
Hand **restoration,** L6900–L6915
    partial prosthesis, L6000–L6020

Hand **restoration** (*Continued*)
    orthosis (WHFO), E1805, E1825, L3800–L3805,
        L3900-L3954
    rims, wheelchair, E0967
Handgrip **(cane, crutch, walker),** A4636
Harness, E0942, E0944, E0945
Headgear **(for positive airway pressure device),**
    K0185
Hearing
    assessment, S0618, V5008, V5010
    devices, V5000–V5299, L8614
    services, V5000–V5999
Heat
    application, E0200–E0239
    lamp, E0200, E0205
    infrared heating pad system, A4639, E0221
    pad, A9273, E0210, E0215, E0237, E0249
Heater **(nebulizer),** E1372
Heavy duty, wheelchair, E1280–E1298, K0006,
    K0007, K0801–K0886
Heel
    elevator, air, E0370
    protector, E0191
    shoe, L3430–L3485
    stabilizer, L3170
Helicopter, **ambulance** (*see also* **Ambulance)**
Helmet
    cervical, L0100, L0110
    head, A8000–A8004
Hemin, J1640
Hemi-wheelchair, E1083–E1086
Hemipelvectomy **prosthesis,** L5280
Hemodialysis **machine,** E1590
Hemodialyzer, **portable,** E1635
Hemofil **M,** J7190
Hemophilia **clotting factor,** J7190–J7198
    NOC, J7199
Hemostats, A4850
Hemostix, A4773
Hepagam B
    IM, J1571
    IV, J1573
Heparin
    infusion pump, dialysis, E1520
    lock flush, J1642
    sodium, J1644
Hepatitis B, vaccine, administration, G0010
Hep-Lock **(U/P),** J1642
Hexalite, A4590
High **osmolar contrast material,** Q9958–Q9964
Hip
    disarticulation prosthesis, L5250, L5270
    orthosis (HO), L1600–L1690
Hip-knee-ankle-foot **orthosis (HKAFO),**
    L2040–L2090
Histrelin
    acetate, J1675
    implant, J9225

◀ New   ← Revised   ✔ Reinstated   d̶e̶l̶e̶t̶e̶d̶ Deleted

HKAFO, L2040–L2090
Home
  glucose, monitor, E0607, E2100, E2101, S1030,
    S1031
  health, aide, G0156, S9122, T1021
  health, clinical, social worker, G0155
  health, nursing, skilled, G0154
  health, occupational, therapist, G0152
  health, physical therapist, G0151
  health, physician, certification, G0179–G0182
  health, respiratory therapy, S5180, S5181
  therapist, speech, S9128
Home Health Agency Services, T0221
HOPPS, C1000–C9999
Hospice **home care,** Q5010
Hospital
  bed, E0250–E0304, E0328, E0329
  observation, G0378, G0379
Hospital ***Outpatient Payment System,*** *C1000–C9999*
Hot water bottle, A9273
Human fibrinogen concentrate, J1680
Humidifier, A7046, E0550–E0563
Hyalgan, J7321
Hyalomatrix, Q4117
Hyaluronan, J7326 ◄
Hyaluronate, sodium, J7317
Hyaluronidase, J3470
  ovine, J3471–J3473
Hydralazine HCl, J0360
Hydraulic patient lift, E0630
Hydrocollator, E0225, E0239
Hydrocolloid dressing, A6234–A6241
Hydrocortisone
  acetate, J1700
  sodium phosphate, J1710
  sodium succinate, J1720
Hydrogel dressing, A6242–A6248, A6231–A6233
Hydromorphone, J1170
Hydroxyprogesterone caproate, J1725 ◄
Hydroxyzine HCl, J3410
Hylan G-F 20, J7325
Hyoscyamine Sulfate, J1980
Hyperbaric oxygen chamber, topical, A4575
~~Hypertonic saline solution, J7130~~

I

Ibandronate sodium, J1740
Ibutilide Fumarate, J1742
Ice
  cap, E0230
  collar, E0230
Idarubicin HCl, J9211
Idursulfase, J1743
Ifosfamide, J9208
Iliac, ***artery, angiography,*** *G0278*
Iloprost, Q4074
Imiglucerase, J1786

Immune globulin
  Flebogamma, J1572
  Gammagard liquid, J1569
  Gammaplex, J1557 ◄
  Gamunex, J1561
  HepaGam B, J1571
  Hizentra, J1559
  NOS, J1566
  Octagam, J1568
  Privigen, J1459
  Rho(D), J2788, J2790
  Rhophylac, J2791
  Subcutaneous, J1562
Immunosuppressive drug, not otherwise
  classified, J7599
Implant
  access system, A4301
  aqueous shunt, L8612
  breast, L8600
  cochlear, L8614, L8619
  collagen, urinary tract, L8603
  dental, D3460, D5925, D6010–D6067,
    D6075–D6199
  dextranomer/hyaluronic acid copolymer, L8604
  ganciclovir, J7310
  hallux, L8642
  urinary tract, L8603, L8606
  infusion pump, programmable, E0783, E0786
  joint, L8630, L8641, L8658
  lacrimal duct, A4262, A4263
  maintenance procedures, D6080
  maxillofacial, D5913–D5937
  metacarpophalangeal joint, L8630
  metatarsal joint, L8641
  neurostimulator pulse generator, L8681–L8688
  not otherwise specified, L8699
  ocular, L8610
  ossicular, L8613
  osteogenesis stimulator, E0749
  percutaneous access system, A4301
  removal, dental, D6100
  repair, dental, D6090
  replacement implantable intraspinal catheter, E0785
  synthetic, urinary, L8606
  vascular graft, L8670
Implantable radiation dosimeter, A4650
Impregnated gauze dressing, A6222–A6230
Incobotulinumtoxin a, J0588 ◄
Incontinence
  appliances and supplies, A4310, A4360, A5071–
    A5075, A5102–A5114, K0280, K0281
  garment, A4520, T4521–T4543
  supply, A4335, A4356–A4358
  treatment system, E0740
  urinary, documentation, G8063, G8067
Indium IN-111
  carpromab pendetide, A9507
  ibritumomab tiuxetan, A9542

◄ New   ← Revised   ✔ Reinstated   ~~deleted~~ Deleted

Indium IN-111 *(Continued)*
  labeled autologous white blood cells, A9570
  labeled autologous platelets, A9571
  oxyquinoline, A9547
  pentetate, A9548
  pentetreotide, A9572
  satumomab, A4642
Infliximab injection, J1745
Influenza
  immunization, documentation, G8482–G8484
  vaccine, administration, G0008
  virus vaccine, Q2035–Q2039
Infusion
  pump, ambulatory, with administrative equipment,
    E0781
  pump, heparin, dialysis, E1520
  pump, implantable, E0782, E0783
  pump, implantable, refill kit, A4220
  pump, insulin, E0784
  pump, mechanical, reusable, E0779, E0780
  pump, uninterrupted infusion of Epiprostenol,
    K0455
  saline, J7030–J7060
  supplies, A4219, A4221, A4222, A4230–A4232,
    E0776–E0791
  therapy, other than chemotherapeutic drugs,
    Q0081
Inhalation solution (*see also* **drug name),** J7608–
    J7699, Q4074
Injection device, needle-free, A4210
Injections (*see also* **drug name),** J0120–J7320
  arthrography, sacroiliac, joint, G0259, G0260
  dental service, D9610, D9630
  supplies for self-administered, A4211
Inlay/onlay dental restoration, D2510–D2664
INR, monitoring, G0248–G0250
Insertion **tray,** A4310–A4316
Insulin, J1815, J1817, S5550–S5571
  ambulatory, external, system, A9274
  treatment, outpatient, G9147
Integra flowable wound matrix, Q4114
Interferon
  Alpha, J9212–J9215
  Beta-1 a, J1826, Q3025–Q3026
  Beta-1 b, J1830
  Gamma, J9216
Intermittent
  assist device with continuous positive airway
    pressure device, E0470–E0472
  limb compression device, E0676
  peritoneal dialysis system, E1592
  positive pressure breathing (IPPB) machine,
    E0500
Interphalangeal **joint, prosthetic implant,** L8658,
    L8659
Interscapular **thoracic prosthesis**
  endoskeletal, L6570
  upper limb, L6350–L6370

Intervention, tobacco, G9016
Intraconazole, J1835
Intraocular
  lenses, V2630–V2632
Intraoral **radiographs, dental,** D0210–D0240
Intrapulmonary **percussive ventilation**
    system, E0481
Intrauterine **copper contraceptive,** J7300
Iodine **Iobenguane sulfate I-131,** A9508
Iodine **I-123 iobenguane,** A9582
Iodine **I-123 ioflupane,** A9584 ◄
Iodine **I-123 sodium iodide,** A9509, A9516
Iodine **I-125 serum albumin,** A9532
  sodium iodide, A9527
  sodium iothalamate, A9554
Iodine **I-131 iodinated serum albumin,** A9524
  sodium iodide capsule, A9517, A9528
  sodium iodide solution, A9529–A9531
  tositumomab, A9544–A9545
Iodine **swabs/wipes,** A4247
IPD
  system, E1592
Ipilimumab, J9228 ◄
IPPB machine, E0500
Ipratropium **bromide, inhalation solution, unit**
    dose, J7644, J7645
Irinotecan, J9206
Iron
  Dextran, J1750
  sucrose, J1756
Irrigation/evacuation **system, bowel**
  control unit, E0350
  disposable supplies for, E0352
Irrigation **solution for bladder calculi,** Q2004
Irrigation **supplies,** A4320–A4322, A4355,
    A4397–A4400
Islet, transplant, G0341–G0343, S2102
Isoetharine **HCl, inhalation solution**
  concentrated, J7647, J7648
  unit dose, J7649, J7650
Isolates, B4150, B4152
Isoproterenol **HCl, inhalation solution**
  concentrated, J7657, J7658
  unit dose, J7659, J7660
Isosulfan **blue,** Q9968
Item, non-covered, A9270
IUD, J7300, S4989
IV pole, each, E0776, K0105
Ixabepilone, J9207

J

Jacket
  scoliosis, L1300, L1310
Jaw, motion, rehabilitation system,
    E1700–E1702
Jenamicin, J1580

◄ New   ← Revised   ✔ Reinstated   ~~deleted~~ Deleted

K

Kanamycin **sulfate,** J1840, J1850
Kartop **patient lift, toilet or bathroom (*see also* Lift),** E0625
Ketorolac **thomethamine,** J1885
Kidney
  ESRD supply, A4650–A4927
  machine, accessories, E1500–E1699
  machine, E1500–E1699
  system, E1510
  wearable artificial, E1632
Kits
  enteral feeding supply (syringe) (pump) (gravity), B4034–B4036
  fistula cannulation (set), A4730
  parenteral nutrition, B4220–B4224
  surgical dressing (tray), A4550
  tracheostomy, A4625
Knee
  arthroscopy, surgical, G0289, S2112, S2300
  disarticulation, prosthesis, L5150, L5160
  joint, miniature, L5826
  orthosis (KO), E1810, L1800–L1885
Knee-ankle-foot **orthosis (KAFO),** L2000–L2039, L2126–L2136
  addition, high strength, lightweight material, L2755
Kyphosis **pad,** L1020, L1025

L

Laboratory
  dental, D0415–D0999
  services, P0000–P9999
Laboratory **tests**
  chemistry, P2028–P2038
  microbiology, P7001
  miscellaneous, P9010–P9615, Q0111–Q0115
  toxicology, P3000–P3001, Q0091
Lacrimal **duct implant**
  permanent, A4263
  temporary, A4262
Lactated **Ringer's infusion,** J7120
Laetrile, J3570
Lancet, A4258, A4259
Lanreotide, J1930
Laronidase, J1931
Larynx, **artificial,** L8500
Laser **blood collection device and accessory,** E0620, A4257
Lead **investigation,** T1029
Lead **wires, per pair,** A4557
Leg
  bag, A4358, A5105, A5112
  extensions for walker, E0158
  rest, elevating, K0195

Leg *(Continued)*
  rest, wheelchair, E0990
  strap, replacement, A5113–A5114
Legg **Perthes orthosis,** L1700–L1755
Lens
  aniseikonic, V2118, V2318
  contact, V2500–V2599
  eye, V2100–V2615, V2700–V2799
  intraocular, V2630–V2632
  low vision, V2600–V2615
  progressive, V2781
Lepirudin, J1945
*Lesion, **destruction, choroid,** G0186*
Leucovorin **calcium,** J0640
Leukocyte **poor blood, each unit,** P9016
Leuprolide **acetate,** J9217, J9218, J9219, J1950
Levalbuterol, **all formulations, inhalation solution**
  concentrated, J7607, J7612
  unit dose, J7614, J7615
Levetiracetam, J1953
Levocarnitine, J1955
Levofloxacin, J1956
Levoleucovorin, J0641
Levonorgestrel, **(contraceptive), implants and supplies,** J7306
Levorphanol **tartrate,** J1960
Lexidronam, A9604
Lidocaine **HCl,** J2001
Lift
  patient (includes seat lift), E0621–E0635
  shoe, L3300–L3334
*Lightweight, **wheelchair,** E1087–E1090, E1240– E1270, E2618*
Lincomycin **HCl,** J2010
Linezolid, J2020
Liquid **barrier, ostomy,** A4363
Lodging, **recipient, escort nonemergency transport,** A0180, A0200
LOPS, G0245–G0247
Lorazepam, J2060
*Loss **of protective sensation,** G0245–G0247*
Low **osmolar contrast material,** Q9965–Q9967
LSO, L0621–L0640
Lubricant, A4402, A4332
Lumbar **flexion,** L0540
Lumbar-sacral **orthosis (LSO),** L0621–L0640
*LVRS, **services,** G0302–G0305*
Lymphocyte **immune globulin,** J7504, J7511

M

Machine
  IPPB, E0500
  kidney, E1500–E1699
Magnesium **sulphate,** J3475
Maintenance **contract,** ESRD, A4890
*Mammography, **screening,** G0202*

◄ New   ← Revised   ✔ Reinstated   ~~deleted~~ Deleted

Mannitol, J2150, J7665←
Mapping, vessel, for hemodialysis access,
  G0365
Marker, tissue, A4648
Mask
  aerosol, K0180
  oxygen, A4620
Mastectomy
  bra, L8000
  form, L8020
  prosthesis, L8030, L8600
  sleeve, L8010
Matristem, Q4118–Q4120
Mattress
  air pressure, E0186
  alternating pressure, E0277
  dry pressure, E0184
  gel pressure, E0196
  hospital bed, E0271, E0272
  non-powered, pressure reducing, E0373
  overlay, E0371–E0372
  powered, pressure reducing, E0277
  water pressure, E0187
Measurement period
  left ventricular function testing, G8682
  not an eligible candidate for left ventricular
    function testing, G8683
  left ventricular function testing not performed, NOS,
    G8685
Mecasermin, J2170
Mechlorethamine **HCl,** J9230
Medicaid, codes, T1000–T9999
Medical **and surgical supplies,** A4206–A8999
Medical **nutritional therapy,** *G0270, G0271*
Medical **services, other,** *M0000–M9999*
Medroxyprogesterone **acetate,** J1051, J1055
Medroxyprogesterone **acetate/estradiol**
    cypionate, J1056
Melphalan
  HCl, J9245
  oral, J8600
Mental, **health, training services,** *G0177*
Meperidine, J2175
  and promethazine, J2180
Mepivacaine **HCl,** J0670
Meropenem, J2185
Mesna, J9209
Metacarpophalangeal **joint, prosthetic implant,**
    L8630, L8631
Metaproterenol **sulfate, inhalation solution**
  concentrated, J7667, J7668
  unit dose, J7669, J7670
Metaraminol **bitartrate,** J0380
Metatarsal **joint, prosthetic implant,** L8641
Meter, **bath conductivity, dialysis,** E1550
Methacholine **chloride,** J7674
Methadone **HCl,** J1230

Methocarbamol, J2800
Methotrexate
  oral, J8610
  sodium, J9250, J9260
Methyldopate **HCl,** J0210
Methylene **blue,** Q9968
Methylprednisolone
  acetate, J1020–J1040
  oral, J7509
  sodium succinate, J2920, J2930
Metoclopramide **HCl,** J2765
Micafungin **sodium,** J2248
Microbiology **test,** P7001
Midazolam **HCl,** J2250
Mileage
  ALS, A0390
  ambulance, A0380, A0390
Milrinone **lactate,** J2260
Mini-bus, **nonemergency transportation,** A0120
Minocycline **hydrochloride,** J2265◄
Mitomycin, J9280
Mitoxantrone **HCl,** J9293
MNT, G0270, G0271
Mobility **device, physician, service,** *G0372*
Modalities, **with office visit,** M0005–M0008
Moisture **exchanger for use with invasive**
    mechanical ventilation, A4483
Moisturizer, **skin,** A6250
Monitor
  blood glucose, E0607
  blood pressure, A4670
  pacemaker, E0610, E0615
Monitoring **feature/device,** A9279
Monitoring, INR, G0248–G0250
Monoclonal **antibodies,** J7505
Morphine **sulfate,** J2270, J2271
  sterile, preservative-free, J2275
Motion, **jaw, rehabilitation system,** *E1700–E1702*
Mouthpiece **(for respiratory equipment),** A4617
Moxifloxacin, J2280
Mucoprotein, **blood,** P2038
Multiaxial **ankle,** L5986
Multidisciplinary **services,** H2000–H2001, T1023–
    T1028
Multiple **post collar, cervical,** L0180–L0200
Multi-Podus **type AFO,** L4396
Muromonab-CD3, J7505
Mycophenolate **mofetil,** J7517
Mycophenolic **acid,** J7518

N

Nabilone, J8650
Nails, **trimming, dystrophic,** *G0127*
Nalbuphine **HCl,** J2300
Naloxone **HCl,** J2310
Naltrexone, J2315

◄ New   ← Revised   ✔ Reinstated   ~~deleted~~ Deleted

Nandrolone
decanoate, J2320
narrowing device, wheelchair, E0969
Nasal
application device, K0183
pillows/seals (for nasal application device), K0184
vaccine inhalation, J3530
Nasogastric **tubing,** B4081, B4082
Natalizumab, J2323
Nebulizer, E0570–E0585
~~aerosol compressor, E0571~~
aerosol mask, A7015
corrugated tubing, disposable, A7010
corrugated tubing, non-disposable, A7011
filter, disposable, A7013
filter, non-disposable, A7014
heater, E1372
large volume, disposable, prefilled, A7008
large volume, disposable, unfilled, A7007
not used with oxygen, durable, glass, A7017
pneumatic, administration set, A7003, A7005, A7006
pneumatic, nonfiltered, A7004
portable, E0570
small volume, A7003–A7005
ultrasonic, E0575
ultrasonic, dome and mouthpiece, A7016
ultrasonic, reservoir bottle, non-disposable, A7009
water collection device, large volume nebulizer, A7012
Needle, A4215
non-coring, A4212
with syringe, A4206–A4209
Negative pressure wound therapy pump, E2402
accessories, A6550
Nelarabine, J9261
Neonatal transport, ambulance, base rate, A0225
Neostigmine methylsulfate, J2710
Nerve, conduction, sensory, test, G0255
Nerve stimulator with batteries, E0765
Nesiritide injection, J2324
Neuromuscular stimulator, E0745
Neurostimulator
battery recharging system, L8695
pulse generator, L8681–L8688
Nitrogen N-13 ammonia, A9526
NMES, E0720–E0749
Nonchemotherapy drug, oral, NOS, J8499
Noncovered services, A9270
Nonemergency transportation, A0080–A0210
Nonimpregnated gauze dressing, A6216–A6221,
A6402–A6404
Nonprescription drug, A9150
Not otherwise classified drug, J3490, J7599, J7699,
J7799, J8499, J8999, J9999, Q0181
NPH, J1820
NPWT, pump, E2402
NTIOL category 3, Q1003
NTIOL category 4, Q1004

NTIOL **category 5,** Q1005
Nursing **care,** T1030–T1031
Nursing service, direct, skilled, outpatient, G0128
Nursing, skilled, home, health, G0154
Nutrition
counseling, dental, D1310, D1320
enteral infusion pump, B9000, B9002
parenteral infusion pump, B9004, B9006
parenteral solution, B4164–B5200
therapy, medical, G0270, G0271

O

Observation
admission, G0379
hospital, G0378
LPN or RN, G0163
Obturator prosthesis
definitive, D5932
interim, D5936
surgical, D5931
Occipital/mandibular support, cervical, L0160
Occult, blood, G0394
Occupational, therapy, G0129, S9129
Octafluoropropane, Q9956
Octagam, J1568
Octreotide acetate, J2353, J2354
Ocular prosthetic implant, L8610
Ofatumumab, J9302
Olanzapine, J2358
Omalizumab, J2357
OnabotulinumtoxinA, J0585
Oncology
disease status, G9063–G9139
practice guidelines, G9056–G9062
visit, G9050–G9055
Ondansetron HCl, J2405 ◀
Ondansetron oral, Q0162 ◀
One arm, drive attachment, K0101
Oprelvekin, J2355
O & P supply/accessory/service, L9900
Oral and maxillofacial surgery, D7000–D7999
Oral device/appliance, E0485–E0486
Oral examination, D0120–D0160
Oral/nasal mask, A7027
nasal pillows, A7029
oral cushion, A7028
Oral, NOS, drug, J8499
Oropharyngeal suction catheter, A4628
Orphenadrine, J2360
Orthodontics, D8000–D8999
Orthopedic shoes
arch support, L3040–L3100
footwear, L3201–L3265, *L3000–L3649*
insert, L3000–L3030
lift, L3300–L3334
miscellaneous additions, L3500–L3595

◀ New　　← Revised　　✔ Reinstated　　~~deleted~~ Deleted

Orthopedic **shoes** *(Continued)*
  positioning device, L3140–L3170
  transfer, L3600–L3649
  wedge, L3340–L3420
Orthotic additions
  carbon graphite lamination, L2755
  fracture, L2180–L2192, L3995
  halo, L0860
  lower extremity, L2200–L2999, L4320
  ratchet lock, L2430
  scoliosis, L1010–L1120, L1210–L1290
  shoe, L3300–L3595, L3649
  spinal, L0970–L0984
  upper limb, L3810–L3890, *L3900, L3901,* L3995
Orthotic devices
  ankle-foot (AFO; *see also* Orthopedic shoes), E1815,
    E1816, E1830, L1900–L1990, L2102–L2116,
    L3160, L4361
  anterior-posterior-lateral, L0700, L0710
  cervical, L0100–L0200
  cervical-thoracic-lumbar-sacral (CTLSO), L0700,
    L0710
  elbow (EO), E1800, E1801, L3700–L3740
  fracture, L2102–L2136, L3980–L3986
  halo, L0810–L0830
  hand, finger, prefabricated, L3923
  hand, (WHFO), E1805, E1825, L3807, L3900–L3954
  hip (HO), L1600–L1690
  hip-knee-ankle-foot (HKAFO), L2040–L2090
  interface material, E1820
  knee (KO), E1810, E1811, L1800–L1885
  knee-ankle-foot (KAFO; *see also* Orthopedic shoes),
    L2000–L2038, L2126–L2136
  Legg Perthes, L1700–L1755
  lumbar, L0625–L0640
  multiple post collar, L0180–L0200
  not otherwise specified, L0999, L1499, L2999,
    L3999, L5999, L7499, L8039, L8239
  pneumatic splint, L4350–L4379
  pronation/supination, E1818
  repair or replacement, L4000–L4210
  replace soft interface material, L4390–L4394
  sacroiliac, L0600–L0620
  scoliosis, L1000–L1499
  shoe, *see* Orthopedic shoes
  shoulder (SO), L1840, L3650, L3674
  shoulder-elbow-wrist-hand (SEWHO), L3960–L3978
  side bar disconnect, L2768
  spinal, cervical, L0100–L0200
  spinal, DME, K0112–K0116
  thoracic, L0210
  ~~thoracic hip-knee-ankle, L1500–L1520~~
  toe, E1830
  wrist-hand-finger (WHFO), E1805, E1806, E1825,
    L3900–L3954
Orthovisc, J7324
Ossicula prosthetic implant, L8613

Osteogenesis stimulator, E0747–E0749, E0760
Osteoporosis
  documentation, G8401
Osteotomy, segmented or subapical, D7944
Ostomy
  accessories, A5093
  belt, A4396
  pouches, A4416–A4434
  skin barrier, A4401–A4449
  supplies, A4361–A4421, A5051–A5149
*Overdoor, **traction,** E0860*
Oxacillin sodium, J2700
Oxaliplatin, J9263
Oxygen
  ambulance, A0422
  battery charger, E1357
  battery pack/cartridge, E1356
  catheter, transtracheal, A7018
  chamber, hyperbaric, topical, A4575
  concentrator, E1390–E1391
  DC power adapter, E1358
  delivery system, topical NOS, E0446
  equipment, E0424–E0486, E1353–E1406
  liquid oxygen system, E0433
  mask, A4620
  medication supplies, A4611–A4627
  rack/stand, E1355
  regulator, E1353
  respiratory equipment/supplies, A4611–A4627,
    E0424–E0480
  supplies and equipment, E0425–E0444, E0455
  tent, E0455
  tubing, A4616
  water vapor enriching system, E1405, E1406
  wheeled cart, E1354
Oxymorphone HCl, J2410
Oxytetracycline HCl, J2460
Oxytocin, J2590

P

Pacemaker monitor, E0610, E0615
Paclitaxel, J9265
Paclitaxel protein-bound particles, J9264
Pad
  correction, CTLSO, L1020–L1060
  gel pressure, E0185, E0196
  heat, *A9273,* E0210, E0215, E0217, E0238, E0249
  orthotic device interface, E1820
  sheepskin, E0188, E0189
  water circulating cold with pump, E0218
  water circulating heat with pump, E0217
  water circulating heat unit, E0249
Pail, for use with commode chair, E0167
Palate, prosthetic implant, L8618
Palifermin, J2425
Paliperidone palmitate, J2426

◄ New   ← Revised   ✔ Reinstated   ~~deleted~~ Deleted

Palonosetron **HCl,** J2469
Pamidronate **disodium,** J2430
Pan, **for use with commode chair,** E0167
Panitumumab, J9303
Papanicolaou **(Pap) screening smear,** P3000, P3001,
   Q0091
Papaverine **HCl,** J2440
Paraffin, A4265
  bath unit, E0235
Parenteral **nutrition**
  administration kit, B4224
  pump, B9004, B9006
  solution, B4164–B5200
  supply kit, B4220, B4222
Paricalcitol, J2501
Parking **fee, nonemergency transport,** A0170
Paste, **conductive,** A4558
Pathology **and laboratory tests, miscellaneous,**
   P9010–P9615
Patient **support system,** E0636
Patient **transfer system,** E1035–E1036
*Payment **adjustment, hardship exemption,** G8642,*
   G8643
*Pediculosis **(lice) treatment,** A9180*
PEFR, **peak expiratory flow rate meter,** A4614
Pegademase **bovine,** J2504
Pegaptanib, J2503
Pegaspargase, J9266
Pegfilgrastim, J2505
Pegloticase, J2507 ◀
Pelvic
  belt/harness/boot, E0944
  traction, E0890, E0900, E0947
Pemetrexed, J9305
Penicillin
  G benzathine/G benzathine and penicillin
    G procaine, J0558, J0561
  G potassium, J2540
  G procaine, aqueous, J2510
Pentamidine **isethionate,** J2545, J7676
Pentastarch, **10% solution,** J2513
Pentazocine **HCl,** J3070
Pentobarbital **sodium,** J2515
Pentostatin, J9268
Percussor, E0480
Percutaneous **access system,** A4301
Perflexane **lipid microspheres,** Q9955
Perflutren **lipid microspheres,** Q9957
Periapical **service,** D3410–D3470
Periodontal **procedures,** D4000–D4999
*Periodontics, **dental,** D4000–D4999*
Peroneal **strap,** L0980
Peroxide, A4244
Perphenazine, J3310
Personal **care services,** T1019–T1021
Pessary, A4561, A4562
PET, G0219, G0235, G0252

*Pharmacologic **therapy,** G8633*
Phenobarbital **sodium,** J2560
Phentolamine **mesylate,** J2760
Phenylephrine **HCl,** J2370
Phenytoin **sodium,** J1165
Phisohex **solution,** A4246
Photofrin, *see* **Porfimer sodium**
Phototherapy **light,** E0202
Phytonadione, J3430
Pillow, **cervical,** E0943
Pin **retention (per tooth),** D2951
Pinworm **examination,** Q0113
Placement
  transcatheter, stent, G0290, G0291, S2211
Plasma
  single donor, fresh frozen, P9017
  multiple donor, pooled, frozen, P9023
Plastazote, L3002, L3252, L3253, L3265, L5654–L5658
Platelet
  concentrate, each unit, P9019
  rich plasma, each unit, P9020
Platform **attachment**
  forearm crutch, E0153
  walker, E0154
Plerixafor, J2562
Plicamycin, J9270
Plumbing, **for home ESRD equipment,** A4870
Pneumatic
  appliance, E0655–E0673, L4350–L4379
  compressor, E0650–E0652
  splint, L4350–L4379
  ventricular assist device, Q0480–Q0505
Pneumatic **nebulizer**
  administration set, small volume, filtered, A7006
  administration set, small volume, nonfiltered, A7003
  administration set, small volume, nonfiltered, non-
    disposable, A7005
  small volume, disposable, A7004
Pneumococcal
  vaccine, administration, G0009
Pontics, D6210–D6252
Porfimer, J9600
Portable
  equipment transfer, R0070–R0076
  gaseous oxygen, K0741, K0742 ◀
  hemodialyzer system, E1635
  liquid oxygen system, E0433
  x-ray equipment, Q0092
Positioning **seat,** T5001
Positive **airway pressure device, accessories,**
   A7030–A7039, E0561–E0562
Positive **expiratory pressure device,** E0484
Post-coital **examination,** Q0115
Postural **drainage board,** E0606
Potassium
  chloride, J3480
  hydroxide (KOH) preparation, Q0112

◀ New   ← Revised   ✔ Reinstated   deleted- Deleted

Pouch
  fecal collection, A4330
  ostomy, A4375–A4378, A5051–A5054, A5061–A5065
  urinary, A4379–A4383, A5071–A5075
Pralatrexate, J9307
Practice, **guidelines, oncology,** *G9056–G9062*
Pralidoxime chloride, J2730
Prednisolone
  acetate, J2650
  oral, J7506, J7510
Prednisone, J7506
Prefabricated crown, D2930–D2933
Preparation kits, dialysis, A4914
Preparatory prosthesis, L5510–L5595
  chemotherapy, J8999
  nonchemotherapy, J8499
Prescribing **privilege, eligible,** *G8644*
Pressure
  alarm, dialysis, E1540
  pad, A4640, E0180–E0199
Preventive dental procedures, D1000–D1999
Privigen, J1459
Procainamide HCl, J2690
Procedure
  HALO, L0810–L0861
  noncovered, G0293, G0294
  scoliosis, L1000–L1499
Prochlorperazine, J0780
Prolotherapy, M0076
Promazine HCl, J2950
Promethazine
  HCl, J2550
  and meperdine, J2180
Prophylaxis
  DVT, documentation, G8218
  thrombosis, deep, vein, documentation, G8218
Propranolol HCl, J1800
Prostate, **cancer, screening,** *G0102, G0103*
Prosthesis
  artificial larynx battery/accessory, L8505
  auricular, D5914
  breast, L8000–L8035, L8600
  dental, D5911–D5960, D5999
  eye, L8610, L8611, V2623–V2629
  fitting, L5400–L5460, L6380–L6388
  foot/ankle one piece system, L5979
  hand, L6000–L6020, L6025
  implants, L8600–L8690
  larynx, L8500
  lower extremity, L5700–L5999, L8640–L8642
  mandible, L8617
  maxilla, L8616
  maxillofacial, provided by a non-physician,
    L8040–L8048
  miscellaneous service, L8499
  obturator, D5931–D5933, D5936
  ocular, V2623–V2629

Prosthesis *(Continued)*
  repair of, L7520, L8049
  socks (shrinker, sheath, stump sock), L8400–L8485
  taxes, orthotic/prosthetic/other, L9999
  tracheo-esophageal, L8507–L8509
  upper extremity, L6000–L6999
  vacuum erection system, L7900
Prosthetic additions
  lower extremity, L5610–L5999
  upper extremity, L6600–L7405
Prosthodontic procedure
  fixed, D6200–D6999
  removable, D5000–D5899
Protamine sulfate, J2720
Protectant, skin, A6250
Protector, heel or elbow, E0191
Protein C Concentrate, J2724
Protirelin, J2725
Pulp capping, D3110, D3120
Pulpotomy, D3220
  partial, D3222
  vitality test, D0460
Pulse generator, E2120
Pump
  alternating pressure pad, E0182
  ambulatory infusion, E0781
  ambulatory insulin, E0784
  blood, dialysis, E1620
  breast, E0602–E0604
  enteral infusion, B9000, B9002
  external infusion, E0779
  heparin infusion, E1520
  implantable infusion, E0782, E0783
  implantable infusion, refill kit, A4220
  infusion, supplies, A4230, A4232
  negative pressure wound therapy, E2402
  parenteral infusion, B9004, B9006
  suction, portable, E0600
  water circulating pad, E0236
  wound, negative, pressure, E2402
Purification system, E1610, E1615
Pyridoxine HCl, J3415

Q

Quad cane, E0105
Quinupristin/dalfopristin, J2770

R

Rack/stand, oxygen, E1355
Radiesse, Q2026
Radioelements for brachytherapy, Q3001
Radiograph, dental, D0210–D0340
Radiology service, R0070–R0076
Radiological, **supplies,** *A4641, A4642*

◀ New   ← Revised   ✔ Reinstated   ~~deleted~~ Deleted

Radiopharmaceutical **diagnostic imaging agent,** A4641, A4642, A9500, A9532
Radiopharmaceutical, **therapeutic,** A9600, A9605
*Radiosurgery, **stereotactic,** G0173, G0251, G0339, G0340*
Rail
  bathtub, E0241, E0242, E0246
  bed, E0305, E0310
  toilet, E0243
Ranibizumab, J2778
Rasburicase, J2783
Reaching/grabbing **device,** A9281
Reagent **strip,** A4252
Recement
  crown, D2920
  inlay, D2910
Reciprocating **peritoneal dialysis system,** E1630
Reclast, J3488
*Reclining, **wheelchair,** E1014, E1050–E1070, E1100–E1110*
Reconstruction, angiography, G0288
Red **blood cells,** P9021, P9022
Regadenoson, J2785
Regular **insulin,** J1820
Regulator, **oxygen,** E1353
Rehabilitation
  cardiac, S9472, S9473
  program, H2001
  psychosocial, H2017, H2018
  system, jaw, motion, E1700–E1702
  vestibular, S9476
*Removal, **cerumen,** G0268*
*Renal, **artery,** angiography, G0275*
Repair
  contract, ESRD, A4890
  maxillofacial prosthesis, L8049
  orthosis, L4000–L4130
  prosthetic, L7510
Replacement
  battery, A4630
  pad (alternating pressure), A4640
  tanks, dialysis, A4880
  tip for cane, crutches, walker, A4637
  underarm pad for crutches, A4635
*Reporting, **asthma measures group,** G8645, G8646*
Resin **dental restoration,** D2330–D2387
RespiGam, *see* **Respiratory syncytial virus immune globulin**
Respiratory
  DME, A7000–A7527
  equipment, E0424–E0601
  function, therapeutic, procedure, G0237–G0239, S5180, S5181
  supplies, A4604–A4629
Restorative **dental procedure,** D2000–D2999
Restraint, **any type,** E0710
Reteplase, J2993

Rho(D) **immune globulin, human,** J2788, J2790, J2791, J2792
Rib **belt, thoracic,** A4572, L0220
Rilanocept, J2793
RimabotulinumtoxinB, J0587
Ringers **lactate infusion,** J7120
Ring, **ostomy,** A4404
*Risk-adjusted **functional status***
  elbow, wrist or hand, G8667–G8670
  hip, G8651-G8654
  knee, G8647–G8650
  lower leg, foot or ankle, G8655–G8658
  lumbar spine, G8659–G8662
  neck, cranium, mandible, thoracic spine, ribs, or other, G8671–G8674
  shoulder, G8663–G8666
Risperidone, J2794
Rituximab, J9310
Robin-Aids, L6000, L6010, L6020, L6855, L6860
Rocking **bed,** E0462
Rollabout **chair,** E1031
Romidepsin, J9315
Romiplostim, J2796
Root **canal therapy,** D3310–D3353
Ropivacaine **HCl,** J2795
Rubidium **Rb-82,** A9555

S

Sacral **nerve stimulation test lead,** A4290
Safety **equipment,** E0700
  vest, wheelchair, E0980
Saline
  ~~hypertonic, J7130~~
  infusion, J7030–J7060
  solution, J7030–J7050, A4216–A4218
Saliva
  analysis, A0418
  artificial, A9155
  collection and preparation, D0417
Sargramostim **(GM-CSF),** J2820
Scoliosis, L1000–L1499
  additions, L1010–L1120, L1210–L1290
Screening
  cancer, cervical or vaginal, G0101
  colorectal, cancer, G0104–G0106, G0120–G0122, G0328, S3890
  cytopathology cervical or vaginal, G0123, G0124, G0141–G0148
  dysphagia, documentation, G8232, V5364
  enzyme immunoassay, G0432
  glaucoma, G0117, G0118
  infectious agent antibody detection, G0433, G0435
  language, V5363
  prostate, cancer, G0102, G0103
  speech, V5362
Sculptra, Q2027

◄ New   ← Revised   ✔ Reinstated   ~~deleted~~ Deleted

◀ **New**   ← **Revised**   ✔ **Reinstated**   ~~deleted~~ **Deleted**

Status
  disease, oncology, G9063–G9139
Stent, transcatheter, placement, G0290, G0291, S2211
Sterile **cefuroxime sodium,** J0697
Sterile **water,** A4216–A4217
Stereotactic, radiosurgery, G0173, G0251, G0339, G0340
Stimulators
  neuromuscular, E0744, E0745
  osteogenesis, electrical, E0747–E0749
  ultrasound, E0760
  salivary reflex, E0755
  stoma absorptive cover, A5083
  transcutaneous, electric, nerve, A4595, E0720–E0749
Stockings
  gradient, compression, A6530–A6549
  surgical, A4490–A4510
Stomach **tube,** B4083
Stool, guaiac, G0394
Streptokinase, J2995
Streptomycin, J3000
Streptozocin, J9320
Strip, **blood glucose test,** A4253, A4772
  urine reagent, A4250
Strontium-89 **chloride, supply of,** A9600
Study, bone density, G0130
Stump **sock,** L8470–L8485
Stylet, A4212
Substance/Alcohol, assessment, G0396, G0397, H0001, H0003, H0049
Succinylcholine **chloride,** J0330
Suction **pump**
  gastric, home model, E2000
  portable, E0600
  respiratory, home model, E0600
Sumatriptan **succinate,** J3030
Supartz, J7321
Supply/accessory/service, A9900
Supplies
  cast, A4580, A4590, Q4001–Q4051
  contraceptive, A4267–A4269
  dialysis, A4650–A4927
  DME, other, A4630–A4640
  enteral, therapy, B4000–B9999
  infusion, A4221, A4222, A4230–A4232, E0776–E0791
  ostomy, A4361–A4434, A5051–A5093, A5120–A5200
  parenteral, therapy, B4000–B9999
  radiological, A4641, A4642
  respiratory, A4604–A4629
  splint, Q4051
  surgical, miscellaneous, A4649
  urinary, external, A4356–A4358
Support
  arch, L3040–L3090
  cervical, L0100–L0200

Support *(Continued)*
  spinal, L0960
  stockings, L8100–L8239
Surgery, **oral,** D7000–D7999
Surgical
  arthroscopy, knee, G0289, S2112, S2113
  boot, L3208–L3211
  brush, dialysis, A4910
  dressing, A6196–A6406
  procedure, noncovered, G0293, G0294
  stocking, A4490–A4510
  supplies, A4649
  tray, A4550
Swabs, **betadine or iodine,** A4247
Syringe, A4213
  with needle, A4206–A4209
Synvisc **and Synvisc-One,** J7325
System
  external, ambulatory insulin, A9274
  rehabilitation, jaw, motion, E1700–E1702
  transport, E1035–E1039

T

Tables, **bed,** E0274, E0315
Tacrolimus
  oral, J7507
  parenteral, J7525
Tape, A4450–A4452
Taxi, **non emergency transportation,** A0100
Team, conference, G0175, G9007, S0220, S0221
Technetium **TC 99M**
  Arcitumomab, A9568
  Bicisate, A9557
  Depreotide, A9536
  Disofenin, A9510
  Exametazine, A9521
  Exametazine labeled autologous white blood cells, A9569
  Fanolesomab, A9566
  Glucepatate, A9550
  Labeled red blood cells, A9560
  Macroaggregated albumin, A9540
  Mebrofenin, A9537
  Mertiatide, A9562
  Oxidronate, A9561
  Pentetate, A9539, A9567
  Pertechnetate, A9512
  Pyrophosphate, A9538
  Sestamibi, A9500
  Succimer, A9551
  Sulfur colloid, A9541
  Teboroxime, A9501
  Tetrofosmin, A9502
TEEV, J0900
Telavancin, J3095
Telehealth, Q3014

◄ New   ← Revised   ✔ Reinstated   ~~deleted~~ Deleted

Telehealth **transmission,** T1014
Televancin, J3095
Temozolomide
  injection, J9328
  oral, J8700
*Temporary **codes,** Q0000–Q9999, S0009–S9999*
Temporomandibular **joint,** D0320, D0321
Temsirolimus, J9330
Tenecteplase, J3101
Teniposide, Q2017
TENS, A4595, E0720–E0749
Tent, **oxygen,** E0455
Terbutaline **sulfate,** J3105
  inhalation solution, concentrated, J7680
  inhalation solution, unit dose, J7681
Teriparatide, J3110
Terminal **devices,** L6700–L6895
Test
  occult, blood, G0394
  sensory, nerve, conduction, G0255
Testosterone
  aqueous, J3140
  cypionate and estradiol cypionate, J1060
  enanthate, J3120, J3130
  enanthate and estradiol valerate, J0900
  propionate, J3150
  suspension, J3140
Tetanus **immune globulin, human,** J1670
Tetracycline, J0120
Thallous **Chloride TL 201,** A9505
Theophylline, J2810
Therapeutic **lightbox,** A4634, E0203
Therapy
  ACE/ARB, G8468–G8475
  activity, G0176
  electromagnetic, G0295, G0329
  endodontic, D3222–D3330
  enteral, supplies, B4000–B9999
  medical, nutritional, G0270, G0271
  occupational, H5300, *G0129, S9129*
  occupational, health, G0152
  respiratory, function, procedure, G0237–G0239,
    S5180, S5181
  parenteral, supplies, B4000–B9999
  speech, home, G0153, S9128
  wound, negative, pressure, pump, E2402
Theraskin, Q4121
Thermometer, A4931–A4932
  dialysis, A4910
Thiamine **HCl,** J3411
Thiethylperazine **maleate,** J3280
Thiotepa, J9340
~~Thoracic-hip-knee-ankle (THKAO), L1500–L1520~~
Thoracic-lumbar-sacral **orthosis (TLSO)**
  scoliosis, L1200–L1290
  spinal, L0430–L0492
Thoracic **orthosis,** L0210
Thymol **turbidity, blood,** P2033

Thyrotropin **Alfa,** J3240
Tigecycline, J3243
Tinzarparin **sodium,** J1655
Tip **(cane, crutch, walker) replacement,** A4637
Tire, **wheelchair,** E0999
Tirofiban, J3246
Tissue **marker,** A4648
TLSO, L0430–L0492, L1200–L1290
Tobacco
  intervention, G9016
Tobramycin
  inhalation solution, unit dose, J7682, J7685
  sulfate, J3260
Tocilizumab, J2362
*Toe **device,** E1831*
Toilet **accessories,** E0167–E0179, E0243, E0244, E0625
Tolazoline **HCl,** J2670
Toll, **non emergency transport,** A0170
Tomographic **radiograph, dental,** D0322
Topical **hyperbaric oxygen chamber,** A4575
Topotecan, J8705, J9351
Torsemide, J3265
*Tositumomab, **administration and supply,** G3001*
Tracheostoma **heat moisture exchange system,**
  A7501–A7509
Tracheostomy
  care kit, A4629
  filter, A4481
  speaking valve, L8501
  supplies, A4623, A4629, A7523–A7524
  tube, A7520–A7522
Tracheotomy **mask or collar,** A7525–A7526
Traction
  cervical, E0855, E0856
  extremity, E0870–E0880
  device, ambulatory, E0830
  equipment, E0840–E0948
  pelvic, E0890, E0900, E0947
Training
  diabetes, outpatient, G0108, G0109
  home health or hospice, G0164
  services, mental, health, G0177
*Transcatheter, **placement, stent,** G0290, G0291, S2211*
Transcutaneous **electrical nerve stimulator**
  (TENS), E0720–E0770
Transducer **protector, dialysis,** E1575
Transfer **(shoe orthosis),** L3600–L3640
Transfer **system with seat,** E1035
Transplant
  islet, G0341–G0343, S2102
Transparent **film (for dressing),** A6257–A6259
Transport
  chair, E1035–E1039
  system, E1035–E1039
  x-ray, R0070–R0076
Transportation
  ambulance, A0021–A0999, Q3019, Q3020
  corneal tissue, V2785

◄ **New**   ← **Revised**   ✔ **Reinstated**   ~~deleted~~ **Deleted**

Transportation *(Continued)*
  EKG (portable), R0076
  handicapped, A0130
  non emergency, A0080–A0210, T2001–T2005
  service, including ambulance, A0021–A0999, T2006
  taxi, non emergency, A0100
  toll, non emergency, A0170
  volunteer, non emergency, A0080, A0090
  x-ray (portable), R0070, R0075
Transtracheal oxygen catheter, A7018
Trapeze bar, E0910–E0912, E0940
Trauma, response, team, G0390
Tray
  insertion, A4310–A4316
  irrigation, A4320
  surgical (*see also* kits), A4550
  wheelchair, E0950
Treatment
  pediculosis (lice), A9180
  services, behavioral health, H0002–H2037
Treprostinil, J3285
Triamcinolone, J3301–J3303
  acetonide, J3300, J3301
  diacetate, J3302
  hexacetonide, J3303
  inhalation solution, concentrated, J7683
  inhalation solution, unit dose, J7684
Triflupromazine HCl, J3400
Trifocal, glass or plastic, V2300–V2399
Trigeminal division block anesthesia, D9212
Trimethobenzamide HCl, J3250
Trimetrexate glucuoronate, J3305
Trimming, nails, dystrophic, G0127
Triptorelin pamoate, J3315
Trismus appliance, D5937
Truss, L8300–L8330
Tube/Tubing
  anchoring device, A5200
  blood, A4750, A4755
  drainage extension, A4331
  gastrostomy, B4087, B4088
  irrigation, A4355
  larynectomy, A4622
  nasogastric, B4081, B4082
  oxygen, A4616
  serum clotting time, A4771
  stomach, B4083
  suction pump, each, A7002
  tire, K0091, K0093, K0095, K0097
  tracheostomy, A4622
  urinary drainage, K0280

U

Ultrasonic nebulizer, E0575
Ultrasound, G0389, S8055, S9024
Ultraviolet, cabinet/system, E0691–E0694

Ultraviolet light therapy system, A4633, E0691–E0694
Unclassified drug, J3490
Underpads, disposable, A4554
Unipuncture control system, dialysis, E1580
Upper extremity addition, locking elbow, L6693
Upper extremity fracture orthosis, L3980–L3999
Upper limb prosthesis, L6000–L7499
Urea, J3350
Ureterostomy supplies, A4454–A4590
Urethral suppository, Alprostadil, J0275
Urinal, E0325, E0326
Urinary
  catheter, A4338–A4346, A4351–A4353
  collection and retention (supplies), A4310–A4360
  incontinence, documentation, G8063, G8067
  supplies, external, A4335, A4356–A4358
  tract implant, collagen, L8603
  tract implant, synthetic, L8606
Urine
  sensitivity study, P7001
  tests, A4250
Urofollitropin, J3355
Urokinase, J3364, J3365
Ustekinumab, J3357
U-V lens, V2755

V

Vabra aspirator, A4480
Vaccination, administration
  hepatitis B, G0010
  influenza virus, G0008
  pneumococcal, G0009
Vaccine
  administration, influenza, G0008
  administration, pneumococcal, G0009
  hepatitis B, administration, G0010
Vaginal
  cancer, screening, G0101
  cytopathology, G0123, G0124, G0141–G0148
Vancomycin HCl, J3370
Vaporizer, E0605
Vascular
  catheter (appliances and supplies), A4300–A4306
  graft material, synthetic, L8670
Vasoxyl, J3390
Velaglucerase alfa, J3385
Venous pressure clamp, dialysis, A4918
Ventilator
  battery, A4611–A4613
  moisture exchanger, disposable, A4483
  negative pressure, E0460
  volume, stationary or portable, E0450, E0461–E0464
Ventricular assist device, Q0478–Q0506
Verteporfin, J3396

◄ New	← Revised	✔ Reinstated	~~deleted~~ Deleted

Vest, **safety, wheelchair,** E0980
Vinblastine **sulfate,** J9360
Vincristine **sulfate,** J9370
Vinorelbine **tartrate,** J9390
Vision **service,** V2020–V2799
Visit, emergency department, G0380–G0384
Vitamin **B-12 cyanocobalamin,** J3420
Vitamin **K,** J3430
Voice
  amplifier, L8510
  prosthesis, L8511–L8514
Von **Willebrand Factor Complex, human,** J7183,
  J7187
Voriconazole, J3465

W

Waiver, T2012–T2050
Walker, E0130–E0149
  accessories, A4636, A4637
  attachments, E0153–E0159
Walking splint, L4386
Washer, Gravlee jet, A4470
Water
  dextrose, J7042, J7060, J7070
  distilled (for nebulizer), A7018
  pressure pad/mattress, E0187, E0198
  purification system (ESRD), E1610, E1615
  softening system (ESRD), E1625
  sterile, A4714
WBC/CBC, G0306
Wedges, **shoe,** L3340–L3420
Wellness visit; annual, G0438, G0439
Wet **mount,** Q0111
Wheel **attachment, rigid pickup walker,** E0155
Wheelchair, E0950–E1298, K0001–K0108, *K0801–*
  K0899
  accessories, E0192, E0950–E1030, E1065–E1069,
    E2211–E2230, E2300–E2399
  amputee, E1170–E1200
  back, fully reclining, manual, E1226
  component or accessory, not otherwise specified,
    K0108
  cushions, E2601–E2625
  heavy duty, E1280–E1298, K0006, K0007, K0801–
    K0886
  lightweight, E1087–E1090, E1240–E1270, E2618
  narrowing device, E0969
  power add-on, E0983–E0984
  reclining, fully, E1014, E1050–E1070, E1100–E1110
  semi-reclining, E1100, E1110
  shock absorber, E1015–E1018
  specially sized, E1220, E1230
  standard, E1130, K0001
  stump support system, K0551
  tire, E0999
  transfer board or device, E0705

Wheelchair *(Continued)*
  tray, K0107
  van, non-emergency, A0130
  youth, E1091
WHFO **with inflatable air chamber,** L3807
WHO, **wrist extension,** L3914
Whirlpool **equipment,** E1300–E1310
Wig, A9282
Wipes, A4245, A4247
Wound
  cleanser, A6260
  closure, adhesive, G0168
  cover
    alginate dressing, A6196–A6198
    collagen dressing, A6020–A6024
    foam dressing, A6209–A6214
    hydrocolloid dressing, A6234–A6239
    hydrogel dressing, A6242–A6247
    non-contact wound warming cover, and
      accessory, E0231, E0232
    specialty absorptive dressing, A6251–A6256
  filler
    alginate dressing, A6199
    collagen based, A6010
    foam dressing, A6215
    hydrocolloid dressing, A6240, A6241
    hydrogel dressing, A6248
    not elsewhere classified, A6261, A6262
  matrix, Q4114
  pouch, A6154
  therapy, negative, pressure, pump, E2402
Wrist
  disarticulation prosthesis, L6050, L6055
  hand/finger orthosis (WHFO), E1805, E1825,
    L3800–L3954

X

Xenon **Xe 133,** A9558
Xylocaine **HCl,** J2000
X-ray
  equipment, portable, Q0092, R0070, R0075
  single, energy, absorptiometry (SEXA), G0130
  transport, R0070–R0076

Y

Yttrium **Y-90 ibritumomab,** A9543

Z

Ziconotide, J2278
Zidovudine, J3485
Ziprasidone **mesylate,** J3486
Zoledronic **acid,** J3487
Zometa, J3487

2012
TABLE OF DRUGS

IA	Intra-arterial administration
IV	Intravenous administration
IM	Intramuscular administration
IT	Intrathecal
SC	Subcutaneous administration
INH	Administration by inhaled solution
VAR	Various routes of administration
OTH	Other routes of administration
ORAL	Administered orally

Intravenous administration includes all methods, such as gravity infusion, injections, and timed pushes. The "VAR" posting denotes various routes of administration and is used for drugs that are commonly administered into joints, cavities, tissues, or topical applications, in addition to other parenteral administrations. Listings posted with "OTH" indicate other administration methods, such as suppositories or catheter injections.

Blue typeface terms are added by publisher.

DRUG NAME	DOSAGE	METHOD OF ADMINISTRATION	HCPCS CODE
A			
Abatacept	10 mg		**J0129**
Abbokinase	5,000 IU vial	IV	J3364
	250,000 IU vial	IV	J3365
Abbokinase, Open Cath	5,000 IU vial	IV	J3364
Abciximab	10 mg	IV	**J0130**
Abelcet	10 mg	IV	J0287, J0288, J0289
Abilify	0.25 mg		J0400
Ablavar	1 ml		A9583
ABLC	50 mg	IV	J0285
AbobotulinumtoxintypeA	5 units		**J0586**
Abraxane	1 mg		J9264
Acetaminophen	10 mg		**J0131** ◀
Acetazolamide sodium	up to 500 mg	IM, IV	J1120
Acetylcysteine			
injection	100 mg		**J0132**
unit dose form	per gram	INH	**J7604, J7608**
Achromycin	up to 250 mg	IM, IV	J0120
Actemra	1 mg		J3262
ACTH	up to 40 units	IV, IM, SC	J0800
Acthar	up to 40 units	IV, IM, SC	J0800
Acthib			J3490
Acthrel	1 mcg		J0795
Actimmune	0.25 mg	SC	J1830
	3 million units	SC	J9216
Activase	1 mg	IV	J2997
Acyclovir	5 mg		**J0133**
			J8499
Adagen	25 IU		J2504

◀ New	← Revised	✔ Reinstated	~~deleted~~ Deleted	

DRUG NAME	DOSAGE	METHOD OF ADMINISTRATION	HCPCS CODE
Adalimumab	20 mg		**J0135**
Adenocard	6 mg	IV	J0150
	30 mg	IV	J0152
Adenoscan	30 mg	IV	**J0152**
Adenosine	6 mg	IV	**J0150**
	30 mg	IV	**J0152**
Adrenalin Chloride	up to 1 ml ampule	SC, IM	J0171
Adrenalin, epinephrine	0.1 mg	SC, IM	**J0171**
Adriamycin, PFS, RDF	10 mg	IV	J9000
Adrucil	500 mg	IV	J9190
Advate	per IU		J7192
Agalsidase beta	1 mg	IV	**J0180**
Aggrastat	0.25 mg	IM, IV	J3246
Aglucosidase alfa	10 mg	IV	J0220
A-hydroCort	up to 50 mg	IV, IM, SC	J1710
	up to 100 m		J1720
Akineton	per 5 mg	IM, IV	J0190
Alatrofloxacin mesylate, injection	100 mg	IV	**J0200**
Albuminar-5	50 ml		P9041
	250 ml		P9045
Albuminar-25	20 ml		P9046
	50 ml		P9047
Albumin-Zlb	50 ml, 5%		P9041
	250 ml, 5%		P9045
	50 ml, 25%		P9047
Albunex	250 ml		P9045
Alburx	50 ml		P9041
	250 ml		P9045
	20 ml		P9046
Albutein	20 ml		P9041
	250 ml		P9045
	20 ml		P9046
	50 ml		P9047
Albuterol	0.5 mg	INH	**J7620**
concentrated form	1 mg	INH	**J7610, J7611**
unit dose form	1 mg	INH	**J7609, J7613**
Aldesleukin	per single use vial	IM, IV	J9015
Aldomet	up to 250 mg	IV	J0210
Aldurazyme	0.1 mg		J1931
Alefacept	0.5 mg		**J0215**
Alemtuzumab	10 mg		**J9010**
Alferon N	250,000 IU	IM	J9215

◄ New   ← Revised   ✔ Reinstated   ~~deleted~~ Deleted

DRUG NAME	DOSAGE	METHOD OF ADMINISTRATION	HCPCS CODE	
Alglucerase	per 10 units	IV	J0205	
Alglucosidase alfa	10 mg	IV	J0220, J0221	←
Alimta	10 mg		J9305	
Alkaban-AQ	1 mg	IV	J9360	
Alkeran	2 mg	ORAL	J8600	
	50 mg	IV	J9245	
Allopurinol Sodium			J9999	
Aloxi	25 mcg		J2469	
Alpha 1-proteinase inhibitor, human	10 mg	IV	J0256 , J0257	←
Alphanate			J7186	
Alphanate	per IU		J7190, J7193, J7194	
Alprostadil				
injection	1.25 mcg	OTH injection	J0270	
urethral suppository	EA	OTH	J0275	
Alteplase recombinant	1 mg	IV	J2997	
Alupent	per 10 mg	INH	J7667, J7668	
noncompounded, unit dose	10 mg	INH	J7669	
AmBisome	10 mg	IV	J0289	
Amcort	per 5 mg	IM	J3302	
A-methaPred	up to 40 mg	IM, IV	J2920	
	up to 125 mg	IM, IV	J2930	
Amevive	0.5 mg		J0215	
Amgen	1 mcg	SC	J9212	
Amifostine	500 mg	IV	J0207	
Amikin	100 mg	IM, IV	J0278	
Amikacin sulfate	100 mg	IM, IV	J0278	
Aminocaproic Acid			J3490	
Aminolevalinic acid HCl	unit dose (354 mg)	OTH	J7308	
Aminolevulinate	1 gm	OTH	J7309	
Amiodarone HCl	30 mg	IV	J0282	
Amitriptyline HCl	up to 20 mg	IM	J1320	
Amobarbital	up to 125 mg	IM, IV	J0300	
Amphadase	up to 150 units		J3470	
Amphocin	50 mg	IV	J0285	
Amphotec	10 mg	IV	J0288	
Amphotericin B	50 mg	IV	J0285	
Amphotericin B, lipid complex	10 mg	IV	J0287–J0289	
Ampicillin				
sodium	up to 500 mg	IM, IV	J0290	
sodium/sulbactam sodium	per 1.5 gm	IM, IV	J0295	
Amygdalin			J3570	

◀ New   ← Revised   ✔ Reinstated   ~~deleted~~ Deleted

DRUG NAME	DOSAGE	METHOD OF ADMINISTRATION	HCPCS CODE
Amytal	up to 125 mg	IM, IV	J0300
Anabolin LA 100	up to 50 mg	IM	J2320
Anadulafungin	1 mg	IV	**J0348**
Ancef	500 mg	IV, IM	J0690
Andrest 90-4	up to 1 cc	IM	J0900
Andro-Cyp	up to 100 mg	IM	J1070
	1 cc, 200 mg	IM	J1080
Andro-Cyp 200	up to 100 mg	IM	J1070
	1 cc, 200 mg	IM	J1080
Andro L.A. 200	up to 100 mg	IM	J3120
	up to 200 mg	IM	J3130
Andro-Estro 90-4	up to 1 cc	IM	J0900
Andro/Fem	up to 1 ml	IM	J1060
Androgyn L.A	up to 1 cc	IM	J0900
Androlone-50	up to 50 mg		J2320
Androlone-D 100	up to 50 mg	IM	J2320
Andronaq-50	up to 50 mg	IM	J3140
Andronaq-LA	up to 100 mg	IM	J1070
	1 cc, 200 mg	IM	J1080
Andronate-200	up to 100 mg	IM	J1070
	1 cc, 200 mg	IM	J1080
Andronate-100	up to 100 mg	IM	J1070
	1 cc, 200 mg	IM	J1080
Andropository 100	up to 100 mg	IM	J3120
	up to 200 mg	IM	J3130
Andryl 200	up to 100 mg	IM	J3120
	up to 200 mg	IM	J3130
Anectine	up to 20 mg	IM, IV	J0330
Anergan 25	up to 50 mg	IM, IV	J2550
	12.5 mg	ORAL	Q0169
	25 mg	ORAL	Q0170
Anergan 50	up to 50 mg	IM, IV	J2550
	12.5 mg	ORAL	Q0169
	25 mg	ORAL	Q0170
Angiomax	1 mg		J0583
Anistreplase	30 units	IV	**J0350**
Antiflex	up to 60 mg		J2360
Anti-Inhibitor	per IU	IV	**J7198**
Antispas	up to 20 mg	IM	J0500
Antithrombin III (human)	per IU	IV	**J7197**
Antithrombin recombinant	50 IU		**J7196**
Antizol	15 mg		J1451

◄ New   ← Revised   ✔ Reinstated   ~~deleted~~ Deleted

DRUG NAME	DOSAGE	METHOD OF ADMINISTRATION	HCPCS CODE
Anzemet	10 mg	IV	J1260
	50 mg	ORAL	S0174
	100 mg	ORAL	Q0180
Apidra	per 50 units		J1817
	per 5 units		J1815
A.P.L.	per 1,000 USP units	IM	J0725
Apokyn	1 mg		J0364
Apomorphine Hydrochloride	1 mg		J0364
Apresoline	up to 20 mg	IV, IM	J0360
Aprotinin	10,000 kiu		J0365
AquaMEPHYTON	per 1 mg	IM, SC, IV	J3430
Aralast	10 mg	IV	J0256
Aralen	up to 250 mg	IM	J0390
Aramine	per 10 mg	IV, IM, SC	J0380
Aranesp			
ESRD use	1 mcg		J0882
Non-ESRD use	1 mcg		J0881
Arbutamine	1 mg	IV	J0395
Arcalyst	1 mg		J2793
Aredia	per 30 mg	IV	J2430
Arfonad, see Trimethaphan camsylate			
Arformoterol tartrate	15 mcg		J7605
Aridol	25% in 50 ml	IV	J2150
	5 mg	INH	J7665
Arimidex			J8999
Aripiprazole	0.25 mg		J0400
Aristocort Forte	per 5 mg	IM	J3302
Aristocort Intralesional	per 5 mg	IM	J3302
Aristopan	per 5 mg		J3303
Aristospan Intra-Articular	per 5 mg	VAR	J3303
Aristospan Intralesional	per 5 mg	VAR	J3303
Arixtra	per 0.5 m		J1652
Aromasin			J8999
Arranon	50 mg		J9261
Arrestin	up to 200 mg	IM	J3250
	250 mg	ORAL	Q0173
Arsenic trioxide	1 mg	IV	J9017
Arzerra	10 mg		J9302
Asparaginase	10,000 units	IV, IM	J9020
Astramorph PF	up to 10 mg	IM, IV, SC	J2270
	100 mg	IM, IV, SC	J2271
Atgam	250 mg	IV	J7504

◄ New   ← Revised   ✔ Reinstated   ~~deleted~~ Deleted

DRUG NAME	DOSAGE	METHOD OF ADMINISTRATION	HCPCS CODE
Ativan	2 mg	IM, IV	J2060
Atropine			
concentrated form	per mg	INH	J7635
unit dose form	per mg	INH	J7636
sulfate	0.01 mg, per mg	IV, IM, SC	J0461, J7636
Atrovent	per mg	INH	J7644, J7645
Atryn	50 IU		J7196
Aurothioglucose	up to 50 mg	IM	J2910
Autologous cultured chondrocytes implant			J7330
Autoplex T	per IU	IV	J7198, J7199
Avastin	10 mg		J9035
Avelox	100 mg		J2280
Avonex	11 mcg	IM	Q3025
	11 mcg	SC	Q3026
	33 mcg	IM	J1826
Azacitidine	1 mg		J9025
Azasan	50 mg		J7500
Azathioprine	50 mg	ORAL	J7500
Azathioprine			
parenteral	100 mg	IV	J7501
dihydrate	1 gm	ORAL	Q0144
injection	500 mg	IV	J0456
Azithromycin Bihydrate	500 mg		J0456
B			
Baci-RX			J3490
Baciim			J3490
Bacitracin			J3490
Baclofen	10 mg	IT	J0475
Baclofen for intrathecal trial	50 mcg	OTH	J0476
Bacteriostatic	10 ml		A4216
Bactocill	up to 250 mg	IM, IV	J2700
BAL in oil	per 100 mg	IM	J0470
Banflex	up to 60 mg	IV, IM	J2360
Basiliximab	20 mg	IV	J0480
Bayhep B			J3590
BayRho-D	50 mcg		J2788
BCG (Bacillus Calmette and Guérin), live	per vial	IV	J9031
Bebulin VH	per IU		J7194
Beclomethasone inhalation solution, unit dose form	per mg	INH	J7622, J7624
Belimumab	10 mg		J0490 ◄
Bena-D 10	up to 50 mg	IV, IM	J1200
Bena-D 50	up to 50 mg	IV, IM	J1200

◄ New   ← Revised   ✔ Reinstated   ~~deleted~~ Deleted

2012 TABLE OF DRUGS A–B

DRUG NAME	DOSAGE	METHOD OF ADMINISTRATION	HCPCS CODE
Benadryl	up to 50 mg	IV, IM	J1200
Benahist 10	up to 50 mg	IV, IM	J1200
Benahist 50	up to 50 mg	IV, IM	J1200
Ben-Allergin-50	up to 50 mg	IV, IM	J1200
	50 mg	ORAL	Q0163
Bendamustine HCl	1 mg		J9033
Benefix	per IU	IV	J7195
Benlysta	10 mg		J0490
Benoject-10	up to 50 mg	IV, IM	J1200
Benoject-50	up to 50 mg	IV, IM	J1200
Bentyl	up to 20 mg	IM	J0500
Benzacot	up to 200 mg		J3250
Benzocaine			J3490
Benztropine mesylate	per 1 mg	IM, IV	J0515
Berinert, see C-1 esterase inhibitor			
Berubigen	up to 1,000 mcg	IM, SC	J3420
Betalin 12	up to 1,000 mcg	IM, SC	J3420
Betameth	per 4 mg	IM, IV	J0702
Betamethasone acetate & betamethasone sodium phosphate	per 3 mg	IM	J0702
Betamethasone inhalation solution, unit dose form	per mg	INH	J7624
Betaseron	0.25 mg	SC	J1830
Bethanechol chloride	up to 5 mg	SC	J0520
Bevacizumab	10 mg		J9035
Bicillin C-R	100,000 units		J0558
Bicillin C-R 900/300	100,000 units	IM	J0558, J0561
Bicillin L-A	100,000 units	IM	J0561
BiCNU	100 mg	IV	J9050
Biperiden lactate	per 5 mg	IM, IV	J0190
Bitolterol mesylate			
concentrated form	per mg	INH	J7628
unit dose form	per mg	INH	J7629
Bivalirudin	1 mg		J0583
Blenoxane	15 units	IM, IV, SC	J9040
Bleomycin sulfate	15 units	IM, IV, SC	J9040
Boniva	1 mg		J1740
Bortezomib	0.1 mg		J9041
Botox	1 unit		J0585
Bravelle	75 IU		J3355
Brethine			
concentrated form	per 1 mg	INH	J7680
unit dose	per 1 mg	INH	J7681
	up to 1 mg	SC, IV	J3105

◄ New   ← Revised   ✔ Reinstated   ~~deleted~~ Deleted

DRUG NAME	DOSAGE	METHOD OF ADMINISTRATION	HCPCS CODE
Brevital Sodium			J3490
Bricanyl Subcutaneous	up to 1 mg	SC, IV	J3105
Brompheniramine maleate	per 10 mg	IM, SC, IV	**J0945**
Broncho Saline	10 ml		A4216
Bronkephrine, see Ethylnorepinephrine HCl			
Bronkosol			
concentrated form	per mg	INH	J7647, J7648
unit dose form	per mg	INH	J7649, J7650
Brovana			J7605, J7699
Budesonide inhalation solution			
concentrated form	0.25 mg	INH	**J7633, J7634**
unit dose form	0.5 mg	INH	**J7626, J7627**
Bumetanide			J3490
Buminate	50 ml		P9041
	250 ml		P9045
	20 ml		P9046
	50 ml		P9047
Bupivacaine			J3490
Buprenex	0.1 mg		J0592
Buprenorphine Hydrochloride	0.1 mg		**J0592, J3490**
Busulfan	1 mg		**J0594**
	2 mg	ORAL	**J8510**
Butorphanol tartrate	1 mg		**J0595**
C			
C1 Esterase Inhibitor	10 units		**J0597, J0598**
Cabazitaxel	1 mg		**J9043**
Cabergoline	0.25 mg	ORAL	**J8515**
Cafcit	5 mg	IV	J0706
Caffeine citrate	5 mg	IV	**J0706**
Caine-1	10 mg	IV	J2001
Caine-2	10 mg	IV	J2001
Calcijex	0.1 mcg	IM	J0636
Calcimar	up to 400 units	SC, IM	J0630
Calcitonin-salmon	up to 400 units	SC, IM	**J0630**
Calcitriol	0.1 mcg	IM	**J0636**
Calcitriol in almond oil	0.1 mcg		J0636
Calcium Disodium Versenate	up to 1,000 mg	IV, SC, IM	J0600
Calcium gluconate	per 10 ml	IV	**J0610**
Calcium glycerophosphate and calcium lactate	per 10 ml	IM, SC	**J0620**
Calcium glycerophosphate and calcium lactate	10 ml	IM, SC	J0620
Calphosan	per 10 ml	IM, SC	J0620
Campath	10 mg		J9010

◄ New   ← Revised   ✔ Reinstated   ~~deleted~~ Deleted

DRUG NAME	DOSAGE	METHOD OF ADMINISTRATION	HCPCS CODE
Camptosar	20 mg	IV	J9206
Canakinumab	1 mg		J0638
Cancidas	5 mg		J0637
Capecitabine	150 mg	ORAL	J8520
	500 mg	ORAL	J8521
Capsaicin patch	per 10 sq cm	OTH	J7335
Carbocaine with Neo-Cobefrin	per 10 ml	VAR	J0670
Carbocaine	per 10 ml	VAR	J0670
Carboplatin	50 mg	IV	J9045
Carimune	500 mg		J1566
Carmustine	100 mg	IV	J9050
Carnitor	per 1 g	IV	J1955
Carticel			J7330
Caspofungin acetate	5 mg	IV	J0637
Cathflo Activase	1 mg		J2997
Caverject injection	1.25 mcg		J0270
Cayston, see Aztreonam			
Ceenu		ORAL	J8799
Cefadyl	up to 1 g	IV, IM	J0710
Cefazolin sodium	500 mg	IV, IM	J0690
Cefepime hydrochloride	500 mg	IV	J0692
Cefizox	per 500 mg	IM, IV	J0715
Cefotan			J3490
Cefotaxime sodium	per 1 g	IV, IM	J0698
Cefotetan			J3490
Cefoxitin sodium	1 g	IV, IM	J0694
Ceftazidime	per 500 mg	IM, IV	J0713
Cefteroline fosamil	1 mg		J0712
Ceftizoxime sodium	per 500 mg	IV, IM	J0715
	per 250 mg	IV, IM	J0696
Cefuroxime sodium, sterile	per 750 mg	IM, IV	J0697
Celestone Soluspan	per 3 mg	IM	J0702
	per mg	ORAL	J7624
CellCept	250 mg	ORAL	J7517
Cel-U-Jec	per 4 mg	IM, IV	Q0511
Cenacort A-40	per 10 mg	IM	J3301
	per 5 mg		J3302
Cenacort Forte	per 5 mg	IM	J3302
Cephalothin sodium	up to 1 g	IM, IV	J1890
Cephapirin sodium	up to 1 g	IV, IM	J0710
Cerebyx	50 mg		Q2009

◄ New   ← Revised   ✔ Reinstated   ~~deleted~~ Deleted

DRUG NAME	DOSAGE	METHOD OF ADMINISTRATION	HCPCS CODE
Ceredase	per 10 units	IV	J0205
Cerezyme	10 units		J1786
Certolizumab pegol	1 mg		**J0718**
Cerubidine	10 mg	IV	J9150
Cetuximab	10 mg		**J9055**
Chealamide	per 150 mg	IV	J3520
Chloramphenicol sodium succinate	up to 1 g	IV	**J0720**
Chlordiazepoxide HCl	up to 100 mg	IM, IV	**J1990**
Chloromycetin Sodium Succinate	up to 1 g	IV	J0720
Chloroprocaine HCl	per 30 ml	VAR	**J2400**
	10 mg	ORAL	**Q0171**
	25 mg	ORAL	**Q0172**
	up to 50 mg	IM, IV	J3230
Chloroquine HCl	up to 250 mg	IM	**J0390**
Chlorothiazide sodium	per 500 mg	IV	**J1205**
Chlorpromazine HCl	up to 50 mg	IM, IV	**J3230**
Cholografin Meglumine	per ml		Q9961
Chorex-5	per 1,000 USP units	IM	J0725
Chorex-10	per 1,000 USP units	IM	J0725
Chorignon	per 1,000 USP units	IM	J0725
Chorionic gonadotropin	per 1,000 USP units	IM	**J0725**
Choron 10	per 1,000 USP units	IM	J0725
Cidofovir	375 mg	IV	**J0740**
Cimzia	1 mg		J0718
Cinryze	10 units		J0598
Cilastatin sodium, imipenem	per 250 mg	IV, IM	**J0743**
Cimetidine HCl			J3490
Cipro IV	200 mg	IV	J0706
Ciprofloxacin	200 mg	IV	**J0706**
			J3490
Cisplatin, powder or solution	per 10 mg	IV	**J9060**
Cladribine	per mg	IV	**J9065**
Claforan	per 1 gm	IM, IV	J0698
Cleocin Phosphate			J3490
Clincacort	per 5 mg		J3302
Clofarabine	1 mg		**J9027**
Clolar	1 mg		J9027
Clonidine Hydrochloride	1 mg	epidural	**J0735**
Cobal-1000	up to 1,000 mcg		J3420
Cobex	up to 1,000 mcg	IM, SC	J3420
Cobulin-M	up to 1,000 mcg		J3420

◄ New   ← Revised   ✔ Reinstated   ~~deleted~~ Deleted

DRUG NAME	DOSAGE	METHOD OF ADMINISTRATION	HCPCS CODE
Codeine phosphate	per 30 mg	IM, IV, SC	**J0745**
Codimal-A	per 10 mg	IM, SC, IV	J0945
Cogentin	per 1 mg	IM, IV	J0515
Colchicine	per 1 mg	IV	**J0760**
Colistimethate sodium	up to 150 mg	IM, IV	**J0770, S0142**
Collagenase, Clostridium Histolyticum	0.01 mg		**J0775**
Coly-Mycin M	up to 150 mg	IM, IV	J0770
Compa-Z	up to 10 mg	IM, IV	J0780
Compazine	up to 10 mg	IM, IV	J0780, J8498
	5 mg	ORAL	Q0164
	10 mg	ORAL	Q0165
Compro			J8498
Comptosar	20 mg		J9206
Conray	per ml		Q9961
Conray 30	per ml		Q9958
Conray 43	per ml		Q9960
Copaxone	20 mg		J1595
Cophene-B	per 10 mg	IM, SC, IV	J0945
Copper contraceptive, intrauterine		OTH	**J7300**
Cordarone	30 mg	IV	J0282
Corgonject-5	per 1,000 USP units	IM	J0725
Corticorelin ovine triflutate	1 mcg		**J0795**
Corticotropin	up to 40 units	IV, IM, SC	**J0800**
Cortisone Acetate			J3490
Cortrosyn	per 0.25 mg	IM, IV	J0835
Corvert	1 mg		J1742
Cosmegen	0.5 mg	IV	J9120
Cosyntropin	per 0.25 mg	IM, IV	**J0833, J0834**
Cotolone	up to 1 ml		J2650
	per 5 mg		J7510
Cotranzine	up to 10 mg	IM, IV	J0780
Crofab	up to 1 gram		J0840	◄
Cromolyn sodium, unit dose form	per 10 mg	INH	**J7631, J7632**
Crotalidae Polyvalent Immune Fab	up to 1 gram		**J0840**	◄
Crystal B-12	up to 1,000 mcg		J3420
Crysticillin 300 A.S.	up to 600,000 units	IM, IV	J2510
Crysticillin 600 A.S.	up to 600,000 units	IM, IV	J2510
Cubicin	1 mg		J0878
Cyano	up to 1,000 mcg		J3420
Cyanocobalamin	up to 1,000 mcg		J3420
Cyclophosphamide	100 mg	IV	**J9070**
oral	25 mg	ORAL	**J8530**

◄ New   ← Revised   ✔ Reinstated   ~~deleted~~ Deleted

DRUG NAME	DOSAGE	METHOD OF ADMINISTRATION	HCPCS CODE
Cyclosporin A	250 mg		J7516
Cyclosporine	25 mg	ORAL	J7515
	100 mg	ORAL	J7502
parenteral	250 mg	IV	J7516
Cymetra	1 cc		Q4112
Cyomin	up to 1,000 mcg		J3420
Cysto-Cornray LI	per ml		Q9958
Cystografin	per ml		Q9958
Cystografin-Dilute	per ml		Q9958
Cytarabine	100 mg	SC, IV	J9100
Cytarabine liposome	10 mg		J9098
CytoGam	per vial		J0850
Cytomegalovirus immune globulin intravenous (human)	per vial	IV	J0850
Cytosar-U	100 mg	SC, IV	J9100
Cytovene	500 mg	IV	J1570
Cytoxan	100 mg	IV	J9070
D			
D-5-W, infusion	1000 cc	IV	J7070
Dacarbazine	100 mg	IV	J9130
Daclizumab	25 mg	IV	J7513
Dactinomycin	0.5 mg	IV	J9120
Dalalone	1 mg	IM, IV, OTH	J1100
Dalalone L.A	1 mg	IM	J1094
Dalteparin sodium	per 2500 IU	SC	J1645
Daptomycin	1 mg		J0878
Darbepoetin Alfa	1 mcg		J0881, J0882
Daunorubicin citrate, liposomal formulation	10 mg	IV	J9151
Daunorubicin HCl	10 mg	IV	J9150
Daunoxome	10 mg	IV	J9151
DDAVP	1 mcg	IV, SC	J2597
Debioclip Kit	3.75 mg		J3310
Decadron Phosphate	1 mg	IM, IV, OTH	J1100
Decadron	1 mg	IM, IV, OTH	J1100
	0.25 mg		J8540
Decadron-LA	1 mg	IM	J1094
Deca-Durabolin	up to 50 mg	IM	J2320
Decaject	1 mg	IM, IV, OTH	J1100
Decaject-L.A.	1 mg	IM	J1094
Decitabine	1 mg		J0894
Decolone-50	up to 50 mg	IM	J2320
Decolone-100	up to 50 mg	IM	J2320

◄ New   ← Revised   ✔ Reinstated   ~~deleted~~ Deleted

DRUG NAME	DOSAGE	METHOD OF ADMINISTRATION	HCPCS CODE
De-Comberol	up to 1 ml	IM	J1060
Decongest	per 10 mg		Q0163
Deferoxamine mesylate	500 mg	IM, SC, IV	J0895
Definity	per ml		J3490, Q9957
Degarelix	1 mg		J9155
Dehist	per 10 mg	IM, SC, IV	J0945
Deladumone OB	up to 1 cc	IM	J0900
Deladumone	up to 1 cc	IM	J0900
Delatest	up to 100 mg	IM	J3120
	up to 200 mg	IM	J3130
Delatestadiol	up to 1 cc	IM	J0900
Delatestryl	up to 100 mg	IM	J3120
	up to 200 mg	IM	J3130
Delta-Cortef	5 mg	ORAL	J7510
Deltasone	5 mg		J7506
Delestrogen	up to 10 mg	IM	J1380
Demadex	10 mg/ml	IV	J3265
Demerol HCl	per 100 mg	IM, IV, SC	J2175
Denileukin diftitox	300 mcg		J9160
Denosumab	1 mg		J0897
DepAndro 100	up to 100 mg	IM	J1070
	1 cc, 200 mg	IM	J1080
	up to 100 mg		J3150
DepAndro 200	up to 100 mg	IM	J1070
	1 cc, 200 mg	IM	J1080
DepAndrogyn	up to 1 ml	IM	J1060
DepGynogen	up to 5 mg	IM	J1000
DepoCyt	10 mg		J9098
DepMedalone 40	20 mg	IM	J1020
	40 mg	IM	J1030
	80 mg	IM	J1040
DepMedalone 80	20 mg	IM	J1020
	40 mg	IM	J1030
	80 mg	IM	J1040
Depo-estradiol cypionate	up to 5 mg	IM	J1000
Depogen	up to 5 mg	IM	J1000
Depoject	20 mg	IM	J1020
	40 mg	IM	J1030
	80 mg	IM	J1040
Depo-Medrol	20 mg	IM	J1020
	40 mg	IM	J1030
	80 mg	IM	J1040

◀ New   ← Revised   ✔ Reinstated   ~~deleted~~ Deleted

DRUG NAME	DOSAGE	METHOD OF ADMINISTRATION	HCPCS CODE
Depopred-40	20 mg	IM	J1020
	40 mg	IM	J1030
	80 mg	IM	J1040
Depopred-80	20 mg	IM	J1020
	40 mg	IM	J1030
	80 mg	IM	J1040
Depo-Provera	50 mg	IM	J1051
	150 mg	IM	J1055
Depotest	up to 100 mg	IM	J1070
	1 cc, 200 mg	IM	J1080
Depo-Testadiol	up to 1 ml	IM	J1060
Depotestrogen	up to 1 ml	IM	J1060
Depo-Testosterone	1 cc, 200 mg	IM	J1080
	up to 100 mg	IM	J1070, J3120
Dermagraft	per square centimeter		Q4106
Desferal Mesylate	500 mg	IM, SC, IV	J0895
Desmopressin acetate	1 mcg	IV, SC	J2597
Dexacen LA-8	1 mg	IM	J1094
Dexacen-4	1 mg	IM, IV, OTH	J1100
Dexamethasone			
concentrated form	per mg	INH	J7637
intravitreal implant	0.1 mg	OTH	J7312
unit form	per mg	INH	J7638
oral	0.25 mg	ORAL	J8540
	1 mg		J1100
Dexamethasone acetate	1 mg	IM	J1094
Dexamethasone sodium phosphate	1 mg	IM, IV, OTH	J1100, J7638
Dexasone	1 mg	IM, IV, OTH	J1100
Dexasone L.A.	1 mg	IM	J1094
Dexferrum	50 mg		J1750
Dexone	0.25 mg	ORAL	J8540
	1 mg	IM, IV, OTH	J1100
Dexone LA	1 mg	IM	J1094
Dexpak	0.25 mg	ORAL	J8540
Dexrazoxane hydrochloride	250 mg	IV	J1190
Dextran 40	500 ml	IV	J7100
Dextran 70	500 ml		J7110
Dextran 75	500 ml	IV	J7110
Dextrose 5%/normal saline solution	500 ml = 1 unit	IV	J7042
Dextrose/water (5%)	500 ml = 1 unit	IV	J7060
D.H.E. 45	per 1 mg		J1110
Diamox	up to 500 mg	IM, IV	J1120

◄ New   ← Revised   ✔ Reinstated   ~~deleted~~ Deleted

DRUG NAME	DOSAGE	METHOD OF ADMINISTRATION	HCPCS CODE
Diazepam	up to 5 mg	IM, IV	**J3360**
Diazoxide	up to 300 mg	IV	**J1730**
Dibent	up to 20 mg	IM	J0500
Dicyclocot	up to 20 mg		J0500
Dicyclomine HCl	up to 20 mg	IM	**J0500**
Didronel	per 300 mg	IV	J1436
Diethylstilbestrol diphosphate	250 mg	IV	**J9165**
Diflucan	200 mg	IV	J1450
Digibind	per vial		J1162
DigiFab	per vial		J1162
Digoxin	up to 0.5 mg	IM, IV	**J1160**
Digoxin immune fab (ovine)	per vial		**J1162**
Dihydrex	up to 50 mg	IV, IM	J1200
	50 mg	ORAL	Q0163
Dihydroergotamine mesylate	per 1 mg	IM, IV	**J1110**
Dilantin	per 50 mg	IM, IV	J1165
Dilaudid	up to 4 mg	SC, IM, IV	J1170
	250 mg	OTH	S0092
Dilocaine	10 mg	IV	J2001
Dilomine	up to 20 mg	IM	J0500
Dilor	up to 500 mg	IM	J1180
Dimenhydrinate	up to 50 mg	IM, IV	**J1240**
Dimercaprol	per 100 mg	IM	**J0470**
Dimethyl sulfoxide	50%, 50 ml	OTH	**J1212**
Dinate	up to 50 mg	IM, IV	J1240
Dioval	up to 10 mg	IM	J1380
Dioval 40	up to 10 mg	IM	J1380
Dioval XX	up to 10 mg	IM	J1380
Diphenacen-50	up to 50 mg	IV, IM	J1200
	50 mg	ORAL	Q0163
Diphenhydramine HCl			
injection	up to 50 mg	IV, IM	**J1200**
oral	50 mg	ORAL	**Q0163**
Diprivan			J3490
Dipyridamole	per 10 mg	IV	**J1245**
Disotate	per 150 mg	IV	J3520
Di-Spaz	up to 20 mg	IM	J0500
Ditate-DS	up to 1 cc	IM	J0900
Diruril	per 500 mg	IV	J1205
Diuril Sodium	per 500 mg	IV	J1205
Dizac	up to 5 mg		J3360

◄ New   ← Revised   ✔ Reinstated   ~~deleted~~ Deleted

DRUG NAME	DOSAGE	METHOD OF ADMINISTRATION	HCPCS CODE
D-Med 80	20 mg	IM	J1020
	40 mg	IM	J1030
	80 mg	IM	J1040
DMSO, Dimethyl sulfoxide 50%	50 ml	OTH	J1212
Dobutamine HCl	per 250 mg	IV	J1250
Dobutrex	per 250 mg	IV	J1250
Docetaxel	20 mg	IV	J9170
Dolasetron mesylate			
injection	10 mg	IV	J1260
tablets	100 mg	ORAL	Q0180
Dolophine HCl	up to 10 mg	IM, SC	J1230
Dommanate	up to 50 mg	IM, IV	J1240
Donbax	10 mg		J1267
Dopamine	40 mg		J1265
Dopamine in D5W	40 mg		J1265
Dopamine HCl	40 mg		J1265
Doribax	10 mg		J1267
Doripenem	10 mg		J1267
Dornase alpha, unit dose form	per mg	INH	J7639
Doxercalciferol	1 mcg	IV	J1270
Doxil	10 mg	IV	J9001
Doxorubicin			
HCl	10 mg	IV	J9000
HCl, all lipid	10 mg	IV	J9001
Dramamine	up to 50 mg	IM, IV	J1240
Dramanate	up to 50 mg	IM, IV	J1240
Dramilin	up to 50 mg	IM, IV	J1240
Dramocen	up to 50 mg	IM, IV	J1240
Dramoject	up to 50 mg	IM, IV	J1240
Dronabinol	2.5 mg	ORAL	Q0167
	5 mg	ORAL	Q0168
Droperidol	up to 5 mg	IM, IV	J1790
Droxia		ORAL	J8799
Drug administered through a metered dose inhaler		INH	J3535
Droperidol and fentanyl citrate	up to 2 ml ampule	IM, IV	J1810
DTIC-Dome	100 mg	IV	J9130
Dua-Gen L.A.	up to 1 cc		J0900
DuoNeb	up to 2.5 mg		J7620
	up to 0.5 mg		J7620
Duoval P.A.	up to 1 cc	IM	J0900
Durabolin, see Nandrolone phenpropionate			

◀ New   ← Revised   ✔ Reinstated   deleted Deleted

DRUG NAME	DOSAGE	METHOD OF ADMINISTRATION	HCPCS CODE
Duraclon	1 mg	epidural	J0735
Dura-Estrin	up to 5 mg	IM	J1000
Duracillin A.S.	up to 600,000 units	IM, IV	J2510
Duragen-10	up to 10 mg	IM	J1380
Duragen-20	up to 10 mg	IM	J1380
Duragen-40	up to 10 mg	IM	J1380
Duralone-40	20 mg	IM	J1020
	40 mg	IM	J1030
	80 mg	IM	J1040
Duralone-80	20 mg	IM	J1020
	40 mg	IM	J1030
	80 mg	IM	J1040
Duralutin, see Hydroxyprogesterone Caproate			
Duramorph	10 mg	IM, IV, SC	J2271
	up to 10 mg	IM, IV, SC	J2270
	500 mg	OTH	S0093
Duratest-100	up to 100 mg	IM	J1070
	1 cc, 200 mg	IM	J1080
Duratest-200	up to 100 mg	IM	J1070
	1 cc, 200 mg	IM	J1080
Duratestrin	up to 1 ml	IM	J1060
Durathate-200	up to 100 mg	IM	J3120
	up to 200 mg	IM	J3130
Dymenate	up to 50 mg	IM, IV	J1240
Dyphylline	up to 500 mg	IM	J1180
Dysport	5 units		J0586
E			
Ecallantide	1 mg		J1290
Eculizumab	10 mg		J1300
Edetate calcium disodium	up to 1,000 mg	IV, SC, IM	J0600
Edetate disodium	per 150 mg	IV	J3520
Edex	per 1.25 millicurie		J0270
Edisylate	up to 10 mg		J0780
Elaprase	1 mg		J1743
Elavil	up to 20 mg	IM	J1320
Elitek	0.5 mg		J2783
Ellence	2 mg		J9178
Elliotts b solution	1 ml	OTH	J9175
Eloxatin	0.5 mg		J9263
Elspar	10,000 units	IV, IM	J9020
Emend	1 mg		J1453
Ememd	5 mg	ORAL	J8501

◀ New   ← Revised   ✔ Reinstated   ~~deleted~~ Deleted

DRUG NAME	DOSAGE	METHOD OF ADMINISTRATION	HCPCS CODE
Emete-Con, see Benzquinamide			
Eminase	30 units	IV	J0350
Enbrel	25 mg	IM, IV	J1438
Endrate ethylenediamine-tetra-acetic acid	per 150 mg	IV	J3520
Enfuvirtide	1 mg		**J1324**
Enovil	up to 20 mg	IM	J1320
Enoxaparin sodium	10 mg	SC	**J1650**
Eovist	1 ml		A9581
Epinephrine, adrenalin	0.1 mg	SC, IM	**J0171**
Epirubicin hydrochloride	2 mg		**J9178, J7799**
Epoetin alfa	1,000 units		**Q4081**
Epogen	1,000 units		J0885
			J0886
			Q4081
Epoprostenol	0.5 mg	IV	**J1325**
Eptifibatide, injection	5 mg	IM, IV	**J1327**
Eraxis	1 mg	IV	J0348
Erbitux	10 mg		J9055
Ergonovine maleate	up to 0.2 mg	IM, IV	**J1330**
Eribulin mesylate	0.1 mg		**J9179**
Ertapenem sodium	500 mg		**J1335**
Erthrocin	500 mg		J1364
Erythromycin lactobionate	500 mg	IV	**J1364**
Estra-D	up to 5 mg	IM	J1000
Estra-L 20	up to 10 mg	IM	J1380
	up to 40 mg	IM	J1370
Estra-L 40	up to 10 mg	IM	J1380
	up to 40 mg	IM	J1370
Estra-Testrin	up to 1 cc	IM	J0900
Estradiol Cypionate	up to 5 mg	IM	J1000, J1056, J1060
Estradiol			
L.A.	up to 10 mg	IM	J1380
	up to 40 mg	IM	J1370
L.A. 20	up to 10 mg	IM	J1380
	up to 40 mg	IM	J1370
L.A. 40	up to 10 mg	IM	J1380
	up to 40 mg	IM	J1370
Estradiol valerate	up to 10 mg	IM	**J1380**
Estragyn 5	per 1 mg		J1435
Estro-Cyp	up to 5 mg	IM	J1000
Estrogen, conjugated	per 25 mg	IV, IM	**J1410**

◄ New   ← Revised   ✔ Reinstated   ~~deleted~~ Deleted

DRUG NAME	DOSAGE	METHOD OF ADMINISTRATION	HCPCS CODE
Estroject L.A.	up to 5 mg	IM	J1000
Estrone	per 1 mg	IM	J1435
Estrone 5	per 1 mg	IM	J1435
Estrone Aqueous	per 1 mg	IM	J1435
Estronol	per 1 mg	IM	J1435
Estronol-L.A.	up to 5 mg	IM	J1000
Etanercept, injection	25 mg	IM, IV	J1438
Ethamolin	100 mg		J1430
Ethanolamine	100 mg		J1430, J3490
Ethyol	500 mg	IV	J0207
Etidronate disodium	per 300 mg	IV	J1436
Etonogestrel implant			J7307
Etopophos	10 mg	IV	J9181
Etoposide	10 mg	IV	J9181
oral	50 mg	ORAL	J8560
Euflexxa			J7323
Everolimus	0.25 mg	ORAL	J8561
Everone	up to 100 mg	IM	J3120
	up to 200 mg	IM	J3130
F			
Fabrazyme	1 mg	IV	J0180
Factor VIIa (coagulation factor, recombinant)	1 mcg	IV	J7189
Factor VIII (anti-hemophilic factor)			
human	per IU	IV	J7190
porcine	per IU	IV	J7191
recombinant	per IU	IV	J7185, J7192
Factor IX			
anti-hemophilic factor, purified, non-recombinant	per IU	IV	J7193
anti-hemophilic factor, recombinant	per IU	IV	J7195
complex	per IU	IV	J7194
Factors, other hemophilia clotting	per IU	IV	J7196
Factrel	per 100 mcg	SC, IV	J1620
Famotidine			J3490
Faraheme	1 mg		Q0138, Q0139
Faslodex	25 mg		J9395
Feiba VH Immuno	per IU	IV	J7196
Fentanyl citrate	0.1 mg	IM, IV	J3010
Ferrlecit	12.5 mg		J2916
Ferumoxytol	1 mg		Q0138, Q0139
Filgrastim (G-CSF)	300 mcg	SC, IV	J1440
	480 mcg	SC, IV	J1441
Firmagon	1 mg		J9155

◀ New　　← Revised　　✔ Reinstated　　~~deleted~~ Deleted

DRUG NAME	DOSAGE	METHOD OF ADMINISTRATION	HCPCS CODE
Flebogamma	500 mg	IV	J1572
	1 cc		J1460
Flexbumin	20 ml		P9046
	50 ml		P9047
Flexoject	up to 60 mg	IV, IM	J2360
Flexon	up to 60 mg	IV, IM	J2360
Flolan	0.5 mg	IV	J1325
Floxuridine	500 mg	IV	J9200
Fluconazole	200 mg	IV	J1450
Fludara	1 mg	ORAL	J8562
	50 mg	IV	J9185
Fludarabine phosphate	50 mg	IV	J9185
Flunisolide inhalation solution, unit dose form	per mg	INH	J7641
Fluocinolone			J7311
Fluorouracil	500 mg	IV	J9190
Flutamide			J8999
Folex	5 mg	IA, IM, IT, IV	J9250
	50 mg	IA, IM, IT, IV	J9260
Folex PFS	5 mg	IA, IM, IT, IV	J9250
	50 mg	IA, IM, IT, IV	J9260
Follutein	per 1,000 USP units	IM	J0725
Folotyn	1 mg		J9307
Fomepizole	15 mg		J1451
Fomivirsen sodium	1.65 mg	Intraocular	J1452
Fondaparinux sodium	0.5 mg		J1652
Formoterol	12 mcg	INH	J7640
Formoterol fumarate	20 mcg		J7606
	12 mcg		J7640
Fortaz	per 500 mg	IM, IV	J0713
Forteo	10 mcg		J3110
Fosaprepitant	1 mg		J1453
Foscarnet sodium	per 1,000 mg	IV	J1455
Foscavir	per 1,000 mg	IV	J1455
Fosphenytoin	50 mg		Q2009
Fragmin	per 2,500 IU		J1645
FUDR	500 mg	IV	J9200
Fulvestrant	25 mg		J9395
Fungizone intravenous	50 mg	IV	J0285
Furomide M.D.	up to 20 mg	IM, IV	J1940
Furosemide	up to 20 mg	IM, IV	J1940
Fuzeon	1 mg		J1324

◀ New   ← Revised   ✔ Reinstated   ~~deleted~~ Deleted

DRUG NAME	DOSAGE	METHOD OF ADMINISTRATION	HCPCS CODE
G			
Gablofen	10 mg		J0475
	50 mcg		J0476
Gadoxetate disodium	1 ml		**A9581**
Gallium nitrate	1 mg		**J1457**
Galsulfase	1 mg		**J1458**
Gamastan	1 cc	IM	**J1460**
	over 10 cc	IM	**J1560**
Gammagard Liquid	500 mg		**J1569**
Gammagard S/D			J1566
Gamma globulin	1 cc	IM	**J1460**
	over 10 cc	IM	**J1560**
Gammaplex	500 mg		**J1557**
GammaGraft	per square centimeter		Q4111
Gammar	1 cc	IM	**J1460**
	over 10 cc	IM	**J1560**
Gammar-IV, see Immune globin intravenous (human)			
Gamulin RH			
immune globulin			J2791
immune globulin, human	1 dose package, 300 mcg	IM	J2790
immune globulin, human, solvent detergent	100 IU	IV	J2792
Gamunex	500 mg		**J1561**
Ganciclovir, implant	4.5 mg	OTH	**J7310**
Ganciclovir sodium	500 mg	IV	**J1570**
Ganirelix			J3490
Ganite	1 mg		J1457
Garamycin, gentamicin	up to 80 mg	IM, IV	**J1580**
Gastrografin	per ml		Q9963
Gastromark	per 100 ml		Q9954
Gatifloxacin	10 mg	IV	**J1590**
Gefitinib	250 mg		**J8565**
Gel-One per dose			**J7326**
Gemcitabine HCl	200 mg	IV	**J9201**
Gemsar	200 mg	IV	J9201
Gemtuzumab ozogamicin	5 mg	IV	**J9300**
Gengraf	100 mg		J7502
	25 mg	ORAL	J7515
	250 mg		J7516
Gentamicin Sulfate	up to 80 mg	IM, IV	J1580
Gentran	500 ml	IV	J7100

◄ New   ← Revised   ✔ Reinstated   ~~deleted~~ Deleted

DRUG NAME	DOSAGE	METHOD OF ADMINISTRATION	HCPCS CODE
Gentran 75	500 ml	IV	J7110
Gentropin	1 mg		J2941
Geodon	10 mg		J3486
Geref Diagnostic	1 mcg		Q0515
Gesterol 50	per 50 mg		J2675
Glassia	10 mg		J0257
Glatiramer Acetate	20 mg		J1595
GlucaGen	per 1 mg		J1610
Glucagon HCl	per 1 mg	SC, IM, IV	J1610
Glukor	per 1,000 USP units	IM	J0725
Glycopyrrolate			
concentrated form	per 1 mg	INH	J7642
unit dose form	per 1 mg	INH	J7643
Gold sodium thiomalate	up to 50 mg	IM	J1600
Gonadorelin HCl	per 100 mcg	SC, IV	J1620
Gonal-F			J3490
Gonic	per 1,000 USP units	IM	J0725
Goserelin acetate implant	per 3.6 mg	SC	J9202
Graftjacket	per square centimeter		Q4107
Graftjacket express	1 cc		Q4113
Granisetron HCl			
injection	100 mcg	IV	J1626
oral	1 mg	ORAL	Q0166
Gynogen L.A. A10	up to 10 mg	IM	J1380
Gynogen L.A. A20	up to 10 mg	IM	J1380
Gynogen L.A. A40	up to 10 mg	IM	J1380
H			
Halaven, see Eribulin mesylate			
Haldol	up to 5 mg	IM, IV	J1630
Haloperidol	up to 5 mg	IM, IV	J1630
Haloperidol decanoate	per 50 mg	IM	J1631
Haloperidol Lactate	up to 5 mg		J1630
Hectoral	1 mcg	IV	J1270
Helixate FS	per IU		J7192
Hemin	1 mg		J1640
Hemofil M	per IU	IV	J7190
Hemophilia clotting factors (e.g., anti-inhibitors)	per IU	IV	J7198
NOC	per IU	IV	J7199
Hepagam B	0.5 ml	IM	J1571
	0.5 ml	IV	J1573
Hep Flush-10	per 10 units		J1642

◀ New   ← Revised   ✔ Reinstated   deleted Deleted

DRUG NAME	DOSAGE	METHOD OF ADMINISTRATION	HCPCS CODE
Hep-Lock	10 units	IV	J1642
Hep-Lock Flush	per 10 units		J1642
Hep-Lock U/P	10 units	IV	J1642
Heparin Combination	per 10 units		J1642
Heparin Lock Flush	per 10 units		J1642
Heparin (Procine) In D5W	per 1,000 units		J1644
Heparin (Procine) In Nacl	per 10 units		J1642
	per 1,000 units		J1644
Heparin (Procine) Lock Flush	per 10 units		J1642
Heparin sodium	1,000 units	IV, SC	J1644
Heparin Sodium (Bovine)	per 1,000 units		J1644
Heparin Sodium Flush	per 10 units		J1642
Heparin sodium (heparin lock flush)	10 units	IV	J1642
Heparin Sodium (Procine)	per 1,000 units		J1644
Herceptin	10 mg	IV	J9355
Hexabrix 320	per ml		Q9967
Hexadrol Phosphate	1 mg	IM, IV, OTH	J1100
Histaject	per 10 mg	IM, SC, IV	J0945
Histerone 50	up to 50 mg	IM	J3140
Histerone 100	up to 50 mg	IM	J3140
Histrelin			
acetate	10 mcg		J1675
implant	50 mg		J9225
Hizentra, see Immune globulin			
Humalog	per 5 units		J1815
	per 50 units		J1817
Human Albumin Grifols	50 ml		P9047
Human fibrinogen concentrate	100 mg		J1680
Humate-P	per IU		J7187
Humatrope	1 mg		J2941
Humira	20 mg		J0135
Humulin	per 5 units		J1815
	per 50 units		J1817
Hyalgan			J7321
Hyaluronic Acid			J3490
Hyaluronidase	up to 150 units	SC, IV	J3470
Hyaluronidase			
ovine	up to 999 units		J3471
ovine	per 1000 units		J3472
recombinant	1 usp		J3473
Hylutin			J3490

◄ New   ← Revised   ✔ Reinstated   ~~deleted~~ Deleted

DRUG NAME	DOSAGE	METHOD OF ADMINISTRATION	HCPCS CODE
Hyate:C	per IU	IV	J7191
Hybolin Improved, see Nandrolone phenpropionate			
Hybolin Decanoate	up to 50 mg	IM	J2320
Hycamtin	0.25 mg	ORAL	J8705
	4 mg	IV	J9351
Hydralazine HCl	up to 20 mg	IV, IM	J0360
Hydrate	up to 50 mg	IM, IV	J1240
Hydrea			J8999
Hydrocortisone acetate	up to 25 mg	IV, IM, SC	J1700
Hydrocortisone sodium phosphate	up to 50 mg	IV, IM, SC	J1710
Hydrocortisone succinate sodium	up to 100 mg	IV, IM, SC	J1720
Hydrocortone Acetate	up to 25 mg	IV, IM, SC	J1700
Hydrocortone Phosphate	up to 50 mg	IM, IV, SC	J1710
Hydromorphone HCl	up to 4 mg	SC, IM, IV	J1170
Hydroxocobalamin	up to 1,000 mcg		J3420
Hydroxyprogesterone Caproate	1 mg		J1725
Hydroxyurea			J8999
Hydroxyzine HCl	up to 25 mg	IM	J3410
Hydroxyzine Pamoate	25 mg	ORAL	Q0177
	50 mg	ORAL	Q0178
Hylan G-F 20			J7322
Hyoscyamine sulfate	up to 0.25 mg	SC, IM, IV	J1980
Hypaque	per ml		Q9961, Q9963
Hypaque Sodium Oral	per ml		Q9958
Hyperhep B			J3590
Hyperrho S/D	300 mcg		J2790
	100 IU		J2792
Hyper-Sal	10 ml		A4216
Hyperstat IV	up to 300 mg	IV	J1730
Hyper-Tet	up to 250 units	IM	J1670
HypRho-D	300 mcg	IM	J2790
			J2791
	50 mcg		J2788
Hyrexin-50	up to 50 mg	IV, IM	J1200
Hyzine-50	up to 25 mg	IM	J3410
I			
Ibandronate sodium	1 mg		J1740
Ibutilide fumarate	1 mg	IV	J1742
Idamycin	5 mg	IV	J9211
Idarubicin HCl	5 mg	IV	J9211
Idursulfase	1 mg		J1743

◄ New   ← Revised   ✔ Reinstated   ~~deleted~~ Deleted

DRUG NAME	DOSAGE	METHOD OF ADMINISTRATION	HCPCS CODE
Ifex	1 g	IV	J9208
Ifosfamide	1 g	IV	J9208
Ilaris	1 mg		J0638
Iletin	per 5 units		J1815
	per 50 units		J1817
Iloprost	20 mcg		Q4074
Ilotycin, see Erythromycin gluceptate			
Imferon	50 mg		J1750, J1752
Imiglucerase	10 units	IV	J1786
Imitrex	6 mg	SC	J3030
Immune globulin			
Flebogamma	500 mg	IV	J1572
Gammagard Liquid	500 mg	IV	J1569
Gammaplex	500 mg		J1557
Gamunex	500 mg	IV	J1561
HepaGam B	0.5 ml	IM	J1571
	0.5 ml	IV	J1573
Hizentra	100 mg		J1559
NOS	500 mg	IV	J1566, J1599
Octagam	500 mg	IV	J1568
Privigen	500 mg	IV	J1459
Rhophylac	100 IU	IM	J2791
Subcutaneous	100 mg		J1562
Immunosuppressive drug, not otherwise classified			J7599
Imuran	50 mg	ORAL	J7500
	100 mg		J7501
Inapsine	up to 5 mg	IM, IV	J1790
Incobotulinumtoxin type A	1 unit		J0558
Increlex	1 mg		J2170
Inderal	up to 1 mg	IV	J1800
Infed	50 mg		J1750
Infergen	1 mcg	SC	J9212
Infliximab, injection	10 mg	IM, IV	J1745
Innohep	1,000 IU	SC	J1655
Innovar	up to 2 ml ampule	IM, IV	J1810
Insulin	5 units	SC	J1815
Insulin-Humalog	per 50 units		J1817
Insulin lispro	50 units	SC	J1817
Intal	per 10 mg	INH	J7631, J7632
Integrilin	5 mg	IM, IV	J1327
Intera-BMWD	per square centimeter		Q4104

◄ **New**   ← **Revised**   ✔ **Reinstated**   deleted **Deleted**

DRUG NAME	DOSAGE	METHOD OF ADMINISTRATION	HCPCS CODE
Integra			
Bilayer Matrix Wound Dressing (BMWD)	per square centimeter		Q4104
Dermal Regeneration Template (DRT)	per square centimeter		Q4105
Flowable Wound Matrix	1 cc		Q4114
Matrix	per square centimeter		Q4108
Interferon alphacon-1, recombinant	1 mcg	SC	J9212
Interferon alfa-2a, recombinant	3 million units	SC, IM	J9213
Interferon alfa-2b, recombinant	1 million units	SC, IM	J9214
Interferon alfa-n3 (human leukocyte derived)	250,000 IU	IM	J9215
Interferon beta-1a	30 mcg	IM	J1826
	11 mcg	IM	Q3025
	11 mcg	SC	Q3026
Interferon beta-1b	0.25 mg	SC	J1830
Interferon gamma-1b	3 million units	SC	J9216
Intrauterine copper contraceptive		OTH	J7300
Intron-A	1 million units		J9214
Invanz	500 mg		J1335
Invega Sustenna	1 mg		J2426
Ipilimumab	1 mg		J9228
Ipratropium bromide, unit dose form	per mg	INH	J7620, J7644, J7645, J3535
Iressa	250 mg	ORAL	J8565
Irinotecan	20 mg	IV	J9206
Iron dextran	50 mg	IV, IM	J1750
Iron sucrose	1 mg	IV	J1756
Irrigation solution for Tx of bladder calculi	per 50 ml	OTH	Q2004
Isocaine HCl	per 10 ml	VAR	J0670
Isoetharine HCl			
concentrated form	per mg	INH	J7647, J7648
unit dose form	per mg	INH	J7649, J7650
Isoproterenol HCl			
concentrated form	per mg	INH	J7657, J7658
unit dose form	per mg	INH	J7659, J7660
Isovue-200	per ml		Q9966
Isovue-250	per ml		Q9966
Isovue-300	per ml		Q9967
Isovue-370	per ml		Q9967
Istodax	1 mg		J9315
Isuprel			
concentrated form	per mg	INH	J7657, J7658
unit dose form	per mg	INH	J7659, J7660

◄ New   ← Revised   ✔ Reinstated   ~~deleted~~ Deleted

DRUG NAME	DOSAGE	METHOD OF ADMINISTRATION	HCPCS CODE
Itraconazole	50 mg	IV	J1835
Ixabepilone	1 mg		J9207
Ixempra	1 mg		J9207
J			
Jenamicin	up to 80 mg	IM, IV	J1580
Jevtana	1 mg		J9043
K			
Kabikinase	per 250,000 IU	IV	J2995
Kalbitor	1 mg		J1290
Kaleinate	per 10 ml	IV	J0610
Kanamycin sulfate	up to 75 mg	IM, IV	J1850
	up to 500 mg	IM, IV	J1840
Kantrex	up to 75 mg	IM, IV	J1850
	up to 500 mg	IM, IV	J1840
Kay-Pred 25	up to 1 ml		J2650
Keflin	up to 1 g	IM, IV	J1890
Kefurox	per 750 mg		J0697
Kefzol	500 mg	IV, IM	J0690
Kenaject-40	per 10 mg	IM	J3301
	1 mg		J3300
Kenalog-10	per 10 mg	IM	J3301
	1 mg		J3300
Kenalog-40	per 10 mg	IM	J3301
	1 mg		J3300
Kepivance	50 mcg		J2425
Keppra	10 mg		J1953
Kestrone 5	per 1 mg	IM	J1435
Ketorolac tromethamine	per 15 mg	IM, IV	J1885
Key-Pred 25	up to 1 ml	IM	J2650
Key-Pred 50	up to 1 ml	IM	J2650
Key-Pred-SP, see Prednisolone sodium phosphate			
K-Flex	up to 60 mg	IV, IM	J2360
Kineret			J3490
Kinlytic	250,000 IU		J3365
Klebcil	up to 75 mg	IM, IV	J1850
	up to 500 mg	IM, IV	J1840
Koate-HP (anti-hemophilic factor)			
human	per IU	IV	J7190
porcine	per IU	IV	J7191
recombinant	per IU	IV	J7192

◄ New   ← Revised   ✔ Reinstated   ~~deleted~~ Deleted

DRUG NAME	DOSAGE	METHOD OF ADMINISTRATION	HCPCS CODE
Kogenate			
human	per IU	IV	**J7190**
porcine	per IU	IV	**J7191**
recombinant	per IU	IV	**J7192**
FS	per IU		J7192
Konakion	per 1 mg	IM, SC, IV	J3430
Konyne-80	per IU	IV	J7194, J7195
Krystexxa	1 mg		J2507
Kytril	1 mg	ORAL	Q0166
	1 mg	IV	S0091
	100 mcg	IV	J1626
L			
Lactated Ringers	up to 1,000 cc		J7120
L.A.E. 20	up to 10 mg	IM	J1380
Laetrile, Amygdalin, vitamin B-17			**J3570**
Lanoxin	up to 0.5 mg	IM, IV	J1160
Lanreotide	1 mg		**J1930**
Lantus	per 5 units		J1815
	per 50 units		J1817
Largon, see Propiomazine HCl			
Laronidase	0.1 mg		**J1931**
Lasix	up to 20 mg	IM, IV	J1940
L-Caine	10 mg	IV	J2001
L-Carnitine	per 1 gm		J1955
Lepirudin	50 mg		**J1945**
Leucovorin calcium	per 50 mg	IM, IV	J0640
Leukeran			J8999
Leukine	50 mcg	IV	J2820
Leuprolide acetate (for depot suspension)	per 3.75 mg	IM	**J1950**
	7.5 mg	IM	**J9217**
Leuprolide acetate	per 1 mg	IM	**J9218**
Leuprolide acetate implant	65 mg		**J9219**
Leustatin	per mg	IV	J9065
Levalbuterol HCl			
concentrated form	0.5 mg	INH	**J7607, J7612**
unit dose form	0.5 mg	INH	**J7614, J7615**
Levaquin I.U.	250 mg	IV	J1956
Levetiracetam	10 mg		**J1953**
Levocarnitine	per 1 gm	IV	**J1955**
Levo-Dromoran	up to 2 mg	SC, IV	J1960

◀ New   ← Revised   ✔ Reinstated   ~~deleted~~ Deleted

DRUG NAME	DOSAGE	METHOD OF ADMINISTRATION	HCPCS CODE
Levofloxacin	250 mg	IV	**J1956**
Levoleucovorin calcium	0.5 mg		**J0641**
Levonorgestrel implant			**J7306**
Levonorgestrel-releasing intrauterine contraceptive system	52 mg	OTH	**J7302**
Levorphanol tartrate	up to 2 mg	SC, IV	**J1960**
Levsin	up to 0.25 mg	SC, IM, IV	J1980
Levulan Kerastick	unit dose (354 mg)	OTH	J7308
Lexiscan	0.1 mg		J2785
Librium	up to 100 mg	IM, IV	J1990
Lidocaine HCl	10 mg	IV	**J2001**
Lidoject-1	10 mg	IV	J2001
Lidoject-2	10 mg	IV	J2001
Lincocin	up to 300 mg	IV	J2010
Lincomycin HCl	up to 300 mg	IV	**J2010**
Linezolid	200 mg	IV	**J2020**
Liquaemin Sodium	1,000 units	IV, SC	J1644
Liquid Pred	5 mg		J7506
Lioresal	10 mg	IT	J0475
			J0476
Lispro	per 5 units		J1815
LMD (10%)	500 ml	IV	J7100
Lovenox	10 mg	SC	J1650
Lorazepam	2 mg	IM, IV	**J2060**
Lucentis	0.1 mg		J2778
Lufyllin	up to 500 mg	IM	J1180
Luminal	up to 120 mg		J2560
Luminal Sodium	up to 120 mg	IM, IV	J2560
Lumizyme	10 mg		J0220, J0221
Lunelle	5 mg/25 mg	IM	J1056
Lupon Depot	7.5 mg		J9217
Lupon Depot-Ped	7.5 mg		J9216
Lupron	per 1 mg	IM	J9218
	per 3.75 mg	IM	J1950
	7.5 mg	IM	J9217
Lymphocyte immune globulin			
anti-thymocyte globulin, equine	250 mg	IV	**J7504**
anti-thymocyte globulin, rabbit	25 mg	IV	**J7511**
Lyophilized			J1566
M			
Macugen	0.3 mg		J2503
Magnesium sulfate	500 mg		**J3475**
Magnevist	per ml		A9579

◀ New   ← Revised   ✔ Reinstated   ~~deleted~~ Deleted

DRUG NAME	DOSAGE	METHOD OF ADMINISTRATION	HCPCS CODE	
Makena	1 mg		J1725	◄
Malulane			J8999	
Mannitol	25% in 50 ml	IV	J2150	
	5 mg	INH	J7665	◄
Marcaine			J3490	
Marinol	2.5 mg	ORAL	Q0167	
	5 mg	ORAL	Q0168	
Marmine	up to 50 mg	IM, IV	J1240	
Maxipime	500 mg	IV	J0692	
MD-76R	per ml		Q9963	
MD Gastroview	per ml		Q9963	
Mecasermin	1 mg		J2170	
Mechlorethamine HCl (nitrogen mustard), HN2	10 mg	IV	J9230	
Medralone 40	20 mg	IM	J1020	
	40 mg	IM	J1030	
	80 mg	IM	J1040	
Medralone 80	20 mg	IM	J1020	
	40 mg	IM	J1030	
	80 mg	IM	J1040	
Medrol	per 4 mg	ORAL	J7509	
Medroxyprogesterone acetate	50 mg	IM	J1051	
	150 mg	IM	J1055	
Medroxyprogesterone acetate/estradiol cypionate	5 mg/25 mg	IM	J1056	
Mefoxin	1 g	IV, IM	J0694	
Megace			J8999	
Megestrol Acetate			J8999	
Melphalan HCl	50 mg	IV	J9245	
Melphalan, oral	2 mg	ORAL	J8600	
Menoject LA	up to 1 ml	IM	J1060	
Mepergan Injection	up to 50 mg	IM, IV	J2180	
Meperidine HCl	per 100 mg	IM, IV, SC	J2175	
Meperidine and promethazine HCl	up to 50 mg	IM, IV	J2180	
Mepivacaine HCl	per 10 ml	VAR	J0670	
Mercaptopurine			J8999	
Meropenem	100 mg		J2185	
Merrem	100 mg		J2185	
Mesna	200 mg	IV	J9209	
Mesnex	200 mg	IV	J9209	
Metaprel				
concentrated form	per 10 mg	INH	J7667, J7668	
unit dose form	per 10 mg	INH	J7669, J7670	

◄ New   ← Revised   ✔ Reinstated   ~~deleted~~ Deleted

DRUG NAME	DOSAGE	METHOD OF ADMINISTRATION	HCPCS CODE
Metaproterenol sulfate			
concentrated form	per 10 mg	INH	**J7667, J7668**
unit dose form	per 10 mg	INH	**J7669, J7670**
Metaraminol bitartrate	per 10 mg	IV, IM, SC	**J0380**
Metastron	per millicurie		A9600
Methacholine chloride	1 mg		**J7674**
Methadone HCl	up to 10 mg	IM, SC	**J1230**
Methergine, see Methylergonovine maleate			
Methocarbamol	up to 10 ml	IV, IM	**J2800**
Methotrexate, oral	2.5 mg	ORAL	**J8610**
Methotrexate sodium	5 mg	IV, IM, IT, IA	**J9250**
	50 mg	IV, IM, IT, IA	**J9260**
Methotrexate LPF	5 mg	IV, IM, IT, IA	J9250
	50 mg	IV, IM, IT, IA	J9260
Methyldopate HCl	up to 250 mg	IV	**J0210**
Methylpred	20 mg		J1020
Methylpred DP	per 4 mg		J7509
Methylprednisolone	40 mg		J1030
Methylprednisolone, oral	per 4 mg	ORAL	**J7509**
Methylprednisolone acetate	20 mg	IM	**J1020**
	40 mg	IM	**J1030**
	80 mg	IM	**J1040**
Methylprednisolone sodium succinate	up to 40 mg	IM, IV	**J2920**
	up to 125 mg	IM, IV	**J2930**
Metoclopramide HCl	up to 10 mg	IV	**J2765**
Metrodin	75 IU		J3355
Metronidazole			J3490
Metvixia, see Aminolevulinate			
Miacalcin	up to 400 units	SC, IM	J0630
Micafungin sodium	1 mg		**J2248**
MicRhoGAM	50 mcg		J2788
Midazolam HCl	per 1 mg	IM, IV	**J2250**
Millipred		ORAL	J8499
Milrinone lactate	5 mg	IV	**J2260**
Minocine	1 mg		J2265
Minocycline Hydrochloride	1 mg		**J2265**
Mio-Rel	up to 60 mg		J2360
Mirena	52 mg	OTH	J7302
Mithracin	2,500 mcg	IV	J9270
Mitomycin	5 mg	IV	**J9280**
Mitoxantrone HCl	per 5 mg	IV	**J9293**
Monocid, see Cefonicic sodium			

◀ New   ← Revised   ✔ Reinstated   ~~deleted~~ Deleted

DRUG NAME	DOSAGE	METHOD OF ADMINISTRATION	HCPCS CODE
Monoclate-P			
human	per IU	IV	J7190
porcine	per IU	IV	J7191
recombinant	per IU	IV	J7192
Monoclonal antibodies, parenteral	5 mg	IV	**J7505**
Monoject Prefill Advanced	10 ml		A4216
Mononine	per IU	IV	J7193
Morphine sulfate	up to 10 mg	IM, IV, SC	**J2270**
	100 mg	IM, IV, SC	**J2271**
preservative-free	per 10 mg	SC, IM, IV	**J2275**
Moxifloxacin	100 mg		**J2280**
Mozobil	1 mg		J2562
M-Prednisol-40	20 mg	IM	J1020
	40 mg	IM	J1030
	80 mg	IM	J1040
M-Prednisol-80	20 mg	IM	J1020
	40 mg	IM	J1030
	80 mg	IM	J1040
Mucomyst			
unit dose form	per gram	INH	J7604, J7608
Mucosol			
injection	100 mg		J0132
unit dose	per gram	INH	J7604, J7608
Muromonab-CD3	5 mg	IV	**J7505**
Muse		OTH	J0275
	1.25 mcg	OTH	J0270
Mustargen	10 mg	IV	J9230
Mutamycin	5 mg	IV	J9280
Mycamine	1 mg		J2248
Mycophenolic acid	180 mg		**J7518**
Mycophenolate Mofetil	250 mg	ORAL	**J7517**
Myfortic	180 mg		J7518
Myleran	1 mg		J0594
	2 mg	ORAL	J8510
Mylotarg	5 mg	IV	J9300
Myobloc	per 100 units	IM	J0587
Myochrysine	up to 50 mg	IM	J1600
Myolin	up to 60 mg	IV, IM	J2360
Myozyme	10 mg		J0220
N			
Nabi-HB			J3590
Nabilone	1 mg	ORAL	**J8650**

◄ **New**   ← **Revised**   ✔ **Reinstated**   ~~deleted~~ **Deleted**

DRUG NAME	DOSAGE	METHOD OF ADMINISTRATION	HCPCS CODE
N-acetyl-L-cysteine	per gram		J7604
Nafcillin			J3490
Naglazyme	1 mg		J1458
Nalbuphine HCl	per 10 mg	IM, IV, SC	J2300
Naloxone HCl	per 1 mg	IM, IV, SC	J2310, J3490
Naltrexone			J3490
Naltrexone, depot form	1 mg		J2315
Nandrobolic L.A.	up to 50 mg	IM	J2320
Nandrolone decanoate	up to 50 mg	IM	J2320
Narcan	1 mg	IM, IV, SC	J2310
Naropin	1 mg		J2795
Nasahist B	per 10 mg	IM, SC, IV	J0945
Nasal vaccine inhalation		INH	J3530
Natalizumab	1 mg		J2323
Natrecor	0.1 mg		J2325
Navane, see Thiothixene			
Navelbine	per 10 mg	IV	J9390
ND Stat	per 10 mg	IM, SC, IV	J0945
Nebcin	up to 80 mg	IM, IV	J3260
	per 300 mg		J7682
NebuPent	per 300 mg	INH	J2545, J7676
	300 mg	IM, IV	S0080
inhalation solution			J7699
Nelarabine	50 mg	IV	J9261
Nembutal Sodium Solution	per 50 mg	IM, IV, OTH	J2515
Neocyten	up to 60 mg	IV, IM	J2360
Neo-Durabolic	up to 50 mg	IM	J2320
Neoral	100 mg		J7502
	25 mg		J7515
Neoquess	up to 20 mg	IM	J0500
Neosar	100 mg	IV	J9070
Neostigmine methylsulfate	up to 0.5 mg	IM, IV, SC	J2710
Neo-Synephrine	up to 1 ml	SC, IM, IV	J2370
Nervidox-6 S	up to 1,000 mcg		J3420
Nervocaine 1%	10 mg	IV	J2001
Nervocaine 2%	10 mg	IV	J2001
Nesacaine	per 30 ml	VAR	J2400
Nesacaine-MPF	per 30 ml	VAR	J2400
Nesiritide	0.1 mg		J2325
Neulasta	6 mg		J2505
Neumega	5 mg	SC	J2355

◄ New   ← Revised   ✔ Reinstated   ~~deleted~~ Deleted

DRUG NAME	DOSAGE	METHOD OF ADMINISTRATION	HCPCS CODE
Neupogen	300 mcg	SC, IV	J1440
	480 mcg	SC, IV	J1441
Neuroforte-R	up to 1,000 mcg		J3420
Neutrexin	per 25 mg	IV	J3305
Nipent	per 10 mg	IV	J9268
Nolvadex			J8999
Nordiflex	1 mg		J2941
Norditropin	1 mg		J2941
Nordryl	up to 50 mg	IV, IM	J1200
	50 mg	ORAL	Q0163
Norflex	up to 60 mg	IV, IM	J2360
Norzine			
injection	up to 10 mg	IM	J3280
oral	10 mg	ORAL	Q0174
Not otherwise classified drugs			J3490
other than inhalation solution administered thru DME			J7799
inhalation solution administered thru DME			J7699
anti-neoplastic			J9999
chemotherapeutic		ORAL	J8999
immunosuppressive			J7599
nonchemotherapeutic		ORAL	J8499
Novantrone	per 5 mg	IV	J9293
Novarel	per 1,000 USP Units		J0725
Novolin	per 5 units		J1815
	per 50 units		J1817
Novolog	per 5 units		J1815
	per 50 units		J1817
Novo Seven	1 mcg	IV	J7189
NPH	5 units	SC	J1815
Nplate	100 units		J0587
	10 mcg		J2796
Nubain	per 10 mg	IM, IV, SC	J2300
Nulicaine	10 mg	IV	J2001
Numorphan	up to 1 mg	IV, SC, IM	J2410
Numorphan H.P.	up to 1 mg	IV, SC, IM	J2410
Nutropin	1 mg		J2941
O			
Oasis Burn Matrix	per square centimeter		Q4103
Oasis Wound Matrix	per square centimeter		Q4102
Octagam	500 mg		J1568
Octreotide Acetate, injection	1 mg	IM	J2353
	25 mcg	IV, SQ	J2354

◀ New   ← Revised   ✔ Reinstated   ~~deleted~~ Deleted

DRUG NAME	DOSAGE	METHOD OF ADMINISTRATION	HCPCS CODE
Oculinum	per unit	IM	J0585
Ofatumumab	10 mg		J9302
Ofirmev	10 mg		J0131
O-Flex	up to 60 mg	IV, IM	J2360
Oforta	10 mg		J8562
Olanzapine	1 mg		J2358
Omalizumab	5 mg		J2357
Omnipaque	per ml		Q9965, Q9967
Omnipen-N	up to 500 mg	IM, IV	J0290
	per 1.5 gm	IM, IV	J0295
Omniscan	per ml		A9579
Omnitrope	1 mg		J2941
OnabotulinumtoxinA	1 unit		J0585
Oncaspar	per single dose vial	IM, IV	J9266
Oncovin	1 mg	IV	J9370
Ondansetron HCl	1 mg	IV	J2405
	1 mg	ORAL	Q0162
Ontak	300 mcg		J9160
Onxol	30 mg		J9265
Opana	up to 1 mg		J2410
Oprelvekin	5 mg	SC	J2355
Optimark	per ml		A9579
Optiray 300	per ml		Q9967
Optiray 320	per ml		Q9967
Optiray 350	per ml		Q9967
Optison	per ml		Q9956
Oraminic II	per 10 mg	IM, SC, IV	J0945
Orfro	up to 60 mg		J2360
Ormazine	10 mg	ORAL	Q0171
	25 mg	ORAL	Q0172
	up to 50 mg	IM, IV	J3230
Orphenadrine citrate	up to 60 mg	IV, IM	J2360
Orphenate	up to 60 mg	IV, IM	J2360
Orencia	10 mg		J0129
Orthoclone OKT3	5 mg		J7505
Orthovisc			J7324
Or-Tyl	up to 20 mg	IM	J0500
Osmitrol			J7799
Ovidrel			J3490
Oxacillin sodium	up to 250 mg	IM, IV	J2700
Oxaliplatin	0.5 mg		J9263

◀ New   ← Revised   ✔ Reinstated   ~~deleted~~ Deleted

DRUG NAME	DOSAGE	METHOD OF ADMINISTRATION	HCPCS CODE
Oxilan 300	per ml		Q9967
Oxilan 350	per ml		Q9967
Oxymorphone HCl	up to 1 mg	IV, SC, IM	J2410
Oxytetracycline HCl	up to 50 mg	IM	J2460
Oxytocin	up to 10 units	IV, IM	J2590
Ozurdex	0.1 mg		J7312
P			
Paclitaxel	30 mg	IV	J9265
Paclitaxel protein-bound particles	1 mg		J9264
Palifermin	50 mcg		J2425
Paliperidone Palmitate	1 mg		J2426
Palonosetron HCl	25 mcg		J2469
Pamidronate disodium	per 30 mg	IV	J2430
Panglobulin NF	500 mg		J1566
Panhematin	1 mg		J1640
Panitumumab	10 mg		J9303
Papaverine HCl	up to 60 mg	IV, IM	J2440
Paragard T 380 A		OTH	J7300
Paraplatin	50 mg	IV	J9045
Paricalcitol, injection	1 mcg	IV, IM	J2501
Pegademase bovine	25 IU		J2504
Pegaptinib	0.3 mg		J2503
Pegaspargase	per single dose vial	IM, IV	J9266
Pegasys			J3490
Pegfilgrastim	6 mg		J2505
Peg-Intron			J3490
Pegloticase	1 mg		J2507
Pemetrexed	10 mg		J9305
Penicillin G benzathine	up to 100,000 units	IM	J0561
Penicillin G benzathine and penicillin G procaine	100,000 units	IM	J0558
Penicillin G potassium	up to 600,000 units	IM, IV	J2540
Penicillin G procaine, aqueous	up to 600,000 units	IM, IV	J2510
Penicillin G Sodium			J3490
Pentam	per 300 mg		J7676
Pentamidine isethionate	per 300 mg	INH	J2545, J7676
Pentastarch, 10%	100 ml		J2513
Pentazocine HCl	30 mg	IM, SC, IV	J3070
Pentobarbital sodium	per 50 mg	IM, IV, OTH	J2515
Pentostatin	per 10 mg	IV	J9268
Peforomist	20 mcg		J7606
Permapen	up to 600,000	IM	J0561

◀ New   ← Revised   ✔ Reinstated   ~~deleted~~ Deleted

DRUG NAME	DOSAGE	METHOD OF ADMINISTRATION	HCPCS CODE
Perphenazine			
injection	up to 5 mg	IM, IV	**J3310**
tablets	4 mg	ORAL	**Q0175**
	8 mg	ORAL	**Q0176**
Persantine IV	per 10 mg	IV	J1245
Pfizerpen	up to 600,000 units	IM, IV	J2540
Pfizerpen A.S.	up to 600,000 units	IM, IV	J2510
Phenadoz			J8498
Phenazine 25	up to 50 mg	IM, IV	J2550
	12.5 mg	ORAL	Q0169
	25 mg	ORAL	Q0170
Phenazine 50	up to 50 mg	IM, IV	J2550
	12.5 mg	ORAL	Q0169
	25 mg	ORAL	Q0170
Phenergan	12.5 mg	ORAL	Q0169
	25 mg	ORAL	Q0170
	up to 50 mg	IM, IV	J2550, J8498
Phenobarbital sodium	up to 120 mg	IM, IV	**J2560**
Phentolamine mesylate	up to 5 mg	IM, IV	**J2760**
Phenylephrine HCl	up to 1 ml	SC, IM, IV	**J2370**
Phenylephrine HCl, other			J7799
Phenytoin sodium	per 50 mg	IM, IV	**J1165**
Photofrin	75 mg	IV	J9600
Phytonadione (Vitamin K)	per 1 mg	IM, SC, IV	**J3430**
Piperacillin/Tazobactam Sodium, injection	1.125 g	IV	**J2543, J3490**
Pitocin	up to 10 units	IV, IM	J2590
Plantinol AQ	10 mg	IV	J9060
Plas+SD	each unit	IV	P9023
Plasma			
cryoprecipitate reduced	each unit		**P9044**
pooled multiple donor, frozen	each unit	IV	**P9023**
Plasbumin	20 ml		P9046
Plasbumin-5	50 ml		P9041
	250 ml		P9045
Plasbumin-25	20 ml		P9046
	50 ml		P9047
Plasmanate	50 ml		P9043, P9047
Plerixafor	1 mg		**J2562**
Plicamycin	2,500 mcg	IV	**J9270**
Polocaine	per 10 ml	VAR	J0670
Poly Bio-Set	per IU		J7192

◀ New   ← Revised   ✔ Reinstated   ~~deleted~~ Deleted

DRUG NAME	DOSAGE	METHOD OF ADMINISTRATION	HCPCS CODE
Polycillin-N	up to 500 mg	IM, IV	J0290
	per 1.5 gm	IM, IV	J0295
Porfimer Sodium	75 mg	IV	J9600
Potassium chloride	per 2 mEq	IV	J3480
Pralatrexate	1 mg		J9307
Pralidoxime chloride	up to 1 g	IV, IM, SC	J2730
Predalone-50	up to 1 ml	IM	J2650
Predcor-25	up to 1 ml	IM	J2650
Predcor-50	up to 1 ml	IM	J2650
Predicort-50	up to 1 ml	IM	J2650
Prelone	5 mg		J7510
Prednicot	5 mg		J7506, J7510
Prednisone	per 5 mg	ORAL	J7506
Prednisolone, oral	5 mg	ORAL	J7510
Prednisolone acetate	up to 1 ml	IM	J2650
Predoject-50	up to 1 ml	IM	J2650
Pregnyl	per 1,000 USP units	IM	J0725
Premarin Intravenous	per 25 mg	IV, IM	J1410
Prescription, chemotherapeutic, not otherwise specified		ORAL	J8999
Prescription, nonchemotherapeutic, not otherwise specified		ORAL	J8499
Prialt	1 mcg		J2278
Primacor	5 mg	IV	J2260
Primatrix	per square centimeter		Q4110
Primaxin	per 250 mg	IV, IM	J0743
Priscoline HCl	up to 25 mg	IV	J2670
Privigen	500 mg		J1459
Pro-Depo, see Hydroxyprogesterone Caproate			
Procainamide HCl	up to 1 g	IM, IV	J2690
Prochlorperazine	up to 10 mg	IM, IV	J0780
			J8498
Prochlorperazine maleate	5 mg	ORAL	Q0164
	10 mg	ORAL	Q0165
			S0183
Procrit			J0885
			J0886
			Q4081
			J3490
Prodrox			
Profasi HP	per 1,000 USP units	IM	J0725
Profilnine Heat-Treated			
non-recombinant	per IU	IV	J7193
recombinant	per IU	IV	J7195
complex	per IU	IV	J7194

◄ New   ← Revised   ✔ Reinstated   ~~deleted~~ Deleted

DRUG NAME	DOSAGE	METHOD OF ADMINISTRATION	HCPCS CODE
Profilnine-SD	per IU		**J7193, J7194, J7195**
Progestaject	per 50 mg		J2675
Progesterone	per 50 mg		**J2675**
Prograf			
oral	per 1 mg	ORAL	J7507
parenteral	5 mg		J7525
Prokine	50 mcg	IV	J2820
Prolastin	10 mg	IV	J0256
Prolastin-C	10 mg		J0256
Proleukin	per single use vial	IM, IV	J9015
Prolixin Decanoate, see Fluphenazine decanoate			
	25 mg	IM, SC	J2680
Promazine HCl	up to 25 mg	IM	**J2950**
Promethazine			J8498
Promethazine HCl			
injection	up to 50 mg	IM, IV	**J2550**
oral	12.5 mg	ORAL	**Q0169**
oral	25 mg	ORAL	**Q0170**
Promethegan			J8498
Pronestyl	up to 1 g	IM, IV	J2690
Proplex T			
non-recombinant	per IU	IV	**J7193**
recombinant	per IU	IV	**J7195**
complex	per IU	IV	**J7194**
Proplex SX-T			
non-recombinant	per IU	IV	**J7193**
recombinant	per IU	IV	**J7195**
complex	per IU	IV	**J7194**
Propofol			J3490
Propranolol HCl	up to 1 mg	IV	**J1800**
Prorex-25			
	up to 50 mg	IM, IV	J2550
	12.5 mg	ORAL	Q0169
	25 mg	ORAL	Q0170
Prorex-50			
	up to 50 mg	IM, IV	J2550
	12.5 mg	ORAL	Q0169
	25 mg	ORAL	Q0170
Prostaphlin	up to 1 g	IM, IV	J2690
Prostigmin	up to 0.5 mg	IM, IV, SC	J2710
Protamine sulfate	per 10 mg	IV	**J2720**

◀ **New**   ← **Revised**   ✔ **Reinstated**   ~~deleted~~ **Deleted**

DRUG NAME	DOSAGE	METHOD OF ADMINISTRATION	HCPCS CODE
Protein C Concentrate	10 IU		**J2724**
Protirelin	per 250 mcg	IV	**J2725**
Prothazine	up to 50 mg	IM, IV	J2550
	12.5 mg	ORAL	Q0169
	25 mg	ORAL	Q0170
Protonix			J3490
Protopam Chloride	up to 1 g	IV, IM, SC	J2730
Proventil			
concentrated form	1 mg	INH	J7610, J7611
unit dose form	1 mg	INH	J7609, J7613
Provocholine	per 1 mg		J7674
Prozine-50	up to 25 mg	IM	J2950
Pulmicort	0.25 mg	INH	J7633
	up to 0.5 mg		J7626
Pulmicort Respules	0.5 mg	INH	J7627, J7626
	per 0.25 mg		J7633
	up to 0.5 mg		J7626
noncompounded, concentrated	0.25 mg	INH	J7626
Pulmozyme	per mg		J7639
Purinethol	50 mg		J8999
Pyridoxine HCl	100 mg		**J3415**
Q			
Quelicin	up to 20 mg	IV, IM	J0330
Quinupristin/dalfopristin	500 mg (150/350)	IV	**J2770**
Qutenza	per 10 square cm		J7335
R			
Ranibizumab	0.1 mg		**J2778**
Ranitidine HCl, injection	25 mg	IV, IM	**J2780**
Rapamune	1 mg	ORAL	J7520
Rasburicase	0.5 mg		**J2783**
Rebetron Kit	1 million units		J9214
Rebif	11 mcg		Q3026
Reclast	1 mg		**J3488**
Recombinate (anti-hemophilic factor)			
human	per IU	IV	J7190
porcine	per IU	IV	J7191
recombinant	per IU	IV	J7192
Recombivax			J3490
Redisol	up to 1,000 mcg	IM, SC	J3420
Regadenoson	0.1 mg		**J2785**
Refacto	per IU		J7192
Refludan	50 mg		J1945

◄ New   ← Revised   ✔ Reinstated   ~~deleted~~ Deleted

DRUG NAME	DOSAGE	METHOD OF ADMINISTRATION	HCPCS CODE
Regitine	up to 5 mg	IM, IV	J2760
Reglan	up to 10 mg	IV	J2765
Regular	5 units	SC	J1815
Relefact TRH	per 250 mcg	IV	J2725
Relion	per 5 units		J1815
	per 50 units		J1817
Remicade	10 mg	IM, IV	J1745
Remodulin	1 mg		J3285
Reno-30	per ml		Q9958
Reno-60	per ml		Q9961
Reno-Dip	per ml		Q9958
Renocal-76	per ml		Q9963
Renografin-60	per ml		Q9961
Reno-M60	per ml		Q9961
ReoPro	10 mg	IV	J0130
Rep-Pred 40	20 mg	IM	J1020
	40 mg	IM	J1030
	80 mg	IM	J1040
Rep-Pred 80	20 mg	IM	J1020
	40 mg	IM	J1030
	80 mg	IM	J1040
Resectisol			J7799
Restall	up to 25 mg		J3410
Retavase	18.1 mg	IV	J2993
Reteplase	18.1 mg	IV	J2993
Retisert			J7311
Retrovir	10 mg	IV	J3485
Rheomacrodex	500 ml	IV	J7100
Rhesonativ	1 dose package/ 300 mcg	IM	J2790
	50 mg		J2788
Rheumatrex Dose Pack	2.5 mg	ORAL	J8610
Rho(D)			
immune globulin			J2791
immune globulin, human	1 dose package/ 300 mcg	IM	J2790
	50 mg		J2788
immune globulin, human, solvent detergent	100	IU, IV	J2792
RhoGAM	1 dose package, 300 mcg	IM	J2790
	50 mg		J2788
Rhophylac	100 IU		J2791

◄ New   ← Revised   ✔ Reinstated   ~~deleted~~ Deleted

DRUG NAME	DOSAGE	METHOD OF ADMINISTRATION	HCPCS CODE
Riastap	100 mg		J1680
Rifadin			J3490
Rifampin			J3490
Rilonacept	1 mg		J2793
RimabotulinumtoxinB	100 units		J0587
Rimso-50	50 ml		J1212
Ringers lactate infusion	up to 1,000 cc	IV	J7120
Risperdal Costa	0.5 mg		J2794
Risperidone	0.5 mg		J2794
Rituxan	100 mg	IV	J9310
Rituximab	100 mg	IV	J9310
Robaxin	up to 10 ml	IV, IM	J2800
Robinul	per mg		J7643
Rocephin	per 250 mg	IV, IM	J0696
Rodex	100 mg		J3415
Roferon-A	3 million units	SC, IM	J9213
Romidepsin	1 mg		J9315
Romiplostim	10 mcg		J2796
Ropivacaine Hydrochloride	1 mg		J2795
Rubex	10 mg	IV	J9000
Rubramin PC	up to 1,000 mcg	IM, SC	J3420
S			
Saizen	1 mg		J2941
Saline solution	10 ml		A4216
5% dextrose	500 ml	IV	J7042
infusion	250 cc	IV	J7050
	1,000 cc	IV	J7030
sterile	500 ml = 1 unit	IV, OTH	J7040
Sandimmune	25 mg	ORAL	J7515
	100 mg	ORAL	J7502
	250 mg	OTH	J7516
Sandoglobulin, see Immune globin intravenous (human)			
Sandostatin, Lar Depot	25 mcg		J2354
	1 mg	IM	J2353
Sargramostim (GM-CSF)	50 mcg	IV	J2820
Selestoject	per 4 mg	IM, IV	J0702
Sensorcaine MPF			J3490
Sermorelin acetate	1 mcg		Q0515
Serostim	1 mg		J2941
Simulect	20 mg		J0480
Sincalide	5 mcg		J2805
Sinografin	per ml		Q9963

◄ New   ← Revised   ✔ Reinstated   ~~deleted~~ Deleted

DRUG NAME	DOSAGE	METHOD OF ADMINISTRATION	HCPCS CODE
Sinusol-B	per 10 mg	IM, SC, IV	J0945
Sirolimus	1 mg	ORAL	**J7520**
Smz-TMP			J3490
Sodium Chloride	1,000 cc		J7030
	10 ml		A4216
	500 ml = 1 unit		J7040
	500 ml		A4217
	250 cc		J7050
inhalation solution			J7699
Sodium Chloride Bacteriostatic	10 ml		A4216
Sodium Chloride Concentrate			J7799
Sodium ferricgluconate in sucrose	12.5 mg		**J2916**
Sodium Hyaluronate			J3490
Euflexxa			**J7323**
Hyalgan			**J7321**
Orthovisc			**J7324**
Supartz			**J7321**
Solganal	up to 50 mg	IM	J2910
Soliris	10 mg		J1300
Solu-Cortef	up to 50 mg	IV, IM, SC	J1710
	100 mg		J1720
Solu-Medrol	up to 40 mg	IM, IV	J2920
	up to 125 mg	IM, IV	J2930
Solurex	1 mg	IM, IV, OTH	J1100
Solurex LA	1 mg	IM	J1094
Somatrem	1 mg		**J2940**
Somatropin	1 mg		**J2941**
Somatulin Depot	1 mg		J1930
Sparine	up to 25 mg	IM	J2950
Spasmoject	up to 20 mg	IM	J0500
Spectinomycin HCl	up to 2 g	IM	**J3320**
Sporanox	50 mg	IV	J1835
Stadol	1 mg		J0595
Staphcillin, see Methicillin sodium			
Stelara, see Ustekinumab			
Sterapred	5 mg		J7506
Stilphostrol	250 mg	IV	J9165
Streptase	250,000 IU	IV	J2995
Streptokinase	per 250,000	IU, IV	**J2995**
Streptomycin Sulfate	up to 1 g	IM	J3000
Streptomycin	up to 1 g	IM	**J3000**
Streptozocin	1 gm	IV	**J9320**

◄ New   ← Revised   ✔ Reinstated   ~~deleted~~ Deleted

DRUG NAME	DOSAGE	METHOD OF ADMINISTRATION	HCPCS CODE
Strontium-89 chloride	per millicurie		A9600
Sublimaze	0.1 mg	IM, IV	J3010
Succinylcholine chloride	up to 20 mg	IV, IM	J0330
Sufenta			J3490
Sufentanil Citrate			J3490
Sumarel Dosepro	6 mg		J3030
Sumatriptan succinate	6 mg	SC	J3030
Supartz			J7321
SurgiMend Inguinal Fenestrated Oval			C9358
SurgiMend Inguinal Rectangle			C9358
SurgiMend Strip			C9358
SurgiMend Thick			C9358
SurgiMend Thin			C9358
Surostrin	up to 20 mg	IV, IM	J0330
Sus-Phrine	up to 1 ml ampule	SC, IM	J0171
Synagis	per 50 mg		C9003
Synercid	500 mg (150/350)	IV	J2770
Synkavite	per 1 mg	IM, SC, IV	J3430
Syntocinon	up to 10 units	IV, IM	J2590
Synvisc and Synvisc-One	1 mg		J7322, J7325
Syrex	10 ml		A4216
Sytobex	1,000 mcg	IM, SC	J3420
T			
Tacrolimus			
oral	per 1 mg	ORAL	J7507
parenteral	5 mg		J7525
Talwin	30 mg	IM, SC, IV	J3070
Tamiflu	per 75 mg		G9035
Tamoxifen Citrate			J8999
Taractan, see Chlorprothixene			
Taxol	30 mg	IV	J9265
Taxotere	20 mg	IV	J9171
Tazicef	per 500 mg		J0713
Tazidime, see Ceftazidime Technetium TC Sestambi	per dose		A9500
			J0713
TEEV	up to 1 cc	IM	J0900
Teflaro	1 mg		J0712
Telavancin	10 mg		J3095
Temodar	5 mg	ORAL	J8700, J9328
Temozolomide	1 mg		J8700
	5 mg	ORAL	J9328
Temsirolimus	1 mg		J9330

◀ **New**   ← **Revised**   ✔ **Reinstated**   ~~deleted~~ **Deleted**

DRUG NAME	DOSAGE	METHOD OF ADMINISTRATION	HCPCS CODE
Tenecteplase	1 mg		**J3101**
Teniposide	50 mg		**Q2017**
Tequin	10 mg	IV	J1590
Terbutaline sulfate	up to 1 mg	SC, IV	**J3105**
concentrated form	per 1 mg	INH	**J7680**
unit dose form	per 1 mg	INH	**J7681**
Teriparatide	10 mcg		**J3110**
Terramycin IM	up to 50 mg	IM	J2460
Testa-C	up to 100 mg	IM	J1070
	1 cc, 200 mg	IM	J1080
Testadiate	up to 1 cc	IM	J0900
Testadiate-Depo	up to 100 mg	IM	J1070
	1 cc, 200 mg	IM	J1080
Testaject-LA	up to 100 mg	IM	J1070
	1 cc, 200 mg	IM	J1080
Testaqua	up to 50 mg	IM	J3140
Test-Estro Cypionates	up to 1 ml	IM	J1060
Test-Estro-C	up to 1 ml	IM	J1060
Testex	up to 100 mg	IM	J3150
Testo AQ	up to 50 mg		J3140
Testoject-50	up to 50 mg	IM	J3140
Testoject-LA	up to 100 mg	IM	J1070
	1 cc, 200 mg	IM	J1080
Testone			
LA 200	up to 100 mg	IM	J3120
	up to 200 mg	IM	J3130
LA 100	up to 100 mg	IM	J3120
	up to 200 mg	IM	J3130
Testosterone	up to 50 mg		J3140
Testosterone Aqueous	up to 50 mg	IM	J3140
Testosterone enanthate and estradiol valerate	up to 1 cc	IM	**J0900**
Testosterone enanthate	up to 100 mg	IM	**J3120**
	up to 200 mg	IM	**J3130**
Testosterone cypionate	up to 100 mg	IM	**J1070**
	1 cc, 200 mg	IM	**J1080**
Testosterone cypionate and estradiol cypionate	up to 1 ml	IM	**J1060**
Testosterone propionate	up to 100 mg	IM	**J3150**
Testosterone suspension	up to 50 mg	IM	**J3140**
Testradiol 90/4	up to 1 cc	IM	J0900
Testrin PA	up to 100 mg	IM	J3120
	up to 200 mg	IM	J3130
Testro AQ	up to 50 mg		J3140

◄ New ← Revised ✔ Reinstated ~~deleted~~ Deleted

DRUG NAME	DOSAGE	METHOD OF ADMINISTRATION	HCPCS CODE
Tetanus immune globulin, human	up to 250 units	IM	J1670
Tetracycline	up to 250 mg	IM, IV	J0120
Tev-Tropin	1 mg		J2941
Thallous Chloride TI–201	per MCI		A9505
Theelin Aqueous	per 1 mg	IM	J1435
Theophylline	per 40 mg	IV	J2810
TheraCys	per vial	IV	J9031
Thiamine HCl	100 mg		J3411
Thiethylenecthiophosphoramide/T	15 mg		J9340
Thiethylperazine maleate			
injection	up to 10 mg	IM	J3280
oral	10 mg	ORAL	Q0174
Thiotepa	15 mg	IV	J9340
Thorazine	10 mg	ORAL	Q0171
	25 mg	ORAL	Q0172
	up to 50 mg		J3230, J8498
Thrombate III	per IU		J7197
Thymoglobulin, see Immune globin, anti-thymocyte			
	25 mg		J7511
Thypinone	per 250 mcg	IV	J2725
Thyrogen	0.9 mg	IM, SC	J3240
Thyrotropin Alfa, injection	0.9 mg	IM, SC	J3240
Tice BCG	per vial	IV	J9031
injection	up to 200 mg	IM	J3250
Ticon			
injection	up to 200 mg	IM	J3250
oral	250 mg	ORAL	Q0173
Tigan			
injection	up to 200 mg	IM	J3250
oral	250 mg	ORAL	Q0173
Tigecycline	1 mg		J3243
Tiject-20	up to 200 mg	IM	J3250
	250 mg	ORAL	Q0173
Timentin			J3490
Tinzaparin	1,000 IU	SC	J1655
Tirofiban Hydrochloride, injection	0.25 mg	IM, IV	J3246
TNKase	1 mg		J3101
Tobi	300 mg	INH	J7682, J7685
Tobramycin, inhalation solution	300 mg	INH	J7682, J7685
Tobramycin sulfate	up to 80 mg	IM, IV	J3260, J7685
Tocilizumab	1 mg		J3262
Tofranil, see Imipramine HCl			

◄ New   ← Revised   ✔ Reinstated   ~~deleted~~ Deleted

DRUG NAME	DOSAGE	METHOD OF ADMINISTRATION	HCPCS CODE
Tolazoline HCl	up to 25 mg	IV	J2670
Topotecan	0.25 mg	ORAL	J8705
	40.1 mg	IV	J9351
Toradol	per 15 mg	IM, IV	J1885
Torecan	10 mg	ORAL	Q0174
	up to 10 mg	IM	J3280
Torisel	1 mg		J9330
Tornalate			
concentrated form	per mg	INH	J7628
unit dose	per mg	INH	J7629
Torsemide	10 mg/ml	IV	J3265
Torsiel	1 mg		J3390
Totacillin-N	up to 500 mg	IM, IV	J0290
	per 1.5 gm	IM, IV	J0295
Trastuzumab	10 mg	IV	J9355
Trasylol	10,000 KIU		J0365
Treanda	1 mg		J9033
Trelstar Depot	3.75 mg		J3315
Trelstar LA	3.75 mg		J3315
Treprostinil	1 mg		J3285
Trexall	2.5 mg	ORAL	J8610
Triethylenethosphoramide	15 mg		J9340
Tri-Kort	1 mg		J3300
	per 10 mg	IM	J3301
Triam-A	1 mg		J3300
	per 10 mg	IM	J3301
Triamcinolone			
concentrated form	per 1 mg	INH	J7683
unit dose	per 1 mg	INH	J7684
Triamcinolone acetonide	1 mg		J3300
	per 10 mg	IM	J3301
Triamcinolone diacetate	per 5 mg	IM	J3302
Triamcinolone hexacetonide	per 5 mg	VAR	J3303
Triamcot	per 5 mg		J3302
Triesence	1 mg		J3300
	per 10 mg	IM	J3301
Triflupromazine HCl	up to 20 mg	IM, IV	J3400
Trilafon	4 mg	ORAL	Q0175
	8 mg	ORAL	Q0176
	up to 5 mg	IM, IV	J3310
Trilog	1 mg		J3300
	per 10 mg	IM	J3301

◄ New   ← Revised   ✔ Reinstated   ~~deleted~~ Deleted

DRUG NAME	DOSAGE	METHOD OF ADMINISTRATION	HCPCS CODE
Trilone	per 5 mg		J3302
Trimethobenzamide HCl			
injection	up to 200 mg	IM	J3250
oral	250 mg	ORAL	Q0173
Trimetrexate glucuronate	per 25 mg	IV	J3305
Triptorelin Pamoate	3.75 mg		J3315
Trisenox	1 mg	IV	J9017
Trobicin	up to 2 g	IM	J3320
Trovan	100 mg	IV	J0200
Truxadryl	50 mg		J1200
Twinrix			J3490
Tysabri	1 mg		J2323
Tyvaso	1.74 mg		J7686
			J7699
U			
Ultra Filtered Plus	50 mcg		J2788
Ultravist 150	per ml		Q9965
Ultravist 240	per ml		Q9966
Ultravist 300	per ml		Q9966
Ultravist 370	per ml		Q9967
Ultrazine-10	up to 10 mg	IM, IV	J0780
Unasyn	per 1.5 gm	IM, IV	J0295
Unclassified drugs (see also Not elsewhere classified)			J3490
Unspecified oral antiemetic			Q0181
Urea	up to 40 g	IV	J3350
Ureaphil	up to 40 g	IV	J3350
Urecholine	up to 5 mg	SC	J0520
Urofollitropin	75 IU		J3355
Urokinase	5,000 IU vial	IV	J3364
	250,000 IU vial	IV	J3365
Ustekinumab	1 mg		J3357
V			
V-Gan 25	up to 50 mg	IM, IV	J2550
	12.5 mg	ORAL	Q0169
	25 mg	ORAL	Q0170
V-Gan 50	up to 50 mg	IM, IV	J2550
	12.5 mg	ORAL	Q0169
	25 mg	ORAL	Q0170
Valcyte			J3490
Valergen 10	10 mg	IM	J1380
Valergen 20	10 mg	IM	J1380
Valergen 40	up to 10 mg	IM	J1380

◄ New   ← Revised   ✔ Reinstated   deleted Deleted

DRUG NAME	DOSAGE	METHOD OF ADMINISTRATION	HCPCS CODE
Valertest No. 1	up to 1 cc	IM	J0900
			J1060
Valertest No. 2	up to 1 cc	IM	J0900
Valium	up to 5 mg	IM, IV	J3360
Valrubicin, intravesical	200 mg	OTH	**J9357**
Valstar	200 mg	OTH	J9357
Vancocin	500 mg	IV, IM	J3370
Vancoled	500 mg	IV, IM	J3370
Vancomycin HCl	500 mg	IV, IM	**J3370**
Vantas	50 mg		J9226
Vasceze	per 10 mg		J1642
Vasceze Sodium Chloride	10 ml		A4216
Vasoxyl, see Methoxamine HCl			
Vectibix	10 mg		J9303
Velaglucerase alfa	100 units		**J3385**
Velban	1 mg	IV	J9360
Velcade	0.1 mg		J9041
Velosulin BR (RDNA)	per 50 units		J1817
Velsar	1 mg	IV	J9360
Venofer	1 mg	IV	J1756
Ventavis	20 mcg		Q4080
Ventolin	0.5 mg	INH	J7620
concentrated form	1 mg	INH	J7610, J7611
unit dose form	1 mg	INH	J7609, J7613
VePesid			
	10 mg	IV	J9181
	50 mg	ORAL	J8560
Veritas Collagen Matrix			J3490
Versed	per 1 mg	IM, IV	J2250
Verteporfin	0.1 mg	IV	**J3396**
Vesprin	up to 20 mg	IM, IV	J3400
VFEND IV	10 mg		J3465
VGan	up to 50 mg		J2550
Viadur	65 mg		J9219
Vibativ	10 mg		J3095
Vidaza	1 mg		J9025
Vinblastine sulfate	1 mg	IV	**J9360**
Vincasar PFS	1 mg	IV	J9370
Vincristine sulfate	1 mg	IV	**J9370**
Vinorelbine tartrate	per 10 mg	IV	**J9390**
Vispaque 320	per ml		Q9967

◄ New   ← Revised   ✔ Reinstated   ~~deleted~~ Deleted

DRUG NAME	DOSAGE	METHOD OF ADMINISTRATION	HCPCS CODE
Vistacot	up to 25 mg		J3410
Vistaject-25	up to 25 mg	IM	J3410
Vistaril	up to 25 mg	IM	J3410
	25 mg	ORAL	Q0177
	50 mg	ORAL	Q0178
Vistide	375 mg	IV	J0740
Visudyne	0.1 mg	IV	J3396
Vita #12	up to 1,000 mcg		J3420
Vitamin B6	100 mg		J2415
Vitamin K, phytonadione, menadione, menadiol sodium diphosphate	per 1 mg	IM, SC, IV	J3430
Vitamin B-12 cyanocobalamin	up to 1,000 mcg	IM, SC	J3420
Vitrase	up to 150 units		J3470
	per 1 USP unit		J3471
	per 1,000 USP units		J3472
Vivaglobulin	100 mg		J1562
Vivitrol	1 mg		J2315
Von Willebrand Factor Complex, human	per IU VWF:RCo	IV	J7187
	per 100 IU VWF:RCo	IV	J7183 ←
Voriconazole	10 mg		J3465
Vpriv	100 units		J3385
Vumon	50 mg		Q2017
W			
Water for injection bacteriostatic	10 ml		A4216
Water for irrigation	500 ml		A4217
Wehamine	up to 50 mg	IM, IV	J1240
Wehdryl	up to 50 mg	IM, IV	J1200
	50 mg	ORAL	Q0163
Wellcovorin	per 50 mg	IM, IV	J0640
Wilate	per IU	IV	J7187
Win Rho SD	100 IU	IV	J2792
Wyamine Sulfate, see Mephentermine sulfate			
Wycillin	up to 600,000 units	IM, IV	J2510
Wydase	up to 150 units	SC, IV	J3470
X			
Xeloda	150 mg	ORAL	J8520
	500 mg	ORAL	J8521
Xeomin	1 unit		J0588 ◄
Xgeva	1 mg		J0897 ◄
Xiaflex	0.01 mg		J0775
Xolair	5 mg		J2357

◄ New   ← Revised   ✔ Reinstated   ~~deleted~~ Deleted

DRUG NAME	DOSAGE	METHOD OF ADMINISTRATION	HCPCS CODE
Xopenex	0.5 mg	INH	J7620
concentrated form	1 mg	INH	J7610, J7611, J7612
unit dose form	1 mg	INH	J7609, J7613, J7614
Xylocaine HCl	10 mg	IV	J2001
Xyntha	per IU IV		J7185, J7192
Y			
Yervoy	1 mg		J9228 ◄
Z			
Zanosar	1 g	IV	J9320
Zantac	25 mg	IV, IM	J2780
Zemaira	10 mg	IV	J0256
Zemplar	1 mcg	IM, IV	J2501
Zenapax	25 mg	IV	J7513
Zetran	up to 5 mg	IM, IV	J3360
Ziconotide	1 mcg		J2278
Zidovudine	10 mg	IV	J3485
Zinacef	per 750 mg	IM, IV	J0697
Ziprasidone Mesylate	10 mg		J3486
Zithromax	1 g	ORAL	Q0144
I.V.	500 mg	IV	J0456
Zithromax Tri-Pak	1 g		Q0144
Zithromax Z-Pak	1 g		Q0144
Zmax	1 g		Q0144
Zofran	1 mg	IV	J2405
	1 mg	ORAL	Q0162 ←
Zoladex	per 3.6 mg	SC	J9202
Zoledronic Acid	1 mg		J3487
Zolicef	500 mg	IV, IM	J0690
Zometa	1 mg		J3487
Zorbtive	1 mg		J2941
Zortress	0.25 mg	ORAL	J8561 ◄
Zosyn	1.125 g	IV	J2543
Zovirax	5 mg		J8499
Zyprexa Relprevv	1 mg		J2358
Zyvox	200 mg	IV	J2020

◄ New   ← Revised   ✔ Reinstated   deleted Deleted

HCPCS 2012: LEVEL II NATIONAL CODES

2012 HCPCS quarterly updates available
on the companion website at:
http://www.codingupdates.com

DISCLAIMER

Every effort has been made to make this text complete and accurate,
but no guarantee, warranty, or representation is made for its accuracy or completeness. This text is based on the Centers for Medicare
and Medicaid Services Healthcare Common Procedure Coding System (HCPCS).

INTRODUCTION

2012 HCPCS quarterly updates available on the companion website at: http://evolve.elsevier.com/Buck/HCPCS/.

The Centers for Medicare and Medicaid Services (CMS) (formerly Health Care Financing Administration [HCFA]) Healthcare Common Procedure Coding System (HCPCS) is a collection of codes and descriptors that represent procedures, supplies, products, and services that may be provided to Medicare beneficiaries and to individuals enrolled in private health insurance programs. The codes are divided as follows:

Level I: Codes and descriptors copyrighted by the American Medical Association's (AMA's) Current Procedural Terminology, ed. 4 (CPT-4). These are 5 position numeric codes representing physician and nonphysician services.

Level II: Includes codes and descriptors copyrighted by the American Dental Association's current dental terminology, seventh edition (CDT-7/8). These are 5 position alpha-numeric codes comprising the D series. All other Level II codes and descriptors are approved and maintained jointly by the alpha-numeric editorial panel (consisting of CMS, the Health Insurance Association of America, and the Blue Cross and Blue Shield Association). These are 5 position alpha-numeric codes representing primarily items and nonphysician services that are not represented in the Level I codes.

Level III: The CMS eliminated Level III local codes. See Program Memorandum AB-02-113.

Headings are provided as a means of grouping similar or closely related items. The placement of a code under a heading does not indicate additional means of classification, nor does it relate to any health insurance coverage categories.

HCPCS also contains modifiers, which are two-position codes and descriptors used to indicate that a service or procedure that has been performed has been altered by some specific circumstance but not changed in its definition or code. Modifiers are grouped by the levels. Level I modifiers and descriptors are copyrighted by the AMA. Level II modifiers are HCPCS modifiers. Modifiers in the D series are copyrighted by the ADA.

HCPCS is designed to promote uniform reporting and statistical data collection of medical procedures, supplies, products, and services.

HCPCS Disclaimer

Inclusion or exclusion of a procedure, supply, product, or service does not imply any health insurance coverage or reimbursement policy.

HCPCS makes as much use as possible of generic descriptions, but the inclusion of brand names to describe devices or drugs is intended only for indexing purposes; it is not meant to convey endorsement of any particular product or drug.

Updating HCPCS

The primary updates are made annually. Quarterly updates are also issued by CMS.

Legend

CMS Updates:
- ▶ New
- → Revised
- ✔ Reinstated
- ✖ Deleted
- ☉ Special coverage instructions
- ◆ Not covered or valid by Medicare
- ✲ Carrier discretion

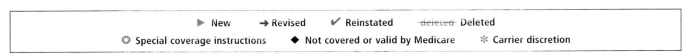

▶ New → Revised ✔ Reinstated deleted Deleted
☉ Special coverage instructions ◆ Not covered or valid by Medicare ✲ Carrier discretion

INTRODUCTION

Publisher Updates:

(PQRS)	PQRS
Qp	Quantity Physician Appendix A
Qh	Quantity Hospital Appendix B
♀	Female only
♂	Male only
A	Age
♿	DMEPOS
A2-Z3	ASC Payment Indicator
A-Y	ASC Status Indicator

Coding Clinic

Do not report HCPCS modifiers with PQRI CPT Category II codes, rather use Category II modifiers (i.e., 1P, 2P, 3P, or 8P) or the claim may be returned or denied.

LEVEL II NATIONAL MODIFIERS

✻ **A1** Dressing for one wound

✻ **A2** Dressing for two wounds

✻ **A3** Dressing for three wounds

✻ **A4** Dressing for four wounds

✻ **A5** Dressing for five wounds

✻ **A6** Dressing for six wounds

✻ **A7** Dressing for seven wounds

✻ **A8** Dressing for eight wounds

✻ **A9** Dressing for nine or more wounds

☼ **AA** Anesthesia services performed personally by anesthesiologist

IOM: 100-04, 12, 90.4

☼ **AD** Medical supervision by a physician: more than four concurrent anesthesia procedures

IOM: 100-04, 12, 90.4

✻ **AE** Registered dietician

✻ **AF** Specialty physician

✻ **AG** Primary physician

☼ **AH** Clinical psychologist

IOM: 100-04, 12, 170

✻ **AI** Principal physician of record

☼ **AJ** Clinical social worker

IOM: 100-04, 12, 170

IOM: 100-04, 12, 150

✻ **AK** Nonparticipating physician

☼ **AM** Physician, team member service

Not assigned for Medicare

✻ **AP** Determination of refractive state was not performed in the course of diagnostic ophthalmological examination

✻ **AQ** Physician providing a service in an unlisted health professional shortage area (HPSA)

✻ **AR** Physician provider services in a physician scarcity area

✻ **AS** Physician assistant, nurse practitioner, or clinical nurse specialist services for assistant at surgery

✻ **AT** Acute treatment (this modifier should be used when reporting service 98940, 98941, 98942)

✻ **AU** Item furnished in conjunction with a urological, ostomy, or tracheostomy supply

✻ **AV** Item furnished in conjunction with a prosthetic device, prosthetic or orthotic

✻ **AW** Item furnished in conjunction with a surgical dressing

✻ **AX** Item furnished in conjunction with dialysis services

▶ ✻ **AY** Item or service furnished to an ESRD patient that is not for the treatment of ESRD

▶ ◆ **AZ** Physician providing a service in a dental health professional shortage area for the purpose of an electronic health record incentive payment

✻ **BA** Item furnished in conjunction with parenteral enteral nutrition (PEN) services

✻ **BL** Special acquisition of blood and blood products

✻ **BO** Orally administered nutrition, not by feeding tube

✻ **BP** The beneficiary has been informed of the purchase and rental options and has elected to purchase the item

✻ **BR** The beneficiary has been informed of the purchase and rental options and has elected to rent the item

✻ **BU** The beneficiary has been informed of the purchase and rental options and after 30 days has not informed the supplier of his/her decision

✻ **CA** Procedure payable only in the inpatient setting when performed emergently on an outpatient who expires prior to admission

(PQRS) PQRS	Qp Quantity Physician Appendix A	Qh Quantity Hospital Appendix B	♀ Female only
♂ Male only	A Age	♿ DMEPOS	A2-Z3 ASC Payment Indicator	A-Y ASC Status Indicator	Coding Clinic

LEVEL II NATIONAL MODIFIERS A1 – CA

81

✳ **CB**   Service ordered by a renal dialysis facility (RDF) physician as part of the ESRD beneficiary's dialysis benefit, is not part of the composite rate, and is separately reimbursable

✳ **CC**   Procedure code change (Use CC when the procedure code submitted was changed either for administrative reasons or because an incorrect code was filed)

☺ **CD**   AMCC test has been ordered by an ESRD facility or MCP physician that is part of the composite rate and is not separately billable

☺ **CE**   AMCC test has been ordered by an ESRD facility or MCP physician that is a composite rate test but is beyond the normal frequency covered under the rate and is separately reimbursable based on medical necessity

☺ **CF**   AMCC test has been ordered by an ESRD facility or MCP physician that is not part of the composite rate and is separately billable

✳ **CG**   Policy criteria applied

✳ **CR**   Catastrophe/Disaster related

▶ ✳ **CS**   Item or service related, in whole or in part, to an illness, injury, or condition that was caused by or exacerbated by the effects, direct or indirect, of the 2010 oil spill in the Gulf of Mexico, including but not limited to subsequent clean-up activities

▶ ✳ **DA**   Oral health assessment by a licensed health professional other than a dentist

✳ **E1**   Upper left, eyelid

✳ **E2**   Lower left, eyelid

✳ **E3**   Upper right, eyelid

✳ **E4**   Lower right, eyelid

☺ **EA**   Erythropoetic stimulating agent (ESA) administered to treat anemia due to anti-cancer chemotherapy

CMS requires claims for non-ESRD ESAs (J0881 and J0885) to include one of three modifiers: EA, EB, EC.

☺ **EB**   Erythropoetic stimulating agent (ESA) administered to treat anemia due to anti-cancer radiotherapy

CMS requires claims for non-ESRD ESAs (J0881 and J0885) to include one of three modifiers: EA, EB, EC.

☺ **EC**   Erythropoetic stimulating agent (ESA) administered to treat anemia not due to anti-cancer radiotherapy or anti-cancer chemotherapy

CMS requires claims for non-ESRD ESAs (J0881 and J0885) to include one of three modifiers: EA, EB, EC.

☺ **ED**   Hematocrit level has exceeded 39% (or hemoglobin level has exceeded 13.0 g/dl) for 3 or more consecutive billing cycles immediately prior to and including the current cycle

☺ **EE**   Hematocrit level has not exceeded 39% (or hemoglobin level has not exceeded 13.0 g/dl) for 3 or more consecutive billing cycles immediately prior to and including the current cycle

☺ **EJ**   Subsequent claims for a defined course of therapy, e.g., EPO, sodium hyaluronate, infliximab

☺ **EM**   Emergency reserve supply (for ESRD benefit only)

✳ **EP**   Service provided as part of Medicaid early periodic screening diagnosis and treatment (EPSDT) program

✳ **ET**   Emergency services

✳ **EY**   No physician or other licensed health care provider order for this item or service

Items billed before a signed and dated order has been received by the supplier must be submitted with an -EY modifier added to each related HCPCS code.

✳ **F1**   Left hand, second digit

✳ **F2**   Left hand, third digit

✳ **F3**   Left hand, fourth digit

✳ **F4**   Left hand, fifth digit

✳ **F5**   Right hand, thumb

✳ **F6**   Right hand, second digit

✳ **F7**   Right hand, third digit

✳ **F8**   Right hand, fourth digit

✳ **F9**   Right hand, fifth digit

✳ **FA**   Left hand, thumb

◆ **FB**   Item provided without cost to provider, supplier or practitioner, or full credit received for replaced device (examples, but not limited to, covered under warranty, replaced due to defect, free samples)

☺ **FC**   Partial credit received for replaced device

▶ **New**   → **Revised**   ✔ **Reinstated**   ~~deleted~~ **Deleted**
☺ **Special coverage instructions**   ◆ **Not covered or valid by Medicare**   ✳ **Carrier discretion**

✳ **FP** Service provided as part of family planning program

✳ **G1** Most recent URR reading of less than 60

✳ **G2** Most recent URR reading of 60 to 64.9

✳ **G3** Most recent URR reading of 65 to 69.9

✳ **G4** Most recent URR reading of 70 to 74.9

✳ **G5** Most recent URR reading of 75 or greater

✳ **G6** ESRD patient for whom less than six dialysis sessions have been provided in a month

✪ **G7** Pregnancy resulted from rape or incest or pregnancy certified by physician as life threatening

IOM: 100-02, 15, 20.1; 100-03, 3, 170.3

✳ **G8** Monitored anesthesia care (MAC) for deep complex, complicated, or markedly invasive surgical procedure

✳ **G9** Monitored anesthesia care for patient who has history of severe cardiopulmonary condition

➔ ✳ **GA** Waiver of liability statement issued as required by payer policy, individual case

An item/service is expected to be denied as not reasonable and necessary and an ABN is on file. Modifier -GA can be used on either a specific or a miscellaneous HCPCS code. Modifiers -GA and -GY should never be reported together on the same line for the same HCPCS code.

✳ **GB** Claim being resubmitted for payment because it is no longer covered under a global payment demonstration

✪ **GC** This service has been performed in part by a resident under the direction of a teaching physician.

IOM: 100-04, 12, 90.4, 100

✳ **GD** Units of service exceeds medically unlikely edit value and represents reasonable and necessary services

✪ **GE** This service has been performed by a resident without the presence of a teaching physician under the primary care exception

✳ **GF** Non-physician (e.g., nurse practitioner (NP), certified registered nurse anesthetist (CRNA), certified registered nurse (CRN), clinical nurse specialist (CNS), physician assistant (PA)) services in a critical access hospital

✳ **GG** Performance and payment of a screening mammogram and diagnostic mammogram on the same patient, same day

✳ **GH** Diagnostic mammogram converted from screening mammogram on same day

✳ **GJ** "Opt out" physician or practitioner emergency or urgent service

✳ **GK** Reasonable and necessary item/service associated with a GA or GZ modifier

An upgrade is defined as an item that goes beyond what is medically necessary under Medicare's coverage requirements. An item can be considered an upgrade even if the physician has signed an order for it. When suppliers know that an item will not be paid in full because it does not meet the coverage criteria stated in the LCD, the supplier can still obtain partial payment at the time of initial determination if the claim is billed using one of the upgrade modifiers (GK or GL). (https://www.cms.gov/manuals/downloads/clm104c01.pdf)

✳ **GL** Medically unnecessary upgrade provided instead of non-upgraded item, no charge, no Advance Beneficiary Notice (ABN)

✳ **GM** Multiple patients on one ambulance trip

✳ **GN** Services delivered under an outpatient speech language pathology plan of care

✳ **GO** Services delivered under an outpatient occupational therapy plan of care

✳ **GP** Services delivered under an outpatient physical therapy plan of care

✳ **GQ** Via asynchronous telecommunications system

✳ **GR** This service was performed in whole or in part by a resident in a department of Veterans Affairs medical center or clinic, supervised in accordance with VA policy

✪ **GS** Dosage of EPO or darbepoetin alfa has been reduced and maintained in response to hematocrit or hemoglobin level

✪ **GT** Via interactive audio and video telecommunication systems

▶ ✳ **GU** Waiver of liability statement issued as required by payer policy, routine notice

LEVEL II NATIONAL MODIFIERS FP – GU

🄟 PQRS	🄠p Quantity Physician Appendix A	🄠h Quantity Hospital Appendix B	♀ Female only
♂ Male only	🄐 Age	♿ DMEPOS	A2-Z3 ASC Payment Indicator A-Y ASC Status Indicator Coding Clinic

83

○ **GV** Attending physician not employed or paid under arrangement by the patient's hospice provider

○ **GW** Service not related to the hospice patient's terminal condition

▶ ✳ **GX** Notice of liability issued, voluntary under payer policy

GX modifier must be submitted with non-covered charges only. This modifier differentiates from the required uses in conjunction with ABN. (https://www.cms.gov/manuals/downloads/clm104c01.pdf)

◆ **GY** Item or service statutorily excluded, does not meet the definition of any Medicare benefit or, for non-Medicare insurers, is not a contract benefit

Examples of "statutorily excluded" include: Infusion drug not administered using a durable infusion pump, a wheelchair that is for use for mobility outside the home or hearing aids. GA and GY should never be coded together on the same line for the same HCPCS code. (https://www.cms.gov/manuals/downloads/clm104c01.pdf)

◆ **GZ** Item or service expected to be denied as not reasonable or necessary

Used when an ABN is not on file and can be used on either a specific or a miscellaneous HCPCS code. It would never be correct to place any combination of GY, GZ or GA modifiers on the same claim line and will result in rejected or denied claim for invalid coding. (https://www.cms.gov/manuals/downloads/clm104c01.pdf)

◆ **H9** Court-ordered

◆ **HA** Child/adolescent program

◆ **HB** Adult program, nongeriatric

◆ **HC** Adult program, geriatric

◆ **HD** Pregnant/parenting women's program

◆ **HE** Mental health program

◆ **HF** Substance abuse program

◆ **HG** Opioid addiction treatment program

◆ **HH** Integrated mental health/substance abuse program

◆ **HI** Integrated mental health and mental retardation/developmental disabilities program

◆ **HJ** Employee assistance program

◆ **HK** Specialized mental health programs for high-risk populations

◆ **HL** Intern

◆ **HM** Less than bachelor degree level

◆ **HN** Bachelors degree level

◆ **HO** Masters degree level

◆ **HP** Doctoral level

◆ **HQ** Group setting

◆ **HR** Family/couple with client present

◆ **HS** Family/couple without client present

◆ **HT** Multi-disciplinary team

◆ **HU** Funded by child welfare agency

◆ **HV** Funded by state addictions agency

◆ **HW** Funded by state mental health agency

◆ **HX** Funded by county/local agency

◆ **HY** Funded by juvenile justice agency

◆ **HZ** Funded by criminal justice agency

✳ **J1** Competitive acquisition program no-pay submission for a prescription number

✳ **J2** Competitive acquisition program, restocking of emergency drugs after emergency administration

✳ **J3** Competitive acquisition program (CAP), drug not available through CAP as written, reimbursed under average sales price methodology

✳ **J4** DMEPOS item subject to DMEPOS competitive bidding program that is furnished by a hospital upon discharge

✳ **JA** Administered intravenously

This modifier is informational only (not a payment modifier) and may be submitted with all injection codes. According to Medicare, reporting this modifier is voluntary. (CMS Pub. 100-04, chapter 8, section 60.2.3.1 and Pub. 100-04, chapter 17, section 80.11)

✳ **JB** Administered subcutaneously

✳ **JC** Skin substitute used as a graft

✳ **JD** Skin substitute not used as a graft

✳ **JW** Drug amount discarded/not administered to any patient

Use JW to identify unused drugs or biologicals from single use vial/package that are appropriately discarded. Bill on separate line for payment of discarded drug/biological.
Coding Clinic: 2010, Q3, P10

✳ **K0** Lower extremity prosthesis functional Level 0 - does not have the ability or potential to ambulate or transfer safely with or without assistance and a prosthesis does not enhance their quality of life or mobility.

▶ New → Revised ✔ Reinstated ~~deleted~~ Deleted

○ Special coverage instructions ◆ Not covered or valid by Medicare ✳ Carrier discretion

✳ **K1** Lower extremity prosthesis functional Level 1 - has the ability or potential to use a prosthesis for transfers or ambulation on level surfaces at fixed cadence. Typical of the limited and unlimited household ambulator.

✳ **K2** Lower extremity prosthesis functional Level 2 - has the ability or potential for ambulation with the ability to traverse low level environmental barriers such as curbs, stairs or uneven surfaces. Typical of the limited community ambulator.

✳ **K3** Lower extremity prosthesis functional Level 3 - has the ability or potential for ambulation with variable cadence. Typical of the community ambulator who has the ability to traverse most environmental barriers and may have vocational, therapeutic, or exercise activity that demands prosthetic utilization beyond simple locomotion.

✳ **K4** Lower extremity prosthesis functional Level 4 - has the ability or potential for prosthetic ambulation that exceeds the basic ambulation skills, exhibiting high impact, stress, or energy levels, typical of the prosthetic demands of the child, active adult, or athlete.

✳ **KA** Add on option/accessory for wheelchair

✳ **KB** Beneficiary requested upgrade for ABN, more than 4 modifiers identified on claim

✳ **KC** Replacement of special power wheelchair interface

✳ **KD** Drug or biological infused through DME

✳ **KE** Bid under round one of the DMEPOS competitive bidding program for use with non-competitive bid base equipment

✳ **KF** Item designated by FDA as Class III device

✳ **KG** DMEPOS item subject to DMEPOS competitive bidding program number 1

✳ **KH** DMEPOS item, initial claim, purchase or first month rental

✳ **KI** DMEPOS item, second or third month rental

✳ **KJ** DMEPOS item, parenteral enteral nutrition (PEN) pump or capped rental, months four to fifteen

✳ **KK** DMEPOS item subject to DMEPOS competitive bidding program number 2

✳ **KL** DMEPOS item delivered via mail

✳ **KM** Replacement of facial prosthesis including new impression/moulage

✳ **KN** Replacement of facial prosthesis using previous master model

✳ **KO** Single drug unit dose formulation

✳ **KP** First drug of a multiple drug unit dose formulation

✳ **KQ** Second or subsequent drug of a multiple drug unit dose formulation

✳ **KR** Rental item, billing for partial month

⊙ **KS** Glucose monitor supply for diabetic beneficiary not treated with insulin

✳ **KT** Beneficiary resides in a competitive bidding area and travels outside that competitive bidding area and receives a competitive bid item

✳ **KU** DMEPOS item subject to DMEPOS competitive bidding program number 3

✳ **KV** DMEPOS item subject to DMEPOS competitive bidding program that is furnished as part of a professional service

✳ **KW** DMEPOS item subject to DMEPOS competitive bidding program number 4

✳ **KX** Requirements specified in the medical policy have been met

✳ **KY** DMEPOS item subject to DMEPOS competitive bidding program number 5

✳ **KZ** New coverage not implemented by managed care

✳ **LC** Left circumflex coronary artery

✳ **LD** Left anterior descending coronary artery

✳ **LL** Lease/rental (use the LL modifier when DME equipment rental is to be applied against the purchase price)

✳ **LR** Laboratory round trip

⊙ **LS** FDA-monitored intraocular lens implant

✳ **LT** Left side (used to identify procedures performed on the left side of the body)

✳ **M2** Medicare secondary payer (MSP)

✳ **MS** Six month maintenance and servicing fee for reasonable and necessary parts and labor which are not covered under any manufacturer or supplier warranty

▶ ✳ **NB** Nebulizer system, any type, FDA-cleared for use with specific drug

✳ **NR** New when rented (use the NR modifier when DME which was new at the time of rental is subsequently purchased)

✳ **NU** New equipment

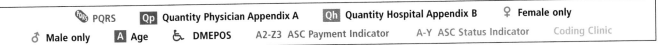

✳ **P1**	A normal healthy patient	
✳ **P2**	A patient with mild systemic disease	
✳ **P3**	A patient with severe systemic disease	
✳ **P4**	A patient with severe systemic disease that is a constant threat to life	
✳ **P5**	A moribund patient who is not expected to survive without the operation	
✳ **P6**	A declared brain-dead patient whose organs are being removed for donor purposes	
◆ **PA**	Surgical or other invasive procedure on wrong body part	
◆ **PB**	Surgical or other invasive procedure on wrong patient	
◆ **PC**	Wrong surgery or other invasive procedure on patient	
▶ ✳ **PD**	Diagnostic or related non diagnostic item or service provided in a wholly owned or operated entity to a patient who is admitted as an inpatient within 3 days	
✳ **PI**	Positron emission tomography (PET) or PET/computed tomography (CT) to inform the initial treatment strategy of tumors that are biopsy proven or strongly suspected of being cancerous based on other diagnostic testing	
✳ **PL**	Progressive addition lenses	
✳ **PS**	Positron emission tomography (PET) or PET/computed tomography (CT) to inform the subsequent treatment strategy of cancerous tumors when the beneficiary's treating physician determines that the PET study is needed to inform subsequent anti-tumor strategy	
▶ ✳ **PT**	Colorectal cancer screening test; converted to diagnostic text or other procedure	

Assign this modifier with the appropriate CPT procedure code for colonoscopy, flexible sigmoidoscopy, or barium enema when the service is initiated as a colorectal cancer screening service but then becomes a diagnostic service. (MLN Matters article MM7012 (PDF, 75 KB)
Coding Clinic: 2011, Q1, P10

⊙ **Q0**	Investigational clinical service provided in a clinical research study that is in an approved clinical research study	
⊙ **Q1**	Routine clinical service provided in a clinical research study that is in an approved clinical research study	
✳ **Q2**	HCFA/ORD demonstration project procedure/service	
✳ **Q3**	Live kidney donor surgery and related services	
✳ **Q4**	Service for ordering/referring physician qualifies as a service exemption	
⊙ **Q5**	Service furnished by a substitute physician under a reciprocal billing arrangement	

IOM: 100-04, 1, 30.2.10

⊙ **Q6**	Service furnished by a locum tenens physician

IOM: 100-04, 1, 30.2.11

✳ **Q7**	One Class A finding
✳ **Q8**	Two Class B findings
✳ **Q9**	One Class B and two Class C findings
✳ **QC**	Single channel monitoring
✳ **QD**	Recording and storage in solid state memory by a digital recorder
✳ **QE**	Prescribed amount of oxygen is less than 1 liter per minute (LPM)
✳ **QF**	Prescribed amount of oxygen exceeds 4 liters per minute (LPM) and portable oxygen is prescribed
✳ **QG**	Prescribed amount of oxygen is greater than 4 liters per minute (LPM)
✳ **QH**	Oxygen conserving device is being used with an oxygen delivery system
⊙ **QJ**	Services/items provided to a prisoner or patient in state or local custody, however, the state or local government, as applicable, meets the requirements in 42 CFR 411.4 (B)
⊙ **QK**	Medical direction of two, three, or four concurrent anesthesia procedures involving qualified individuals

IOM: 100-04, 12, 50K, 90

✳ **QL**	Patient pronounced dead after ambulance called
✳ **QM**	Ambulance service provided under arrangement by a provider of services
✳ **QN**	Ambulance service furnished directly by a provider of services
⊙ **QP**	Documentation is on file showing that the laboratory test(s) was ordered individually or ordered as a CPT-recognized panel other than automated profile codes 80002-80019, G0058, G0059, and G0060.

▶ New   → Revised   ✔ Reinstated   ~~deleted~~ Deleted
⊙ Special coverage instructions   ◆ Not covered or valid by Medicare   ✳ Carrier discretion

P1 – QP   LEVEL II NATIONAL MODIFIERS

☉ **QS**   Monitored anesthesia care service
IOM: 100-04, 12, 30.6, 501

✳ **QT**   Recording and storage on tape by an analog tape recorder

✳ **QW**   CLIA-waived test

✳ **QX**   CRNA service: with medical direction by a physician

☉ **QY**   Medical direction of one certified registered nurse anesthetist (CRNA) by an anesthesiologist
IOM: 100-04, 12, 50K, 90

✳ **QZ**   CRNA service: without medical direction by a physician

➜ ✳ **RA**   Replacement of a DME, orthotic or prosthetic item

Contractors will deny claims for replacement parts when furnished in conjunction with the repair of a capped rental item and billed with modifier -RB, including claims for parts submitted using code E1399, that are billed during the capped rental period (i.e., the last day of the 13th month of continuous use or before). Repair includes all maintenance, servicing, and repair of capped rental DME because it is included in the allowed rental payment amounts. (Pub 100-20 One-Time Notification Centers for Medicare & Medicaid Services, Transmittal: 901, May 13, 2011)

➜ ✳ **RB**   Replacement of a part of a DME, orthotic or prosthetic item furnished as part of a repair

✳ **RC**   Right coronary artery

✳ **RD**   Drug provided to beneficiary, but not administered "incident-to"

✳ **RE**   Furnished in full compliance with FDA-mandated risk evaluation and mitigation strategy (REMS)

✳ **RR**   Rental (use the 'RR' modifier when DME is to be rented)

✳ **RT**   Right side (used to identify procedures performed on the right side of the body)

◆ **SA**   Nurse practitioner rendering service in collaboration with a physician

◆ **SB**   Nurse midwife

➜ ✳ **SC**   Medically necessary service or supply

◆ **SD**   Services provided by registered nurse with specialized, highly technical home infusion training

◆ **SE**   State and/or federally funded programs/ services

✳ **SF**   Second opinion ordered by a professional review organization (PRO) per Section 9401, P.L. 99-272 (100% reimbursement - no Medicare deductible or coinsurance)

✳ **SG**   Ambulatory surgical center (ASC) facility service

◆ **SH**   Second concurrently administered infusion therapy

◆ **SJ**   Third or more concurrently administered infusion therapy

◆ **SK**   Member of high risk population (use only with codes for immunization)

◆ **SL**   State supplied vaccine

◆ **SM**   Second surgical opinion

◆ **SN**   Third surgical opinion

◆ **SQ**   Item ordered by home health

◆ **SS**   Home infusion services provided in the infusion suite of the IV therapy provider

◆ **ST**   Related to trauma or injury

◆ **SU**   Procedure performed in physician's office (to denote use of facility and equipment)

◆ **SV**   Pharmaceuticals delivered to patient's home but not utilized

✳ **SW**   Services provided by a certified diabetic educator

◆ **SY**   Persons who are in close contact with member of high-risk population (use only with codes for immunization)

✳ **T1**   Left foot, second digit

✳ **T2**   Left foot, third digit

✳ **T3**   Left foot, fourth digit

✳ **T4**   Left foot, fifth digit

✳ **T5**   Right foot, great toe

✳ **T6**   Right foot, second digit

✳ **T7**   Right foot, third digit

✳ **T8**   Right foot, fourth digit

✳ **T9**   Right foot, fifth digit

✳ **TA**   Left foot, great toe

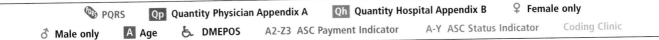

| PQRS | **Qp** Quantity Physician Appendix A | **Qh** Quantity Hospital Appendix B | ♀ Female only |
| ♂ Male only | **A** Age | DMEPOS | A2-Z3 ASC Payment Indicator | A-Y ASC Status Indicator | Coding Clinic |

＊ **TC**   Technical component; Under certain circumstances, a charge may be made for the technical component alone; under those circumstances the technical component charge is identified by adding modifier TC to the usual procedure number; technical component charges are institutional charges and not billed separately by physicians; however, portable x-ray suppliers only bill for technical component and should utilize modifier TC; the charge data from portable x-ray suppliers will then be used to build customary and prevailing profiles.

◆ **TD**   RN

◆ **TE**   LPN/LVN

◆ **TF**   Intermediate level of care

◆ **TG**   Complex/high tech level of care

◆ **TH**   Obstetrical treatment/services, prenatal or postpartum

◆ **TJ**   Program group, child and/or adolescent

◆ **TK**   Extra patient or passenger, non-ambulance

◆ **TL**   Early intervention/individualized family service plan (IFSP)

◆ **TM**   Individualized education program (IEP)

◆ **TN**   Rural/outside providers' customary service area

◆ **TP**   Medical transport, unloaded vehicle

◆ **TQ**   Basic life support transport by a volunteer ambulance provider

◆ **TR**   School-based individual education program (IEP) services provided outside the public school district responsible for the student

＊ **TS**   Follow-up service

◆ **TT**   Individualized service provided to more than one patient in same setting

◆ **TU**   Special payment rate, overtime

◆ **TV**   Special payment rates, holidays/weekends

◆ **TW**   Back-up equipment

◆ **U1**   Medicaid Level of Care 1, as defined by each State

◆ **U2**   Medicaid Level of Care 2, as defined by each State

◆ **U3**   Medicaid Level of Care 3, as defined by each State

◆ **U4**   Medicaid Level of Care 4, as defined by each State

◆ **U5**   Medicaid Level of Care 5, as defined by each State

◆ **U6**   Medicaid Level of Care 6, as defined by each State

◆ **U7**   Medicaid Level of Care 7, as defined by each State

◆ **U8**   Medicaid Level of Care 8, as defined by each State

◆ **U9**   Medicaid Level of Care 9, as defined by each State

◆ **UA**   Medicaid Level of Care 10, as defined by each State

◆ **UB**   Medicaid Level of Care 11, as defined by each State

◆ **UC**   Medicaid Level of Care 12, as defined by each State

◆ **UD**   Medicaid Level of Care 13, as defined by each State

＊ **UE**   Used durable medical equipment

◆ **UF**   Services provided in the morning

◆ **UG**   Services provided in the afternoon

◆ **UH**   Services provided in the evening

◆ **UJ**   Services provided at night

◆ **UK**   Services provided on behalf of the client to someone other than the client (collateral relationship)

＊ **UN**   Two patients served

＊ **UP**   Three patients served

＊ **UQ**   Four patients served

＊ **UR**   Five patients served

＊ **US**   Six or more patients served

→ ＊ **V5**   Vascular catheter (alone or with any other vascular access)

→ ＊ **V6**   Arteriovenous graft (or other vascular access not including a vascular catheter)

→ ＊ **V7**   Arteriovenous fistula only (in use with two needles)

＊ **V8**   Infection present

＊ **V9**   No infection present

＊ **VP**   Aphakic patient

▶ New   → Revised   ✔ Reinstated   ~~deleted~~ Deleted

⊙ Special coverage instructions   ◆ Not covered or valid by Medicare   ＊ Carrier discretion

Ambulance Modifiers

Modifiers that are used on claims for ambulance services are created by combining two alpha characters. Each alpha character, with the exception of X, represents an origin (source) code or a destination code. The pair of alpha codes creates one modifier. The first position alpha-code = origin; the second position alpha-code = destination. On form CMS-1491, used to report ambulance services, Item 12 should contain the origin code and Item 13 should contain the destination code. Origin and destination codes and their descriptions are as follows:

D	Diagnostic or therapeutic site other than P or H when these are used as origin codes
E	Residential, domiciliary, custodial facility (other than an 1819 facility)
G	Hospital-based dialysis facility (hospital or hospital related)
H	Hospital
I	Site of transfer (e.g., airport or helicopter pad) between modes of ambulance transport
J	Non–hospital-based dialysis facility
N	Skilled nursing facility (SNF) (1819 facility)
P	Physician's office (includes HMO non-hospital facility, clinic, etc.)
R	Residence
S	Scene of accident or acute event
X	Destination code only. Intermediate stop at physician's office en route to the hospital (includes non-hospital facility, clinic, etc.)

TRANSPORT SERVICES INCLUDING AMBULANCE (A0000-A0999)

A0021-A099:   Bill local carrier

◆ **A0021**   Ambulance service, outside state per mile, transport (Medicaid only)   E
Cross Reference A0030

◆ **A0080**   Non-emergency transportation, per mile - vehicle provided by volunteer (individual or organization), with no vested interest   E

◆ **A0090**   Non-emergency transportation, per mile - vehicle provided by individual (family member, self, neighbor) with vested interest   E

◆ **A0100**   Non-emergency transportation; taxi   E

◆ **A0110**   Non-emergency transportation and bus, intra or inter state carrier   E

◆ **A0120**   Non-emergency transportation: mini-bus, mountain area transports, or other transportation systems   E

◆ **A0130**   Non-emergency transportation: wheel chair van   E

◆ **A0140**   Non-emergency transportation and air travel (private or commercial), intra or inter state   E

◆ **A0160**   Non-emergency transportation: per mile - caseworker or social worker   E

◆ **A0170**   Transportation: ancillary: parking fees, tolls, other   E

◆ **A0180**   Non-emergency transportation: ancillary: lodging - recipient   E

◆ **A0190**   Non-emergency transportation: ancillary: meals - recipient   E

◆ **A0200**   Non-emergency transportation: ancillary: lodging - escort   E

◆ **A0210**   Non-emergency transportation: ancillary: meals - escort   E

◆ **A0225**   Ambulance service, neonatal transport, base rate, emergency transport, one way   E

◆ **A0380**   BLS mileage (per mile)   E
Cross Reference A0425

✳ **A0382**   BLS routine disposable supplies   A

✳ **A0384**   BLS specialized service disposable supplies; defibrillation (used by ALS ambulances and BLS ambulances in jurisdictions where defibrillation is permitted in BLS ambulances)   A

◆ **A0390**   ALS mileage (per mile)   E
Cross Reference A0425

✳ **A0392**   ALS specialized service disposable supplies; defibrillation (to be used only in jurisdictions where defibrillation cannot be performed in BLS ambulances)   A

✳ **A0394**   ALS specialized service disposable supplies; IV drug therapy   A

✳ **A0396**   ALS specialized service disposable supplies; esophageal intubation   A

✳ **A0398**   ALS routine disposable supplies   A

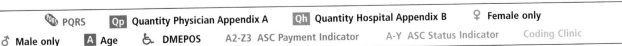

🔲 PQRS	**Qp** Quantity Physician Appendix A	**Qh** Quantity Hospital Appendix B	♀ Female only	
♂ Male only	**A** Age	♿ DMEPOS	A2-Z3 ASC Payment Indicator A-Y ASC Status Indicator	Coding Clinic

✳ **A0420** Ambulance waiting time (ALS or BLS), one half (½) hour increments   A

Waiting Time Table			
UNITS	TIME	UNITS	TIME
1	½ to 1 hr.	6	3 to 3½ hrs.
2	1 to 1½ hrs.	7	3½ to 4 hrs.
3	1½ to 2 hrs.	8	4 to 4½ hrs.
4	2 to 2½ hrs.	9	4½ to 5 hrs.
5	2½ to 3 hrs.	10	5 to 5½ hrs.

✳ **A0422** Ambulance (ALS or BLS) oxygen and oxygen supplies, life sustaining situation   A

✳ **A0424** Extra ambulance attendant, ground (ALS or BLS) or air (fixed or rotary winged); (requires medical review)   A

✳ **A0425** Ground mileage, per statute mile   A

✳ **A0426** Ambulance service, advanced life support, non-emergency transport, Level 1 (ALS1)   A

✳ **A0427** Ambulance service, advanced life support, emergency transport, Level 1 (ALS1-Emergency)   A

✳ **A0428** Ambulance service, basic life support, non-emergency transport (BLS)   A

✳ **A0429** Ambulance service, basic life support, emergency transport (BLS-Emergency)   A

✳ **A0430** Ambulance service, conventional air services, transport, one way (fixed wing)   A

✳ **A0431** Ambulance service, conventional air services, transport, one way (rotary wing)   A

✳ **A0432** Paramedic intercept (PI), rural area, transport furnished by a volunteer ambulance company, which is prohibited by state law from billing third party payers   A

✳ **A0433** Advanced life support, Level 2 (ALS2)   A

✳ **A0434** Specialty care transport (SCT)   A

✳ **A0435** Fixed wing air mileage, per statute mile   A

✳ **A0436** Rotary wing air mileage, per statute mile   A

◆ **A0888** Noncovered ambulance mileage, per mile (e.g., for miles traveled beyond closest appropriate facility)   E
MCM 2125

◆ **A0998** Ambulance response and treatment, no transport   E
IOM: 100-02, 10, 20

☼ **A0999** Unlisted ambulance service   A
IOM: 100-02, 10, 20

MEDICAL AND SURGICAL SUPPLIES (A4000-A9999)

✳ **A4206** Syringe with needle, sterile 1cc or less, each   E
If "incident to" a physician's service, do not bill; otherwise, bill DME/MAC.

✳ **A4207** Syringe with needle, sterile 2cc, each   E
If "incident to" a physician's service, do not bill; otherwise, bill DME/MAC.

✳ **A4208** Syringe with needle, sterile 3cc, each   E
If "incident to" a physician's service, do not bill; otherwise, bill DME/MAC.

✳ **A4209** Syringe with needle, sterile 5cc or greater, each   E
If "incident to" a physician's service, do not bill; otherwise, bill DME/MAC.

◆ **A4210** Needle-free injection device, each   E
IOM: 100-03, 4, 280.1
Bill DME/MAC

☼ **A4211** Supplies for self-administered injections   E
If "incident to" a physican service, do not bill; otherwise, bill DME/MAC.
IOM: 100-02, 15, 50

✳ **A4212** Non-coring needle or stylet with or without catheter   B
Bill local carrier

✳ **A4213** Syringe, sterile, 20 cc or greater, each   E
If "incident to" a physican service, do not bill; otherwise, bill DME/MAC.

✳ **A4215** Needle, sterile, any size, each   E
If "incident to" a physican service, do not bill; otherwise, bill DME/MAC.

▶ New   → Revised   ✔ Reinstated   ~~deleted~~ Deleted
☼ Special coverage instructions   ◆ Not covered or valid by Medicare   ✳ Carrier discretion

⚙ **A4216** Sterile water, saline and/or dextrose diluent/flush, 10 ml ♿   A

If "incident to" a physican service, do not bill; otherwise, bill DME/MAC.

Other: Broncho Saline, Hyper-Sal, Monoject Prefill advanced, Sodium Chloride, Sodium Chloride Bacteriostatic, Syrex, Vasceze Sodium Chloride, Water for Injection Bacteriostatic

IOM: 100-02, 15, 50

⚙ **A4217** Sterile water/saline, 500 ml ♿   A

If "incident to" a physican service, do not bill; otherwise, bill DME/MAC.

Other: Sodium Chloride

IOM: 100-02, 15, 50

DMEPOS Modifier(s): AU

⚙ **A4218** Sterile saline or water, metered dose dispenser, 10 ml   N1   N

If "incident to" a physican service, do not bill; otherwise, bill DME/MAC.

⚙ **A4220** Refill kit for implantable infusion pump   N1   N

Bill local carrier. Do not report with 95990 or 95991 since Medicare payment for these codes includes the refill kit.

IOM: 100-03, 4, 280.1

✳ **A4221** Supplies for maintenance of drug infusion catheter, per week (list drug separately) `Qp` ♿   Y

If "incident to" a physican service, do not bill; otherwise, bill DME/MAC. Includes dressings for catheter site and flush solutions not directly related to drug infusion

✳ **A4222** Infusion supplies for external drug infusion pump, per cassette or bag (list drug separately) ♿   Y

If "incident to" physician service, do not bill; otherwise bill DME/MAC. Includes cassette or bag, diluting solutions, tubing and/or administration supplies, port cap changes, compounding charges, and preparation charges.

✳ **A4223** Infusion supplies not used with external infusion pump, per cassette or bag (list drugs separately)   E

If "incident to" physician service, do not bill; otherwise bill DME/MAC

IOM: 100-03, 4, 280.1

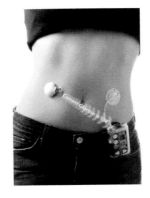

Figure 1 Insulin pump.

⚙ **A4230** Infusion set for external insulin pump, non-needle cannula type   N

If "incident to" physician service, do not bill; otherwise bill DME/MAC. Requires prior authorization and copy of invoice

IOM: 100-03, 4, 280.1

⚙ **A4231** Infusion set for external insulin pump, needle type   N

If "incident to" physician service, do not bill; otherwise bill DME/MAC. Requires prior authorization and copy of invoice

IOM: 100-03, 4, 280.1

◆ **A4232** Syringe with needle for external insulin pump, sterile, 3cc   E

If "incident to" physician service, do not bill; otherwise bill DME/MAC. Reports insulin reservoir for use with external insulin infusion pump (E0784); may be glass or plastic; includes needle for drawing up insulin. Does not include insulin for use in reservoir

IOM: 100-03, 4, 280.1

✳ **A4233** Replacement battery, alkaline (other than J cell), for use with medically necessary home blood glucose monitor owned by patient, each ♿   Y

If "incident to" physician service, do not bill; otherwise bill DME/MAC

DMEPOS Modifier(s): NU   KL

✳ **A4234** Replacement battery, alkaline, J cell, for use with medically necessary home blood glucose monitor owned by patient, each ♿   Y

If "incident to" a physician's service, do not bill; otherwise, bill DME/MAC.

DMEPOS Modifier(s): NU   KL

MEDICAL AND SURGICAL SUPPLIES   A4216 – A4234

✳ **A4235** Replacement battery, lithium, for use with medically necessary home blood glucose monitor owned by patient, each ♿   Y

If "incident to" a physician's service, do not bill; otherwise, bill DME/MAC.

DMEPOS Modifier(s): NU KL

✳ **A4236** Replacement battery, silver oxide, for use with medically necessary home blood glucose monitor owned by patient, each ♿   Y

If "incident to" a physician's service, do not bill; otherwise, bill DME/MAC.

DMEPOS Modifier(s): NU KL

✳ **A4244** Alcohol or peroxide, per pint   E

If "incident to" a physician's service, do not bill; otherwise, bill DME/MAC.

✳ **A4245** Alcohol wipes, per box   E

If "incident to" a physician's service, do not bill; otherwise, bill DME/MAC.

✳ **A4246** Betadine or pHisoHex solution, per pint   E

If "incident to" a physician's service, do not bill; otherwise, bill DME/MAC.

✳ **A4247** Betadine or iodine swabs/wipes, per box   E

If "incident to" a physician's service, do not bill; otherwise, bill DME/MAC.

✳ **A4248** Chlorhexidine containing antiseptic, 1 ml   N1 N

If "incident to" a physician's service, do not bill; otherwise, bill DME/MAC.

◆ **A4250** Urine test or reagent strips or tablets (100 tablets or strips)   E

If "incident to" a physician's service, do not bill; otherwise, bill DME/MAC.

IOM: 100-02, 15, 110

◆ **A4252** Blood ketone test or reagent strip, each   E

Bill DME/MAC

Medicare Statute 1861(n)

✺ **A4253** Blood glucose test or reagent strips for home blood glucose monitor, per 50 strips **Qp** ♿   Y

Bill DME/MAC. Test strips (1 unit = 50 strips); non-insulin treated (every 3 months) 100 test strips (1×/day testing), 100 lancets (1×/day testing); modifier KS

IOM: 100-03, 1, 40.2

DMEPOS Modifier(s): NU KL

✺ **A4255** Platforms for home blood glucose monitor, 50 per box **Qp** ♿   Y

Bill DME/MAC

IOM: 100-03, 1, 40.2

✺ **A4256** Normal, low and high calibrator solution/chips ♿   Y

Bill DME/MAC

IOM: 100-03, 1, 40.2

DMEPOS Modifier(s): KL

✳ **A4257** Replacement lens shield cartridge for use with laser skin piercing device, each ♿   Y

Bill DME/MAC

✺ **A4258** Spring-powered device for lancet, each **Qp** **Qh** ♿   Y

Bill DME/MAC

IOM: 100-03, 1, 40.2

DMEPOS Modifier(s): KL

✺ **A4259** Lancets, per box of 100 **Qp** ♿   Y

Bill DME/MAC

IOM: 100-03, 1, 40.2

DMEPOS Modifier(s): KL

◆ **A4261** Cervical cap for contraceptive use   E

Bill local carrier

Medicare Statute 1862A1 ♀

✺ **A4262** Temporary, absorbable lacrimal duct implant, each   N1 N

Bill local carrier

✺ **A4263** Permanent, long term, non-dissolvable lacrimal duct implant, each   N1 N

Bill local carrier

Bundled if performed in physician office.

IOM: 100-04, 12, 30.4

◆ **A4264** Permanent implantable contraceptive intratubal occlusion device(s) and delivery system ♀   E

Reports the Essure device.

✺ **A4265** Paraffin, per pound ♿   Y

If "incident to" a physician's service, do not bill; otherwise, bill DME/MAC.

IOM: 100-03, 4, 280.1

◆ **A4266** Diaphragm for contraceptive use ♀   E

Bill local carrier

◆ **A4267** Contraceptive supply, condom, male, each ♂   E

Bill local carrier

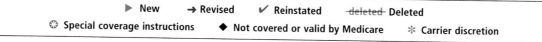

▶ New   → Revised   ✔ Reinstated   ~~deleted~~ Deleted
✺ Special coverage instructions   ◆ Not covered or valid by Medicare   ✳ Carrier discretion

◆ **A4268** Contraceptive supply, condom, female, each ♀   E

Bill local carrier

◆ **A4269** Contraceptive supply, spermicide (e.g., foam, gel), each ♀   E

Bill local carrier

✳ **A4270** Disposable endoscope sheath, each   N1   N

Bill local carrier

✳ **A4280** Adhesive skin support attachment for use with external breast prosthesis, each ♀ ɴ   A

Bill DME/MAC

✳ **A4281** Tubing for breast pump, replacement ♀   E

Bill DME/MAC

✳ **A4282** Adapter for breast pump, replacement ♀   E

Bill DME/MAC

✳ **A4283** Cap for breast pump bottle, replacement ♀   E

Bill DME/MAC

✳ **A4284** Breast shield and splash protector for use with breast pump, replacement ♀   E

Bill DME/MAC

✳ **A4285** Polycarbonate bottle for use with breast pump, replacement ♀   E

Bill DME/MAC

✳ **A4286** Locking ring for breast pump, replacement ♀   E

Bill DME/MAC

✳ **A4290** Sacral nerve stimulation test lead, each   B

Bill local carrier

Vascular Catheters

⚙ **A4300** Implantable access catheter, (e.g., venous, arterial, epidural subarachnoid, or peritoneal, etc.) external access   N1   N

Bill local carrier

IOM: 100-02, 15, 120

✳ **A4301** Implantable access total; catheter, port/reservoir (e.g., venous, arterial, epidural, subarachnoid, peritoneal, etc.)   N1   N

Bill local carrier

✳ **A4305** Disposable drug delivery system, flow rate of 50 ml or greater per hour   N1   N

If "incident to" a physician's service, do not bill; otherwise, bill DME/MAC.

✳ **A4306** Disposable drug delivery system, flow rate of less than 50 ml per hour   N1   N

If "incident to" a physician's service, do not bill; otherwise, bill DME/MAC.

Incontinence Appliances and Care Supplies

A4310-A4355: If provided in the physician's office for a temporary condition, the item is incident to the physician's service and billed to the local carrier. If provided in the physician's office or other place of service for a permanent condition, the item is a prosthetic device and billed to the DME/MAC.

⚙ **A4310** Insertion tray without drainage bag and without catheter (accessories only) ɴ   A

IOM: 100-02, 15, 120

⚙ **A4311** Insertion tray without drainage bag with indwelling catheter, Foley type, two-way latex with coating (Teflon, silicone, silicone elastomer, or hydrophilic, etc.) ɴ   A

IOM: 100-02, 15, 120

⚙ **A4312** Insertion tray without drainage bag with indwelling catheter, Foley type, two-way, all silicone ɴ   A

IOM: 100-02, 15, 120

⚙ **A4313** Insertion tray without drainage bag with indwelling catheter, Foley type, three-way, for continuous irrigation ɴ   A

IOM: 100-02, 15, 120

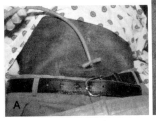
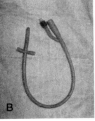

Figure 2 Foley catheter.

MEDICAL AND SURGICAL SUPPLIES   A4268 – A4313

⊛ **A4314** Insertion tray with drainage bag with indwelling catheter, Foley type, two-way latex with coating (Teflon, silicone, silicone elastomer or hydrophilic, etc.)   A

IOM: 100-02, 15, 120

⊛ **A4315** Insertion tray with drainage bag with indwelling catheter, Foley type, two-way, all silicone   A

IOM: 100-02, 15, 120

⊛ **A4316** Insertion tray with drainage bag with indwelling catheter, Foley type, three-way, for continuous irrigation   A

IOM: 100-02, 15, 120

⊛ **A4320** Irrigation tray with bulb or piston syringe, any purpose   A

IOM: 100-02, 15, 120

⊛ **A4321** Therapeutic agent for urinary catheter irrigation   A

⊛ **A4322** Irrigation syringe, bulb, or piston, each   A

IOM: 100-02, 15, 120

⊛ **A4326** Male external catheter with integral collection chamber, any type, each ♂   A

IOM: 100-02, 15, 120

⊛ **A4327** Female external urinary collection device; meatal cup, each ♀   A

IOM: 100-02, 15, 120

⊛ **A4328** Female external urinary collection device; pouch, each ♀   A

IOM: 100-02, 15, 120

⊛ **A4330** Perianal fecal collection pouch with adhesive, each   A

IOM: 100-02, 15, 120

⊛ **A4331** Extension drainage tubing, any type, any length, with connector/adaptor, for use with urinary leg bag or urostomy pouch, each   A

IOM: 100-02, 15, 120

⊛ **A4332** Lubricant, individual sterile packet, each   A

IOM: 100-02, 15, 120

⊛ **A4333** Urinary catheter anchoring device, adhesive skin attachment, each   A

IOM: 100-02, 15, 120

⊛ **A4334** Urinary catheter anchoring device, leg strap, each   A

IOM: 100-02, 15, 120

⊛ **A4335** Incontinence supply; miscellaneous   A

IOM: 100-02, 15, 120

⊛ **A4336** Incontinence supply, urethral insert, any type, each   N1 A

⊛ **A4338** Indwelling catheter; Foley type, two-way latex with coating (Teflon, silicone, silicone elastomer, or hydrophilic, etc.), each   A

IOM: 100-02, 15, 120

⊛ **A4340** Indwelling catheter; specialty type (e.g., coude, mushroom, wing, etc.), each   A

IOM: 100-02, 15, 120

⊛ **A4344** Indwelling catheter, Foley type, two-way, all silicone, each   A

IOM: 100-02, 15, 120

⊛ **A4346** Indwelling catheter; Foley type, three way for continuous irrigation, each   A

IOM: 100-02, 15, 120

⊛ **A4349** Male external catheter, with or without adhesive, disposable, each ♂   A

IOM: 100-02, 15, 120

⊛ **A4351** Intermittent urinary catheter; straight tip, with or without coating (Teflon, silicone, silicone elastomer, or hydrophilic, etc.), each   A

IOM: 100-02, 15, 120

⊛ **A4352** Intermittent urinary catheter; coude (curved) tip, with or without coating (Teflon, silicone, silicone elastomeric, or hydrophilic, etc.), each   A

IOM: 100-02, 15, 120

⊛ **A4353** Intermittent urinary catheter, with insertion supplies   A

IOM: 100-02, 15, 120

⊛ **A4354** Insertion tray with drainage bag but without catheter   A

IOM: 100-02, 15, 120

⊛ **A4355** Irrigation tubing set for continuous bladder irrigation through a three-way indwelling Foley catheter, each   A

IOM: 100-02, 15, 120

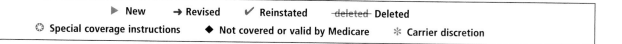

▶ **New**   → **Revised**   ✔ **Reinstated**   ~~deleted~~ **Deleted**

⊛ **Special coverage instructions**   ◆ **Not covered or valid by Medicare**   ✳ **Carrier discretion**

External Urinary Supplies

⊙ **A4356** External urethral clamp or compression device (not to be used for catheter clamp), each ♿ A

If provided in the physician's office for a temporary condition, the item is incident to the physician's service and billed to the local carrier. If provided in the physician's office or other place of service for a permanent condition, the item is a prosthetic device and billed to the DME/MAC.

IOM: 100-02, 15, 120

⊙ **A4357** Bedside drainage bag, day or night, with or without anti-reflux device, with or without tube, each ♿ A

If provided in the physician's office for a temporary condition, the item is incident to the physician's service and billed to the local carrier. If provided in the physician's office or other place of service for a permanent condition, the item is a prosthetic device and billed to the DME/MAC.

IOM: 100-02, 15, 120

⊙ **A4358** Urinary drainage bag, leg or abdomen, vinyl, with or without tube, with straps, each ♿ A

If provided in the physician's office for a temporary condition, the item is incident to the physician's service and billed to the local carrier. If provided in the physician's office or other place of service for a permanent condition, the item is a prosthetic device and billed to the DME/MAC.

IOM: 100-02, 15, 120

⊙ **A4360** Disposable external urethral clamp or compression device, with pad and/or pouch, each ♿ N1 A

Added to the consolidated billing supply code list January 1, 2010.

Ostomy Supplies

A4361-A4434: If provided in the physician's office for a temporary condition, the item is incident to the physician's service and billed to the local carrier. If provided in the physician's office or other place of service for a permanent condition, the item is a prosthetic device and billed to the DME/MAC.

⊙ **A4361** Ostomy faceplate, each ♿ A

IOM: 100-02, 15, 120

⊙ **A4362** Skin barrier; solid, 4 × 4 or equivalent; each ♿ A

IOM: 100-02, 15, 120

⊙ **A4363** Ostomy clamp, any type, replacement only, each ♿ A

⊙ **A4364** Adhesive, liquid or equal, any type, per oz ♿ A

Fee schedule category: Ostomy, tracheostomy, and urologicals items.

IOM: 100-02, 15, 120

✳ **A4366** Ostomy vent, any type, each ♿ A

⊙ **A4367** Ostomy belt, each ♿ A

IOM: 100-02, 15, 120

✳ **A4368** Ostomy filter, any type, each ♿ A

⊙ **A4369** Ostomy skin barrier, liquid (spray, brush, etc), per oz ♿ A

IOM: 100-02, 15, 120

⊙ **A4371** Ostomy skin barrier, powder, per oz ♿ A

IOM: 100-02, 15, 120

⊙ **A4372** Ostomy skin barrier, solid 4 × 4 or equivalent, standard wear, with built-in convexity, each ♿ A

IOM: 100-02, 15, 120

⊙ **A4373** Ostomy skin barrier, with flange (solid, flexible, or accordian), with built-in convexity, any size, each ♿ A

IOM: 100-02, 15, 120

⊙ **A4375** Ostomy pouch, drainable, with faceplate attached, plastic, each ♿ A

IOM: 100-02, 15, 120

⊙ **A4376** Ostomy pouch, drainable, with faceplate attached, rubber, each ♿ A

IOM: 100-02, 15, 120

⊙ **A4377** Ostomy pouch, drainable, for use on faceplate, plastic, each ♿ A

IOM: 100-02, 15, 120

⊙ **A4378** Ostomy pouch, drainable, for use on faceplate, rubber, each ♿ A

IOM: 100-02, 15, 120

⊙ **A4379** Ostomy pouch, urinary, with faceplate attached, plastic, each ♿ A

IOM: 100-02, 15, 120

⊙ **A4380** Ostomy pouch, urinary, with faceplate attached, rubber, each ♿ A

IOM: 100-02, 15, 120

⊙ **A4381** Ostomy pouch, urinary, for use on faceplate, plastic, each ♿ A

IOM: 100-02, 15, 120

⍟ PQRS	**Qp** Quantity Physician Appendix A	**Qh** Quantity Hospital Appendix B	♀ Female only
♂ Male only	**A** Age	♿ DMEPOS	A2-Z3 ASC Payment Indicator	A-Y ASC Status Indicator	Coding Clinic

⊚ **A4382** Ostomy pouch, urinary, for use on faceplate, heavy plastic, each ♿   A

IOM: 100-02, 15, 120

⊚ **A4383** Ostomy pouch, urinary, for use on faceplate, rubber, each ♿   A

IOM: 100-02, 15, 120

⊚ **A4384** Ostomy faceplate equivalent, silicone ring, each ♿   A

IOM: 100-02, 15, 120

⊚ **A4385** Ostomy skin barrier, solid 4 × 4 or equivalent, extended wear, without built-in convexity, each ♿   A

IOM: 100-02, 15, 120

⊚ **A4387** Ostomy pouch closed, with barrier attached, with built-in convexity (1 piece), each ♿   A

IOM: 100-02, 15, 120

⊚ **A4388** Ostomy pouch, drainable, with extended wear barrier attached (1 piece), each ♿   A

IOM: 100-02, 15, 120

⊚ **A4389** Ostomy pouch, drainable, with barrier attached, with built-in convexity (1 piece), each ♿   A

IOM: 100-02, 15, 120

⊚ **A4390** Ostomy pouch, drainable, with extended wear barrier attached, with built-in convexity (1 piece), each ♿   A

IOM: 100-02, 15, 120

⊚ **A4391** Ostomy pouch, urinary, with extended wear barrier attached (1 piece), each ♿   A

IOM: 100-02, 15, 120

⊚ **A4392** Ostomy pouch, urinary, with standard wear barrier attached, with built-in convexity (1 piece), each ♿   A

IOM: 100-02, 15, 120

⊚ **A4393** Ostomy pouch, urinary, with extended wear barrier attached, with built-in convexity (1 piece), each ♿   A

IOM: 100-02, 15, 120

⊚ **A4394** Ostomy deodorant, with or without lubricant, for use in ostomy pouch, per fluid ounce ♿   A

IOM: 100-02, 15, 20

⊚ **A4395** Ostomy deodorant for use in ostomy pouch, solid, per tablet ♿   A

IOM: 100-02, 15, 20

⊚ **A4396** Ostomy belt with peristomal hernia support ♿   A

IOM: 100-02, 15, 120

⊚ **A4397** Irrigation supply; sleeve, each ♿   A

IOM: 100-02, 15, 120

⊚ **A4398** Ostomy irrigation supply; bag, each ♿   A

IOM: 100-02, 15, 120

➜ ⊚ **A4399** Ostomy irrigation supply; cone/catheter, with or without brush ♿   A

IOM: 100-02, 15, 120

⊚ **A4400** Ostomy irrigation set ♿   A

IOM: 100-02, 15, 120

⊚ **A4402** Lubricant, per ounce ♿   A

IOM: 100-02, 15, 120

⊚ **A4404** Ostomy ring, each ♿   A

IOM: 100-02, 15, 120

⊚ **A4405** Ostomy skin barrier, non-pectin based, paste, per ounce ♿   A

IOM: 100-02, 15, 120

⊚ **A4406** Ostomy skin barrier, pectin-based, paste, per ounce ♿   A

IOM: 100-02, 15, 120

⊚ **A4407** Ostomy skin barrier, with flange (solid, flexible, or accordion), extended wear, with built-in convexity, 4 × 4 inches or smaller, each ♿   A

IOM: 100-02, 15, 120

⊚ **A4408** Ostomy skin barrier, with flange (solid, flexible, or accordion), extended wear, with built-in convexity, larger than 4 × 4 inches, each ♿   A

IOM: 100-02, 15, 120

⊚ **A4409** Ostomy skin barrier, with flange (solid, flexible, or accordion), extended wear, without built-in convexity, 4 × 4 inches or smaller, each ♿   A

IOM: 100-02, 15, 120

⊚ **A4410** Ostomy skin barrier, with flange (solid, flexible, or accordion), extended wear, without built-in convexity, larger than 4 × 4 inches, each ♿   A

IOM: 100-02, 15, 120

⊚ **A4411** Ostomy skin barrier, solid 4 × 4 or equivalent, extended wear, with built-in convexity, each ♿   A

⊚ **A4412** Ostomy pouch, drainable, high output, for use on a barrier with flange (2 piece system), without filter, each ♿   A

IOM: 100-02, 15, 120

▶ New   ➜ Revised   ✔ Reinstated   ~~deleted~~ Deleted

⊚ Special coverage instructions   ◆ Not covered or valid by Medicare   ✳ Carrier discretion

⊘ **A4413** Ostomy pouch, drainable, high output, for use on a barrier with flange (2 piece system), with filter, each & ⟍   A

IOM: 100-02, 15, 120

⊘ **A4414** Ostomy skin barrier, with flange (solid, flexible, or accordion), without built-in convexity, 4 × 4 inches or smaller, each &   A

IOM: 100-02, 15, 120

⊘ **A4415** Ostomy skin barrier, with flange (solid, flexible, or accordion), without built-in convexity, larger than 4 × 4 inches, each &   A

IOM: 100-02, 15, 120

∗ **A4416** Ostomy pouch, closed, with barrier attached, with filter (1 piece), each &   A

∗ **A4417** Ostomy pouch, closed, with barrier attached, with built-in convexity, with filter (1 piece), each &   A

∗ **A4418** Ostomy pouch, closed; without barrier attached, with filter (1 piece), each &   A

∗ **A4419** Ostomy pouch, closed; for use on barrier with non-locking flange, with filter (2 piece), each &   A

∗ **A4420** Ostomy pouch, closed; for use on barrier with locking flange (2 piece), each &   A

∗ **A4421** Ostomy supply; miscellaneous   E

⊘ **A4422** Ostomy absorbent material (sheet/pad/crystal packet) for use in ostomy pouch to thicken liquid stomal output, each &   A

IOM: 100-02, 15, 120

∗ **A4423** Ostomy pouch, closed; for use on barrier with locking flange, with filter (2 piece), each &   A

∗ **A4424** Ostomy pouch, drainable, with barrier attached, with filter (1 piece), each &   A

∗ **A4425** Ostomy pouch, drainable; for use on barrier with non-locking flange, with filter (2 piece system), each &   A

∗ **A4426** Ostomy pouch, drainable; for use on barrier with locking flange (2 piece system), each &   A

∗ **A4427** Ostomy pouch, drainable; for use on barrier with locking flange, with filter (2 piece system), each &   A

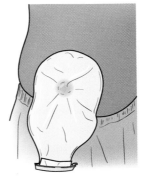

Figure 3 Ostomy pouch.

∗ **A4428** Ostomy pouch, urinary, with extended wear barrier attached, with faucet-type tap with valve (1 piece), each &   A

∗ **A4429** Ostomy pouch, urinary, with barrier attached, with built-in convexity, with faucet-type tap with valve (1 piece), each &   A

∗ **A4430** Ostomy pouch, urinary, with extended wear barrier attached, with built-in convexity, with faucet-type tap with valve (1 piece), each &   A

∗ **A4431** Ostomy pouch, urinary; with barrier attached, with faucet-type tap with valve (1 piece), each &   A

∗ **A4432** Ostomy pouch, urinary; for use on barrier with non-locking flange, with faucet-type tap with valve (2 piece), each &   A

∗ **A4433** Ostomy pouch, urinary; for use on barrier with locking flange (2 piece), each &   A

∗ **A4434** Ostomy pouch, urinary; for use on barrier with locking flange, with faucet-type tap with valve (2 piece), each &   A

Miscellaneous Supplies

⊘ **A4450** Tape, non-waterproof, per 18 square inches &   A

If "incident to" physician service, do not bill separately; otherwise bill DME/MAC. If used with surgical dressings, billed with AW modifier (in addition to appropriate A1-A9 modifier).

IOM: 100-02, 15, 120

DMEPOS Modifier(s): AU, AV, AW

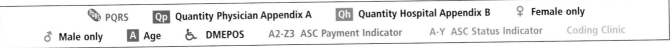

ⓅQRS PQRS	Qp Quantity Physician Appendix A	Qh Quantity Hospital Appendix B		♀ Female only
♂ Male only	A Age	& DMEPOS	A2-Z3 ASC Payment Indicator A-Y ASC Status Indicator	Coding Clinic

⊘ **A4452** Tape, waterproof, per 18 square inches ⅃   A

If "incident to" physician service, do not bill separately; otherwise, bill DME/MAC. If used with surgical dressings, billed with AW modifier (in addition to appropriate A1-A9 modifier).

IOM: 100-02, 15, 120

DMEPOS Modifier(s): AU, AV, AW

⊘ **A4455** Adhesive remover or solvent (for tape, cement or other adhesive), per ounce ⅃   A

If "incident to" a physician service, do not bill; otherwise, bill DME/MAC.

IOM: 100-02, 15, 120

⊘ **A4456** Adhesive remover, wipes, any type, each ⅃   A

Added to the consolidated billing supply code list January 1, 2010. May be reimbursed for male or female clients to home health DME providers and DME medical suppliers in the home setting.

✳ **A4458** Enema bag with tubing, reusable   E

Bill DME/MAC

✳ **A4461** Surgical dressing holder, non-reusable, each ⅃   A

If "incident to" a physician's service, do not bill; otherwise, bill DME/MAC.

✳ **A4463** Surgical dressing holder, reusable, each ⅃   A

If "incident to" a physician's service, do not bill; otherwise, bill DME/MAC.

✳ **A4465** Non-elastic binder for extremity   N

Bill DME/MAC

◆ **A4466** Garment, belt, sleeve or other covering, elastic or similar stretchable material, any type, each   N1   E

⊘ **A4470** Gravlee jet washer `Qp` `Qh`   N

Bill local carrier

IOM: 100-02, 16, 90; 100-03, 4, 230.5

⊘ **A4480** VABRA aspirator `Qp` `Qh`   N

Bill local carrier

IOM: 100-02, 16, 90; 100-03, 4, 230.6

⊘ **A4481** Tracheostoma filter, any type, any size, each ⅃   A

If "incident to" a physician's service, do not bill; otherwise, bill DME/MAC.

IOM: 100-02, 15, 120

⊘ **A4483** Moisture exchanger, disposable, for use with invasive mechanical ventilation ⅃   A

Bill DME/MAC

IOM: 100-02, 15, 120

◆ **A4490** Surgical stockings above knee length, each   E

Bill DME/MAC

IOM: 100-02, 15, 100; 100-02, 15, 110; 100-03, 4, 280.1

◆ **A4495** Surgical stockings thigh length, each   E

Bill DME/MAC

IOM: 100-02, 15, 100; 100-02, 15, 110; 100-03, 4, 280.1

◆ **A4500** Surgical stockings below knee length, each   E

Bill DME/MAC

IOM: 100-02, 15, 100; 100-02, 15, 110; 100-03, 4, 280.1

◆ **A4510** Surgical stockings full length, each   E

Bill DME/MAC

IOM: 100-02, 15, 100; 100-02, 15, 110; 100-03, 4, 280.1

◆ **A4520** Incontinence garment, any type, (e.g. brief, diaper), each   E

Bill DME/MAC

IOM: 100-03, 4, 280.1

⊘ **A4550** Surgical trays   B

Bill local carrier. No longer payable by Medicare; included in practice expense for procedures. Some private payers may pay, most private payers follow Medicare guidelines

IOM: 100-04, 12, 20.3, 30.4

◆ **A4554** Disposable underpads, all sizes   E

Bill DME/MAC

IOM: 100-02, 15, 120; 100-03, 4, 280.1

✳ **A4556** Electrodes, (e.g., apnea monitor), per pair ⅃   Y

If "incident to" a physician's service, do not bill; otherwise, bill DME/MAC.

✳ **A4557** Lead wires, (e.g., apnea monitor), per pair `Qp` `Qh` ⅃   Y

If "incident to" a physician's service, do not bill; otherwise, bill DME/MAC.

▶ New   → Revised   ✔ Reinstated   ~~deleted~~ Deleted

⊘ Special coverage instructions   ◆ Not covered or valid by Medicare   ✳ Carrier discretion

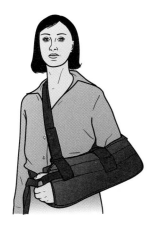

Figure 4 Arm sling.

* **A4558** Conductive gel or paste, for use with electrical device (e.g., TENS, NMES), per oz ♿   Y

If "incident to" a physician's service, do not bill; otherwise, bill DME/MAC.

* **A4559** Coupling gel or paste, for use with ultrasound device, per oz ♿   Y

If "incident to" a physician's service, do not bill; otherwise, bill DME/MAC.

* **A4561** Pessary, rubber, any type Qp Qh ♀ ♿   N

Bill local carrier

* **A4562** Pessary, non rubber, any type Qp Qh ♀ ♿   N

Bill local carrier

* **A4565** Slings   N

Bill local carrier

▶ ◆ **A4566** Shoulder sling or vest design, abduction restrainer, with or without swathe control, prefabricated, includes fitting and adjustment   E

◆ **A4570** Splint   E

Bill local carrier

IOM: 100-02, 6, 10; 100-02, 15, 100; 100-04, 4, 240

◆ **A4575** Topical hyperbaric oxygen chamber, disposable   E

Bill DME/MAC

IOM: 100-03, 1, 20.29

◆ **A4580** Cast supplies (e.g. plaster)   E

Bill local carrier

IOM: 100-02, 6, 10; 100-02, 15, 100; 100-04, 4, 240

◆ **A4590** Special casting material (e.g. fiberglass)   E

Bill local carrier

IOM: 100-02, 6, 10; 100-02, 15, 100; 100-04, 4, 240

☺ **A4595** Electrical stimulator supplies, 2 lead, per month, (e.g. TENS, NMES) ♿   Y

If "incident to" a physician's service, do not bill; otherwise, bill DME/MAC.

IOM: 100-03, 2, 160.13

* **A4600** Sleeve for intermittent limb compression device, replacement only, each   Y

Bill DME/MAC

* **A4601** Lithium ion battery for non-prosthetic use, replacement   Y

Bill DME/MAC

* **A4604** Tubing with integrated heating element for use with positive airway pressure device ♿   Y

Bill DME/MAC

DMEPOS Modifier(s): NU

* **A4605** Tracheal suction catheter, closed system, each ♿   Y

Bill DME/MAC

DMEPOS Modifier(s): NU

* **A4606** Oxygen probe for use with oximeter device, replacement   A

Bill DME/MAC

* **A4608** Transtracheal oxygen catheter, each ♿   Y

Bill DME/MAC

Supplies for Respiratory and Oxygen Equipment

* **A4611** Battery, heavy duty; replacement for patient owned ventilator ♿   Y

Bill DME/MAC

DMEPOS Modifier(s): NU, RR, UE

* **A4612** Battery cables; replacement for patient-owned ventilator ♿   Y

Bill DME/MAC

DMEPOS Modifier(s): NU, RR, UE

* **A4613** Battery charger; replacement for patient-owned ventilator ♿   Y

Bill DME/MAC

DMEPOS Modifier(s): NU, RR, UE

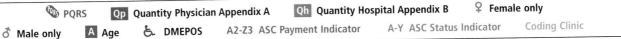

PQRS PQRS	Qp Quantity Physician Appendix A	Qh Quantity Hospital Appendix B	♀ Female only
♂ Male only	A Age ♿ DMEPOS	A2-Z3 ASC Payment Indicator	A-Y ASC Status Indicator Coding Clinic

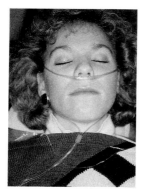

Figure 5 Nasal cannula.

* **A4614** Peak expiratory flow rate meter, hand held `Qp` `Qh` ♿   Y

If "incident to" a physician's service, do not bill; otherwise, bill DME/MAC.

☼ **A4615** Cannula, nasal ♿   Y

If "incident to" a physician's service, do not bill; otherwise, bill DME/MAC.

IOM: 100-03, 2, 160.6; 100-04, 20, 100.2

☼ **A4616** Tubing (oxygen), per foot ♿   Y

If "incident to" a physician's service, do not bill; otherwise, bill DME/MAC.

IOM: 100-03, 2, 160.6; 100-04, 20, 100.2

☼ **A4617** Mouth piece ♿   Y

If "incident to" a physician's service, do not bill; otherwise, bill DME/MAC.

IOM: 100-03, 2, 160.6; 100-04, 20, 100.2

☼ **A4618** Breathing circuits ♿   Y

If "incident to" a physician's service, do not bill; otherwise, bill DME/MAC.

IOM: 100-03, 2, 160.6; 100-04, 20, 100.2

DMEPOS Modifier(s): NU, RR, UE

→ ☼ **A4619** Face tent ♿   Y

If "incident to" a physician's service, do not bill; otherwise, bill DME/MAC.

IOM: 100-03, 2, 160.6; 100-04, 20, 100.2

DMEPOS Modifier(s): NU

☼ **A4620** Variable concentration mask ♿   Y

If "incident to" a physician's service, do not bill; otherwise, bill DME/MAC.

IOM: 100-03, 2, 160.6; 100-04, 20, 100.2

☼ **A4623** Tracheostomy, inner cannula ♿   A

If "incident to" a physician's service, do not bill; otherwise, bill DME/MAC.

IOM: 100-02, 15, 120; 100-03, 1, 20.9

* **A4624** Tracheal suction catheter, any type, other than closed system, each ♿   Y

If "incident to" a physician's service, do not bill; otherwise, bill DME/MAC.

DMEPOS Modifier(s): NU

Sterile suction catheters are medically necessary only for tracheostomy suctioning. Limitations include three suction catheters per day when covered for medically necessary tracheostomy suctioning. Assign DX V44.0 or V55.0 on the claim form. (CMS Manual System, Pub. 100-3, NCD manual, Chapter 1, Section 280-1)

☼ **A4625** Tracheostomy care kit for new tracheostomy ♿   A

If "incident to" a physician's service, do not bill; otherwise, bill DME/MAC.

IOM: 100-02, 15, 120

Dressings used with tracheostomies are included in the allowance for the code. This starter kit is covered after a surgical tracheostomy. (https://www.noridianmedicare.com/dme/coverage/docs/lcds/current_lcds/tracheostomy_care_supplies.htm)

☼ **A4626** Tracheostomy cleaning brush, each ♿   A

If "incident to" a physician's service, do not bill; otherwise, bill DME/MAC.

IOM: 100-02, 15, 120

◆ **A4627** Spacer, bag, or reservoir, with or without mask, for use with metered dose inhaler   E

If "incident to" a physician's service, do not bill; otherwise, bill DME/MAC.

IOM: 100-02, 15, 110

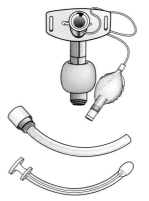

Figure 6 Tracheostomy cannula.

▶ New   → Revised   ✔ Reinstated   ~~deleted~~ Deleted

☼ Special coverage instructions   ◆ Not covered or valid by Medicare   ✳ Carrier discretion

✱ **A4628**   Oropharyngeal suction catheter, each ♿   Y

If "incident to" a physician's service, do not bill; otherwise, bill DME/MAC.

DMEPOS Modifier(s): NU

No more than three catheters per week are covered for medically necessary oropharyngeal suctioning because the catheters can be reused if cleansed and disinfected. (MS Manual System, Pub. 100-3, NCD manual, Chapter 1, Section 280-1)

✿ **A4629**   Tracheostomy care kit for established tracheostomy ♿   A

If "incident to" a physician's service, do not bill; otherwise, bill DME/MAC.

IOM: 100-02, 15, 120

DMEPOS Modifier(s): NU

Supplies for Other Durable Medical Equipment

A4630-A4640:   Bill DME/MAC

✿ **A4630**   Replacement batteries, medically necessary, transcutaneous electrical stimulator, owned by patient ♿   Y

IOM: 100-03, 3, 160.7

✱ **A4633**   Replacement bulb/lamp for ultraviolet light therapy system, each ♿   Y

DMEPOS Modifier(s): NU

✱ **A4634**   Replacement bulb for therapeutic light box, tabletop model   A

✿ **A4635**   Underarm pad, crutch, replacement, each ♿   Y

IOM: 100-03, 4, 280.1

DMEPOS Modifier(s): NU, RR, UE

✿ **A4636**   Replacement, handgrip, cane, crutch, or walker, each ♿   Y

IOM: 100-03, 4, 280.1

DMEPOS Modifier(s): NU, KE, RR, UE

✿ **A4637**   Replacement, tip, cane, crutch, walker, each ♿   Y

IOM: 100-03, 4, 280.1

DMEPOS Modifier(s): NU, KE, RR, UE

✱ **A4638**   Replacement battery for patient-owned ear pulse generator, each ♿   Y

DMEPOS Modifier(s): NU, RR, UE

✱ **A4639**   Replacement pad for infrared heating pad system, each ♿   Y

DMEPOS Modifier(s): NU

✿ **A4640**   Replacement pad for use with medically necessary alternating pressure pad owned by patient `Qp` `Qh` ♿   Y

IOM: 100-03, 4, 280.1; 100-08, 5, 5.2.3

DMEPOS Modifier(s): NU, RR, UE

Supplies for Radiological Procedures

✱ **A4641**   Radiopharmaceutical, diagnostic, not otherwise classified   N1   N

Bill local carrier. Is not an applicable tracer for PET scans

✱ **A4642**   Indium In-111 satumomab pendetide, diagnostic, per study dose, up to 6 millicuries `Qp` `Qh`   N1   N

Bill local carrier

Miscellaneous Supplies

✱ **A4648**   Tissue marker, implantable, any type, each   N1   N

Bill local carrier

✱ **A4649**   Surgical supply; miscellaneous   N

Bill local carrier if incident to a physician's service (not separately payable) or if supply for implanted prosthetic device or implanted DME. If other, bill DME/MAC.

✱ **A4650**   Implantable radiation dosimeter, each `Qp` `Qh`   N1   N

Bill local carrier

✿ **A4651**   Calibrated microcapillary tube, each   A

Bill DME/MAC

IOM: 100-04, 3, 40.3

✿ **A4652**   Microcapillary tube sealant   A

Bill DME/MAC

IOM: 100-04, 3, 40.3

Supplies for Dialysis

A4653-A4932:   Bill DME/MAC

✱ **A4653**   Peritoneal dialysis catheter anchoring device, belt, each   A

✿ **A4657**   Syringe, with or without needle, each   N

IOM: 100-04, 8, 90.3.2

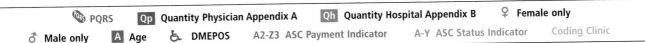

⊕ **A4660** Sphygmomanometer/blood pressure apparatus with cuff and stethoscope `Qp` `Qh`   N

IOM: 100-04, 8, 90.3.2

⊕ **A4663** Blood pressure cuff only `Qp` `Qh`   N

IOM: 100-04, 8, 90.3.2

◆ **A4670** Automatic blood pressure monitor   E

IOM: 100-04, 8, 90.3.2

⊕ **A4671** Disposable cycler set used with cycler dialysis machine, each   B

IOM: 100-04, 8, 90.3.2

⊕ **A4672** Drainage extension line, sterile, for dialysis, each   B

IOM: 100-04, 8, 90.3.2

⊕ **A4673** Extension line with easy lock connectors, used with dialysis   B

IOM: 100-04, 8, 90.3.2

⊕ **A4674** Chemicals/antiseptics solution used to clean/sterilize dialysis equipment, per 8 oz   B

IOM: 100-04, 8, 90.3.2

⊕ **A4680** Activated carbon filters for hemodialysis, each   N

IOM: 100-04, 8, 90.3.2

⊕ **A4690** Dialyzers (artificial kidneys), all types, all sizes, for hemodialysis, each   N

IOM: 100-04, 8, 90.3.2

⊕ **A4706** Bicarbonate concentrate, solution, for hemodialysis, per gallon   N

IOM: 100-04, 8, 90.3.2

⊕ **A4707** Bicarbonate concentrate, powder, for hemodialysis, per packet   N

IOM: 100-04, 8, 90.3.2

⊕ **A4708** Acetate concentrate solution, for hemodialysis, per gallon   N

IOM: 100-04, 8, 90.3.2

⊕ **A4709** Acid concentrate, solution, for hemodialysis, per gallon   N

IOM: 100-04, 8, 90.3.2

⊕ **A4714** Treated water (deionized, distilled, or reverse osmosis) for peritoneal dialysis, per gallon   N

IOM: 100-03, 4, 230.7; 100-04, 3, 40.3

⊕ **A4719** "Y set" tubing for peritoneal dialysis   N

IOM: 100-04, 8, 90.3.2

⊕ **A4720** Dialysate solution, any concentration of dextrose, fluid volume greater than 249cc, but less than or equal to 999cc, for peritoneal dialysis   N

Do not use AX modifier

IOM: 100-04, 8, 90.3.2

⊕ **A4721** Dialysate solution, any concentration of dextrose, fluid volume greater than 999cc but less than or equal to 1999cc, for peritoneal dialysis   N

IOM: 100-04, 8, 90.3.2

⊕ **A4722** Dialysate solution, any concentration of dextrose, fluid volume greater than 1999cc but less than or equal to 2999cc, for peritoneal dialysis   N

IOM: 100-04, 8, 90.3.2

⊕ **A4723** Dialysate solution, any concentration of dextrose, fluid volume greater than 2999cc but less than or equal to 3999cc, for peritoneal dialysis   N

IOM: 100-04, 8, 90.3.2

⊕ **A4724** Dialysate solution, any concentration of dextrose, fluid volume greater than 3999cc but less than or equal to 4999cc for peritoneal dialysis   N

IOM: 100-04, 8, 90.3.2

⊕ **A4725** Dialysate solution, any concentration of dextrose, fluid volume greater than 4999cc but less than or equal to 5999cc, for peritoneal dialysis   N

IOM: 100-04, 8, 90.3.2

⊕ **A4726** Dialysate solution, any concentration of dextrose, fluid volume greater than 5999cc, for peritoneal dialysis   N

IOM: 100-04, 8, 90.3.2

✳ **A4728** Dialysate solution, non-dextrose containing, 500 ml   B

⊕ **A4730** Fistula cannulation set for hemodialysis, each   N

IOM: 100-04, 8, 90.3.2

⊕ **A4736** Topical anesthetic, for dialysis, per gram   N

IOM: 100-04, 8, 90.3.2

⊕ **A4737** Injectable anesthetic, for dialysis, per 10 ml   N

IOM: 100-04, 8, 90.3.2

⊕ **A4740** Shunt accessory, for hemodialysis, any type, each   N

IOM: 100-04, 8, 90.3.2

⊕ **A4750** Blood tubing, arterial or venous, for hemodialysis, each   N

IOM: 100-04, 8, 90.3.2

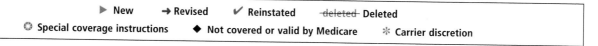

▶ New   → Revised   ✔ Reinstated   ~~deleted~~ Deleted
⊕ Special coverage instructions   ◆ Not covered or valid by Medicare   ✳ Carrier discretion

A4755 Blood tubing, arterial and venous combined, for hemodialysis, each   N

IOM: 100-04, 8, 90.3.2

A4760 Dialysate solution test kit, for peritoneal dialysis, any type, each   N

IOM: 100-04, 8, 90.3.2

A4765 Dialysate concentrate, powder, additive for peritoneal dialysis, per packet   N

IOM: 100-04, 8, 90.3.2

A4766 Dialysate concentrate, solution, additive for peritoneal dialysis, per 10 ml   N

IOM: 100-04, 8, 90.3.2

A4770 Blood collection tube, vacuum, for dialysis, per 50   N

IOM: 100-04, 8, 90.3.2

A4771 Serum clotting time tube, for dialysis, per 50   N

IOM: 100-04, 8, 90.3.2

A4772 Blood glucose test strips, for dialysis, per 50   N

IOM: 100-04, 8, 90.3.2

A4773 Occult blood test strips, for dialysis, per 50   N

IOM: 100-04, 8, 90.3.2

A4774 Ammonia test strips, for dialysis, per 50   N

IOM: 100-04, 8, 90.3.2

A4802 Protamine sulfate, for hemodialysis, per 50 mg   N

IOM: 100-04, 8, 90.3.2

A4860 Disposable catheter tips for peritoneal dialysis, per 10   N

IOM: 100-04, 8, 90.3.2

A4870 Plumbing and/or electrical work for home hemodialysis equipment   N

IOM: 100-04, 8, 90.3.2

A4890 Contracts, repair and maintenance, for hemodialysis equipment   N

IOM: 100-02, 15, 110.2

A4911 Drain bag/bottle, for dialysis, each   N

A4913 Miscellaneous dialysis supplies, not otherwise specified   N

Items not related to dialysis must not be billed with the miscellaneous codes A4913 or E1699.

A4918 Venous pressure clamp, for hemodialysis, each   N

A4927 Gloves, non-sterile, per 100   N

A4928 Surgical mask, per 20   N

A4929 Tourniquet for dialysis, each   N

A4930 Gloves, sterile, per pair   N

✳ A4931 Oral thermometer, reusable, any type, each   N

✳ A4932 Rectal thermometer, reusable, any type, each   E

Additional Ostomy Supplies

A5051-A5093: If provided in the physician's office for a temporary condition, the item is incident to the physician's service and billed to the local carrier. If provided in the physician's office or other place of service for a permanent condition, the item is a prosthetic device and billed to the DME/MAC.

A5051 Ostomy pouch, closed; with barrier attached (1 piece), each ⅃   A

IOM: 100-02, 15, 120

A5052 Ostomy pouch, closed; without barrier attached (1 piece), each ⅃   A

IOM: 100-02, 15, 120

A5053 Ostomy pouch, closed; for use on faceplate, each ⅃   A

IOM: 100-02, 15, 120

A5054 Ostomy pouch, closed; for use on barrier with flange (2 piece), each ⅃   A

IOM: 100-02, 15, 120

A5055 Stoma cap ⅃   A

IOM: 100-02, 15, 120

▶ **A5056** Ostomy pouch, drainable, with extended wear barrier attached, with filter, (1 piece), each   A

IOM: 100-02, 15, 120

▶ **A5057** Ostomy pouch, drainable, with extended wear barrier attached, with built in convexity, with filter, (1 piece), each   A

IOM: 100-02, 15, 120

✳ A5061 Ostomy pouch, drainable; with barrier attached, (1 piece), each ⅃   A

IOM: 100-02, 15, 120

A5062 Ostomy pouch, drainable; without barrier attached (1 piece), each ⅃   A

IOM: 100-02, 15, 120

A5063 Ostomy pouch, drainable; for use on barrier with flange (2 piece system), each ⅃   A

IOM: 100-02, 15, 120

ⓟ PQRS	Qp Quantity Physician Appendix A	Qh Quantity Hospital Appendix B	♀ Female only
♂ Male only A Age ⅃ DMEPOS A2-Z3 ASC Payment Indicator A-Y ASC Status Indicator Coding Clinic			

MEDICAL AND SURGICAL SUPPLIES   A4755 – A5063

103

⊛ **A5071**   Ostomy pouch, urinary; with barrier attached (1 piece), each ♿   A

IOM: 100-02, 15, 120

⊛ **A5072**   Ostomy pouch, urinary; without barrier attached (1 piece), each ♿   A

IOM: 100-02, 15, 120

⊛ **A5073**   Ostomy pouch, urinary; for use on barrier with flange (2 piece), each ♿   A

IOM: 100-02, 15, 120

⊛ **A5081**   Continent device; plug for continent stoma ♿   A

IOM: 100-02, 15, 120

⊛ **A5082**   Continent device; catheter for continent stoma ♿   A

IOM: 100-02, 15, 120

＊ **A5083**   Continent device, stoma absorptive cover for continent stoma ♿   A

⊛ **A5093**   Ostomy accessory; convex insert ♿   A

IOM: 100-02, 15, 120

Additional Incontinence Appliances/Supplies

A5102-A5114:   If provided in the physician's office for a temporary condition, the item is incident to the physician's service and billed to the local carrier. If provided in the physician's office or other place of service for a permanent condition, the item is a prosthetic device and billed to the DME/MAC.

⊛ **A5102**   Bedside drainage bottle with or without tubing, rigid or expandable, each ♿   A

IOM: 100-02, 15, 120

⊛ **A5105**   Urinary suspensory, with leg bag, with or without tube, each ♿   A

IOM: 100-02, 15, 120

➔ ⊛ **A5112**   Urinary drainage bag, leg bag, leg or abdomen, latex, with or without tube, with straps, each ♿   A

IOM: 100-02, 15, 120

⊛ **A5113**   Leg strap; latex, replacement only, per set ♿   A

IOM: 100-02, 15, 120

⊛ **A5114**   Leg strap; foam or fabric, replacement only, per set ♿   A

IOM: 100-02, 15, 120

Supplies for Either Incontinence or Ostomy Appliances

A5120-A5200:   If provided in the physician's office for a temporary condition, the item is incident to the physician's service and billed to the local carrier. If provided in the physician's office or other place of service for a permanent condition, the item is a prosthetic device and billed to the DME/MAC.

⊛ **A5120**   Skin barrier, wipes or swabs, each ♿   A

IOM: 100-02, 15, 120

DMEPOS Modifier(s): AU, AV

⊛ **A5121**   Skin barrier; solid, 6×6 or equivalent, each ♿   A

IOM: 100-02, 15, 120

⊛ **A5122**   Skin barrier; solid, 8×8 or equivalent, each ♿   A

IOM: 100-02, 15, 120

⊛ **A5126**   Adhesive or non-adhesive; disk or foam pad ♿   A

IOM: 100-02, 15, 120

⊛ **A5131**   Appliance cleaner, incontinence and ostomy appliances, per 16 oz ♿   A

IOM: 100-02, 15, 120

⊛ **A5200**   Percutaneous catheter/tube anchoring device, adhesive skin attachment ♿   A

IOM: 100-02, 15, 120

Diabetic Shoes, Fitting, and Modifications

A5500-A5513:   Bill DME/MAC

⊛ **A5500**   For diabetics only, fitting (including follow-up), custom preparation and supply of off-the-shelf depth-inlay shoe manufactured to accommodate multi-density insert(s), per shoe **Qp** **Qh** ♿   Y

IOM: 100-02, 15, 140

⊛ **A5501**   For diabetics only, fitting (including follow-up), custom preparation and supply of shoe molded from cast(s) of patient's foot (custom-molded shoe), per shoe **Qp** **Qh** ♿   Y

Covered when patient has foot deformity that cannot be accommodated by depth shoe

IOM: 100-02, 15, 140

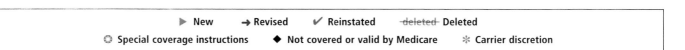

▶ New   ➔ Revised   ✔ Reinstated   ~~deleted~~ Deleted
⊛ Special coverage instructions   ◆ Not covered or valid by Medicare   ＊ Carrier discretion

⚙ **A5503**　For diabetics only, modification (including fitting) of off-the-shelf depth-inlay shoe or custom-molded shoe with roller or rigid rocker bottom, per shoe `Qp` `Qh` ☇ 　　　　Y

IOM: 100-02, 15, 140

⚙ **A5504**　For diabetics only, modification (including fitting) of off-the-shelf depth-inlay shoe or custom-molded shoe with wedge(s), per shoe `Qp` `Qh` ☇ 　　　　Y

IOM: 100-02, 15, 140

⚙ **A5505**　For diabetics only, modification (including fitting) of off-the-shelf depth-inlay shoe or custom-molded shoe with metatarsal bar, per shoe `Qp` `Qh` ☇ 　　　　Y

IOM: 100-02, 15, 140

⚙ **A5506**　For diabetics only, modification (including fitting) of off-the-shelf depth-inlay shoe or custom-molded shoe with off-set heel(s), per shoe `Qp` `Qh` ☇ 　　　　Y

IOM: 100-02, 15, 140

⚙ **A5507**　For diabetics only, not otherwise specified modification (including fitting) of off-the-shelf depth-inlay shoe or custom-molded shoe, per shoe `Qp` `Qh` ☇ 　　　　Y

Only used for not otherwise specified therapeutic modifications to shoe or for repairs to a diabetic shoe(s)

IOM: 100-02, 15, 140

⚙ **A5508**　For diabetics only, deluxe feature of off-the-shelf depth-inlay shoe or custom-molded shoe, per shoe `Qp` 　　　　Y

⚙ **A5510**　For diabetics only, direct formed, compression molded to patient's foot without external heat source, multiple-density insert(s) prefabricated, per shoe `Qp` 　　　　E

IOM: 100-02, 15, 140

✳ **A5512**　For diabetics only, multiple density insert, direct formed, molded to foot after external heat source of 230 degrees Fahrenheit or higher, total contact with patient's foot, including arch, base layer minimum of 1/4 inch material of shore a 35 durometer or 3/16 inch material of shore a 40 durometer (or higher), prefabricated, each ☇ 　　　　Y

✳ **A5513**　For diabetics only, multiple density insert, custom molded from model of patient's foot, total contact with patient's foot, including arch, base layer minimum of 3/16 inch material of shore a 35 durometer (or higher), includes arch filler and other shaping material, custom fabricated, each ☇ 　　　　Y

Dressings

A6010-A6512:　Bill local carrier if incident to a physician's service (not separately payable) or if supply for implanted prosthetic device or implanted DME. If other, bill DME/MAC.

◆ **A6000**　Non-contact wound warming wound cover for use with the non-contact wound warming device and warming card 　　　　E

Bill DME/MAC

IOM: 100-02, 16, 20

⚙ **A6010**　Collagen based wound filler, dry form, sterile, per gram of collagen ☇ 　　　　A

IOM: 100-02, 15, 100

→ ⚙ **A6011**　Collagen based wound filler, gel/paste, per gram of collagen ☇ 　　　　A

IOM: 100-02, 15, 100

⚙ **A6021**　Collagen dressing, sterile, pad size 16 sq. in. or less, each ☇ 　　　　A

IOM: 100-02, 15, 100

⚙ **A6022**　Collagen dressing, sterile, pad size more than 16 sq. in. but less than or equal to 48 sq. in., each ☇ 　　　　A

IOM: 100-02, 15, 100

⚙ **A6023**　Collagen dressing, sterile, pad size more than 48 sq. in., each ☇ 　　　　A

IOM: 100-02, 15, 100

⚙ **A6024**　Collagen dressing wound filler, sterile, per 6 inches ☇ 　　　　A

IOM: 100-02, 15, 100

✳ **A6025**　Gel sheet for dermal or epidermal application, (e.g., silicone, hydrogel, other), each 　　　　E

Only for gel sheets for treatment of keloids or other scars

If used for the treatment of keloids or other scars, a silicone gel sheet will not meet the definition of the surgical dressing benefit and will be denied as noncovered.

⚙ **A6154** Wound pouch, each ♿ A

Waterproof collection device with drainable port that adheres to skin around wound. Usual dressing change is up to 3 × per week.

IOM: 100-02, 15, 100

⚙ **A6196** Alginate or other fiber gelling dressing, wound cover, sterile, pad size 16 sq. in. or less, each dressing ♿ A

IOM: 100-02, 15, 100

⚙ **A6197** Alginate or other fiber gelling dressing, wound cover, sterile, pad size more than 16 sq. in., but less than or equal to 48 sq. in., each dressing ♿ A

IOM: 100-02, 15, 100

⚙ **A6198** Alginate or other fiber gelling dressing, wound cover, sterile, pad size more than 48 sq. in., each dressing A

IOM: 100-02, 15, 100

⚙ **A6199** Alginate or other fiber gelling dressing, wound filler, sterile, per 6 inches ♿ A

IOM: 100-02, 15, 100

⚙ **A6203** Composite dressing, sterile, pad size 16 sq. in. or less, with any size adhesive border, each dressing ♿ A

Usual composite dressing change is up to 3 times per week, one wound cover per dressing change.

IOM: 100-02, 15, 100

⚙ **A6204** Composite dressing, sterile, pad size more than 16 sq. in. but less than or equal to 48 sq. in., with any size adhesive border, each dressing ♿ A

Usual composite dressing change is up to 3 times per week, one wound cover per dressing change.

IOM: 100-02, 15, 100

⚙ **A6205** Composite dressing, sterile, pad size more than 48 sq. in., with any size adhesive border, each dressing A

Usual composite dressing change is up to 3 times per week, one wound cover per dressing change.

IOM: 100-02, 15, 100

⚙ **A6206** Contact layer, sterile, 16 sq. in. or less, each dressing A

Contact layers are porous to allow wound fluid to pass through for absorption by separate overlying dressing and are not intended to be changed with each dressing change. Usual dressing change is up to once per week.

IOM: 100-02, 15, 100

⚙ **A6207** Contact layer, sterile, more than 16 sq. in. but less than or equal to 48 sq. in., each dressing ♿ A

Contact layer dressings are used to line the entire wound; they are not intended to be changed with each dressing change. Usual dressing change is up to once per week.

IOM: 100-02, 15, 100

⚙ **A6208** Contact layer, sterile, more than 48 sq. in., each dressing A

Contact layer dressings are used to line the entire wound; they are not intended to be changed with each dressing change. Usual dressing change is up to once per week.

IOM: 100-02, 15, 100

⚙ **A6209** Foam dressing, wound cover, sterile, pad size 16 sq. in. or less, without adhesive border, each dressing ♿ A

Made of open cell, medical grade expanded polymer; with nonadherent property over wound site

IOM: 100-02, 15, 100

⚙ **A6210** Foam dressing, wound cover, sterile, pad size more than 16 sq. in. but less than or equal to 48 sq. in., without adhesive border, each dressing ♿ A

Foam dressings are covered items when used on full thickness wounds (e.g., stage III or IV ulcers) with moderate to heavy exudates. Usual dressing change for a foam wound cover when used as primary dressing is up to 3 times per week. When foam wound cover is used as a secondary dressing for wounds with very heavy exudates, dressing change may be up to 3 times per week. Usual dressing change for foam wound fillers is up to once per day (A6209-A6215).

IOM: 100-02, 15, 100

▶ New → Revised ✔ Reinstated ~~deleted~~ Deleted
⚙ Special coverage instructions ◆ Not covered or valid by Medicare ✳ Carrier discretion

⊚ **A6211** Foam dressing, wound cover, sterile, pad size more than 48 sq. in., without adhesive border, each dressing ♿   A

IOM: 100-02, 15, 100

⊚ **A6212** Foam dressing, wound cover, sterile, pad size 16 sq. in. or less, with any size adhesive border, each dressing ♿   A

IOM: 100-02, 15, 100

⊚ **A6213** Foam dressing, wound cover, sterile, pad size more than 16 sq. in. but less than or equal to 48 sq. in., with any size adhesive border, each dressing   A

IOM: 100-02, 15, 100

⊚ **A6214** Foam dressing, wound cover, sterile, pad size more than 48 sq. in., with any size adhesive border, each dressing ♿   A

IOM: 100-02, 15, 100

⊚ **A6215** Foam dressing, wound filler, sterile, per gram   A

IOM: 100-02, 15, 100

⊚ **A6216** Gauze, non-impregnated, non-sterile, pad size 16 sq. in. or less, without adhesive border, each dressing ♿   A

IOM: 100-02, 15, 100

⊚ **A6217** Gauze, non-impregnated, non-sterile, pad size more than 16 sq. in. but less than or equal to 48 sq. in., without adhesive border, each dressing ♿   A

IOM: 100-02, 15, 100

⊚ **A6218** Gauze, non-impregnated, non-sterile, pad size more than 48 sq. in., without adhesive border, each dressing   A

IOM: 100-02, 15, 100

⊚ **A6219** Gauze, non-impregnated, sterile, pad size 16 sq. in. or less, with any size adhesive border, each dressing ♿   A

IOM: 100-02, 15, 100

⊚ **A6220** Gauze, non-impregnated, sterile, pad size more than 16 sq. in. but less than or equal to 48 sq. in., with any size adhesive border, each dressing ♿   A

IOM: 100-02, 15, 100

⊚ **A6221** Gauze, non-impregnated, sterile, pad size more than 48 sq. in., with any size adhesive border, each dressing   A

IOM: 100-02, 15, 100

⊚ **A6222** Gauze, impregnated with other than water, normal saline, or hydrogel, sterile, pad size 16 sq. in. or less, without adhesive border, each dressing ♿   A

Substances may have been incorporated into dressing material (i.e., iodinated agents, petrolatum, zinc paste, crystalline sodium chloride, chlorhexadine gluconate [CHG], bismuth tribromophenate [BTP], water, aqueous saline, hydrogel, or agents)

IOM: 100-02, 15, 100

⊚ **A6223** Gauze, impregnated with other than water, normal saline, or hydrogel, sterile, pad size more than 16 sq. in. but less than or equal to 48 sq. in., without adhesive border, each dressing ♿   A

IOM: 100-02, 15, 100

⊚ **A6224** Gauze, impregnated with other than water, normal saline, or hydrogel, sterile, pad size more than 48 square inches, without adhesive border, each dressing ♿   A

IOM: 100-02, 15, 100

⊚ **A6228** Gauze, impregnated, water or normal saline, sterile, pad size 16 sq. in. or less, without adhesive border, each dressing   A

IOM: 100-02, 15, 100

⊚ **A6229** Gauze, impregnated, water or normal saline, sterile, pad size more than 16 sq. in. but less than or equal to 48 sq. in., without adhesive border, each dressing ♿   A

IOM: 100-02, 15, 100

⊚ **A6230** Gauze, impregnated, water or normal saline, sterile, pad size more than 48 sq. in., without adhesive border, each dressing   A

IOM: 100-02, 15, 100

⊚ **A6231** Gauze, impregnated, hydrogel, for direct wound contact, sterile, pad size 16 sq. in. or less, each dressing ♿   A

IOM: 100-02, 15, 100

⊚ **A6232** Gauze, impregnated, hydrogel, for direct wound contact, sterile, pad size greater than 16 sq. in., but less than or equal to 48 sq. in., each dressing ♿   A

IOM: 100-02, 15, 100

⟨PQRS⟩ PQRS	Qp **Quantity Physician Appendix A**	Qh **Quantity Hospital Appendix B**	♀ **Female only**
♂ **Male only** A **Age** ♿ **DMEPOS**	A2-Z3 ASC Payment Indicator	A-Y ASC Status Indicator	Coding Clinic

⚙ **A6233** Gauze, impregnated, hydrogel, for direct wound contact, sterile, pad size more than 48 sq. in., each dressing ♿ A

IOM: 100-02, 15, 100

⚙ **A6234** Hydrocolloid dressing, wound cover, sterile, pad size 16 sq. in. or less, without adhesive border, each dressing ♿ A

This type of dressing is usually used on wounds with light to moderate exudate with an average of three dressing changes a week.

IOM: 100-02, 15, 100

⚙ **A6235** Hydrocolloid dressing, wound cover, sterile, pad size more than 16 sq. in. but less than or equal to 48 sq. in., without adhesive border, each dressing ♿ A

IOM: 100-02, 15, 100

⚙ **A6236** Hydrocolloid dressing, wound cover, sterile, pad size more than 48 sq. in., without adhesive border, each dressing ♿ A

IOM: 100-02, 15, 100

⚙ **A6237** Hydrocolloid dressing, wound cover, sterile, pad size 16 sq. in. or less, with any size adhesive border, each dressing ♿ A

IOM: 100-02, 15, 100

⚙ **A6238** Hydrocolloid dressing, wound cover, sterile, pad size more than 16 sq. in. but less than or equal to 48 sq. in., with any size adhesive border, each dressing ♿ A

IOM: 100-02, 15, 100

⚙ **A6239** Hydrocolloid dressing, wound cover, sterile, pad size more than 48 sq. in., with any size adhesive border, each dressing A

IOM: 100-02, 15, 100

⚙ **A6240** Hydrocolloid dressing, wound filler, paste, sterile, per ounce ♿ A

IOM: 100-02, 15, 100

⚙ **A6241** Hydrocolloid dressing, wound filler, dry form, sterile, per gram ♿ A

IOM: 100-02, 15, 100

⚙ **A6242** Hydrogel dressing, wound cover, sterile, pad size 16 sq. in. or less, without adhesive border, each dressing ♿ A

Considered medically necessary when used on full thickness wounds with minimal or no exudate (e.g., stage III or IV ulcers)

Usually up to one dressing change per day is considered medically necessary, but if well documented and medically necessary, the payer may allow more frequent dressing changes.

IOM: 100-02, 15, 100

⚙ **A6243** Hydrogel dressing, wound cover, sterile, pad size more than 16 sq. in. but less than or equal to 48 sq. in., without adhesive border, each dressing ♿ A

IOM: 100-02, 15, 100

⚙ **A6244** Hydrogel dressing, wound cover, sterile, pad size more than 48 sq. in., without adhesive border, each dressing ♿ A

IOM: 100-02, 15, 100

⚙ **A6245** Hydrogel dressing, wound cover, sterile, pad size 16 sq. in. or less, with any size adhesive border, each dressing ♿ A

Coverage of a non-elastic gradient compression wrap is limited to one per 6 months per leg.

IOM: 100-02, 15, 100

⚙ **A6246** Hydrogel dressing, wound cover, sterile, pad size more than 16 sq. in. but less than or equal to 48 sq. in., with any size adhesive border, each dressing ♿ A

IOM: 100-02, 15, 100

⚙ **A6247** Hydrogel dressing, wound cover, sterile, pad size more than 48 sq. in., with any size adhesive border, each dressing ♿ A

IOM: 100-02, 15, 100

⚙ **A6248** Hydrogel dressing, wound filler, gel, per fluid ounce ♿ A

IOM: 100-02, 15, 100

⚙ **A6250** Skin sealants, protectants, moisturizers, ointments, any type, any size A

IOM: 100-02, 15, 100

⚙ **A6251** Specialty absorptive dressing, wound cover, sterile, pad size 16 sq. in. or less, without adhesive border, each dressing ♿ A

IOM: 100-02, 15, 100

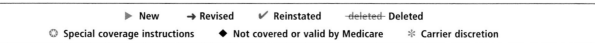

▶ New   → Revised   ✔ Reinstated   ~~deleted~~ Deleted
⚙ Special coverage instructions   ◆ Not covered or valid by Medicare   ✳ Carrier discretion

◎ **A6252** Specialty absorptive dressing, wound cover, sterile, pad size more than 16 sq. in. but less than or equal to 48 sq. in., without adhesive border, each dressing 👤   A

IOM: 100-02, 15, 100

◎ **A6253** Specialty absorptive dressing, wound cover, sterile, pad size more than 48 sq. in., without adhesive border, each dressing 👤   A

IOM: 100-02, 15, 100

◎ **A6254** Specialty absorptive dressing, wound cover, sterile, pad size 16 sq. in. or less, with any size adhesive border, each dressing 👤   A

IOM: 100-02, 15, 100

◎ **A6255** Specialty absorptive dressing, wound cover, sterile, pad size more than 16 sq. in. but less than or equal to 48 sq. in., with any size adhesive border, each dressing 👤   A

IOM: 100-02, 15, 100

◎ **A6256** Specialty absorptive dressing, wound cover, sterile, pad size more than 48 sq. in., with any size adhesive border, each dressing   A

Considered medically necessary when used for moderately or highly exudative wounds (e.g., stage III or IV ulcers)

IOM: 100-02, 15, 100

◎ **A6257** Transparent film, sterile, 16 sq. in. or less, each dressing 👤   A

Considered medically necessary when used on open partial thickness wounds with minimal exudate or closed wounds

IOM: 100-02, 15, 100

◎ **A6258** Transparent film, sterile, more than 16 sq. in. but less than or equal to 48 sq. in., each dressing 👤   A

IOM: 100-02, 15, 100

◎ **A6259** Transparent film, sterile, more than 48 sq. in., each dressing 👤   A

IOM: 100-02, 15, 100

➔ ◎ **A6260** Wound cleansers, any type, any size   A

IOM: 100-02, 15, 100

➔ ◎ **A6261** Wound filler, gel/paste, per fluid ounce, not otherwise specified   A

Units of service for wound fillers are 1 gram, 1 fluid ounce, 6 inch length, or 1 yard depending on product

IOM: 100-02, 15, 100

➔ ◎ **A6262** Wound filler, dry form, per gram, not otherwise specified   A

Dry forms (e.g., powder, granules, beads) are used to eliminate dead space in an open wound.

IOM: 100-02, 15, 100

◎ **A6266** Gauze, impregnated, other than water, normal saline, or zinc paste, sterile, any width, per linear yard 👤   A

IOM: 100-02, 15, 100

◎ **A6402** Gauze, non-impregnated, sterile, pad size 16 sq. in. or less, without adhesive border, each dressing 👤   A

IOM: 100-02, 15, 100

◎ **A6403** Gauze, non-impregnated, sterile, pad size more than 16 sq. in., less than or equal to 48 sq. in., without adhesive border, each dressing 👤   A

IOM: 100-02, 15, 100

◎ **A6404** Gauze, non-impregnated, sterile, pad size more than 48 sq. in., without adhesive border, each dressing   A

IOM: 100-02, 15, 100

✳ **A6407** Packing strips, non-impregnated, sterile, up to 2 inches in width, per linear yard 👤   A

IOM: 100-02, 15, 100

◎ **A6410** Eye pad, sterile, each 👤   A

IOM: 100-02, 15, 100

◎ **A6411** Eye pad, non-sterile, each 👤   A

IOM: 100-02, 15, 100

✳ **A6412** Eye patch, occlusive, each   A

◆ **A6413** Adhesive bandage, first-aid type, any size, each   E

First aid type bandage is a wound cover with a pad size of less than 4 square inches.

Medicare Statute 1861(s)(5)

✳ **A6441** Padding bandage, non-elastic, non-woven/non-knitted, width greater than or equal to three inches and less than five inches, per yard 👤   A

✳ **A6442** Conforming bandage, non-elastic, knitted/woven, non-sterile, width less than three inches, per yard 👤   A

Non-elastic, moderate or high compression that is typically sustained for one week

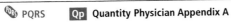 PQRS   **Qp** Quantity Physician Appendix A   **Qh** Quantity Hospital Appendix B   ♀ **Female only**

♂ **Male only**   **A** Age   👤 **DMEPOS**   A2-Z3 ASC Payment Indicator   A-Y ASC Status Indicator   Coding Clinic

❋ **A6443** Conforming bandage, non-elastic, knitted/woven, non-sterile, width greater than or equal to three inches and less than five inches, per yard ♿   A

❋ **A6444** Conforming bandage, non-elastic, knitted/woven, non-sterile, width greater than or equal to five inches, per yard ♿   A

❋ **A6445** Conforming bandage, non-elastic, knitted/woven, sterile, width less than three inches, per yard ♿   A

❋ **A6446** Conforming bandage, non-elastic, knitted/woven, sterile, width greater than or equal to three inches and less than five inches, per yard ♿   A

❋ **A6447** Conforming bandage, non-elastic, knitted/woven, sterile, width greater than or equal to five inches, per yard ♿   A

❋ **A6448** Light compression bandage, elastic, knitted/woven, width less than three inches, per yard ♿   A

Used to hold wound cover dressings in place over a wound. Example is an ACE type elastic bandage.

❋ **A6449** Light compression bandage, elastic, knitted/woven, width greater than or equal to three inches and less than five inches, per yard ♿   A

❋ **A6450** Light compression bandage, elastic, knitted/woven, width greater than or equal to five inches, per yard ♿   A

❋ **A6451** Moderate compression bandage, elastic, knitted/woven, load resistance of 1.25 to 1.34 foot pounds at 50% maximum stretch, width greater than or equal to three inches and less than five inches, per yard ♿   A

Elastic bandages that produce moderate compression that is typically sustained for one week

Medicare considers coverage if part of a multi-layer compression bandage system for the treatment of a venous stasis ulcer. Do not assign for strains or sprains.

❋ **A6452** High compression bandage, elastic, knitted/woven, load resistance greater than or equal to 1.35 foot pounds at 50% maximum stretch, width greater than or equal to three inches and less than five inches, per yard ♿   A

Elastic bandages that produce high compression that is typically sustained for one week

❋ **A6453** Self-adherent bandage, elastic, non-knitted/non-woven, width less than three inches, per yard ♿   A

❋ **A6454** Self-adherent bandage, elastic, non-knitted/non-woven, width greater than or equal to three inches and less than five inches, per yard ♿   A

❋ **A6455** Self-adherent bandage, elastic, non-knitted/non-woven, width greater than or equal to five inches, per yard ♿   A

❋ **A6456** Zinc paste impregnated bandage, non-elastic, knitted/woven, width greater than or equal to three inches and less than five inches, per yard ♿   A

❋ **A6457** Tubular dressing with or without elastic, any width, per linear yard ♿   A

❂ **A6501** Compression burn garment, bodysuit (head to foot), custom fabricated Qp Qh ♿   A

Garments used to reduce hypertrophic scarring and joint contractures following burn injury

IOM: 100-02, 15, 100

❂ **A6502** Compression burn garment, chin strap, custom fabricated Qp Qh ♿   A

IOM: 100-02, 15, 100

❂ **A6503** Compression burn garment, facial hood, custom fabricated Qp Qh ♿   A

IOM: 100-02, 15, 100

❂ **A6504** Compression burn garment, glove to wrist, custom fabricated Qp Qh ♿   A

IOM: 100-02, 15, 100

❂ **A6505** Compression burn garment, glove to elbow, custom fabricated Qp Qh ♿   A

IOM: 100-02, 15, 100

❂ **A6506** Compression burn garment, glove to axilla, custom fabricated Qp Qh ♿   A

IOM: 100-02, 15, 100

❂ **A6507** Compression burn garment, foot to knee length, custom fabricated Qp Qh ♿   A

IOM: 100-02, 15, 100

❂ **A6508** Compression burn garment, foot to thigh length, custom fabricated Qp Qh ♿   A

IOM: 100-02, 15, 100

▶ New   → Revised   ✔ Reinstated   ~~deleted~~ Deleted

❂ Special coverage instructions   ◆ Not covered or valid by Medicare   ❋ Carrier discretion

⊕ **A6509** Compression burn garment, upper trunk to waist including arm openings (vest), custom fabricated `Qp` `Qh`   A

IOM: 100-02, 15, 100

⊕ **A6510** Compression burn garment, trunk, including arms down to leg openings (leotard), custom fabricated `Qp` `Qh`   A

IOM: 100-02, 15, 100

⊕ **A6511** Compression burn garment, lower trunk including leg openings (panty), custom fabricated `Qp` `Qh`   A

IOM: 100-02, 15, 100

⊕ **A6512** Compression burn garment, not otherwise classified   A

IOM: 100-02, 15, 100

✳ **A6513** Compression burn mask, face and/or neck, plastic or equal, custom fabricated `Qp` `Qh`   B

Bill DME/MAC

GRADIENT COMPRESSION STOCKINGS (A6530-A6549)

A6530-A6549: Bill DME/MAC

➔ ◆ **A6530** Gradient compression stocking, below knee, 18–30 mmHg, each   E

IOM: 100-03, 4, 280.1

⊕ **A6531** Gradient compression stocking, below knee, 30–40 mmHg, each   A

Covered when used in treatment of open venous stasis ulcer. Modifiers A1-A9 are not assigned. Must be billed with AW, RT, or LT

IOM: 100-02, 15, 100

DMEPOS Modifier(s): AW

⊕ **A6532** Gradient compression stocking, below knee, 40–50 mmHg, each   A

Covered when used in treatment of open venous stasis ulcer. Modifiers A1-A9 are not assigned. Must be billed with AW, RT, or LT

IOM: 100-02, 15, 100

DMEPOS Modifier(s): AW

➔ ◆ **A6533** Gradient compression stocking, thigh length, 18–30 mmHg, each   E

IOM: 100-02, 15, 130; 100-03, 4, 280.1

➔ ◆ **A6534** Gradient compression stocking, thigh length, 30–40 mmHg, each   E

IOM: 100-02, 15, 130; 100-03, 4, 280.1

➔ ◆ **A6535** Gradient compression stocking, thigh length, 40–50 mmHg, each   E

IOM: 100-02, 15, 130; 100-03, 4, 280.1

➔ ◆ **A6536** Gradient compression stocking, full length/chap style, 18–30 mmHg, each   E

IOM: 100-02, 15, 130; 100-03, 4, 280.1

➔ ◆ **A6537** Gradient compression stocking, full length/chap style, 30–40 mmHg, each   E

IOM: 100-02, 15, 130; 100-03, 4, 280.1

➔ ◆ **A6538** Gradient compression stocking, full length/chap style, 40–50 mmHg, each   E

IOM: 100-02, 15, 130; 100-03, 4, 280.1

➔ ◆ **A6539** Gradient compression stocking, waist length, 18–30 mmHg, each   E

IOM: 100-02, 15, 130; 100-03, 4, 280.1

➔ ◆ **A6540** Gradient compression stocking, waist length, 30–40 mmHg, each   E

IOM: 100-02, 15, 130; 100-03, 4, 280.1

➔ ◆ **A6541** Gradient compression stocking, waist length, 40–50 mmHg, each   E

IOM: 100-02, 15, 130; 100-03, 4, 280.1

➔ ◆ **A6544** Gradient compression stocking, garter belt   E

IOM: 100-02, 15, 130; 100-03, 4, 280.1

➔ ⊕ **A6545** Gradient compression wrap, non-elastic, below knee, 30-50 mm hg, each `Qp` `Qh`   A

Modifiers -RT and/or -LT must be appended. When assigned for bilateral items (left/right) on the same date of service, bill both items on the same claim line using -RT/-LT modifiers and 2 units of service.

IOM: 10-02, 15, 100

DMEPOS Modifier(s): AW

➔ ◆ **A6549** Gradient compression stocking/ sleeve, not otherwise specified   E

IOM: 100-02, 15, 130; 100-03, 4, 280.1

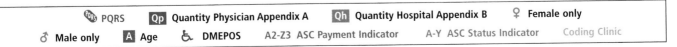

⊛ PQRS   `Qp` Quantity Physician Appendix A   `Qh` Quantity Hospital Appendix B   ♀ Female only
♂ Male only   A Age   & DMEPOS   A2-Z3 ASC Payment Indicator   A-Y ASC Status Indicator   Coding Clinic

WOUND CARE (A6550)

* **A6550** Wound care set, for negative pressure wound therapy electrical pump, includes all supplies and accessories ♿ Y

    Bill DME/MAC

RESPIRATORY DURABLE MEDICAL EQUIPMENT, INEXPENSIVE AND ROUTINELY PURCHASED (A7000-A7509)

* **A7000** Canister, disposable, used with suction pump, each ♿ Y

    Bill DME/MAC

    DMEPOS Modifier(s): NU, KE

* **A7001** Canister, non-disposable, used with suction pump, each ♿ Y

    Bill DME/MAC

    DMEPOS Modifier(s): NU

* **A7002** Tubing, used with suction pump, each ♿ Y

    Bill DME/MAC

    DMEPOS Modifier(s): NU

* **A7003** Administration set, with small volume nonfiltered pneumatic nebulizer, disposable ♿ Y

    Bill DME/MAC

    DMEPOS Modifier(s): NU

* **A7004** Small volume nonfiltered pneumatic nebulizer, disposable ♿ Y

    Bill DME/MAC

    DMEPOS Modifier(s): NU

* **A7005** Administration set, with small volume nonfiltered pneumatic nebulizer, non-disposable ♿ Y

    Bill DME/MAC

    DMEPOS Modifier(s): NU

* **A7006** Administration set, with small volume filtered pneumatic nebulizer ♿ Y

    Bill DME/MAC

    DMEPOS Modifier(s): NU

* **A7007** Large volume nebulizer, disposable, unfilled, used with aerosol compressor ♿ Y

    Bill DME/MAC

    DMEPOS Modifier(s): NU

* **A7008** Large volume nebulizer, disposable, prefilled, used with aerosol compressor ♿ Y

    Bill DME/MAC

    DMEPOS Modifier(s): NU

* **A7009** Reservoir bottle, nondisposable, used with large volume ultrasonic nebulizer ♿ Y

    Bill DME/MAC

    DMEPOS Modifier(s): NU

* **A7010** Corrugated tubing, disposable, used with large volume nebulizer, 100 feet ♿ Y

    Bill DME/MAC

    DMEPOS Modifier(s): NU

* **A7011** Corrugated tubing, non-disposable, used with large volume nebulizer, 10 feet Y

    Bill DME/MAC

* **A7012** Water collection device, used with large volume nebulizer ♿ Y

    Bill DME/MAC

    DMEPOS Modifier(s): NU

→ * **A7013** Filter, disposable, used with aerosol compressor or ultrasonic generator ♿ Y

    Bill DME/MAC

    DMEPOS Modifier(s): NU

* **A7014** Filter, non-disposable, used with aerosol compressor or ultrasonic generator ♿ Y

    Bill DME/MAC

    DMEPOS Modifier(s): NU

* **A7015** Aerosol mask, used with DME nebulizer ♿ Y

    Bill DME/MAC

    DMEPOS Modifier(s): NU

* **A7016** Dome and mouthpiece, used with small volume ultrasonic nebulizer ♿ Y

    Bill DME/MAC

    DMEPOS Modifier(s): NU

☺ **A7017** Nebulizer, durable, glass or autoclavable plastic, bottle type, not used with oxygen Qp Qh ♿ Y

    Bill DME/MAC

    IOM: 100-03, 4, 280.1

    DMEPOS Modifier(s): NU, RR, UE

* **A7018** Water, distilled, used with large volume nebulizer, 1000 ml ♿ Y

    Bill DME/MAC

▶ New   → Revised   ✔ Reinstated   deleted Deleted
☺ Special coverage instructions   ◆ Not covered or valid by Medicare   * Carrier discretion

▶ ✳ **A7020** Interface for cough stimulating device, includes all components, replacement only Qp Qh ♿ Y

Bill DME/MAC

DMEPOS Modifier(s): NU

✳ **A7025** High frequency chest wall oscillation system vest, replacement for use with patient owned equipment, each Qp Qh ♿ Y

Bill DME/MAC

DMEPOS Modifier(s): NU

✳ **A7026** High frequency chest wall oscillation system hose, replacement for use with patient owned equipment, each Qp Qh ♿ Y

Bill DME/MAC

DMEPOS Modifier(s): NU

✳ **A7027** Combination oral/nasal mask, used with continuous positive airway pressure device, each Qp Qh ♿ Y

Bill DME/MAC

DMEPOS Modifier(s): NU

✳ **A7028** Oral cushion for combination oral/nasal mask, replacement only, each ♿ Y

Bill DME/MAC

DMEPOS Modifier(s): NU

✳ **A7029** Nasal pillows for combination oral/nasal mask, replacement only, pair ♿ Y

Bill DME/MAC

DMEPOS Modifier(s): NU

✳ **A7030** Full face mask used with positive airway pressure device, each ♿ Y

Bill DME/MAC

DMEPOS Modifier(s): NU

✳ **A7031** Face mask interface, replacement for full face mask, each ♿ Y

Bill DME/MAC

DMEPOS Modifier(s): NU

✳ **A7032** Cushion for use on nasal mask interface, replacement only, each ♿ Y

Bill DME/MAC

DMEPOS Modifier(s): NU

✳ **A7033** Pillow for use on nasal cannula type interface, replacement only, pair ♿ Y

Bill DME/MAC

DMEPOS Modifier(s): NU

✳ **A7034** Nasal interface (mask or cannula type) used with positive airway pressure device, with or without head strap ♿ Y

Bill DME/MAC

DMEPOS Modifier(s): NU

✳ **A7035** Headgear used with positive airway pressure device Qp Qh ♿ Y

Bill DME/MAC

DMEPOS Modifier(s): NU

✳ **A7036** Chinstrap used with positive airway pressure device Qp Qh ♿ Y

Bill DME/MAC

DMEPOS Modifier(s): NU

✳ **A7037** Tubing used with positive airway pressure device ♿ Y

Bill DME/MAC

DMEPOS Modifier(s): NU

✳ **A7038** Filter, disposable, used with positive airway pressure device ♿ Y

Bill DME/MAC

DMEPOS Modifier(s): NU

✳ **A7039** Filter, non disposable, used with positive airway pressure device Qp ♿ Y

Bill DME/MAC

DMEPOS Modifier(s): NU

✳ **A7040** One way chest drain valve Qp Qh ♿ A

Bill local carrier

✳ **A7041** Water seal drainage container and tubing for use with implanted chest tube Qp Qh ♿ A

Bill local carrier

✳ **A7042** Implanted pleural catheter, each Qp Qh ♿ N

Bill local carrier

✳ **A7043** Vacuum drainage bottle and tubing for use with implanted catheter Qp Qh ♿ A

Bill local carrier

✳ **A7044** Oral interface used with positive airway pressure device, each ♿ Y

Bill DME/MAC

DMEPOS Modifier(s): NU

⟲ PQRS	Qp **Quantity Physician Appendix A**	Qh **Quantity Hospital Appendix B**	♀ **Female only**
♂ **Male only**	A **Age**	♿ **DMEPOS**	A2-Z3 **ASC Payment Indicator**	A-Y **ASC Status Indicator**	Coding Clinic

⚙ **A7045** Exhalation port with or without swivel used with accessories for positive airway devices, replacement only ♿ Y

Bill DME/MAC

IOM: 100-03, 4, 230.17

DMEPOS Modifier(s): NU, RR, UE

⚙ **A7046** Water chamber for humidifier, used with positive airway pressure device, replacement, each ♿ Y

Bill DME/MAC

IOM: 100-03, 4, 230.17

DMEPOS Modifier(s): NU

⚙ **A7501** Tracheostoma valve, including diaphragm, each ♿ A

Bill DME/MAC

IOM: 100-02, 15, 120

⚙ **A7502** Replacement diaphragm/faceplate for tracheostoma valve, each ♿ A

Bill DME/MAC

IOM: 100-02, 15, 120

⚙ **A7503** Filter holder or filter cap, reusable, for use in a tracheostoma heat and moisture exchange system, each ♿ A

Bill DME/MAC

IOM: 100-02, 15, 120

⚙ **A7504** Filter for use in a tracheostoma heat and moisture exchange system, each ♿ A

Bill DME/MAC

IOM: 100-02, 15, 120

⚙ **A7505** Housing, reusable without adhesive, for use in a heat and moisture exchange system and/or with a tracheostoma valve, each ♿ A

Bill DME/MAC

IOM: 100-02, 15, 120

⚙ **A7506** Adhesive disc for use in a heat and moisture exchange system and/or with tracheostoma valve, any type, each ♿ A

Bill DME/MAC

IOM: 100-02, 15, 120

⚙ **A7507** Filter holder and integrated filter without adhesive, for use in a tracheostoma heat and moisture exchange system, each ♿ A

Bill DME/MAC

IOM: 100-02, 15, 120

⚙ **A7508** Housing and integrated adhesive, for use in a tracheostoma heat and moisture exchange system and/or with a tracheostoma valve, each ♿ A

Bill DME/MAC

IOM: 100-02, 15, 120

⚙ **A7509** Filter holder and integrated filter housing, and adhesive, for use as a tracheostoma heat and moisture exchange system, each ♿ A

Bill DME/MAC

IOM: 100-02, 15, 120

✳ **A7520** Tracheostomy/laryngectomy tube, non-cuffed, polyvinylchloride (PVC), silicone or equal, each ♿ A

Bill DME/MAC

✳ **A7521** Tracheostomy/laryngectomy tube, cuffed, polyvinylchloride (PVC), silicone or equal, each ♿ A

Bill DME/MAC

✳ **A7522** Tracheostomy/laryngectomy tube, stainless steel or equal (sterilizable and reusable), each ♿ A

Bill DME/MAC

✳ **A7523** Tracheostomy shower protector, each A

Bill DME/MAC

✳ **A7524** Tracheostoma stent/stud/button, each ♿ A

Bill DME/MAC

✳ **A7525** Tracheostomy mask, each ♿ A

Bill DME/MAC

✳ **A7526** Tracheostomy tube collar/holder, each ♿ A

Bill DME/MAC

✳ **A7527** Tracheostomy/laryngectomy tube plug/stop, each ♿ A

Bill DME/MAC

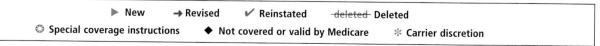

▶ New → Revised ✔ Reinstated ~~deleted~~ Deleted
⚙ Special coverage instructions ◆ Not covered or valid by Medicare ✳ Carrier discretion

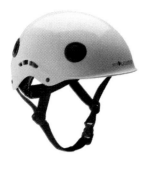

Figure 7 Helmet.

HELMETS (A8000-A8004)

A8000-8004: Bill DME/MAC

✳ **A8000** Helmet, protective, soft, prefabricated, includes all components and accessories ♿   Y

DMEPOS Modifier(s): NU, RR, UE

✳ **A8001** Helmet, protective, hard, prefabricated, includes all components and accessories ♿   Y

DMEPOS Modifier(s): NU, RR, UE

✳ **A8002** Helmet, protective, soft, custom fabricated, includes all components and accessories ♿   Y

DMEPOS Modifier(s): NU, RR, UE

✳ **A8003** Helmet, protective, hard, custom fabricated, includes all components and accessories ♿   Y

DMEPOS Modifier(s): NU, RR, UE

✳ **A8004** Soft interface for helmet, replacement only ♿   Y

DMEPOS Modifier(s): NU, RR, UE

ADMINISTRATIVE, MISCELLANEOUS, AND INVESTIGATIONAL (A9000-A9999)

NOTE: The following codes do not imply that codes in other sections are necessarily covered.

✪ **A9150** Non-prescription drugs   B

Bill local carrier

IOM: 100-02, 15, 50

◆ **A9152** Single vitamin/mineral/trace element, oral, per dose, not otherwise specified   E

Bill local carrier

◆ **A9153** Multiple vitamins, with or without minerals and trace elements, oral, per dose, not otherwise specified   E

Bill local carrier

✳ **A9155** Artificial saliva, 30 ml   B

Bill local carrier

◆ **A9180** Pediculosis (lice infestation) treatment, topical, for administration by patient/caretaker   E

Bill local carrier

◆ **A9270** Non-covered item or service   E

Bill DME/MAC

IOM: 100-02, 16, 20

▶ ◆ **A9272** Mechanical wound suction, disposable, includes dressing, all accessories and components, each   E

◆ **A9273** Hot water bottle, ice cap or collar, heat and/or cold wrap, any type   Y

◆ **A9274** External ambulatory insulin delivery system, disposable, each, includes all supplies and accessories   E

Bill DME/MAC

◆ **A9275** Home glucose disposable monitor, includes test strips   E

Bill DME/MAC

◆ **A9276** Sensor; invasive (e.g. subcutaneous), disposable, for use with interstitial continuous glucose monitoring system, one unit = 1 day supply   E

Bill DME/MAC

Medicare Statute 1861(n)

◆ **A9277** Transmitter; external, for use with interstitial continuous glucose monitoring system   E

Bill DME/MAC

Medicare Statute 1861(n)

◆ **A9278** Receiver (monitor); external, for use with interstitial continuous glucose monitoring system   E

Bill DME/MAC

Medicare Statute 1861(n)

◆ **A9279** Monitoring feature/device, stand-alone or integrated, any type, includes all accessories, components and electronics, not otherwise classified   E

Bill DME/MAC

◆ **A9280** Alert or alarm device, not otherwise classified E

Bill DME/MAC

Medicare Statute 1861

◆ **A9281** Reaching/grabbing device, any type, any length, each E

Bill DME/MAC

Medicare Statute 1862 SSA

◆ **A9282** Wig, any type, each E

Bill DME/MAC

Medicare Statute 1862 SSA

◆ **A9283** Foot pressure off loading/supportive device, any type, each E

Bill DME/MAC

Medicare Statute 1862A(i)13

☼ **A9284** Spirometer, non-electronic, includes all accessories `Qp` `Qh` N

Bill DME/MAC

◆ **A9300** Exercise equipment E

Bill DME/MAC

IOM: 100-02, 15, 110.1; 100-03, 4, 280.1

Supplies for Radiology Procedures (Radiopharmaceuticals)

A9500-9700: Bill local carrier

✳ **A9500** Technetium Tc-99m sestamibi, diagnostic, per study dose N1 N
`Qp` `Qh`

Should be filed on same claim as procedure code reporting radiopharmaceutical. Verify with payer definition of a "study."

Coding Clinic: 2006, Q2, P5

✳ **A9501** Technetium Tc-99m teboroxime, diagnostic, per study dose `Qp` `Qh` N1 N

✳ **A9502** Technetium Tc-99m tetrofosmin, diagnostic, per study dose `Qp` `Qh` N1 N

Coding Clinic: 2006, Q2, P5

✳ **A9503** Technetium Tc-99m medronate, diagnostic, per study dose, up to 30 millicuries `Qp` `Qh` N1 N

✳ **A9504** Technetium Tc-99m apcitide, diagnostic, per study dose, up to 20 millicuries `Qp` `Qh` N1 N

✳ **A9505** Thallium Tl-201 thallous chloride, diagnostic, per millicurie N1 N

✳ **A9507** Indium In-111 capromab pendetide, diagnostic, per study dose, up to 10 millicuries `Qp` `Qh` N1 N

✳ **A9508** Iodine I-131 iobenguane sulfate, diagnostic, per 0.5 millicurie N1 N

✳ **A9509** Iodine I-123 sodium iodide, diagnostic, per millicurie N1 N

✳ **A9510** Technetium Tc-99m disofenin, diagnostic, per study dose, up to 15 millicuries `Qp` `Qh` N1 N

✳ **A9512** Technetium Tc-99m pertechnetate, diagnostic, per millicurie N1 N

✳ **A9516** Iodine I-123 sodium iodide, diagnostic, per 100 microcuries, up to 999 microcuries N1 N

✳ **A9517** Iodine I-131 sodium iodide capsule(s), therapeutic, per millicurie K

✳ **A9521** Technetium Tc-99m exametazime, diagnostic, per study dose, up to 25 millicuries `Qp` `Qh` N1 N

✳ **A9524** Iodine I-131 iodinated serum albumin, diagnostic, per 5 microcuries N1 N

✳ **A9526** Nitrogen N-13 ammonia, diagnostic, per study dose, up to 40 millicuries `Qp` `Qh` N1 N

✳ **A9527** Iodine I-125, sodium iodide solution, therapeutic, per millicurie H2 U

✳ **A9528** Iodine I-131 sodium iodide capsule(s), diagnostic, per millicurie N1 N

✳ **A9529** Iodine I-131 sodium iodide solution, diagnostic, per millicurie N1 N

✳ **A9530** Iodine I-131 sodium iodide solution, therapeutic, per millicurie K

✳ **A9531** Iodine I-131 sodium iodide, diagnostic, per microcurie (up to 100 microcuries) N1 N

✳ **A9532** Iodine I-125 serum albumin, diagnostic, per 5 microcuries N1 N

✳ **A9536** Technetium Tc-99m depreotide, diagnostic, per study dose, up to 35 millicuries `Qp` `Qh` N1 N

✳ **A9537** Technetium Tc-99m mebrofenin, diagnostic, per study dose, up to 15 millicuries `Qp` `Qh` N1 N

✳ **A9538** Technetium Tc-99m pyrophosphate, diagnostic, per study dose, up to 25 millicuries `Qp` `Qh` N1 N

✳ **A9539** Technetium Tc-99m pentetate, diagnostic, per study dose, up to 25 millicuries `Qp` `Qh` N1 N

✳ **A9540** Technetium Tc-99m macroaggregated albumin, diagnostic, per study dose, up to 10 millicuries `Qp` `Qh` N1 N

▶ New → Revised ✔ Reinstated ~~deleted~~ Deleted

☼ Special coverage instructions ◆ Not covered or valid by Medicare ✳ Carrier discretion

✳ **A9541** Technetium Tc-99m sulfur colloid, diagnostic, per study dose, up to 20 millicuries `Qp` `Qh` N1 N

✳ **A9542** Indium In-111 ibritumomab tiuxetan, diagnostic, per study dose, up to 5 millicuries `Qp` `Qh` N1 N

Specifically for diagnostic use.

✳ **A9543** Yttrium Y-90 ibritumomab tiuxetan, therapeutic, per treatment dose, up to 40 millicuries `Qp` `Qh` K

Specifically for therapeutic use.

✳ **A9544** Iodine I-131 tositumomab, diagnostic, per study dose `Qp` `Qh` N1 N

✳ **A9545** Iodine I-131 tositumomab, therapeutic, per treatment dose `Qp` `Qh` K

✳ **A9546** Cobalt Co-57/58, cyanocobalamin, diagnostic, per study dose, up to 1 microcurie `Qp` `Qh` N1 N

✳ **A9547** Indium In-111 oxyquinoline, diagnostic, per 0.5 millicurie N1 N

✳ **A9548** Indium In-111 pentetate, diagnostic, per 0.5 millicurie N1 N

✳ **A9550** Technetium Tc-99m sodium gluceptate, diagnostic, per study dose, up to 25 millicuries `Qp` `Qh` N1 N

✳ **A9551** Technetium Tc-99m succimer, diagnostic, per study dose, up to 10 millicuries `Qp` `Qh` N1 N

✳ **A9552** Fluorodeoxyglucose F-18 FDG, diagnostic, per study dose, up to 45 millicuries `Qp` `Qh` N1 N

Coding Clinic: 2008, Q3, P7

✳ **A9553** Chromium Cr-51 sodium chromate, diagnostic, per study dose, up to 250 microcuries `Qp` `Qh` N1 N

✳ **A9554** Iodine I-125 sodium Iothalamate, diagnostic, per study dose, up to 10 microcuries `Qp` `Qh` N1 N

✳ **A9555** Rubidium Rb-82, diagnostic, per study dose, up to 60 millicuries `Qp` `Qh` N1 N

✳ **A9556** Gallium Ga-67 citrate, diagnostic, per millicurie N1 N

✳ **A9557** Technetium Tc-99m bicisate, diagnostic, per study dose, up to 25 millicuries `Qp` `Qh` N1 N

✳ **A9558** Xenon Xe-133 gas, diagnostic, per 10 millicuries N1 N

✳ **A9559** Cobalt Co-57 cyanocobalamin, oral, diagnostic, per study dose, up to 1 microcurie `Qp` `Qh` N1 N

✳ **A9560** Technetium Tc-99m labeled red blood cells, diagnostic, per study dose, up to 30 millicuries `Qp` `Qh` N1 N

Coding Clinic: 2008, Q3, P7

✳ **A9561** Technetium Tc-99m oxidronate, diagnostic, per study dose, up to 30 millicuries `Qp` `Qh` N1 N

✳ **A9562** Technetium Tc-99m mertiatide, diagnostic, per study dose, up to 15 millicuries `Qp` `Qh` N1 N

✳ **A9563** Sodium phosphate P-32, therapeutic, per millicurie K

✳ **A9564** Chromic phosphate P-32 suspension, therapeutic, per millicurie K

✳ **A9566** Technetium Tc-99m fanolesomab, diagnostic, per study dose, up to 25 millicuries `Qp` `Qh` N1 N

✳ **A9567** Technetium Tc-99m pentetate, diagnostic, aerosol, per study dose, up to 75 millicuries `Qp` `Qh` N1 N

✳ **A9568** Technetium TC-99m arcitumomab, diagnostic, per study dose, up to 45 millicuries N1 N

✳ **A9569** Technetium Tc-99m exametazime labeled autologous white blood cells, diagnostic, per study dose `Qp` `Qh` N1 N

✳ **A9570** Indium In-111 labeled autologous white blood cells, diagnostic, per study dose `Qp` `Qh` N1 N

✳ **A9571** Indium In-111 labeled autologous platelets, diagnostic, per study dose `Qp` `Qh` N1 N

✳ **A9572** Indium In-111 pentetreotide, diagnostic, per study dose, up to 6 millicuries N1 N

✳ **A9576** Injection, gadoteridol, (ProHance Multipack), per ml N1 N

✳ **A9577** Injection, gadobenate dimeglumine (MultiHance), per ml N1 N

✳ **A9578** Injection, gadobenate dimeglumine (MultiHance Multipack), per ml N1 N

✳ **A9579** Injection, gadolinium-based magnetic resonance contrast agent, not otherwise specified (NOS), per ml N1 N

NDC: Magnevist, Omniscan, Optimark, Prohance

✳ **A9580** Sodium fluoride F-18, diagnostic, per study dose, up to 30 millicuries `Qp` `Qh` N1 N

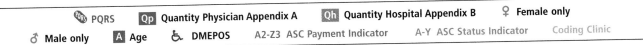

✳ **A9581** Injection, gadoxetate disodium, 1 ml N1 N

Local Medicare contractors may require the use of modifier JW to identify unused product from single-dose vials that are appropriately discarded.

✳ **A9582** Iodine I-123 iobenguane, diagnostic, per study dose, up to 15 millicuries Qp Qh N1 N

Molecular imaging agent that assists in the identification of rare neuroendocrine tumors.

✳ **A9583** Injection, gadofosveset trisodium, 1 ml N1 N

NDC: Ablavar

▶ ✳ **A9584** Iodine 1-123 ioflupane, diagnostic, per study dose, up to 5 millicuries K2 G

▶ ✳ **A9585** Injection, gadobutrol, 0.1 ml N1 N

✳ **A9600** Strontium Sr-89 chloride, therapeutic, per millicurie K

✳ **A9604** Samarium SM-153 lexidronam, therapeutic, per treatment dose, up to 150 millicuries Qp Qh K

✪ **A9698** Non-radioactive contrast imaging material, not otherwise classified, per study N1 N

IOM: 100-04, 12, 70; 100-04, 13, 20

✳ **A9699** Radiopharmaceutical, therapeutic, not otherwise classified N

✪ **A9700** Supply of injectable contrast material for use in echocardiography, per study Qp Qh B

IOM: 100-04, 12, 30.4

Miscellaneous Service Component

✳ **A9900** Miscellaneous DME supply, accessory, and/or service component of another HCPCS code Y

Local carrier if used with implanted DME. If other, bill DME/MAC.

On DMEPOS fee schedule as a payable replacement for miscellaneous implanted or non-implanted items.

✳ **A9901** DME delivery, set up, and/or dispensing service component of another HCPCS code A

Bill DME/MAC

✳ **A9999** Miscellaneous DME supply or accessory, not otherwise specified Y

Local carrier if used with implanted DME. If other, bill DME/MAC.

On DMEPOS fee schedule as a payable replacement for miscellaneous implanted or non-implanted items.

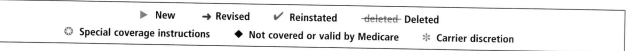

▶ **New** → **Revised** ✔ **Reinstated** ~~deleted~~ **Deleted**
✪ **Special coverage instructions** ◆ **Not covered or valid by Medicare** ✳ **Carrier discretion**

ENTERAL AND PARENTERAL THERAPY (B4000-B9999)

Enteral Formulae and Enteral Medical Supplies

B4034-B4162: Bill DME/MAC

→ ⊛ **B4034** Enteral feeding supply kit; syringe fed, per day, includes but not limited to feeding/flushing syringe, administration set tubing, dressings, tape   Y

Dressings used with gastrostomy tubes for enteral nutrition (covered under the prosthetic device benefit) are included in the payment.

IOM: 100-02, 15, 120; 100-03, 3, 180.2; 100-04, 20, 100.2.2

PEN: On Fee Schedule

→ ⊛ **B4035** Enteral feeding supply kit; pump fed, per day, includes but not limited to feeding/flushing syringe, administration set tubing, dressings, tape   Y

IOM: 100-02, 15, 120; 100-03, 3, 180.2; 100-04, 20, 100.2.2

PEN: On Fee Schedule

→ ⊛ **B4036** Enteral feeding supply kit; gravity fed, per day, includes but not limited to feeding/flushing syringe, administration set tubing, dressings, tape   Y

IOM: 100-02, 15, 120; 100-03, 3, 180.2; 100-04, 20, 100.2.2

PEN: On Fee Schedule

⊛ **B4081** Nasogastric tubing with stylet   Y

More than 3 nasogastric tubes (B4081-B4083), or 1 gastrostomy/jejunostomy tube (B4087-B4088) every three months is rarely medically necessary

IOM: 100-02, 15, 120; 100-03, 3, 180.2; 100-04, 20, 100.2.2

PEN: On Fee Schedule

⊛ **B4082** Nasogastric tubing without stylet   Y

IOM: 100-02, 15, 120; 100-03, 3, 180.2; 100-04, 20, 100.2.2

PEN: On Fee Schedule

⊛ **B4083** Stomach tube - Levine type   Y

IOM: 100-02, 15, 120; 100-03, 3, 180.2; 100-04, 20, 100.2.2

PEN: On Fee Schedule

✳ **B4087** Gastrostomy/jejunostomy tube, standard, any material, any type, each   A

PEN: On Fee Schedule

✳ **B4088** Gastrostomy/jejunostomy tube, low-profile, any material, any type, each   A

PEN: On Fee Schedule

◆ **B4100** Food thickener, administered orally, per ounce   E

⊛ **B4102** Enteral formula, for adults, used to replace fluids and electrolytes (e.g. clear liquids), 500 ml = 1 unit **A**   Y

IOM: 100-03, 3, 180.2

⊛ **B4103** Enteral formula, for pediatrics, used to replace fluids and electrolytes (e.g. clear liquids), 500 ml = 1 unit **A**   Y

IOM: 100-03, 3, 180.2

⊛ **B4104** Additive for enteral formula (e.g. fiber)   E

IOM: 100-03, 3, 180.2

⊛ **B4149** Enteral formula, manufactured blenderized natural foods with intact nutrients, includes proteins, fats, carbohydrates, vitamins and minerals, may include fiber, administered through an enteral feeding tube, 100 calories = 1 unit   Y

Produced to meet unique nutrient needs for specific disease conditions; medical record must document specific condition and need for special nutrient

IOM: 100-02, 15, 120; 100-03, 3, 180.2; 100-04, 20, 100.2.2

PEN: On Fee Schedule

⊛ **B4150** Enteral formulae, nutritionally complete with intact nutrients, includes proteins, fats, carbohydrates, vitamins, and minerals, may include fiber, administered through an enteral feeding tube, 100 calories = 1 unit   Y

IOM: 100-02, 15, 120; 100-03, 3, 180.2; 100-04, 20, 100.2.2

PEN: On Fee Schedule

⊛ **B4152** Enteral formula, nutritionally complete, calorically dense (equal to or greater than 1.5 kcal/ml) with intact nutrients, includes proteins, fats, carbohydrates, vitamins and minerals, may include fiber, administered through an enteral feeding tube, 100 calories = 1 unit   Y

IOM: 100-02, 15, 120; 100-03, 3, 180.2; 100-04, 20, 100.2.2

PEN: On Fee Schedule

PQRS PQRS   **Qp** Quantity Physician Appendix A   **Qh** Quantity Hospital Appendix B   ♀ Female only

♂ Male only   **A** Age   ♿ DMEPOS   A2-Z3 ASC Payment Indicator   A-Y ASC Status Indicator   Coding Clinic

⊗ **B4153** Enteral formula, nutritionally complete, hydrolyzed proteins (amino acids and peptide chain), includes fats, carbohydrates, vitamins and minerals, may include fiber, administered through an enteral feeding tube, 100 calories = 1 unit Y

If 2 enteral nutrition products described by same HCPCS code and provided at same time billed on single claim line with units of service reflecting total calories of both nutrients

IOM: 100-02, 15, 120; 100-03, 3, 180.2; 100-04, 20, 100.2.2

PEN: On Fee Schedule

⊗ **B4154** Enteral formula, nutritionally complete, for special metabolic needs, excludes inherited disease of metabolism, includes altered composition of proteins, fats, carbohydrates, vitamins and/or minerals, may include fiber, administered through an enteral feeding tube, 100 calories = 1 unit Y

IOM: 100-02, 15, 120; 100-03, 3, 180.2; 100-04, 20, 100.2.2

PEN: On Fee Schedule

⊗ **B4155** Enteral formula, nutritionally incomplete/modular nutrients, includes specific nutrients, carbohydrates (e.g. glucose polymers), proteins/amino acids (e.g. glutamine, arginine), fat (e.g. medium chain triglycerides) or combination, administered through an enteral feeding tube, 100 calories = 1 unit Y

IOM: 100-02, 15, 120; 100-03, 3, 180.2; 100-04, 20, 100.2.2

PEN: On Fee Schedule

⊗ **B4157** Enteral formula, nutritionally complete, for special metabolic needs for inherited disease of metabolism, includes proteins, fats, carbohydrates, vitamins and minerals, may include fiber, administered through an enteral feeding tube, 100 calories = 1 unit Y

IOM: 100-03, 3, 180.2

⊗ **B4158** Enteral formula, for pediatrics, nutritionally complete with intact nutrients, includes proteins, fats, carbohydrates, vitamins and minerals, may include fiber and/or iron, administered through an enteral feeding tube, 100 calories = 1 unit A Y

Bill DME/MAC

IOM: 100-03, 3, 180.2

⊗ **B4159** Enteral formula, for pediatrics, nutritionally complete soy based with intact nutrients, includes proteins, fats, carbohydrates, vitamins and minerals, may include fiber and/or iron, administered through an enteral feeding tube, 100 calories = 1 unit A Y

IOM: 100-03, 3, 180.2

⊗ **B4160** Enteral formula, for pediatrics, nutritionally complete calorically dense (equal to or greater than 0.7 kcal/ml) with intact nutrients, includes proteins, fats, carbohydrates, vitamins and minerals, may include fiber, administered through an enteral feeding tube, 100 calories = 1 unit A Y

IOM: 100-03, 3, 180.2

⊗ **B4161** Enteral formula, for pediatrics, hydrolyzed/amino acids and peptide chain proteins, includes fats, carbohydrates, vitamins and minerals, may include fiber, administered through an enteral feeding tube, 100 calories = 1 unit A Y

IOM: 100-03, 3, 180.2

⊗ **B4162** Enteral formula, for pediatrics, special metabolic needs for inherited disease of metabolism, includes proteins, fats, carbohydrates, vitamins and minerals, may include fiber, administered through an enteral feeding tube, 100 calories = 1 unit A Y

IOM: 100-03, 3, 180.2

▶ New → Revised ✔ Reinstated deleted Deleted
⊗ Special coverage instructions ◆ Not covered or valid by Medicare ✳ Carrier discretion

Parenteral Nutritional Solutions and Supplies

B4164-B5200:   Bill DME/MAC

⊛ **B4164**   Parenteral nutrition solution: carbohydrates (dextrose), 50% or less (500 ml = 1 unit) - homemix   Y

IOM: 100-02, 15, 120; 100-03, 3, 180.2; 100-04, 20, 100.2.2

PEN: On Fee Schedule

⊛ **B4168**   Parenteral nutrition solution; amino acid, 3.5%, (500 ml = 1 unit) - homemix   Y

IOM: 100-02, 15, 120; 100-03, 3, 180.2; 100-04, 20, 100.2.2

PEN: On Fee Schedule

⊛ **B4172**   Parenteral nutrition solution; amino acid, 5.5% through 7%, (500 ml = 1 unit) - homemix   Y

IOM: 100-02, 15, 120; 100-03, 3, 180.2; 100-04, 20, 100.2.2

⊛ **B4176**   Parenteral nutrition solution; amino acid, 7% through 8.5%, (500 ml = 1 unit) - homemix   Y

IOM: 100-02, 15, 120; 100-03, 3, 180.2; 100-04, 20, 100.2.2

PEN: On Fee Schedule

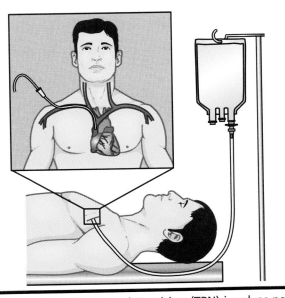

Figure 8   Total Parenteral Nutrition (TPN) involves percutaneous placement of central venous catheter into vena cava or right atrium.

⊛ **B4178**   Parenteral nutrition solution: amino acid, greater than 8.5%, (500 ml = 1 unit) - homemix   Y

IOM: 100-02, 15, 120; 100-03, 3, 180.2; 100-04, 20, 100.2.2

PEN: On Fee Schedule

⊛ **B4180**   Parenteral nutrition solution; carbohydrates (dextrose), greater than 50% (500 ml = 1 unit) - home mix   Y

IOM: 100-02, 15, 120; 100-03, 3, 180.2; 100-04, 20, 100.2.2

PEN: On Fee Schedule

⊛ **B4185**   Parenteral nutrition solution, per 10 grams lipids   B

PEN: On Fee Schedule

⊛ **B4189**   Parenteral nutrition solution; compounded amino acid and carbohydrates with electrolytes, trace elements, and vitamins, including preparation, any strength, 10 to 51 grams of protein - premix   Y

IOM: 100-02, 15, 120; 100-03, 3, 180.2; 100-04, 20, 100.2.2

PEN: On Fee Schedule

⊛ **B4193**   Parenteral nutrition solution; compounded amino acid and carbohydrates with electrolytes, trace elements, and vitamins, including preparation, any strength, 52 to 73 grams of protein - premix   Y

IOM: 100-02, 15, 120; 100-03, 3, 180.2; 100-04, 20, 100.2.2

PEN: On Fee Schedule

⊛ **B4197**   Parenteral nutrition solution; compounded amino acid and carbohydrates with electrolytes, trace elements and vitamins, including preparation, any strength, 74 to 100 grams of protein - premix   Y

IOM: 100-02, 15, 120; 100-03, 3, 180.2; 100-04, 20, 100.2.2

PEN: On Fee Schedule

⊛ **B4199**   Parenteral nutrition solution; compounded amino acid and carbohydrates with electrolytes, trace elements and vitamins, including preparation, any strength, over 100 grams of protein - premix   Y

IOM: 100-02, 15, 120; 100-03, 3, 180.2; 100-04, 20, 100.2.2

PEN: On Fee Schedule

⊛ **B4216** Parenteral nutrition; additives (vitamins, trace elements, heparin, electrolytes) homemix per day   Y

IOM: 100-02, 15, 120; 100-03, 3, 180.2; 100-04, 20, 100.2.2

PEN: On Fee Schedule

⊛ **B4220** Parenteral nutrition supply kit; premix, per day   Y

IOM: 100-02, 15, 120; 100-03, 3, 180.2; 100-04, 20, 100.2.2

PEN: On Fee Schedule

⊛ **B4222** Parenteral nutrition supply kit; home mix, per day   Y

IOM: 100-02, 15, 120; 100-03, 3, 180.2; 100-04, 20, 100.2.2

PEN: On Fee Schedule

⊛ **B4224** Parenteral nutrition administration kit, per day   Y

Dressings used with parenteral nutrition (covered under the prosthetic device benefit) are included in the payment. (www.cms.gov/medicare-coverage-database/)

IOM: 100-02, 15, 120; 100-03, 3, 180.2; 100-04, 20, 100.2.2

PEN: On Fee Schedule

⊛ **B5000** Parenteral nutrition solution: compounded amino acid and carbohydrates with electrolytes, trace elements, and vitamins, including preparation, any strength, renal - Amirosyn-RF, NephrAmine, RenAmine - premix   Y

IOM: 100-02, 15, 120; 100-03, 3, 180.2; 100-04, 20, 100.2.2

PEN: On Fee Schedule

⊛ **B5100** Parenteral nutrition solution: compounded amino acid and carbohydrates with electrolytes, trace elements, and vitamins, including preparation, any strength, hepatic - FreAmine HBC, HepatAmine - premix   Y

IOM: 100-02, 15, 120; 100-03, 3, 180.2; 100-04, 20, 100.2.2

PEN: On Fee Schedule

⊛ **B5200** Parenteral nutrition solution; compounded amino acid and carbohydrates with electrolytes, trace elements, and vitamins, including preparation, any strength, stress - branch chain amino acids - premix   Y

Bill DME/MAC

IOM: 100-02, 15, 120; 100-03, 3, 180.2; 100-04, 20, 100.2.2

Enteral and Parenteral Pumps

B9000-B9999:   Bill DME/MAC

⊛ **B9000** Enteral nutrition infusion pump - without alarm   Y

Pump will be denied as not medically necessary if medical necessity of pump is not documented

IOM: 100-02, 15, 120; 100-03, 3, 180.2; 100-04, 20, 100.2.2

PEN: On Fee Schedule, DMEPOS Modifier(s): NU, RR, UE

⊛ **B9002** Enteral nutrition infusion pump - with alarm   Y

IOM: 100-02, 15, 120; 100-03, 3, 180.2; 100-04, 20, 100.2.2

PEN: On Fee Schedule, DMEPOS Modifier(s): NU, RR, UE

⊛ **B9004** Parenteral nutrition infusion pump, portable   Y

IOM: 100-02, 15, 120; 100-03, 3, 180.2; 100-04, 20, 100.2.2

PEN: On Fee Schedule, DMEPOS Modifier(s): NU, RR, UE

⊛ **B9006** Parenteral nutrition infusion pump, stationary   Y

IOM: 100-02, 15, 120; 100-03, 3, 180.2; 100-04, 20, 100.2.2

PEN: On Fee Schedule, DMEPOS Modifier(s): NU, RR, UE

⊛ **B9998** NOC for enteral supplies   Y

IOM: 100-02, 15, 120; 100-03, 3, 180.2; 100-04, 20, 100.2.2

⊛ **B9999** NOC for parenteral supplies   Y

Determine if an alternative HCPCS Level II or a CPT code better describes the service being reported. This code should be reported only if a more specific code is unavailable.

IOM: 100-02, 15, 120; 100-03, 3, 180.2; 100-04, 20, 100.2.2

▶ New   → Revised   ✔ Reinstated   deleted Deleted

⊛ Special coverage instructions   ◆ Not covered or valid by Medicare   ✳ Carrier discretion

122

CMS HOSPITAL OUTPATIENT PAYMENT SYSTEM (C1000-C9999)

NOTE: C codes are used ONLY as a part of Hospital Outpatient Prospective Payment System (OPPS) and are not to be used to report other services. C codes are updated quarterly by the Centers for Medicare and Medicaid Services.

⊛ **C1300** Hyperbaric oxygen under pressure, full body chamber, per 30-minute interval   S

Medicare Statute 1833(t)

Coding Clinic: 2005, Q1, P6

⊛ **C1713** Anchor/Screw for opposing bone-to-bone or soft tissue-to-bone (implantable)   N1   N

Medicare Statute 1833(t)

Coding Clinic: 2010, Q2, P3

⊛ **C1714** Catheter, transluminal atherectomy, directional   N1   N

Medicare Statute 1833(t)

⊛ **C1715** Brachytherapy needle   N1   N

Medicare Statute 1833(t)

⊛ **C1716** Brachytherapy source, non-stranded, gold-198, per source   H2   U

Medicare Statute 1833(t)

⊛ **C1717** Brachytherapy source, non-stranded, high dose rate iridium 192, per source   H2   U

Medicare Statute 1833(t)

⊛ **C1719** Brachytherapy source, non-stranded, non-high dose rate iridium-192, per source   H2   U

Medicare Statute 1833(t)

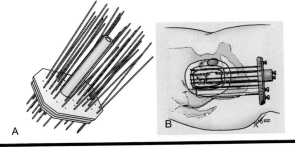

Figure 9 **A.** Brachytherapy device. **B.** Brachytherapy device inserted.

⊛ **C1721** Cardioverter-defibrillator, dual chamber (implantable) **Qh**   N1   N

Related CPT codes: 33224, 33240, 33249.

Medicare Statute 1833(t)

⊛ **C1722** Cardioverter-defibrillator, single chamber (implantable) **Qh**   N1   N

Related CPT codes: 33240, 33249.

Medicare Statute 1833(t)

Coding Clinic: 2006, Q2, P9

⊛ **C1724** Catheter, transluminal atherectomy, rotational   N1   N

Medicare Statute 1833(t)

⊛ **C1725** Catheter, transluminal angioplasty, non-laser (may include guidance, infusion/perfusion capability)   N1   N

Medicare Statute 1833(t)

⊛ **C1726** Catheter, balloon dilatation, non-vascular   N1   N

Medicare Statute 1833(t)

⊛ **C1727** Catheter, balloon tissue dissector, non-vascular (insertable)   N1   N

Medicare Statute 1833(t)

⊛ **C1728** Catheter, brachytherapy seed administration   N1   N

Medicare Statute 1833(t)

⊛ **C1729** Catheter, drainage   N1   N

Medicare Statute 1833(t)

⊛ **C1730** Catheter, electrophysiology, diagnostic, other than 3D mapping (19 or fewer electrodes)   N1   N

Medicare Statute 1833(t)

⊛ **C1731** Catheter, electrophysiology, diagnostic, other than 3D mapping (20 or more electrodes)   N1   N

Medicare Statute 1833(t)

⊛ **C1732** Catheter, electrophysiology, diagnostic/ablation, 3D or vector mapping   N1   N

Medicare Statute 1833(t)

⊛ **C1733** Catheter, electrophysiology, diagnostic/ablation, other than 3D or vector mapping, other than cool-tip   N1   N

Medicare Statute 1833(t)

▶ ⊛ **C1749** Endoscope, retrograde imaging/illumination colonoscope device (implantable) **Qh**   J7   H

Medicare Statute 1833(t)

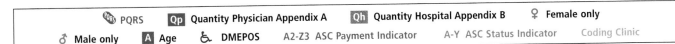

| 🄥 PQRS | **Qp** Quantity Physician Appendix A | **Qh** Quantity Hospital Appendix B | ♀ Female only |
| ♂ Male only | **A** Age | ♿ DMEPOS | A2-Z3 ASC Payment Indicator | A-Y ASC Status Indicator | Coding Clinic |

⊛ **C1750** Catheter, hemodialysis/peritoneal, long-term `Qh`   N1 N

Medicare Statute 1833(t)

⊛ **C1751** Catheter, infusion, inserted peripherally, centrally, or midline (other than hemodialysis)   N1 N

Medicare Statute 1833(t)

⊛ **C1752** Catheter, hemodialysis/peritoneal, short-term `Qh`   N1 N

Medicare Statute 1833(t)

⊛ **C1753** Catheter, intravascular ultrasound `Qh`   N1 N

Medicare Statute 1833(t)

⊛ **C1754** Catheter, intradiscal   N1 N

Medicare Statute 1833(t)

⊛ **C1755** Catheter, instraspinal `Qh`   N1 N

Medicare Statute 1833(t)

⊛ **C1756** Catheter, pacing, transesophageal `Qh`   N1 N

Medicare Statute 1833(t)

⊛ **C1757** Catheter, thrombectomy/ embolectomy   N1 N

Medicare Statute 1833(t)

⊛ **C1758** Catheter, ureteral `Qh`   N1 N

Medicare Statute 1833(t)

⊛ **C1759** Catheter, intracardiac echocardiography   N1 N

Medicare Statute 1833(t)

⊛ **C1760** Closure device, vascular (implantable/ insertable)   N1 N

Medicare Statute 1833(t)

⊛ **C1762** Connective tissue, human (includes fascia lata)   N1 N

Medicare Statute 1833(t)

Coding Clinic: 2003, Q3, P12

⊛ **C1763** Connective tissue, non-human (includes synthetic)   N1 N

Medicare Statute 1833(t)

Coding Clinic: 2010, Q4, P3; Q2, P3; 2003, Q3, P12

⊛ **C1764** Event recorder, cardiac (implantable) `Qh`   N1 N

Medicare Statute 1833(t)

⊛ **C1765** Adhesion barrier   N1 N

Medicare Statute 1833(t)

⊛ **C1766** Introducer/sheath, guiding, intracardiac electrophysiological, steerable, other than peel-away   N1 N

Medicare Statute 1833(t)

⊛ **C1767** Generator, neurostimulator (implantable), nonrechargeable `Qh`   N1 N

Related CPT codes: 61885, 61886, 63685, 64590.

Medicare Statute 1833(t)

Coding Clinic: 2007, Q1, P8

⊛ **C1768** Graft, vascular `Qh`   N1 N

Medicare Statute 1833(t)

⊛ **C1769** Guide wire   N1 N

Medicare Statute 1833(t)

Coding Clinic: 2007, Q2, P7-8

⊛ **C1770** Imaging coil, magnetic reasonance (insertable) `Qh`   N1 N

Medicare Statute 1833(t)

⊛ **C1771** Repair device, urinary, incontinence, with sling graft `Qh`   N1 N

Medicare Statute 1833(t)

Coding Clinic: 2008, Q3, P7

⊛ **C1772** Infusion pump, programmable (implantable) `Qh`   N1 N

Medicare Statute 1833(t)

⊛ **C1773** Retrieval device, insertable (used to retrieve fractured medical devices)   N1 N

Medicare Statute 1833(t)

⊛ **C1776** Joint device (implantable)   N1 N

Medicare Statute 1833(t)

Coding Clinic: 2010, Q3, P6; 2008, Q4, P10

⊛ **C1777** Lead, cardioverter-defibrillator, endocardial single coil (implantable) `Qh`   N1 N

Related CPT codes: 33216, 33217, 33249.

Medicare Statute 1833(t)

Coding Clinic: 2006, Q2, P9

⊛ **C1778** Lead, neurostimulator (implantable)   N1 N

Related CPT codes: 43647, 63650, 63655, 63663, 63664, 64553, 64555, 64560, 64561, 64565, 64573, 64575, 64577, 64580, 64581.

Medicare Statute 1833(t)

Coding Clinic: 2007, Q1, P8

⊛ **C1779** Lead, pacemaker, trasvenous VDD single pass   N1 N

Related CPT codes: 33206, 33207, 33208, 33210, 33211, 33214, 33216, 33217, 33249.

Medicare Statute 1833(t)

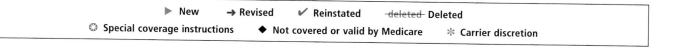

▶ New   → Revised   ✔ Reinstated   ~~deleted~~ Deleted
⊛ Special coverage instructions   ◆ Not covered or valid by Medicare   ❋ Carrier discretion

⚙ **C1780**   Lens, intraocular (new
technology) Qh   N1 N

Medicare Statute 1833(t)

⚙ **C1781**   Mesh (implantable)   N1 N

Medicare Statute 1833(t)

Coding Clinic: 2010, Q2, P2-3

⚙ **C1782**   Morcellator Qh   N1 N

Medicare Statute 1833(t)

⚙ **C1783**   Ocular implant, aqueous drainage
assist device Qh   N1 N

Medicare Statute 1833(t)

⚙ **C1784**   Ocular device, intraoperative, detached
retina   N1 N

Medicare Statute 1833(t)

⚙ **C1785**   Pacemaker, dual chamber, rate-
responsive (implantable) Qh   N1 N

Related CPT codes: 33206, 33207,
33208, 33213, 33214, 33224.

Medicare Statute 1833(t)

⚙ **C1786**   Pacemaker, single chamber, rate-
responsive (implantable) Qh   N1 N

Related CPT codes: 33206, 33207, 33212.

Medicare Statute 1833(t)

⚙ **C1787**   Patient programmer,
neurostimulator Qh   N1 N

Medicare Statute 1833(t)

⚙ **C1788**   Port, indwelling
(implantable) Qh   N1 N

Medicare Statute 1833(t)

⚙ **C1789**   Prosthesis, breast
(implantable) ♀ Qh   N1 N

Medicare Statute 1833(t)

⚙ **C1813**   Prosthesis, penile,
inflatable ♂ Qh   N1 N

Medicare Statute 1833(t)

⚙ **C1814**   Retinal tamponade device,
silicone oil Qh   N1 N

Medicare Statute 1833(t)

Coding Clinic: 2006, Q2, P9

⚙ **C1815**   Prosthesis, urinary sphincter
(implantable) Qh   N1 N

Medicare Statute 1833(t)

⚙ **C1816**   Receiver and/or transmitter,
neurostimulator
(implantable) Qh   N1 N

Medicare Statute 1833(t)

⚙ **C1817**   Septal defect implant system,
intracardiac Qh   N1 N

Medicare Statute 1833(t)

⚙ **C1818**   Integrated
keratoprosthesic Qh   N1 N

Medicare Statute 1833(t)

⚙ **C1819**   Surgical tissue localization and excision
device (implantable)   N1 N

Medicare Statute 1833(t)

⚙ **C1820**   Generator, neurostimulator
(implantable), with rechargeable
battery and charging
system Qh   N1 N

Related CPT codes: 61885, 61886,
63685, 64590.

Medicare Statute 1833(t)

⚙ **C1821**   Interspinous process distraction device
(implantable)   N1 N

Medicare Statute 1833(t)

▶ ⚙ **C1830**   Powered bone marrow biopsy
needle   J7 H

Medicare Statute 1833(t)

▶ ⚙ **C1840**   Lens, intraocular (telescopic) J7 H

Medicare Statute 1833(t)

⚙ **C1874**   Stent, coated/covered, with delivery
system   N1 N

Medicare Statute 1833(t)

⚙ **C1875**   Stent, coated/covered, without delivery
system   N1 N

Medicare Statute 1833(t)

⚙ **C1876**   Stent, non-coated/non-covered, with
delivery system   N1 N

Medicare Statute 1833(t)

⚙ **C1877**   Stent, non-coated/non-covered, without
delivery system   N1 N

Medicare Statute 1833(t)

⚙ **C1878**   Material for vocal cord medialization,
synthetic (implantable) Qh   N1 N

Medicare Statute 1833(t)

⚙ **C1879**   Tissue marker (implantable)   N1 N

Medicare Statute 1833(t)

⚙ **C1880**   Vena cava filter Qh   N1 N

Medicare Statute 1833(t)

⚙ **C1881**   Dialysis access system
(implantable) Qh   N1 N

Medicare Statute 1833(t)

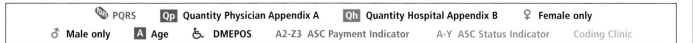

⊛ **C1882**   Cardioverter-defibrillator, other than single or dual chamber (implantable) **Qh**   N1   N

Related CPT codes: 33224, 33240, 33249.

Medicare Statute 1833(t)

Coding Clinic: 2006, Q2, P9

⊛ **C1883**   Adaptor/Extension, pacing lead or neurostimulator lead (implantable)   N1   N

Medicare Statute 1833(t)

Coding Clinic: 2007, Q1, P8

⊛ **C1884**   Embolization protective system   N1   N

Medicare Statute 1833(t)

⊛ **C1885**   Catheter, transluminal angioplasty, laser   N1   N

Medicare Statute 1833(t)

▶ ⊛ **C1886**   Catheter, extravascular tissue ablation, any modality (insertable)   H

Medicare Statute 1833(t)

⊛ **C1887**   Catheter, guiding (may include infusion/perfusion capability)   N1   N

Medicare Statute 1833(t)

⊛ **C1888**   Catheter, ablation, non-cardiac, endovascular (implantable) **Qh**   N1   N

Medicare Statute 1833(t)

⊛ **C1891**   Infusion pump, non-programmable, permanent (implantable) **Qh**   N1   N

Medicare Statute 1833(t)

⊛ **C1892**   Introducer/sheath, guiding, intracardiac electrophysiological, fixed-curve, peel-away   N1   N

Medicare Statute 1833(t)

⊛ **C1893**   Introducer/sheath, guiding, intracardiac electrophysiological, fixed-curve, other than peel-away   N1   N

Medicare Statute 1833(t)

⊛ **C1894**   Introducer/sheath, other than guiding, other than intracardiac electrophysiological, non-laser   N1   N

Medicare Statute 1833(t)

⊛ **C1895**   Lead, cardioverter-defibrillator, endocardial dual coil (implantable) **Qh**   N1   N

Related CPT codes: 33216, 33217, 33249.

Medicare Statute 1833(t)

Coding Clinic: 2006, Q2, P9

⊛ **C1896**   Lead, cardioverter-defibrillator, other than endocardial single or dual coil (implantable) **Qh**   N1   N

Related CPT codes: 33216, 33217, 33249.

Medicare Statute 1833(t)

⊛ **C1897**   Lead, neurostimulator test kit (implantable) **Qh**   N1   N

Related CPT codes: 43647, 63650, 63655, 63663, 63664, 64553, 64555, 64560, 64561, 64565, 64575, 64577, 64580, 64581.

Medicare Statute 1833(t)

Coding Clinic: 2007, Q1, P8

⊛ **C1898**   Lead, pacemaker, other than transvenous VDD single pass   N1   N

Related CPT codes: 33206, 33207, 33208, 33210, 33211, 33214, 33216, 33217, 33249.

Medicare Statute 1833(t)

Coding Clinic: 2002, Q3, P8

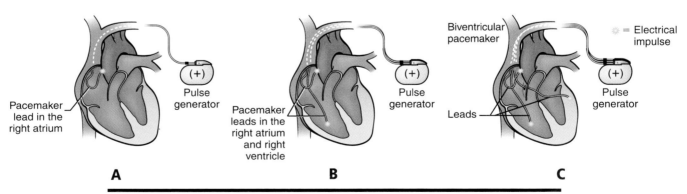

Figure 10   A. Single pacemaker. B. Dual pacemaker. C. Biventricular pacemaker.

▶ New   → Revised   ✔ Reinstated   ~~deleted~~ Deleted
⊛ Special coverage instructions   ◆ Not covered or valid by Medicare   ✳ Carrier discretion

✪ **C1899** Lead, pacemaker/cardioverter-
defibrillator combination
(implantable) `Qh`   N1   N

Related CPT codes: 33216, 33217,
33249.

Medicare Statute 1833(t)

✪ **C1900** Lead, left ventricular coronary venous
system `Qh`   N1   N

Related CPT codes: 33224, 33225.

Medicare Statute 1833(t)

✪ **C2614** Probe, percutaneous lumbar
discectomy `Qh`   N1   N

Medicare Statute 1833(t)

✪ **C2615** Sealant, pulmonary, liquid `Qh`   N1   N

Medicare Statute 1833(t)

✪ **C2616** Brachytherapy source, non-stranded,
yttrium-90, per source `Qh`   H2   U

Medicare Statute 1833(t)

✪ **C2617** Stent, non-coronary, temporary,
without delivery system   N1   N

Medicare Statute 1833(t)

✪ **C2618** Probe, cryoablation   N1   N

Medicare Statute 1833(t)

✪ **C2619** Pacemaker, dual chamber,
non rate-responsive
(implantable) `Qh`   N1   N

Related CPT codes: 33206, 33207,
33208, 33213, 33214, 33224.

Medicare Statute 1833(t)

✪ **C2620** Pacemaker, single chamber,
non rate-responsive
(implantable) `Qh`   N1   N

Related CPT codes: 33206, 33207,
33212, 33224.

Medicare Statute 1833(t)

✪ **C2621** Pacemaker, other than single or dual
chamber (implantable) `Qh`   N1   N

Related CPT codes: 33206, 33207,
33208, 33212, 33213, 33214, 33224.

Medicare Statute 1833(t)

Coding Clinic: 2002, Q3, P8

✪ **C2622** Prosthesis, penile,
non-inflatable ♂ `Qh`   N1   N

Medicare Statute 1833(t)

✪ **C2625** Stent, non-coronary, temporary, with
delivery system   N1   N

Medicare Statute 1833(t)

✪ **C2626** Infusion pump, non-programmable,
temporary (implantable) `Qh`   N1   N

Medicare Statute 1833(t)

✪ **C2627** Catheter, suprapubic/
cystoscopic `Qh`   N1   N

Medicare Statute 1833(t)

✪ **C2628** Catheter, occlusion   N1   N

Medicare Statute 1833(t)

✪ **C2629** Introducer/Sheath, other
than guiding, intracardiac
electrophysiological, laser   N1   N

Medicare Statute 1833(t)

✪ **C2630** Catheter, electrophysiology, diagnostic/
ablation, other than 3D or vector
mapping, cool-tip   N1   N

Medicare Statute 1833(t)

✪ **C2631** Repair device, urinary, incontinence,
without sling graft   N1   N

Medicare Statute 1833(t)

✪ **C2634** Brachytherapy source, non-stranded,
high activity, iodine-125, greater than
1.01 mci (NIST), per source   H2   U

Medicare Statute 1833(t)

✪ **C2635** Brachytherapy source, non-stranded,
high activity, paladium-103, greater than
2.2 mci (NIST), per source   H2   U

Medicare Statute 1833(t)

✪ **C2636** Brachytherapy linear source,
non-stranded, paladium-103,
per 1 mm   H2   U

✪ **C2637** Brachytherapy source, non-stranded,
Ytterbium-169, per source   B

Medicare Statute 1833(t)

✪ **C2638** Brachytherapy source, stranded,
iodine-125, per source   H2   U

Medicare Statute 1833(t)(2)

✪ **C2639** Brachytherapy source, non-stranded,
iodine-125, per source   H2   U

Medicare Statute 1833(t)(2)

✪ **C2640** Brachytherapy source, stranded,
palladium-103, per source   H2   U

Medicare Statute 1833(t)(2)

✪ **C2641** Brachytherapy source, non-stranded,
palladium-103, per source   H2   U

Medicare Statute 1833(t)(2)

✪ **C2642** Brachytherapy source, stranded,
cesium-131, per source   H2   U

Medicare Statute 1833(t)(2)

✪ **C2643** Brachytherapy source, non-stranded,
cesium-131, per source   H2   U

Medicare Statute 1833(t)(2)

✪ **C2698** Brachytherapy source, stranded, not
otherwise specified, per source   H2   U

Medicare Statute 1833(t)(2)

PQRS	`Qp` Quantity Physician Appendix A	`Qh` Quantity Hospital Appendix B	♀ Female only
♂ Male only	`A` Age DMEPOS A2-Z3 ASC Payment Indicator	A-Y ASC Status Indicator	Coding Clinic

⊛ **C2699** Brachytherapy source, non-stranded, not otherwise specified, per source   H2   U

Medicare Statute 1833(t)(2)

⊛ **C8900** Magnetic resonance angiography with contrast, abdomen Qh   Z2   Q3

Medicare Statute 1833(t)(2)

⊛ **C8901** Magnetic resonance angiography without contrast, abdomen Qh   Z2   Q3

Medicare Statute 1833(t)(2)

⊛ **C8902** Magnetic resonance angiography without contrast followed by with contrast, abdomen Qh   Z2   Q3

Medicare Statute 1833(t)(2)

⊛ **C8903** Magnetic resonance imaging with contrast, breast; unilateral Qh   Z2   Q3

Medicare Statute 1833(t)(2)

⊛ **C8904** Magnetic resonance imaging without contrast, breast; unilateral Qh   Z2   Q3

Medicare Statute 1833(t)(2)

⊛ **C8905** Magnetic resonance imaging without contrast followed by with contrast, breast; unilateral Qh   Z2   Q3

Medicare Statute 1833(t)(2)

⊛ **C8906** Magnetic resonance imaging with contrast, breast; bilateral Qh   Z2   Q3

Medicare Statute 1833(t)(2)

⊛ **C8907** Magnetic resonance imaging without contrast, breast; bilateral Qh   Z2   Q3

Medicare Statute 1833(t)(2)

⊛ **C8908** Magnetic resonance imaging without contrast followed by with contrast, breast; bilateral Qh   Z2   Q3

Medicare Statute 1833(t)(2)

⊛ **C8909** Magnetic resonance angiography with contrast, chest (excluding myocardium) Qh   Z2   Q3

Medicare Statute 1833(t)(2)

⊛ **C8910** Magnetic resonance angiography without contrast, chest (excluding myocardium) Qh   Z2   Q3

Medicare Statute 1833(t)(2)

⊛ **C8911** Magnetic resonance angiography without contrast followed by with contrast, chest (excluding myocardium) Qh   Z2   Q3

Medicare Statute 1833(t)(2)

⊛ **C8912** Magnetic resonance angiography with contrast, lower extremity Qh   Z2   Q3

Medicare Statute 1833(t)(2)

⊛ **C8913** Magnetic resonance angiography without contrast, lower extremity Qh   Z2   Q3

Medicare Statute 1833(t)(2)

⊛ **C8914** Magnetic resonance angiography without contrast followed by with contrast, lower extremity Qh   Z2   Q3

Medicare Statute 1833(t)(2)

⊛ **C8918** Magnetic resonance angiography with contrast, pelvis Qh   Z2   Q3

Medicare Statute 1833(t)(2)

⊛ **C8919** Magnetic resonance angiography without contrast, pelvis Qh   Z2   Q3

Medicare Statute 1833(t)(2)

⊛ **C8920** Magnetic resonance angiography without contrast followed by with contrast, pelvis Qh   Z2   Q3

Medicare Statute 1833(t)(2)

⊛ **C8921** Transthoracic echocardiography with contrast, or without contrast followed by with contrast, for congenital cardiac anomalies; complete Qh   S

Medicare Statute 1833(t)(2)

⊛ **C8922** Transthoracic echocardiography with contrast, or without contrast followed by with contrast, for congenital cardiac anomalies; follow-up or limited study Qh   S

Medicare Statute 1833(t)(2)

⊛ **C8923** Transthoracic echocardiography with contrast, or without contrast followed by with contrast, real-time with image documentation (2D), includes M-mode recording, when performed, complete, without spectral or color Doppler echocardiography Qh   S

Medicare Statute 1833(t)(2)

⊛ **C8924** Transthoracic echocardiography with contrast, or without contrast followed by with contrast, real-time with image documentation (2D), includes M-mode recording, when performed, follow-up or limited study Qh   S

Medicare Statute 1833(t)(2)

⊛ **C8925** Transesophageal echocardiography (TEE) with contrast, or without contrast followed by with contrast, real time with image documentation (2D) (with or without M-mode recording); including probe placement, image acquisition, interpretation and report Qh   S

Medicare Statute 1833(t)(2)

▶ New   → Revised   ✔ Reinstated   ~~deleted~~ Deleted

⊛ Special coverage instructions   ◆ Not covered or valid by Medicare   ✳ Carrier discretion

⊙ **C8926** Transesophageal echocardiography (TEE) with contrast, or without contrast followed by with contrast, for congenital cardiac anomalies; including probe placement, image acquisition, interpretation and report **Qh**   S

Medicare Statute 1833(t)(2)

⊙ **C8927** Transesophageal echocardiography (TEE) with contrast, or without contrast followed by with contrast, for monitoring purposes, including probe placement, real time 2-dimensional image acquisition and interpretation leading to ongoing (continuous) assessment of (dynamically changing) cardiac pumping function and to therapeutic measures on an immediate time basis **Qh**   S

Medicare Statute 1833(t)(2)

⊙ **C8928** Transthoracic echocardiography with contrast, or without contrast followed by with contrast, real-time with image documentation (2D), includes M-mode recording, when performed, during rest and cardiovascular stress test using treadmill, bicycle exercise and/or pharmacologically induced stress, with interpretation and report **Qh**   S

Medicare Statute 1833(t)(2)

⊙ **C8929** Transthoracic echocardiography with contrast, or without contrast followed by with contrast, real-time with image documentation (2D), includes M-mode recording, when performed, complete, with spectral Doppler echocardiography, and with color flow Doppler echocardiography **Qh**   S

Medicare Statute 1833(t)(2)

⊙ **C8930** Transthoracic echocardiography, with contrast, or without contrast followed by with contrast, real-time with image documentation (2D), includes M-mode recording, when performed, during rest and cardiovascular stress test using treadmill, bicycle exercise and/or pharmacologically induced stress, with interpretation and report; including performance of continuous electrocardiographic monitoring, with physician supervision **Qh**   S

Medicare Statute 1833(t)(2)

▶ ⊙ **C8931** Magnetic resonance angiography with contrast, spinal canal and contents **Qh**   Z2 Q3

Medicare Statute 1833(t)

▶ ⊙ **C8932** Magnetic resonance angiography without contrast, spinal canal and contents **Qh**   Z2 Q3

Medicare Statute 1833(t)

▶ ⊙ **C8933** Magnetic resonance angiography without contrast followed by with contrast, spinal canal and contents **Qh**   Z2 Q3

Medicare Statute 1833(t)

▶ ⊙ **C8934** Magnetic resonance angiography with contrast, upper extremity **Qh**   Z2 Q3

Medicare Statute 1833(t)

▶ ⊙ **C8935** Magnetic resonance angiography without contrast, upper extremity **Qh**   Z2 Q3

Medicare Statute 1833(t)

▶ ⊙ **C8936** Magnetic resonance angiography without contrast followed by with contrast, upper extremity **Qh**   Z2 Q3

Medicare Statute 1833(t)

⊙ **C8957** Intravenous infusion for therapy/diagnosis; initiation of prolonged infusion (more than 8 hours), requiring use of portable or implantable pump **Qh**   S

Medicare Statute 1833(t)

Coding Clinic: 2008, Q3, P8

⊙ **C9113** Injection, pantoprazole sodium, per vial   N1 N

Medicare Statute 1833(t)

⊙ **C9121** Injection, argatroban, per 5 mg   K2 K

Medicare Statute 1833(t)

✳ **C9248** Injection, clevidipine butyrate, 1 mg   K2 K

Medicare Statute 1833(t)

⊙ **C9250** Human plasma fibrin sealant, vapor-heated, solvent-detergent (ARTISS), 2ml   K2 K

Example of diagnosis codes to be reported with C9250: 941.00–949.5.

621MMA

⊙ **C9254** Injection, lacosamide, 1 mg   K2 K

621MMA

⊙ **C9257** injection, bevacizumab, 0.25 mg   K2 K

Medicare Statute 1833(t)

~~C9270~~ ~~Injection, immune globulin (Gammaplex), intravenous, non-lyophilized (e.g. liquid), 500 mg~~   ✖

~~C9272~~ ~~Injection, denosumab, 1 mg~~   ✖

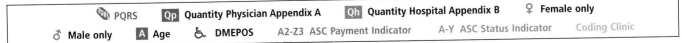

PQRS   **Qp** Quantity Physician Appendix A   **Qh** Quantity Hospital Appendix B   ♀ Female only

♂ Male only   **A** Age   ⅙ DMEPOS   A2-Z3 ASC Payment Indicator   A-Y ASC Status Indicator   Coding Clinic

C9273 Sipuleucel-T, minimum of 50 million autologous CD54+ cells activated with PAP-GM-CSF, including leukapheresis and all other preparatory procedures, per infusion ✳

C9274 Crotalidae polyvalent immune fab (Ovine), 1 vial ✳

▶ ☺ **C9275** Injection, hexaminolevulinate hydrochloride, 100 mg, per study dose K2 G

Medicare Statute 1833(t)

Coding Clinic: 2011, Q1, P6

C9276 Injection, cabazitaxel, 1 mg ✳

C9277 Injection, alglucosidase alfa (Lumizyme), 1 mg ✳

C9278 Injection, incobotulinumtoxin a, 1 unit ✳

▶ ☺ **C9279** Injection, ibuprofen, 100 mg K2 G

Medicare Statute 1833(t)

Coding Clinic: 2011, Q1, P6

C9280 Injection, eribulin mesylate, 1 mg ✳

C9281 Injection, pegloticase, 1 mg ✳

C9282 Injection, ceftaroline fosamil, 10 mg ✳

C9283 Injection, acetaminophen, 10 mg ✳

C9284 Injection, ipilimumab, 1mg ✳

▶ ☺ **C9285** Lidocaine 70 mg/tetracaine 70 mg, per patch K2 G

Medicare Statute 1833(t)

▶ ☺ **C9286** Injection, belatacept, 1 mg K2 G

Medicare Statute 1833(t)

▶ ☺ **C9287** Injection, brentuximab vedotin, 1 mg K2 G

Medicare Statute 1833(t)

☺ **C9352** Microporous collagen implantable tube (NeuraGen Nerve Guide), per centimeter length N1 N

621MMA

☺ **C9353** Microporous collagen implantable slit tube (NeuraWrap Nerve Protector), per centimeter length N1 N

621MMA

☺ **C9354** Acellular pericardial tissue matrix of non-human origin (Veritas), per square centimeter N1 N

621MMA

☺ **C9355** Collagen nerve cuff (NeuroMatrix), per 0.5 centimeter length N1 N

621MMA

☺ **C9356** Tendon, porous matrix of cross-linked collagen and glycosaminoglycan matrix (TenoGlide Tendon Protector Sheet), per square centimeter N1 N

621MMA

☺ **C9358** Dermal substitute, native, non-denatured collagen, fetal bovine origin (SurgiMend Collagen Matrix), per 0.5 square centimeters K2 K

621MMA

☺ **C9359** Porous purified collagen matrix bone void filler (Integra Mozaik Osteoconductive Scaffold Putty, Integra OS Osteoconductive Scaffold Putty), per 0.5 cc N1 N

Medicare Statute 1833(t)

☺ **C9360** Dermal substitute, native, non-denatured collagen, neonatal bovine origin (SurgiMend Collagen Matrix), per 0.5 square centimeters K2 K

621MMA

☺ **C9361** Collagen matrix nerve wrap (NeuroMend Collagen Nerve Wrap), per 0.5 centimeter length N1 N

621MMA

☺ **C9362** Porous purified collagen matrix bone void filler (Integra Mozaik Osteoconductive Scaffold Strip), per 0.5 cc N1 N

621MMA

Coding Clinic: 2010, Q2, P8

☺ **C9363** Skin substitute, Integra Meshed Bilayer Wound Matrix, per square centimeter K2 K

621MMA

Coding Clinic: 2010, Q2, P8

☺ **C9364** Porcine implant, Permacol, per square centimeter N1 N

621MMA

C9365 Oasis ultri tri-layer matrix, per square centimeter ✳

▶ ☺ **C9366** Epifix, per square centimeter K2 G

Medicare Statute 1833(t)

▶ ☺ **C9367** Skin substitute, endoform dermal template, per square centimeter K2 G

Medicare Statute 1833(t)(6)

☺ **C9399** Unclassified drugs or biologicals K7 A

621MMA

Coding Clinic: 2010, Q3, P8

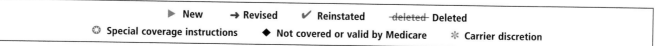

▶ New → Revised ✔ Reinstated deleted Deleted

☺ Special coverage instructions ◆ Not covered or valid by Medicare ✳ Carrier discretion

C9406 ~~Iodine i 123 ioflupane, diagnostic, per study dose, up to 5 millicuries~~ ✖

⚙ **C9716** Creations of thermal anal lesions by radiofrequency energy `Qh` T

Medicare Statute 1833(t)

⚙ **C9724** Endoscopic full-thickness plication in the gastric cardia using endoscopic plication system (EPS); includes endoscopy `Qh` T

Medicare Statute 1833(t)

⚙ **C9725** Placement of endorectal intracavitary applicator for high intensity brachytherapy `Qh` T

Medicare Statute 1833(t)

⚙ **C9726** Placement and removal (if performed) of applicator into breast for radiation therapy `Qh` T

Medicare Statute 1833(t)

⚙ **C9727** Insertion of implants into the soft palate; minimum of three implants `Qh` T

Medicare Statute 1833(t)

✳ **C9728** Placement of interstitial device(s) for radiation therapy/surgery guidance (e.g., fiducial markers, dosimeter), for other than the following sites (any approach): abdomen, pelvis, prostate, retroperitoneum, thorax, single or multiple `Qh` X

Medicare Statute 1833(t)

C9729 ~~Percutaneous laminotomy/ laminectomy (intralaminar approach) for decompression of neural elements (with ligamentous resection, discectomy, facetectomy and/or foraminotomy, when performed) any method under indirect image guidance, with the use of an endoscope when performed, single or multiple levels, unilateral or bilateral; lumbar~~ ✖

C9730 ~~Bronchoscopic bronchial thermoplasty with imaging guidance (if performed), radiofrequency ablation of airway smooth muscle, 1 lobe~~ ✖

C9731 ~~Bronchoscopic bronchial thermoplasty with imaging guidance (if performed), radiofrequency ablation of airway smooth muscle, 2 or more lobes~~ ✖

▶ ⚙ **C9732** Insertion of ocular telescope prosthesis including removal of crystalline lens T

Medicare Statute 1833(t)

▶ ⚙ **C9800** Dermal injection procedure(s) for facial lipodystrophy syndrome (LDS) and provision of radiesse or sculptra dermal filler, including all items and supplies T

Temporary office-based destination

Medicare Statute 1833(t)

Coding Clinic: 2010, Q3, P8, 10

⚙ **C9898** Radiolabeled product provided during a hospital inpatient stay `Qh` N

⚙ **C9899** Implanted prosthetic device, payable only for inpatients who do not have inpatient coverage A

Medicare Statute 1833(t)

ⓅⓆⓇⓈ PQRS	`Qp` **Quantity Physician Appendix A**	`Qh` **Quantity Hospital Appendix B**	♀ **Female only**
♂ **Male only**	`A` **Age**	♿ **DMEPOS**	A2-Z3 **ASC Payment Indicator**	A-Y **ASC Status Indicator**	Coding Clinic

131

CMS HOSPITAL OUTPATIENT PAYMENT SYSTEM   C9716 – C9899

DENTAL PROCEDURES (D0000-D9999)

Diagnostic

D0120-D0363: Bill local carrier

◆ **D0120** Periodic oral evaluation E

Medicare Statute 1862A(12)

◆ **D0140** Limited oral evaluation - problem focused E

Medicare Statute 1862A(12)

◆ **D0145** Oral evaluation for a patient under three years of age and counseling with primary caregiver A E

Medicare Statute 1862A(12)

☺ **D0150** Comprehensive oral evaluation - new or established patient S

IOM: 100-02, 15, 150; 100-02, 16, 140; 100-03, 4, 260.6

◆ **D0160** Detailed and extensive oral evaluation - problem focused, by report E

Medicare Statute 1862A(12)

◆ **D0170** Re-evaluation-limited, problem focused (established patient; not post-operative visit) E

Medicare Statute 1862A(12)

◆ **D0180** Comprehensive periodontal evaluation - new or established patient E

Medicare Statute 1862A(12)

◆ **D0210** Intraoral-complete series (including bitewings) E

Cross Reference CPT 70320

◆ **D0220** Intraoral-periapical-first film E

Cross Reference CPT 70300

◆ **D0230** Intraoral-periapical-each additional film E

Cross Reference CPT 70310

☺ **D0240** Intraoral-occlusal film S

IOM: 100-02, 15, 150; 100-02, 16, 140

☺ **D0250** Extraoral-first film S

IOM: 100-02, 15, 150; 100-02, 16, 140

☺ **D0260** Extraoral-each additional film S

IOM: 100-02, 15, 150; 100-02, 16, 140

☺ **D0270** Bitewing-single film S

IOM: 100-02, 15, 150; 100-02, 16, 140

☺ **D0272** Bitewings-two films S

IOM: 100-02, 15, 150; 100-02, 16, 140

◆ **D0273** Bitewings - three films E

Medicare Statute 1862A(12)

☺ **D0274** Bitewings-four films S

IOM: 100-02, 15, 150; 100-02, 16, 140

☺ **D0277** Vertical bitewings - 7 to 8 films S

IOM: 100-02, 15, 150; 100-02, 16, 140

◆ **D0290** Posterior-anterior or lateral skull and facial bone survey film E

Cross Reference 70150

◆ **D0310** Sialography E

Cross Reference 70390

◆ **D0320** Temporomandibular joint arthrogram, including injection E

Cross Reference 70332

◆ **D0321** Other temporomandibular joint films, by report E

Cross Reference 76499

◆ **D0322** Tomographic survey E

Cross Reference CPT
IOM: 100-03, 4, 260.6

◆ **D0330** Panoramic film E

Cross Reference 70320

◆ **D0340** Cephalometric film E

Cross Reference 70350

◆ **D0350** Oral/facial photographic images E

◆ **D0360** Cone beam CT - craniofacial data capture E

Medicare Statute 1862A(12)

◆ **D0362** Cone beam - two-dimensional image reconstruction using existing data, includes multiple images E

Medicare Statute 1862A(12)

◆ **D0363** Cone beam - three-dimensional image reconstruction using existing data, includes multiple images E

Medicare Statute 1862A(12)

Tests and Examinations

D0415-D0999: Bill local carrier

◆ **D0415** Collection of microorganisms for culture and sensitivity E

Medicare Statute 1862A(12)
Cross Reference D0410

☺ **D0416** Viral culture B

◆ **D0417** Collection and preparation of saliva sample for laboratory diagnostic testing E

▶ **New**   → **Revised**   ✔ **Reinstated**   ~~deleted~~ **Deleted**
☺ **Special coverage instructions**   ◆ **Not covered or valid by Medicare**   ✳ **Carrier discretion**

◆ **D0418** Analysis of saliva sample E

☺ **D0421** Genetic test for susceptibility to oral diseases B

◆ **D0425** Caries susceptibility tests E

Medicare Statute 1862A(12)

Cross Reference D0420

☺ **D0431** Adjunctive pre-diagnostic test that aids in detection of mucosal abnormalities including premalignant and malignant lesions, not to include cytology or biopsy procedures B

☺ **D0460** Pulp vitality tests S

IOM: 100-02, 15, 150; 100-02, 16, 140; 100-03, 4, 260.6

◆ **D0470** Diagnostic casts E

Medicare Statute 1862A(12)

☺ **D0472** Accession of tissue, gross examination, preparation and transmission of written report B

IOM: 100-02, 15, 150; 100-02, 16, 140; 100-03, 4, 260.6

☺ **D0473** Accession of tissue, gross and microscopic examination, preparation and transmission of written report B

IOM: 100-02, 15, 150; 100-02, 16, 140; 100-03, 4, 260.6

☺ **D0474** Accession of tissue, gross and microscopic examination, including assessment of surgical margins for presence of disease, preparation and transmission of written report B

IOM: 100-02, 15, 150; 100-02, 16, 140; 100-03, 4, 260.6

☺ **D0475** Decalcification procedure B

☺ **D0476** Special stains for microorganisms B

☺ **D0477** Special stains, not for microorganisms B

☺ **D0478** Immunohistochemical stains B

☺ **D0479** Tissue in-situ hybridization, including interpretation B

☺ **D0480** Accession of exfoliative cytologic smears, microscopic examination, preparation and transmission of written report B

IOM: 100-02, 15, 150; 100-02, 16, 140; 100-03, 4, 260.6

☺ **D0481** Electron microscopy – diagnostic B

☺ **D0482** Direct immunofluorescence B

☺ **D0483** Indirect immunofluorescence B

☺ **D0484** Consultation on slides prepared elsewhere B

☺ **D0485** Consultation, including preparation of slides from biopsy material supplied by referring source B

◆ **D0486** Laboratory accession of transepithelial cytologic sample, microscopic examination, preparation and transmission of written report E

Medicare Statute 1862A(12)

☺ **D0502** Other oral pathology procedures, by report B

IOM: 100-02, 15, 150; 100-02, 16, 140; 100-03, 4, 260.6

☺ **D0999** Unspecified diagnostic procedure, by report B

IOM: 100-02, 15, 150; 100-02, 16, 140; 100-03, 4, 260.6

Preventative

D1110-D1555: Bill local carrier

◆ **D1110** Prophylaxis-adult **A** E

Medicare Statute 1862A(12)

◆ **D1120** Prophylaxis-child **A** E

Medicare Statute 1862A(12)

◆ **D1203** Topical application of fluoride-child **A** E

Medicare Statute 1862A(12)

◆ **D1204** Topical application of fluoride-adult **A** E

Medicare Statute 1862A(12)

◆ **D1206** Topical fluoride varnish; therapeutic application for moderate to high caries risk patients E

Medicare Statute 1862A(12)

◆ **D1310** Nutritional counseling for the control of dental disease E

IOM: 100-02, 16, 10

◆ **D1320** Tobacco counseling for the control and prevention of oral disease E

IOM: 100-02, 16, 10

◆ **D1330** Oral hygiene instruction E

IOM: 100-02, 16, 10

◆ **D1351** Sealant-per tooth E

Medicare Statute 1862A(12)

◆ **D1352** Preventive resin restoration in a moderate to high caries risk patient — permanent tooth E

⊛ **D1510**   Space maintainer-fixed unilateral   S
IOM: 100-02, 16, 140; 100-04, 4, 20.5

⊛ **D1515**   Space maintainer-fixed bilateral   S
IOM: 100-02, 15, 150; 100-02, 16, 140

⊛ **D1520**   Space maintainer-removable unilateral   S
IOM: 100-02, 15, 150; 100-02, 16, 140

⊛ **D1525**   Space maintainer-removable bilateral   S
IOM: 100-02, 15, 150; 100-02, 16, 140

⊛ **D1550**   Recementation of space maintainer   S
IOM: 100-02, 15, 150; 100-02, 16, 140

◆ **D1555**   Removal of fixed space maintainer   E
Medicare Statute 1862A(12)

Restorative

D2140-D2999:   Bill local carrier

◆ **D2140**   Amalgam-one surface, primary or permanent   E
Medicare Statute 1862A(12)

◆ **D2150**   Amalgam-two surfaces, primary or permanent   E
Medicare Statute 1862A(12)

◆ **D2160**   Amalgam-three surfaces, primary or permanent   E
Medicare Statute 1862A(12)

◆ **D2161**   Amalgam-four or more surfaces, primary or permanent   E
Medicare Statute 1862A(12)

◆ **D2330**   Resin-one surface, anterior   E
Medicare Statute 1862A(12)

◆ **D2331**   Resin-two surfaces, anterior   E
Medicare Statute 1862A(12)

◆ **D2332**   Resin-three surfaces, anterior   E
Medicare Statute 1862A(12)

◆ **D2335**   Resin-four or more surfaces or involving incisal angle (anterior)   E
Medicare Statute 1862A(12)

◆ **D2390**   Resin-based composite crown, anterior   E
Medicare Statute 1862A(12)

◆ **D2391**   Resin-based composite - one surface, posterior   E
Medicare Statute 1862A(12)

◆ **D2392**   Resin-based composite - two surfaces, posterior   E
Medicare Statute 1862A(12)

◆ **D2393**   Resin-based composite - three surfaces, posterior   E
Medicare Statute 1862A(12)

◆ **D2394**   Resin-based composite - four or more surfaces, posterior   E
Medicare Statute 1862A(12)

◆ **D2410**   Gold foil-one surface   E
Medicare Statute 1862A(12)

◆ **D2420**   Gold foil-two surfaces   E
Medicare Statute 1862A(12)

◆ **D2430**   Gold foil-three surfaces   E
Medicare Statute 1862A(12)

◆ **D2510**   Inlay-metallic-one surface   E
Medicare Statute 1862A(12)

◆ **D2520**   Inlay-metallic-two surfaces   E
Medicare Statute 1862A(12)

◆ **D2530**   Inlay-metallic-three or more surfaces   E
Medicare Statute 1862A(12)

◆ **D2542**   Onlay-metallic-two surfaces   E
Medicare Statute 1862A(12)

◆ **D2543**   Onlay - metallic - three surfaces   E
Medicare Statute 1862A(12)

◆ **D2544**   Onlay - metallic - four or more surfaces   E
Medicare Statute 1862A(12)

◆ **D2610**   Inlay-porcelain/ceramic-one surface   E
Medicare Statute 1862A(12)

◆ **D2620**   Inlay-porcelain/ceramic-two surfaces   E
Medicare Statute 1862A(12)

◆ **D2630**   Inlay-porcelain/ceramic-three or more surfaces   E
Medicare Statute 1862A(12)

◆ **D2642**   Onlay - porcelain/ceramic - two surfaces   E
Medicare Statute 1862A(12)

◆ **D2643**   Onlay - porcelain/ceramic - three surfaces   E
Medicare Statute 1862A(12)

◆ **D2644**   Onlay - porcelain/ceramic - four or more surfaces   E
Medicare Statute 1862A(12)

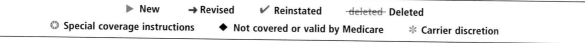

▶ New   → Revised   ✔ Reinstated   ~~deleted~~ Deleted
⊛ Special coverage instructions   ◆ Not covered or valid by Medicare   ✳ Carrier discretion

◆ **D2650** Inlay - resin-based composite - one surface   E

Medicare Statute 1862A(12)

◆ **D2651** Inlay - resin-based composite - two surfaces   E

Medicare Statute 1862A(12)

◆ **D2652** Inlay - resin-based composite - three or more surfaces   E

Medicare Statute 1862A(12)

◆ **D2662** Onlay - resin-based composite - two surfaces   E

Medicare Statute 1862A(12)

◆ **D2663** Onlay - resin-based composite - three surfaces   E

Medicare Statute 1862A(12)

◆ **D2664** Onlay - resin-based composite - four or more surfaces   E

Medicare Statute 1862A(12)

◆ **D2710** Crown - resin-based composite (indirect)   E

Medicare Statute 1862A(12)

◆ **D2712** Crown - 3/4 resin-based composite (indirect)   E

Medicare Statute 1862A(12)

◆ **D2720** Crown-resin with high noble metal   E

Medicare Statute 1862A(12)

◆ **D2721** Crown-resin with predominantly base metal   E

Medicare Statute 1862A(12)

◆ **D2722** Crown-resin with noble metal   E

Medicare Statute 1862A(12)

◆ **D2740** Crown-porcelain/ceramic substrate   E

Medicare Statute 1862A(12)

◆ **D2750** Crown-porcelain fused to high noble metal   E

Medicare Statute 1862A(12)

◆ **D2751** Crown-porcelain fused to predominantly base metal   E

Medicare Statute 1862A(12)

◆ **D2752** Crown-porcelain fused to noble metal   E

Medicare Statute 1862A(12)

◆ **D2780** Crown - 3/4 cast high noble metal   E

Medicare Statute 1862A(12)

◆ **D2781** Crown - 3/4 cast predominantly base metal   E

Medicare Statute 1862A(12)

◆ **D2782** Crown - 3/4 cast noble metal   E

Medicare Statute 1862A(12)

◆ **D2783** Crown - 3/4 porcelain/ceramic   E

Medicare Statute 1862A(12)

◆ **D2790** Crown-full cast high noble metal   E

Medicare Statute 1862A(12)

◆ **D2791** Crown-full cast predominantly base metal   E

Medicare Statute 1862A(12)

◆ **D2792** Crown-full cast noble metal   E

Medicare Statute 1862A(12)

◆ **D2794** Crown-titanium   E

Medicare Statute 1862A(12)

◆ **D2799** Provisional crown   E

Medicare Statute 1862A(12)

◆ **D2910** Recement inlay, onlay or partial coverage restoration   E

Medicare Statute 1862A(12)

◆ **D2915** Recement cast or prefabricated post and core   E

Medicare Statute 1862A(12)

◆ **D2920** Recement crown   E

Medicare Statute 1862A(12)

◆ **D2930** Prefabricated stainless steel crown-primary tooth   E

Medicare Statute 1862A(12)

◆ **D2931** Prefabricated stainless steel crown-permanent tooth   E

Medicare Statute 1862A(12)

◆ **D2932** Prefabricated resin crown   E

Medicare Statute 1862A(12)

◆ **D2933** Prefabricated stainless steel crown with resin window   E

Medicare Statute 1862A(12)

◆ **D2934** Prefabricated esthetic coated stainless steel crown - primary tooth   E

Medicare Statute 1862A(12)

◆ **D2940** Protective restoration   E

Medicare Statute 1862A(12)

◆ **D2950** Core build-up, including any pins   E

Medicare Statute 1862A(12)

◆ **D2951** Pin retention-per tooth, in addition to restoration   E

Medicare Statute 1862A(12)

◆ **D2952** Post and core in addition to crown, indirectly fabricated   E

Medicare Statute 1862A(12)

◆ **D2953** Each additional indirectly fabricated post - same tooth   E

Medicare Statute 1862A(12)

◆ **D2954** Prefabricated post and core in addition to crown   E

Medicare Statute 1862A(12)

◆ **D2955** Post removal (not in conjuction with endodontic therapy)   E

Medicare Statute 1862A(12)

◆ **D2957** Each additional prefabricated post - same tooth   E

Medicare Statute 1862A(12)

◆ **D2960** Labial veneer (laminate)-chairside   E

Medicare Statute 1862A(12)

◆ **D2961** Labial veneer (resin laminate)- laboratory   E

Medicare Statute 1862A(12)

◆ **D2962** Labial veneer (porcelain laminate)- laboratory   E

Medicare Statute 1862A(12)

❂ **D2970** Temporary crown (fractured tooth)   E

IOM: 100-02, 15, 150; 100-02, 16, 140

◆ **D2971** Additional procedures to construct new crown under existing partial denture framework   E

Medicare Statute 1862A(12)

◆ **D2975** Coping   E

Medicare Statute 1862A(12)

◆ **D2980** Crown repair, by report   E

Medicare Statute 1862A(12)

❂ **D2999** Unspecified restorative procedure, by report   S

Endodontics

D3110-D3999: Bill local carrier

◆ **D3110** Pulp cap-direct (excluding final restoration)   E

Medicare Statute 1862A(12)

◆ **D3120** Pulp cap-indirect (excluding final restoration)   E

Medicare Statute 1862A(12)

◆ **D3220** Therapeutic pulpotomy (excluding final restoration) removal of pulp coronal to the dentinocemental junction and application of medicament   E

Medicare Statute 1862A(12)

◆ **D3221** Pulpal debridement, primary and permanent teeth   E

Medicare Statute 1862A(12)

◆ **D3222** Partial pulpotomy for apexogenesis- permanent tooth with incomplete root development   E

Medicare Statute 1862A(12)

◆ **D3230** Pulpal therapy (resorbable filling)- anterior, primary tooth (excluding final restoration)   E

Medicare Statute 1862A(12)

◆ **D3240** Pulpal therapy (resorbable filling)- posterior, primary tooth (excluding final restoration)   E

Medicare Statute 1862A(12)

◆ **D3310** Endodontic therapy, anterior tooth (excluding final restoration)   E

Medicare Statute 1862A(12)

◆ **D3320** Endodontic therapy bicuspid tooth (excluding final restoration)   E

Medicare Statute 1862A(12)

◆ **D3330** Endodontic therapy molar (excluding final restoration)   E

Medicare Statute 1862A(12)

◆ **D3331** Treatment of root canal obstruction; non-surgical access   E

Medicare Statute 1862A(12)

◆ **D3332** Incomplete endodontic therapy; inoperable, unrestorable or fractured tooth   E

Medicare Statute 1862A(12)

◆ **D3333** Internal root repair of perforation defects   E

Medicare Statute 1862A(12)

◆ **D3346** Retreatment of previous root canal therapy-anterior   E

Medicare Statute 1862A(12)

◆ **D3347** Retreatment of previous root canal therapy-bicuspid   E

Medicare Statute 1862A(12)

◆ **D3348** Retreatment of previous root canal therapy-molar   E

Medicare Statute 1862A(12)

◆ **D3351** Apexification/recalcification/pulpal regeneration-initial visit (apical closure/ calcific repair of perforations, root resorption, pulp space disinfection, etc.)   E

Medicare Statute 1862A(12)

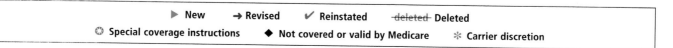

▶ New   → Revised   ✔ Reinstated   ̶d̶e̶l̶e̶t̶e̶d̶ Deleted

❂ Special coverage instructions   ◆ Not covered or valid by Medicare   ✳ Carrier discretion

◆ **D3352** Apexification/recalcification/pulpal regeneration-interim medication replacement (apical closure/calcific repair of perforations, root resorption, pulp space disinfection, etc.)   E

Medicare Statute 1862A(12)

◆ **D3353** Apexification/recalcification-final visit (includes completed root canal therapy-apical closure/calcific repair of perforations, root resorption, etc.)   E

Medicare Statute 1862A(12)

◆ **D3354** Pulpal regeneration - (completion of regenerative treatment in an immature permanent tooth with a necrotic pulp); does not include final restoration   E

◆ **D3410** Apicoectomy/periradicular surgery - anterior   E

Medicare Statute 1862A(12)

◆ **D3421** Apicoectomy/periradicular surgery-bicuspid (first root)   E

Medicare Statute 1862A(12)

◆ **D3425** Apicoectomy/periradicular surgery-molar (first root)   E

Medicare Statute 1862A(12)

◆ **D3426** Apicoectomy/periradicular surgery (each additional root)   E

Medicare Statute 1862A(12)

◆ **D3430** Retrograde filling-per root   E

Medicare Statute 1862A(12)

◆ **D3450** Root amputation-per root   E

Medicare Statute 1862A(12)

۞ **D3460** Endodontic endosseous implant   S

IOM: 100-02, 15, 150; 100-02, 16, 140

◆ **D3470** Intentional replantation (including necessary splinting)   E

Medicare Statute 1862A(12)

◆ **D3910** Surgical procedure for isolation of tooth with rubber dam   E

Medicare Statute 1862A(12)

◆ **D3920** Hemisection (including any root removal), not including root canal therapy   E

Medicare Statute 1862A(12)

◆ **D3950** Canal preparation and fitting of preformed dowel or post   E

Medicare Statute 1862A(12)

۞ **D3999** Unspecified endodontic procedure, by report   S

IOM: 100-02, 15, 150; 100-02, 16, 140

Periodontics

D4210-D4999: Bill local carrier

◆ **D4210** Gingivectomy or gingivoplasty - four or more contiguous teeth or tooth bounded spaces per quadrant   E

Cross Reference CPT 41820

◆ **D4211** Gingivectomy or gingivoplasty - one to three contiguous teeth or tooth bounded spaces per quadrant   E

Cross Reference CPT

◆ **D4230** Anatomical crown exposure - four or more contiguous teeth per quadrant   E

Medicare Statute 1862A(12)

◆ **D4231** Anatomical crown exposure - one to three teeth per quadrant   E

Medicare Statute 1862A(12)

◆ **D4240** Gingival flap procedure, including root planing - four or more contiguous teeth or tooth bounded spaces per quadrant   E

Medicare Statute 1862A(12)

◆ **D4241** Gingival flap procedure, including root planing - one to three contiguous teeth or tooth bounded spaces per quadrant   E

Medicare Statute 1862A(12)

◆ **D4245** Apically positioned flap   E

Medicare Statute 1862A(12)

◆ **D4249** Clinical crown lengthening-hard tissue   E

Medicare Statute 1862A(12)

۞ **D4260** Osseous surgery (including flap entry and closure) - four or more contiguous teeth or tooth bounded spaces per quadrant   S

IOM: 100-2, 15, 150; 100-02, 16, 140

◆ **D4261** Osseous surgery (including flap entry and closure) - one to three contiguous teeth or tooth bounded spaces per quadrant   E

Medicare Statute 1862A(12)

۞ **D4263** Bone replacement graft - first site in quadrant   S

IOM: 100-02, 15, 150; 100-02, 16, 140; 100-03, 4, 260.6

۞ **D4264** Bone replacement graft - each additional site in quadrant   S

IOM: 100-02, 15, 150; 100-2, 16, 140; 100-3, 4, 260.6

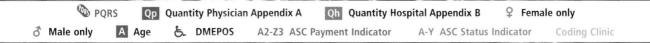
DENTAL PROCEDURES   D3352 – D4264

◆ **D4265** Biologic materials to aid in soft and osseous tissue regeneration   E

Medicare Statute 1862A(12)

◆ **D4266** Guided tissue regeneration - resorbable barrier, per site   E

Medicare Statute 1862A(12)

◆ **D4267** Guided tissue regeneration - nonresorbable barrier, per site, (includes membrane removal)   E

Medicare Statute 1862A(12)

☼ **D4268** Surgical revision procedure, per tooth   S

IOM: 100-02; 15, 150; 100-02, 16, 140

☼ **D4270** Pedicle soft tissue graft procedure   S

IOM: 100-02, 15, 150; 100-02, 16, 140

☼ **D4271** Free soft tissue graft procedure (including donor site surgery)   S

IOM: 100-02, 15, 150; 100-02, 16, 140

☼ **D4273** Subepithelial connective tissue graft procedures, per tooth   S

IOM:100-02, 15, 150; 100-02, 16, 140; 100-03, 4, 260.6

◆ **D4274** Distal or proximal wedge procedure (when not performed in conjuction with surgical procedures in the same anatomical area)   E

Medicare Statute 1862A(12)

◆ **D4275** Soft tissue allograft   E

Medicare Statute 1862A(12)

◆ **D4276** Combined connective tissue and double pedicle graft, per tooth   E

Medicare Statute 1862A(12)

◆ **D4320** Provisional splinting-intracoronal   E

Medicare Statute 1862A(12)

◆ **D4321** Provisional splinting-extracoronal   E

Medicare Statute 1862A(12)

◆ **D4341** Periodontal scaling and root planing - four or more teeth per quadrant   E

Medicare Statute 1862A(12)

◆ **D4342** Periodontal scaling and root planing - one to three teeth, per quadrant   E

Medicare Statute 1862A(12)

☼ **D4355** Full mouth debridement to enable comprehensive evaluation and diagnosis   S

IOM: 100-02, 15, 150; 100-02, 16, 140

☼ **D4381** Localized delivery of antimicrobial agents via a controlled release vehicle into diseased crevicular tissue, per tooth, by report   S

IOM: 100-02, 15, 150; 100-02, 16, 140

◆ **D4910** Periodontal maintenance   E

Medicare Statute 1862A(12)

◆ **D4920** Unscheduled dressing change (by someone other than treating dentist)   E

Medicare Statute 1862A(12)

◆ **D4999** Unspecified periodontal procedure, by report   E

Medicare Statute 1862A(12)

Prosthodontics (removable)

D5110-D5899: Bill local carrier

◆ **D5110** Complete denture – maxillary   E

Medicare Statute 1862A(12)

◆ **D5120** Complete denture – mandibular   E

Medicare Statute 1862A(12)

◆ **D5130** Immediate denture – maxillary   E

Medicare Statute 1862A(12)

◆ **D5140** Immediate denture – mandibular   E

Medicare Statute 1862A(12)

◆ **D5211** Upper partial-resin base (including any conventional clasps, rests and teeth)   E

Medicare Statute 1862A(12)

◆ **D5212** Lower partial-resin base (including any conventional clasps, rests and teeth)   E

Medicare Statute 1862A(12)

◆ **D5213** Maxillary partial denture - cast metal framework with resin denture bases (including any conventional clasps, rests and teeth)   E

Medicare Statute 1862A(12)

◆ **D5214** Mandibular partial denture - cast metal framework with resin denture bases (including any conventional clasps, rests and teeth)   E

Medicare Statute 1862A(12)

◆ **D5225** Maxillary partial denture - flexible base (including any clasps, rests and teeth)   E

Medicare Statute 1862A(12)

▶ New	→ Revised	✔ Reinstated	~~deleted~~ Deleted
☼ Special coverage instructions	◆ Not covered or valid by Medicare	✳ Carrier discretion	

◆ **D5226** Mandibular partial denture - flexible base (including any clasps, rests and teeth)   E
Medicare Statute 1862A(12)

◆ **D5281** Removable unilateral partial denture-one piece cast metal (including clasps and teeth)   E
Medicare Statute 1862A(12)

◆ **D5410** Adjust complete denture – maxillary   E
Medicare Statute 1862A(12)

◆ **D5411** Adjust complete denture – mandibular   E
Medicare Statute 1862A(12)

◆ **D5421** Adjust partial denture – maxillary   E
Medicare Statute 1862A(12)

◆ **D5422** Adjust partial denture – mandibular   E
Medicare Statute 1862A(12)

◆ **D5510** Repair broken complete denture base   E
Medicare Statute 1862A(12)

◆ **D5520** Replace missing or broken teeth-complete denture (each tooth)   E
Medicare Statute 1862A(12)

◆ **D5610** Repair resin denture base   E
Medicare Statute 1862A(12)

◆ **D5620** Repair cast framework   E
Medicare Statute 1862A(12)

◆ **D5630** Repair or replace broken clasp   E
Medicare Statute 1862A(12)

◆ **D5640** Replace broken teeth-per tooth   E
Medicare Statute 1862A(12)

◆ **D5650** Add tooth to existing partial denture   E
Medicare Statute 1862A(12)

◆ **D5660** Add clasp to existing partial denture   E
Medicare Statute 1862A(12)

◆ **D5670** Replace all teeth and acrylic on cast metal framework (maxillary)   E
Medicare Statute 1862A(12)

◆ **D5671** Replace all teeth and acrylic on cast metal framework (mandibular)   E
Medicare Statute 1862A(12)

◆ **D5710** Rebase complete maxillary denture   E
Medicare Statute 1862A(12)

◆ **D5711** Rebase complete mandibular denture   E
Medicare Statute 1862A(12)

◆ **D5720** Rebase maxillary partial denture   E
Medicare Statute 1862A(12)

◆ **D5721** Rebase mandibular partial denture   E
Medicare Statute 1862A(12)

◆ **D5730** Reline complete maxillary denture (chairside)   E
Medicare Statute 1862A(12)

◆ **D5731** Reline lower complete mandibular denture (chairside)   E
Medicare Statute 1862A(12)

◆ **D5740** Reline maxillary partial denture (chairside)   E
Medicare Statute 1862A(12)

◆ **D5741** Reline mandibular partial denture (chairside)   E
Medicare Statute 1862A(12)

◆ **D5750** Reline complete maxillary denture (laboratory)   E
Medicare Statute 1862A(12)

◆ **D5751** Reline complete mandibular denture (laboratory)   E
Medicare Statute 1862A(12)

◆ **D5760** Reline maxillary partial denture (laboratory)   E
Medicare Statute 1862A(12)

◆ **D5761** Reline mandibular partial denture (laboratory)   E
Medicare Statute 1862A(12)

◆ **D5810** Interim complete denture (maxillary)   E
Medicare Statute 1862A(12)

◆ **D5811** Interim complete denture (mandibular)   E
Medicare Statute 1862A(12)

◆ **D5820** Interim partial denture (maxillary)   E
Medicare Statute 1862A(12)

◆ **D5821** Interim partial denture (mandibular)   E
Medicare Statute 1862A(12)

◆ **D5850** Tissue conditioning, maxillary   E
Medicare Statute 1862A(12)

◆ **D5851** Tissue conditioning, mandibular   E
Medicare Statute 1862A(12)

◆ **D5860** Overdenture-complete, by report   E
Medicare Statute 1862A(12)

◆ **D5861** Overdenture-partial, by report   E
Medicare Statute 1862A(12)

DENTAL PROCEDURES D5226 – D5861

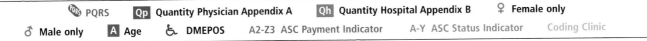

◆ **D5862**   Precision attachment, by report   E

Medicare Statute 1862A(12)

◆ **D5867**   Replacement of replaceable part of semi-precision or precision attachment (male or female component)   E

Medicare Statute 1862A(12)

◆ **D5875**   Modification of removable prosthesis following implant surgery   E

Medicare Statute 1862A(12)

◆ **D5899**   Unspecified removable prosthodontic procedure, by report   E

Medicare Statute 1862A(12)

Maxillofacial Prosthetics

D5911-D5999:   Bill local carrier

☉ **D5911**   Facial moulage (sectional)   S

IOM: 100-02, 15, 150; 100-02, 16, 140

☉ **D5912**   Facial moulage (complete)   S

IOM: 100-02, 15, 150

◆ **D5913**   Nasal prosthesis   E

Cross Reference CPT 21087

◆ **D5914**   Auricular prosthesis   E

Cross Reference CPT 21086

◆ **D5915**   Orbital prosthesis   E

Cross Reference CPT L8611

◆ **D5916**   Ocular prosthesis   E

Cross Reference CPT, V2623, V2629

◆ **D5919**   Facial prosthesis   E

Cross Reference CPT 21088

◆ **D5922**   Nasal septal prosthesis   E

Cross Reference CPT 30220

◆ **D5923**   Ocular prosthesis, interim   E

Cross Reference CPT 92330

◆ **D5924**   Cranial prosthesis   E

Cross Reference CPT 62143

◆ **D5925**   Facial augmentation implant prosthesis   E

Cross Reference CPT 21208

◆ **D5926**   Nasal prosthesis, replacement   E

Cross Reference CPT 21087

◆ **D5927**   Auricular prosthesis, replacement   E

Cross Reference CPT 21086

◆ **D5928**   Orbital prosthesis, replacement   E

Cross Reference CPT 67550

◆ **D5929**   Facial prosthesis, replacement   E

Cross Reference CPT 21088

◆ **D5931**   Obturator prosthesis, surgical   E

Cross Reference CPT 21079

◆ **D5932**   Obturator prosthesis, definitive   E

Cross Reference CPT 21080

◆ **D5933**   Obturator prosthesis, modification   E

Cross Reference CPT 21080

◆ **D5934**   Mandibular resection prosthesis with guide flange   E

Cross Reference CPT 21081

◆ **D5935**   Mandibular resection prosthesis without guide flange   E

Cross Reference CPT 21081

◆ **D5936**   Obturator/prosthesis, interim   E

Cross Reference CPT 21079

◆ **D5937**   Trismus appliance (not for tm treatment)   E

IOM: 100-02, 15, 150

☉ **D5951**   Feeding aid   E

IOM: 100-02, 15, 150; 100-02, 16, 140

◆ **D5952**   Speech aid prosthesis, pediatric   E

Cross Reference CPT 21084

◆ **D5953**   Speech aid prosthesis, adult   E

Cross Reference CPT 21084

◆ **D5954**   Palatal augmentation prosthesis   E

Cross Reference CPT 21082

◆ **D5955**   Palatal lift prosthesis, definitive   E

Cross Reference CPT 21083

◆ **D5958**   Palatal lift prosthesis, interim   E

Cross Reference CPT 21083

◆ **D5959**   Palatal lift prosthesis, modification   E

Cross Reference CPT 21083

◆ **D5960**   Speech aid prosthesis, modification   E

Cross Reference CPT 21084

◆ **D5982**   Surgical stent   E

Cross Reference CPT 21085

☉ **D5983**   Radiation carrier   S

IOM: 100-02, 15, 150; 100-02, 16, 140

☉ **D5984**   Radiation shield   S

IOM: 100-02, 15, 150; 100-02, 16, 140

☉ **D5985**   Radiation cone locator   S

IOM: 100-02, 15, 150; 100-02, 16, 140

◆ **D5986**   Fluoride gel carrier   E

Medicare Statute 1862A(12)

▶ **New**   → **Revised**   ✔ **Reinstated**   deleted **Deleted**

☉ **Special coverage instructions**   ◆ **Not covered or valid by Medicare**   ✳ **Carrier discretion**

◎ **D5987**   Commissure splint   S

IOM: 100-02, 15, 150; 100-02, 16, 140

◆ **D5988**   Surgical splint   E

Cross Reference CPT

◆ **D5991**   Topical medicament carrier   E

Medicare Statute 1862A(12)

◆ **D5992**   Adjust maxillofacial prosthetic appliance, by report   E

◆ **D5993**   Maintenance and cleaning of a maxillofacial prosthesis (extra or intraoral) other than required adjustments, by report   E

◆ **D5999**   Unspecified maxillofacial prosthesis, by report   E

Cross Reference CPT

Implant Services

D6010-D6199:   Bill local carrier

FPD = fixed partial denture

◆ **D6010**   Surgical placement of implant body: endosteal implant   E

Cross Reference CPT 21248

◆ **D6012**   Surgical placement of interim implant body for transitional prosthesis: endosteal implant   E

Medicare Statute 1862A(12)

◆ **D6040**   Surgical placement: eposteal implant   E

Cross Reference CPT 21245

◆ **D6050**   Surgical placement: transosteal implant   E

Cross Reference CPT 21244

◆ **D6053**   Implant/abutment supported removable denture for completely edentulous arch   E

IOM: 100-02, 15, 150

◆ **D6054**   Implant/abutment supported removable denture for partially edentulous arch   E

IOM: 100-02, 15, 150

◆ **D6055**   Connecting bar — implant supported or abutment supported   E

IOM: 100-02, 15, 150

◆ **D6056**   Prefabricated abutment - includes placement   E

IOM: 100-02, 15, 150

◆ **D6057**   Custom abutment - includes placement   E

IOM: 100-02, 15, 150

◆ **D6058**   Abutment supported porcelain/ceramic crown   E

IOM: 100-02, 15, 150

◆ **D6059**   Abutment supported porcelain fused to metal crown (high noble metal)   E

IOM: 100-02, 15, 150

◆ **D6060**   Abutment supported porcelain fused to metal crown (predominantly base metal)   E

IOM: 100-02, 15, 150

◆ **D6061**   Abutment supported porcelain fused to metal crown (noble metal)   E

IOM: 100-02, 15, 150

◆ **D6062**   Abutment supported cast metal crown (high noble metal)   E

IOM: 100-02, 15, 150

◆ **D6063**   Abutment supported cast metal crown (predominantly base metal)   E

IOM: 100-02, 15, 150

◆ **D6064**   Abutment supported cast metal crown (noble metal)   E

IOM: 100-02, 15, 150

◆ **D6065**   Implant supported porcelain/ceramic crown   E

IOM: 100-02, 15, 150

◆ **D6066**   Implant supported porcelain fused to metal crown (titanium, titanium alloy, high noble metal)   E

IOM: 100-02, 15, 150

◆ **D6067**   Implant supported metal crown (titanium, titanium alloy, high noble metal)   E

IOM: 100-02, 15, 150

◆ **D6068**   Abutment supported retainer for porcelain/ceramic FPD   E

IOM: 100-02, 15, 150

◆ **D6069**   Abutment supported retainer for porcelain fused to metal FPD (high noble metal)   E

IOM: 100-02, 15, 150

◆ **D6070**   Abutment supported retainer for porcelain fused to metal FPD (predominantly base metal)   E

IOM: 100-02, 15, 150

◆ **D6071**   Abutment supported retainer for porcelain fused to metal FPD (noble metal)   E

IOM: 100-02, 15, 150

◆ **D6072**   Abutment supported retainer for cast metal FPD (high noble metal)   E

IOM: 100-02, 15, 150

| 🏅 PQRS | Qp Quantity Physician Appendix A | Qh Quantity Hospital Appendix B | ♀ Female only |
| ♂ Male only | A Age | 🦽 DMEPOS | A2-Z3 ASC Payment Indicator | A-Y ASC Status Indicator | Coding Clinic |

DENTAL PROCEDURES   D5987 – D6072

141

◆ **D6073** Abutment supported retainer for cast metal FPD (predominantly base metal)   E

IOM: 100-02, 15, 150

◆ **D6074** Abutment supported retainer for cast metal FPD (noble metal)   E

IOM: 100-02, 15, 150

◆ **D6075** Implant supported retainer for ceramic FPD   E

IOM: 100-02, 15, 150

◆ **D6076** Implant supported retainer for porcelain fused to metal FPD (titanium, titanium alloy, or high noble metal)   E

IOM: 100-02, 15, 150

◆ **D6077** Implant supported retainer for cast metal FPD (titanium, titanium alloy, or high noble metal)   E

IOM: 100-02, 15, 150

◆ **D6078** Implant/abutment supported fixed denture for completely edentulous arch   E

IOM: 100-02, 15, 150

◆ **D6079** Implant/abutment supported fixed denture for partially edentulous arch   E

IOM: 100-02, 15, 150

◆ **D6080** Implant maintenance procedures, including: removal of prosthesis, cleansing of prosthesis and abutmen reinsertion of prosthesis   E

IOM: 100-02, 15, 150

◆ **D6090** Repair implant supported prosthesis by report   E

Cross Reference CPT 21299

◆ **D6091** Replacement of semi-precision or precision attachment (male or female component) of implant/abutment supported prosthesis, per attachment   E

Medicare Statute 1862A(12)

◆ **D6092** Recement implant/abutment supported crown   E

Medicare Statute 1862A(12)

◆ **D6093** Recement implant/abutment supported fixed partial denture   E

Medicare Statute 1862A(12)

◆ **D6094** Abutment supported crown - (titanium)   E

Medicare Statute 1862A(12)

◆ **D6095** Repair implant abutment, by report   E

Cross Reference CPT 21299

◆ **D6100** Implant removal, by report   E

Cross Reference CPT 21299

◆ **D6190** Radiographic/surgical implant index, by report   E

Medicare Statute 1862A(12)

◆ **D6194** Abutment supported retainer crown for FPD - (titanium)   E

Medicare Statute 1862A(12)

◆ **D6199** Unspecified implant procedure, by report   E

Cross Reference CPT 21299

Prosthodontics, fixed

D6205-D6999:   Bill local carrier

◆ **D6205** Pontic - indirect resin based composite   E

Medicare Statute 1862A(12)

◆ **D6210** Pontic-cast high noble metal   E

Medicare Statute 1862A(12)

◆ **D6211** Pontic-cast predominantly base metal   E

Medicare Statute 1862A(12)

◆ **D6212** Pontic-cast noble metal   E

Medicare Statute 1862A(12)

◆ **D6214** Pontic – titanium   E

Medicare Statute 1862A(12)

◆ **D6240** Pontic-porcelain fused to high noble metal   E

Medicare Statute 1862A(12)

◆ **D6241** Pontic-porcelain fused to predominantly base metal   E

Medicare Statute 1862A(12)

◆ **D6242** Pontic-porcelain fused to noble metal   E

Medicare Statute 1862A(12)

IOM: 100-02, 15, 150

◆ **D6245** Pontic - porcelain/ceramic   E

IOM: 100-02, 15, 150

◆ **D6250** Pontic-resin with high noble metal   E

Medicare Statute 1862A(12)

◆ **D6251** Pontic-resin with predominantly base metal   E

Medicare Statute 1862A(12)

◆ **D6252** Pontic-resin with noble metal   E

Medicare Statute 1862A(12)

▶ New   → Revised   ✔ Reinstated   ~~deleted~~ Deleted

○ Special coverage instructions   ◆ Not covered or valid by Medicare   ✳ Carrier discretion

◆ **D6253** Provisional pontic   E
Medicare Statute 1862A(12)

◆ **D6254** Interim pontic   E

◆ **D6545** Retainer-cast metal for resin bonded fixed prosthesis   E
Medicare Statute 1862A(12)

◆ **D6548** Retainer - porcelain/ceramic for resin bonded fixed prosthesis   E
IOM: 100-02, 15, 150

◆ **D6600** Inlay-porcelain/ceramic, two surfaces   E
IOM: 100-02, 15, 150

◆ **D6601** Inlay - porcelain/ceramic, three or more surfaces   E
IOM: 100-02, 15, 150

◆ **D6602** Inlay - cast high noble metal, two surfaces   E
IOM: 100-02, 15, 150

◆ **D6603** Inlay - cast high noble metal, three or more surfaces   E
IOM: 100-02, 15, 150

◆ **D6604** Inlay - cast predominantly base metal, two surfaces   E
IOM: 100-02, 15, 150

◆ **D6605** Inlay - cast predominantly base metal, three or more surfaces   E
IOM: 100-02, 15, 150

◆ **D6606** Inlay - cast noble metal, two surfaces   E
IOM: 100-02, 15, 150

◆ **D6607** Inlay - cast noble metal, three or more surfaces   E
IOM: 100-02, 15, 150

◆ **D6608** Onlay - porcelain/ceramic, two surfaces   E
IOM: 100-02, 15, 150

◆ **D6609** Onlay - porcelain/ceramic, three or more surfaces   E
IOM: 100-02, 15, 150

◆ **D6610** Onlay - cast high noble metal, two surfaces   E
IOM: 100-02, 15, 150

◆ **D6611** Onlay - cast high noble metal, three or more surfaces   E
IOM: 100-02, 15, 150

◆ **D6612** Onlay - cast predominantly base metal, two surfaces   E
IOM: 100-02, 15, 150

◆ **D6613** Onlay - cast predominantly base metal, three or more surfaces   E
IOM: 100-02, 15, 150

◆ **D6614** Onlay - cast noble metal, two surfaces   E
IOM: 100-02, 15, 150

◆ **D6615** Onlay - cast noble metal, three or more surfaces   E
IOM: 100-02, 15, 150

◆ **D6624** Inlay – titanium   E
Medicare Statute 1862A(12)

◆ **D6634** Onlay – titanium   E
Medicare Statute 1862A(12)

◆ **D6710** Crown - indirect resin based composite   E
Medicare Statute 1862A(12)

◆ **D6720** Crown-resin with high noble metal   E
Medicare Statute 1862A(12)

◆ **D6721** Crown-resin with predominantly base metal   E
Medicare Statute 1862A(12)

◆ **D6722** Crown-resin with noble metal   E
Medicare Statute 1862A(12)

◆ **D6740** Crown - porcelain/ceramic   E
IOM: 100-02, 15, 150

◆ **D6750** Crown-porcelain fused to high noble metal   E
Medicare Statute 1862A(12)

◆ **D6751** Crown-porcelain fused to predominantly base metal   E
Medicare Statute 1862A(12)

◆ **D6752** Crown-porcelain fused to noble metal   E
Medicare Statute 1862A(12)

◆ **D6780** Crown-3/4 cast high noble metal   E
Medicare Statute 1862A(12)

◆ **D6781** Crown - 3/4 cast predominantly based metal   E
IOM: 100-02, 15, 150

◆ **D6782** Crown - 3/4 cast noble metal   E
IOM: 100-02, 15, 150

◆ **D6783** Crown - 3/4 porcelain/ceramic   E
IOM: 100-02, 15, 150

◆ **D6790** Crown-full cast high noble metal   E
Medicare Statute 1862A(12)

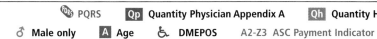

◆ **D6791** Crown-full cast predominantly base metal   E

Medicare Statute 1862A(12)

◆ **D6792** Crown-full cast noble metal   E

Medicare Statute 1862A(12)

◆ **D6793** Provisional retainer crown   E

Medicare Statute 1862A(12)

◆ **D6794** Crown - titanium   E

Medicare Statute 1862A(12)

◆ **D6795** Interim retainer crown   E

⊙ **D6920** Connector bar   S

IOM: 100-02, 15, 150; 100-02, 16, 140; 100-03, 4, 260.6

◆ **D6930** Recement bridge   E

Medicare Statute 1862A(12)

◆ **D6940** Stress breaker   E

Medicare Statute 1862A(12)

◆ **D6950** Precision attachment   E

Medicare Statute 1862A(12)

◆ **D6970** Post and core in addition to fixed partial denture retainer, indirectly fabricated   E

Medicare Statute 1862A(12)

◆ **D6972** Prefabricated post and core in addition to bridge retainer   E

Medicare Statute 1862A(12)

◆ **D6973** Core build up for retainer, including any pins   E

Medicare Statute 1862A(12)

◆ **D6975** Coping-metal   E

Medicare Statute 1862A(12)

◆ **D6976** Each additional indirectly fabricated post - same tooth   E

IOM: 100-02, 15, 150

◆ **D6977** Each additional prefabricated post - same tooth   E

IOM: 100-02, 15, 150

◆ **D6980** Bridge repair, by report   E

Medicare Statute 1862A(12)

◆ **D6985** Pediatric partial denture, fixed **A**   E

Medicare Statute 1862A(12)

◆ **D6999** Unspecified fixed prosthodontic procedure, by report   E

Medicare Statute 1862A(12)

Oral and Maxillofacial Surgery

D7111-D7999: Bill local carrier

⊙ **D7111** Extraction, coronal remnants - deciduous tooth   S

IOM: 100-02, 16, 140

🔵 ⊙ **D7140** Extraction, erupted tooth or exposed root (elevation and/or forceps removal)   S

IOM: 100-02, 16, 140

🔵 ⊙ **D7210** Surgical removal of erupted tooth requiring removal of bone and/or section of tooth, and elevation of mucoperiosteal flap   S

IOM: 100-02, 15, 150; 100-02, 16, 140

⊙ **D7220** Removal of impacted tooth-soft tissue   S

IOM: 100-02, 15, 150; 100-02, 16, 140

⊙ **D7230** Removal of impacted tooth-partially bony   S

IOM: 100-02, 15, 150; 100-02, 16, 140

⊙ **D7240** Removal of impacted tooth-completely bony   S

IOM: 100-02, 15, 150; 100-02, 16, 140

⊙ **D7241** Removal of impacted tooth-completely bony, with unusual surgical complications   S

IOM: 100-02, 15, 150; 100-02, 16, 140

⊙ **D7250** Surgical removal of residual tooth roots (cutting procedure)   S

IOM: 100-02, 15, 150; 100-02, 16, 140

◆ **D7251** Coronectomy — intentional partial tooth removal   E

⊙ **D7260** Oral antral fistula closure   S

IOM: 100-02, 15, 150; 100-02, 16, 140

⊙ **D7261** Primary closure of a sinus perforation   S

IOM: 100-02, 16, 140

◆ **D7270** Tooth reimplantation and/or stabilization of accidentally evulsed or displaced tooth   E

Medicare Statute 1862A(12)

◆ **D7272** Tooth transplantation (includes reimplantation from one site to another and splinting and/or stabilization)   E

Medicare Statute 1862A(12)

◆ **D7280** Surgical access of an unerupted tooth   E

Medicare Statute 1862A(12)

▶ New   → Revised   ✔ Reinstated   ~~deleted~~ Deleted

⊙ Special coverage instructions   ◆ Not covered or valid by Medicare   ✳ Carrier discretion

◆ **D7282** Mobilization of erupted or malpositioned tooth to aid eruption E

Medicare Statute 1862A(12)

❂ **D7283** Placement of device to facilitate eruption of impacted tooth B

◆ **D7285** Biopsy of oral tissue - hard (bone, tooth) E

Cross Reference CPT 20220, 20225, 20240, 20245

◆ **D7286** Biopsy of oral tissue – soft E

Cross Reference CPT 40808

◆ **D7287** Exfoliative cytological sample collection E

❂ **D7288** Brush biopsy - transepithelial sample collection B

◆ **D7290** Surgical repositioning of teeth E

Medicare Statute 1862A(12)

❂ **D7291** Transseptal fiberotomy/supra crestal fiberotomy, by report S

IOM: 100-02, 15, 150; 100-02, 16, 140

◆ **D7292** Surgical placement: temporary anchorage device [screw retained plate] requiring surgical flap E

Medicare Statute 1862A(12)

◆ **D7293** Surgical placement: temporary anchorage device requiring surgical flap E

Medicare Statute 1862A(12)

◆ **D7294** Surgical placement: temporary anchorage device without surgical flap E

Medicare Statute 1862A(12)

◆ **D7295** Harvest of bone for use in autogenous grafting procedure E

◆ **D7310** Alveoloplasty in conjunction with extractions - four or more teeth or tooth spaces, per quadrant E

Cross Reference CPT 41874

◆ **D7311** Alveoloplasty in conjunction with extractions - one to three teeth or tooth spaces, per quadrant E

Medicare Statute 1862A(12)

◆ **D7320** Alveoloplasty not in conjunction with extractions - four or more teeth or tooth spaces, per quadrant E

Cross Reference CPT 41870

❂ **D7321** Alveoloplasty not in conjunction with extractions - one to three teeth or tooth spaces, per quadrant B

◆ **D7340** Vestibuloplasty-ridge extension (second epithelialization) E

Cross Reference CPT 40840, 40842, 40843, 40844

◆ **D7350** Vestibuloplasty-ridge extension (including soft tissue grafts, muscle re-attachments, revision of soft tissue attachment, and management of hypertrophied and hyperplastic tissue) E

Cross Reference CPT 40845

◆ **D7410** Excision of benign lesion up to 1.25 cm E

Cross Reference CPT

◆ **D7411** Excision of benign lesion greater than 1.25 cm E

◆ **D7412** Excision of benign lesion, complicated E

◆ **D7413** Excision of malignant lesion up to 1.25 cm E

◆ **D7414** Excision of malignant lesion greater than 1.25 cm E

◆ **D7415** Excision of malignant lesion, complicated E

◆ **D7440** Excision of malignant tumor-lesion diameter up to 1.25 cm E

Cross Reference CPT

◆ **D7441** Excision of malignant tumor-lesion diameter greater than 1.25 cm E

Cross Reference CPT

◆ **D7450** Removal of benign odontogenic cyst or tumor-lesion diameter up to 1.25 cm E

Cross Reference CPT

◆ **D7451** Removal of benign odontogenic cyst or tumor-lesion diameter greater than 1.25 cm E

Cross Reference CPT

◆ **D7460** Removal of benign nonodontogenic cyst or tumor-lesion diameter up to 1.25 cm E

Cross Reference CPT

◆ **D7461** Removal of benign nonodontogenic cyst or tumor-lesion diameter greater than 1.25 cm E

Cross Reference CPT

◆ **D7465** Destruction of lesion(s) by physical or chemical methods, by report E

Cross Reference CPT 41850

◆ **D7471** Removal of lateral exostosis (maxilla or mandible) E

Cross Reference CPT 21031, 21032

🄿 PQRS	**Qp** Quantity Physician Appendix A	**Qh** Quantity Hospital Appendix B	♀ Female only
♂ Male only	**A** Age	🦽 DMEPOS	A2-Z3 ASC Payment Indicator A-Y ASC Status Indicator Coding Clinic

◆ **D7472**   Removal of torus palatinus   E

◆ **D7473**   Removal of torus mandibularis   E

◆ **D7485**   Surgical reduction of osseous tuberosity   E

◆ **D7490**   Radical resection of maxilla or mandible   E

Cross Reference CPT 21095

◆ **D7510**   Incision and drainage of abscess-intraoral soft tissue   E

Cross Reference CPT 41800

⊚ **D7511**   Incision and drainage of abscess - intraoral soft tissue-complicated (includes drainage of multiple fascial spaces)   B

◆ **D7520**   Incision and drainage of abscess-extraoral soft tissue   E

Cross Reference CPT 41800

⊚ **D7521**   Incision and drainage of abscess - extraoral soft tissue - complicated (includes drainage of multiple fascial spaces)   B

◆ **D7530**   Removal of foreign body from mucosa, skin, or subcutaneous alveolar tissue   E

Cross Reference CPT 41805, 41828

◆ **D7540**   Removal of reaction-producing foreign bodies-musculoskeletal system   E

Cross Reference CPT 20520, 41800, 41806

◆ **D7550**   Partial ostectomy/sequestrectomy for removal of non-vital bone   E

Cross Reference CPT 20999

◆ **D7560**   Maxillary sinusotomy for removal of tooth fragment or foreign body   E

Cross Reference CPT 31020

◆ **D7610**   Maxilla-open reduction (teeth immobilized if present)   E

Cross Reference CPT

◆ **D7620**   Maxilla-closed reduction (teeth immobilized if present)   E

Cross Reference CPT

◆ **D7630**   Mandible-open reduction (teeth immobilized if present)   E

Cross Reference CPT

◆ **D7640**   Mandible-closed reduction (teeth immobilized if present)   E

Cross Reference CPT

◆ **D7650**   Malar and/or zygomatic arch-open reduction   E

Cross Reference CPT

◆ **D7660**   Malar and/or zygomatic arch-closed reduction   E

Cross Reference CPT

◆ **D7670**   Alveolus - closed reduction, may include stabilization of teeth   E

Cross Reference CPT

◆ **D7671**   Alveolus - open reduction, may include stabilization of teeth   E

◆ **D7680**   Facial bones-complicated reduction with fixation and multiple surgical approaches   E

Cross Reference CPT

◆ **D7710**   Maxilla-open reduction   E

Cross Reference CPT 21346

◆ **D7720**   Maxilla-closed reduction   E

Cross Reference CPT 21345

◆ **D7730**   Mandible-open reduction   E

Cross Reference CPT 21461, 21462

◆ **D7740**   Mandible-closed reduction   E

Cross Reference CPT 21455

◆ **D7750**   Malar and/or zygomatic arch-open reduction   E

Cross Reference CPT 21360, 21365

◆ **D7760**   Malar and/or zygomatic arch-closed reduction   E

Cross Reference CPT 21355

◆ **D7770**   Alveolus - open reduction stabilization of teeth   E

Cross Reference CPT 21422

◆ **D7771**   Alveolus, closed reduction stabilization of teeth   E

◆ **D7780**   Facial bones-complicated reduction with fixation and multiple surgical approaches   E

Cross Reference CPT 21433, 21435

◆ **D7810**   Open reduction of dislocation   E

Cross Reference CPT 21490

◆ **D7820**   Closed reduction of dislocation   E

Cross Reference CPT 21480

◆ **D7830**   Manipulation under anesthesia   E

Cross Reference CPT 00190

◆ **D7840**   Condylectomy   E

Cross Reference CPT 21050

◆ **D7850**   Surgical discectomy; with/without implant   E

Cross Reference CPT 21060

◆ **D7852**   Disc repair   E

Cross Reference CPT 21299

▶ New   → Revised   ✔ Reinstated   ~~deleted~~ Deleted

⊚ Special coverage instructions   ◆ Not covered or valid by Medicare   ✷ Carrier discretion

◆ **D7854**   Synovectomy   E
Cross Reference CPT 21299

◆ **D7856**   Myotomy   E
Cross Reference CPT 21299

◆ **D7858**   Joint reconstruction   E
Cross Reference CPT 21242, 21243

◆ **D7860**   Arthrotomy   E
IOM: 100-02, 15, 150; 100-02, 16, 140

◆ **D7865**   Arthroplasty   E
Cross Reference CPT 21240

◆ **D7870**   Arthrocentesis   E
Cross Reference CPT 21060

◆ **D7871**   Non-arthroscopic lysis and lavage   E
Medicare Statute 1862A(12)

◆ **D7872**   Arthroscopy-diagnosis, with or without
              biopsy   E
Cross Reference CPT 29800

◆ **D7873**   Arthroscopy-surgical: lavage and lysis
              of adhesions   E
Cross Reference CPT 29804

◆ **D7874**   Arthroscopy-surgical: disc repositioning
              and stabilization   E
Cross Reference CPT 29804

◆ **D7875**   Arthroscopy-surgical: synovectomy   E
Cross Reference CPT 29804

◆ **D7876**   Arthroscopy-surgical: discectomy   E
Cross Reference CPT 29804

◆ **D7877**   Arthroscopy-surgical: debridement   E
Cross Reference CPT 29804

◆ **D7880**   Occlusal orthotic appliance   E
Cross Reference CPT 21499

◆ **D7899**   Unspecified TMD therapy, by
              report   E
Cross Reference CPT 21499

◆ **D7910**   Suture of recent small wounds up to
              5 cm   E
Cross Reference CPT 12011, 12013

◆ **D7911**   Complicated suture-up to 5 cm   E
Cross Reference CPT 12051, 12052

◆ **D7912**   Complicated suture-greater than
              5 cm   E
Cross Reference CPT 13132

◆ **D7920**   Skin graft (identify defect covered,
              location, and type of graft)   E
Cross Reference CPT

⊛ **D7940**   Osteoplasty-for orthognathic
              deformities   S
IOM: 100-02, 15, 150; 100-02, 16, 140

◆ **D7941**   Osteotomy - mandibular rami   E
*Cross Reference CPT 21193, 21195,
21196*

◆ **D7943**   Osteotomy - mandibular rami with
              bone graft; includes obtaining the
              graft   E
Cross Reference CPT 21194

◆ **D7944**   Osteotomy-segmented or subapical   E
Cross Reference CPT 21198, 21206

◆ **D7945**   Osteotomy-body of mandible   E
*Cross Reference CPT 21193, 21194,
21195, 21196*

◆ **D7946**   Lefort I (maxilla-total)   E
Cross Reference CPT 21147

◆ **D7947**   Lefort I (maxilla-segmented)   E
Cross Reference CPT 21145, 21146

◆ **D7948**   Lefort II or lefort III (osteoplasty of
              facial bones for midface hypoplasia or
              retrusion)-without bone graft   E
Cross Reference CPT 21150

◆ **D7949**   Lefort II or lefort III-with bone
              graft   E
Cross Reference CPT

◆ **D7950**   Osseous, osteoperiosteal, or cartilage
              graft of the mandible or maxilla -
              autogenous or nonautogenous, by
              report   E
Cross Reference CPT 21247

◆ **D7951**   Sinus augmentation with bone or bone
              substitutes   E
Medicare Statute 1862A(12)

◆ **D7953**   Bone replacement graft for ridge
              preservation - per site   E
Medicare Statute 1862A(12)

◆ **D7955**   Repair of maxillofacial soft and/or hard
              tissue defect   E
Cross Reference CPT 21299

◆ **D7960**   Frenulectomy also known as
              frenectomy or frenotomy-separate
              procedure not incidental to another
              procedure   E
*Cross Reference CPT 40819, 41010,
41115*

◆ **D7963**   Frenuloplasty   E
Medicare Statute 1862A(12)

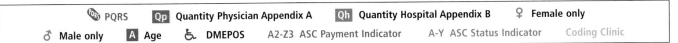

Ⓟ PQRS   Qp **Quantity Physician Appendix A**   Qh **Quantity Hospital Appendix B**   ♀ **Female only**

♂ **Male only**   Ⓐ **Age**   ♿ **DMEPOS**   A2-Z3 **ASC Payment Indicator**   A-Y **ASC Status Indicator**   Coding Clinic

◆ **D7970** Excision of hyperplastic tissue-per arch   E

Cross Reference CPT

◆ **D7971** Excision of pericoronal gingival   E

Cross Reference CPT 41821

◆ **D7972** Surgical reduction of fibrous tuberosity   E

◆ **D7980** Sialolithotomy   E

Cross Reference CPT 42330, 42335, 42340

◆ **D7981** Excision of salivary gland, by report   E

Cross Reference CPT 42408

◆ **D7982** Sialodochoplasty   E

Cross Reference CPT 42500

◆ **D7983** Closure of salivary fistula   E

Cross Reference CPT 42600

◆ **D7990** Emergency tracheotomy   E

Cross Reference CPT 21070

◆ **D7991** Coronoidectomy   E

Cross Reference CPT 21070

◆ **D7995** Synthetic graft-mandible or facial bones, by report   E

Cross Reference CPT 21299

◆ **D7996** Implant-mandible for augmentation purposes (excluding alveolar ridge), by report   E

Cross Reference CPT 21299

◆ **D7997** Appliance removal (not by dentist who placed appliance), includes removal of archbar   E

Medicare Statute 1862A(12)

◆ **D7998** Intraoral placement of a fixation device not in conjunction with a fracture   E

Medicare Statute 1862A(12)

◆ **D7999** Unspecified oral surgery procedure, by report   E

Cross Reference CPT 21299

Orthodontics

D8010-D8999: Bill local carrier

◆ **D8010** Limited orthodontic treatment of the primary dentition   E

Medicare Statute 1862A(12)

◆ **D8020** Limited orthodontic treatment of the transitional dentition   E

Medicare Statute 1862A(12)

◆ **D8030** Limited orthodontic treatment of the adolescent dentition **A**   E

Medicare Statute 1862A(12)

◆ **D8040** Limited orthodontic treatment of the adult dentition **A**   E

Medicare Statute 1862A(12)

◆ **D8050** Interceptive orthodontic treatment of the primary dentition   E

Medicare Statute 1862A(12)

◆ **D8060** Interceptive orthodontic treatment of the transitional dentition   E

Medicare Statute 1862A(12)

◆ **D8070** Comprehensive orthodontic treatment of the transitional dentition   E

Medicare Statute 1862A(12)

◆ **D8080** Comprehensive orthodontic treatment of the adolescent dentition **A**   E

Medicare Statute 1862A(12)

◆ **D8090** Comprehensive orthodontic treatment of the adult dentition **A**   E

Medicare Statute 1862A(12)

◆ **D8210** Removable appliance therapy   E

Medicare Statute 1862A(12)

◆ **D8220** Fixed appliance therapy   E

Medicare Statute 1862A(12)

◆ **D8660** Pre-orthodontic visit   E

Medicare Statute 1862A(12)

◆ **D8670** Periodic orthodontic treatment visit (as part of contract)   E

Medicare Statute 1862A(12)

◆ **D8680** Orthodontic retention (removal of appliances, construction and placement of retainer(s))   E

Medicare Statute 1862A(12)

◆ **D8690** Orthodontic treatment (alternative billing to a contract fee)   E

Medicare Statute 1862A(12)

◆ **D8691** Repair of orthodontic appliance   E

Medicare Statute 1862A(12)

◆ **D8692** Replacement of lost or broken retainer   E

Medicare Statute 1862A(12)

◆ **D8693** Rebonding or recementing; and/or repair, as required, of fixed retainers   E

Medicare Statute 1862A(12)

◆ **D8999** Unspecified orthodontic procedure, by report   E

Medicare Statute 1862A(12)

▶ New   → Revised   ✔ Reinstated   ~~deleted~~ Deleted

☼ Special coverage instructions   ◆ Not covered or valid by Medicare   ✳ Carrier discretion

Adjunctive General Services

D9110-D9999: Bill local carrier

⊕ **D9110**   Palliative (emergency) treatment of dental pain-minor procedures   N

IOM: 100-02, 15, 150; 100-02, 16, 140

◆ **D9120**   Fixed partial denture sectioning   E

Medicare Statute 1862A(12)

◆ **D9210**   Local anesthesia not in conjunction with operative or surgical procedures   E

Cross Reference CPT 90784

◆ **D9211**   Regional block anesthesia   E

Cross Reference CPT 01995

◆ **D9212**   Trigeminal division block anesthesia   E

Cross Reference CPT 64400

◆ **D9215**   Local anesthesia in conjunction with operative or surgical procedures   E

Cross Reference CPT 90784

◆ **D9220**   Deep sedation/general anesthesia-first 30 minutes   E

Cross Reference CPT

◆ **D9221**   Deep sedation/general anesthesia-each additional 15 minutes   E

IOM: 100-02, 15, 150; 100-02, 16, 140

⊕ **D9230**   Inhalation of nitrous oxide/analgesia, anxiolysis   N

IOM: 100-02, 15, 150; 100-02, 16, 140

◆ **D9241**   Intravenous conscious sedation/ analgesia - first 30 minutes   E

Cross Reference CPT 90784

◆ **D9242**   Intravenous conscious sedation/ analgesia - each additional 15 minutes   E

Cross Reference CPT 90784

⊕ **D9248**   Non-intravenous conscious sedation   N

◆ **D9310**   Consultation - diagnostic service provided by dentist or physician other than requesting dentist or physician   E

Cross Reference CPT

◆ **D9410**   House/extended care facility call   E

Cross Reference CPT

◆ **D9420**   Hospital or ambulatory surgical center call   E

Cross Reference CPT

◆ **D9430**   Office visit for observation (during regularly scheduled hours) no other services performed   E

Cross Reference CPT

◆ **D9440**   Office visit-after regularly scheduled hours   E

Cross Reference CPT 99050

◆ **D9450**   Case presentation, detailed and extensive treatment planning   E

◆ **D9610**   Therapeutic parenteral drug, single administration   E

◆ **D9612**   Therapeutic parenteral drugs, two or more administrations, different medications   E

Medicare Statute 1862A(12)

⊕ **D9630**   Other drugs and/or medicaments, by report   S

IOM: 100-02, 15, 150; 100-02, 16, 140

◆ **D9910**   Application of desensitizing medicament   E

Medicare Statute 1862A(12)

◆ **D9911**   Application of desensitizing resin for cervical and/or root surface, per tooth   E

Medicare Statute 1862A(12)

◆ **D9920**   Behavior management, by report   E

Medicare Statute 1862A(12)

⊕ **D9930**   Treatment of complications (postsurgical) - unusual circumstances, by report   S

IOM: 100-02, 15, 150; 100-02, 16, 140

⊕ **D9940**   Occlusal guards, by report   S

IOM: 100-02, 15, 150; 100-02, 16, 140

◆ **D9941**   Fabrication of athletic mouthguard   E

Medicare Statute 1862A(12)

Cross Reference CPT 21089

◆ **D9942**   Repair and/or reline of occlusal guard   E

Medicare Statute 1862A(12)

⊕ **D9950**   Occlusion analysis-mounted case   S

IOM: 100-02, 15, 150; 100-02, 16, 140

⊕ **D9951**   Occlusal adjustment-limited   S

IOM: 100-02, 15, 150; 100-02, 16, 140

⊕ **D9952**   Occlusal adjustment-complete   S

IOM: 100-02, 15, 150; 100-02, 16, 140

◆ **D9970**   Enamel microabrasion   E

Medicare Statute 1862A(12)

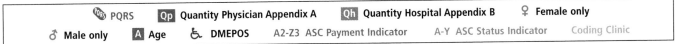

PQRS   **Qp** Quantity Physician Appendix A   **Qh** Quantity Hospital Appendix B   ♀ **Female only**

♂ **Male only**   **A** Age   ♿ **DMEPOS**   A2-Z3 ASC Payment Indicator   A-Y ASC Status Indicator   Coding Clinic

◆ **D9971** Odontoplasty 1 - 2 teeth; includes removal of enamel projections   E
Medicare Statute 1862A(12)

◆ **D9972** External bleaching - per arch   E
Medicare Statute 1862A(12)

◆ **D9973** External bleaching - per tooth   E
Medicare Statute 1862A(12)

◆ **D9974** Internal bleaching - per tooth   E
Medicare Statute 1862A(12)

◆ **D9999** Unspecified adjunctive procedure, by report   E
Cross Reference CPT 21499

▶ New   → Revised   ✔ Reinstated   ~~deleted~~ Deleted
✪ Special coverage instructions   ◆ Not covered or valid by Medicare   ✳ Carrier discretion

DURABLE MEDICAL EQUIPMENT
(E0100-E9999)

Canes

E0100-E0105   Bill DME/MAC

⊛ **E0100**   Cane, includes canes of all materials, adjustable or fixed, with tip **Qp** 🦽   Y

IOM: 100-02, 15, 110.1; 100-03, 4, 280.1; 100-03, 4, 280.2

DMEPOS Modifier(s): NU, RR, UE

⊛ **E0105**   Cane, quad or three prong, includes canes of all materials, adjustable or fixed, with tips **Qp** 🦽   Y

IOM: 100-02, 15, 110.1; 100-03, 4, 280.1; 100-03, 4, 280.2

DMEPOS Modifier(s): NU, RR, UE

Crutches

E0110-E0118:   Bill DME/MAC

⊛ **E0110**   Crutches, forearm, includes crutches of various materials, adjustable or fixed, pair, complete with tips and handgrips **Qp** 🦽   Y

Crutches are covered when prescribed for a patient who is normally ambulatory but suffers from a condition that impairs ambulation. Provides minimal to moderate weight support while ambulating.

IOM: 100-02, 15, 110.1; 100-03, 4, 280.1

DMEPOS Modifier(s): NU, RR, UE

⊛ **E0111**   Crutch forearm, includes crutches of various materials, adjustable or fixed, each, with tips and handgrips **Qp** 🦽   Y

IOM: 100-02, 15, 110.1; 100-03, 4, 280.1

DMEPOS Modifier(s): NU, RR, UE

⊛ **E0112**   Crutches, underarm, wood, adjustable or fixed, pair, with pads, tips, and handgrips **Qp** 🦽   Y

IOM: 100-02, 15, 110.1; 100-03, 4, 280.1

DMEPOS Modifier(s): NU, RR, UE

⊛ **E0113**   Crutch underarm, wood, adjustable or fixed, each, with pad, tip, and handgrip **Qp** 🦽   Y

IOM: 100-02, 15, 110.1; 100-03, 4, 280.1

DMEPOS Modifier(s): NU, RR, UE

⊛ **E0114**   Crutches, underarm, other than wood, adjustable or fixed, pair, with pads, tips and handgrips **Qp** 🦽   Y

IOM: 100-02, 15, 110.1; 100-03, 4, 280.1

DMEPOS Modifier(s): NU, RR, UE

⊛ **E0116**   Crutch, underarm, other than wood, adjustable or fixed, with pad, tip, handgrip, with or without shock absorber, each **Qp** 🦽   Y

IOM: 100-02, 15, 110.1; 100-03, 4, 280.1

DMEPOS Modifier(s): NU, RR, UE

⊛ **E0117**   Crutch, underarm, articulating, spring assisted, each **Qp** 🦽   Y

IOM: 100-02, 15, 110.1

DMEPOS Modifier(s): NU, RR, UE

✳ **E0118**   Crutch substitute, lower leg platform, with or without wheels, each **Qp**   E

Walkers

E0130-E0155:   Bill DME/MAC

⊛ **E0130**   Walker, rigid (pickup), adjustable or fixed height **Qp** 🦽   Y

Standard walker criteria for payment: Individual has a mobility limitation that significantly impairs ability to participate in mobility-related activities of daily living that cannot be adequately or safely addressed by a cane. The patient is able to use the walker safely; the functional mobility deficit can be resolved with use of a standard walker.

IOM: 100-02, 15, 110.1; 100-03, 4, 280.1

DMEPOS Modifier(s): NU, RR, UE

⊛ **E0135**   Walker, folding (pickup), adjustable or fixed height **Qp** 🦽   Y

IOM: 100-02, 15, 110.1; 100-03, 4, 280.1

DMEPOS Modifier(s): NU, RR, UE

⊛ **E0140**   Walker, with trunk support, adjustable or fixed height, any type **Qp** 🦽   Y

IOM: 100-02, 15, 110.1; 100-03, 4, 280.1

DMEPOS Modifier(s): NU, RR, UE

⊛ **E0141**   Walker, rigid, wheeled, adjustable or fixed height **Qp** 🦽   Y

IOM: 100-02, 15, 110.1; 100-03, 4, 280.1

DMEPOS Modifier(s): NU, RR, UE

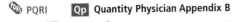

🅠 PQRI	**Qp** Quantity Physician Appendix B	**Qh** Quantity Hospital Appendix C	♀ Female only
♂ Male only	**A** Age	🦽 DMEPOS	A2-Z3 ASC Payment Indicator	A-Y ASC Status Indicator	Coding Clinic

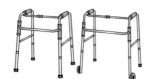

Figure 11 Walkers.

⊛ **E0143** Walker, folding, wheeled, adjustable or fixed height Qp ⅃   Y

IOM: 100-02, 15, 110.1; 100-03, 4, 280.1

DMEPOS Modifier(s): NU, RR, UE

⊛ **E0144** Walker, enclosed, four sided framed, rigid or folding, wheeled, with posterior seat Qp ♿   Y

IOM: 100-02, 15, 110.1; 100-03, 4, 280.1

DMEPOS Modifier(s): NU, RR, UE

⊛ **E0147** Walker, heavy duty, multiple braking system, variable wheel resistance Qp ⅃   Y

IOM: 100-02, 15, 110.1; 100-03, 4, 280.1

DMEPOS Modifier(s): NU, RR, UE

✳ **E0148** Walker, heavy duty, without wheels, rigid or folding, any type, each Qp ⅃   Y

Heavy-duty walker is labeled as capable of supporting more than 300 pounds

DMEPOS Modifier(s): NU, RR, UE

✳ **E0149** Walker, heavy duty, wheeled, rigid or folding, any type Qp ⅃   Y

Heavy-duty walker is labeled as capable of supporting more than 300 pounds

DMEPOS Modifier(s): NU, RR, UE

✳ **E0153** Platform attachment, forearm crutch, each Qp ♿   Y

DMEPOS Modifier(s): NU, RR, UE

✳ **E0154** Platform attachment, walker, each Qp ⅃   Y

DMEPOS Modifier(s): NU, RR, UE

✳ **E0155** Wheel attachment, rigid pick-up walker, per pair Qp ⅃   Y

DMEPOS Modifier(s): NU, RR, UE

Attachments

E0156-E0159:   Bill DME/MAC

✳ **E0156** Seat attachment, walker Qp ⅃   Y

DMEPOS Modifier(s): NU, RR, UE

✳ **E0157** Crutch attachment, walker, each Qp ⅃   Y

DMEPOS Modifier(s): NU, RR, UE

✳ **E0158** Leg extensions for walker, per set of four (4) Qp ⅃   Y

Leg extensions are considered medically necessary DME for patients 6 feet tall or more

DMEPOS Modifier(s): NU, RR, UE

✳ **E0159** Brake attachment for wheeled walker, replacement, each ⅃   Y

DMEPOS Modifier(s): NU, RR, UE

Commodes

E0160-E0175:   Bill DME/MAC

⊛ **E0160** Sitz type bath or equipment, portable, used with or without commode ⅃   Y

IOM: 100-03, 4, 280.1

DMEPOS Modifier(s): NU, RR, UE

⊛ **E0161** Sitz type bath or equipment, portable, used with or without commode, with faucet attachment/ s ⅃   Y

IOM: 100-03, 4, 280.1

DMEPOS Modifier(s): NU, RR, UE

⊛ **E0162** Sitz bath chair ⅃   Y

IOM: 100-03, 4, 280.1

DMEPOS Modifier(s): NU, RR, UE

⊛ **E0163** Commode chair, mobile or stationary, with fixed arms Qp ⅃   Y

IOM: 100-02, 15, 110.1; 100-03, 4, 280.1

DMEPOS Modifier(s): NU, RR, UE

⊛ **E0165** Commode chair, mobile or stationary, with detachable arms Qp ⅃   Y

IOM: 100-02, 15, 110.1; 100-03, 4, 280.1

DMEPOS Modifier(s): RR

⊛ **E0167** Pail or pan for use with commode chair, replacement only Qp ⅃   Y

IOM: 100-03, 4, 280.1

DMEPOS Modifier(s): NU, RR, UE

✳ **E0168** Commode chair, extra wide and/or heavy duty, stationary or mobile, with or without arms, any type, each Qp ⅃   Y

DMEPOS Modifier(s): NU, RR, UE

✳ **E0170** Commode chair with integrated seat lift mechanism, electric, any type Qp ⅃   Y

DMEPOS Modifier(s): RR

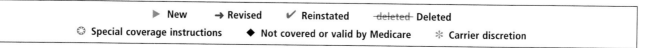

▶ New   → Revised   ✔ Reinstated   deleted Deleted

⊛ Special coverage instructions   ◆ Not covered or valid by Medicare   ✳ Carrier discretion

✳ **E0171** Commode chair with integrated seat lift mechanism, non-electric, any type Qp   Y

DMEPOS Modifier(s): RR

◆ **E0172** Seat lift mechanism placed over or on top of toilet, any type   E

Medicare Statute 1861 SSA

✳ **E0175** Foot rest, for use with commode chair, each Qp   Y

DMEPOS Modifier(s): NU, RR, UE

Decubitus Care Equipment

E0181-E0199: Bill DME/MAC

❂ **E0181** Powered pressure reducing mattress overlay/pad, alternating, with pump, includes heavy duty Qp   Y

Requires the provider to determine medical necessity compliance. To demonstrate the requirements in the medical policy were met, attach -KX.

IOM: 100-03, 4, 280.1; 100-08, 5, 5.2.3

DMEPOS Modifier(s): RR

❂ **E0182** Pump for alternating pressure pad, for replacement only Qp   Y

IOM: 100-03, 4, 280.1; 100-08, 5, 5.2.3

DMEPOS Modifier(s): RR

❂ **E0184** Dry pressure mattress Qp   Y

IOM: 100-03, 4, 280.1; 100-08, 5, 5.2.3

DMEPOS Modifier(s): NU, RR, UE

❂ **E0185** Gel or gel-like pressure pad for mattress, standard mattress length and width Qp   Y

IOM: 100-03, 4, 280.1; 100-08, 5, 5.2.3

DMEPOS Modifier(s): NU, RR, UE

❂ **E0186** Air pressure mattress Qp   Y

IOM: 100-03, 4, 280.1

DMEPOS Modifier(s): RR

❂ **E0187** Water pressure mattress Qp   Y

IOM: 100-03, 4, 280.1

DMEPOS Modifier(s): RR

❂ **E0188** Synthetic sheepskin pad Qp   Y

IOM: 100-03, 4, 280.1; 100-08, 5, 5.2.3

DMEPOS Modifier(s): NU, RR, UE

❂ **E0189** Lambswool sheepskin pad, any size Qp   Y

IOM: 100-03, 4, 280.1; 100-08, 5, 5.2.3

DMEPOS Modifier(s): NU, RR, UE

❂ **E0190** Positioning cushion/pillow/wedge, any shape or size, includes all components and accessories   E

IOM: 100-02, 15, 110.1

✳ **E0191** Heel or elbow protector, each   Y

DMEPOS Modifier(s): NU, RR, UE

✳ **E0193** Powered air flotation bed (low air loss therapy) Qp   Y

DMEPOS Modifier(s): RR

❂ **E0194** Air fluidized bed Qp   Y

IOM: 100-03, 4, 280.1

DMEPOS Modifier(s): RR

❂ **E0196** Gel pressure mattress Qp   Y

IOM: 100-03, 4, 280.1

DMEPOS Modifier(s): RR

❂ **E0197** Air pressure pad for mattress, standard mattress length and width Qp   Y

IOM: 100-03, 4, 280.1

DMEPOS Modifier(s): NU, RR, UE

❂ **E0198** Water pressure pad for mattress, standard mattress length and width Qp   Y

IOM: 100-03, 4, 280.1

DMEPOS Modifier(s): NU, RR, UE

❂ **E0199** Dry pressure pad for mattress, standard mattress length and width Qp   Y

IOM: 100-03, 4, 280.1

DMEPOS Modifier(s): NU, RR, UE

Heat/Cold Application

E0200-E0239: Bill DME/MAC

❂ **E0200** Heat lamp, without stand (table model), includes bulb, or infrared element Qp   Y

Covered when medical review determines patient's medical condition is one for which application of heat by heat lamp is therapeutically effective

IOM: 100-02, 15, 110.1; 100-03, 4, 280.1

DMEPOS Modifier(s): NU, RR, UE

✳ **E0202** Phototherapy (bilirubin) light with photometer Qp   Y

DMEPOS Modifier(s): RR

◆ **E0203** Therapeutic lightbox, minimum 10,000 lux, table top model   E

IOM: 100-03, 4, 280.1

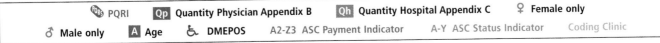

DURABLE MEDICAL EQUIPMENT   E0171 – E0203

⊗ **E0205** Heat lamp, with stand, includes bulb, or infrared element Qp & Y

IOM: 100-02, 15, 110.1; 100-03, 4, 280.1

DMEPOS Modifier(s): NU, RR, UE

⊗ **E0210** Electric heat pad, standard Qp & Y

Flexible device containing electric resistive elements producing heat; has fabric cover to prevent burns; with or without timing devices for automatic shut-off

IOM: 100-03, 4, 280.1

DMEPOS Modifier(s): NU, RR, UE

⊗ **E0215** Electric heat pad, moist Qp & Y

Flexible device containing electric resistive elements producing heat. Must have component that will absorb and retain liquid (water)

IOM: 100-03, 4, 280.1

DMEPOS Modifier(s): NU, RR, UE

⊗ **E0217** Water circulating heat pad with pump Qp & Y

Consists of flexible pad containing series of channels through which water is circulated by means of electrical pumping mechanism and heated in external reservoir

IOM: 100-03, 4, 280.1

DMEPOS Modifier(s): NU, RR, UE

⊗ **E0218** Water circulating cold pad with pump Qp Y

IOM: 100-03, 4, 280.1

✳ **E0221** Infrared heating pad system Y

⊗ **E0225** Hydrocollator unit, includes pads Qp & Y

IOM: 100-02, 15, 230; 100-03, 4, 280.1

DMEPOS Modifier(s): NU, RR, UE

◆ **E0231** Non-contact wound warming device (temperature control unit, AC adapter and power cord) for use with warming card and wound cover E

IOM: 100-02, 16, 20

◆ **E0232** Warming card for use with the non-contact wound warming device and non-contact wound warming wound cover E

IOM: 100-02, 16, 20

⊗ **E0235** Paraffin bath unit, portable (see medical supply code A4265 for paraffin) Qp & Y

Ordered by physician and patient's condition expected to be relieved by long term use of modality

IOM: 100-02, 15, 230; 100-03, 4, 280.1

DMEPOS Modifier(s): RR

⊗ **E0236** Pump for water circulating pad Qp & Y

IOM: 100-03, 4, 280.1

DMEPOS Modifier(s): RR

⊗ **E0239** Hydrocollator unit, portable Qp & Y

IOM: 100-02, 15, 230; 100-03, 4, 280.1

DMEPOS Modifier(s): NU, RR, UE

Bath and Toilet Aids

E0240-E0249: Bill DME/MAC

◆ **E0240** Bath/shower chair, with or without wheels, any size E

IOM: 100-03, 4, 280.1

◆ **E0241** Bath tub wall rail, each E

IOM: 100-02, 15, 110.1; 100-03, 4, 280.1

◆ **E0242** Bath tub rail, floor base E

IOM: 100-02, 15, 110.1; 100-03, 4, 280.1

◆ **E0243** Toilet rail, each E

IOM: 100-02, 15, 110.1; 100-03, 4, 280.1

◆ **E0244** Raised toilet seat E

IOM: 100-03, 4, 280.1

◆ **E0245** Tub stool or bench E

IOM: 100-03, 4, 280.1

✳ **E0246** Transfer tub rail attachment E

⊗ **E0247** Transfer bench for tub or toilet with or without commode opening E

IOM: 100-03, 4, 280.1

⊗ **E0248** Transfer bench, heavy duty, for tub or toilet with or without commode opening E

IOM: 100-03, 4, 280.1

✳ **E0249** Pad for water circulating heat unit, for replacement only Qp & Y

Describes durable replacement pad used with water circulating heat pump system

IOM: 100-03, 4, 280.1

DMEPOS Modifier(s): NU, RR, UE

▶ New   → Revised   ✔ Reinstated   deleted Deleted
⊗ Special coverage instructions   ◆ Not covered or valid by Medicare   ✳ Carrier discretion

Hospital Beds and Accessories

E0250-E0373: Bill DME/MAC

⊛ **E0250** Hospital bed, fixed height, with any type side rails, with mattress Qp ⅄   Y
IOM: 100-02, 15, 110.1; 100-03, 4, 280.7
DMEPOS Modifier(s): RR

⊛ **E0251** Hospital bed, fixed height, with any type side rails, without mattress Qp ⅄   Y
IOM:100-02, 15, 110.1; 100-03, 4, 280.7
DMEPOS Modifier(s): RR

⊛ **E0255** Hospital bed, variable height, hi-lo, with any type side rails, with mattress Qp ⅄   Y
IOM: 100-02, 15, 110.1; 100-03, 4, 280.7
DMEPOS Modifier(s): RR

⊛ **E0256** Hospital bed, variable height, hi-lo, with any type side rails, without mattress Qp ⅄   Y
IOM: 100-02, 15, 110.1; 100-03, 4, 280.7
DMEPOS Modifier(s): RR

⊛ **E0260** Hospital bed, semi-electric (head and foot adjustment), with any type side rails, with mattress Qp ⅄   Y
IOM: 100-02, 15, 110.1; 100-03, 4, 280.7
DMEPOS Modifier(s): RR

⊛ **E0261** Hospital bed, semi-electric (head and foot adjustment), with any type side rails, without mattress Qp ⅄   Y
IOM: 100-02, 15, 110.1; 100-03, 4, 280.7
DMEPOS Modifier(s): RR

⊛ **E0265** Hospital bed, total electric (head, foot and height adjustments), with any type side rails, with mattress Qp ⅄   Y
IOM: 100-02, 15, 110.1; 100-03, 4, 280.7
DMEPOS Modifier(s): RR

⊛ **E0266** Hospital bed, total electric (head, foot and height adjustments), with any type side rails, without mattress Qp ⅄   Y
IOM: 100-02, 15, 110.1; 100-03, 4, 280.7
DMEPOS Modifier(s): RR

◆ **E0270** Hospital bed, institutional type includes: oscillating, circulating and Stryker frame, with mattress Qp   E
IOM: 100-03, 4, 280.1

⊛ **E0271** Mattress, innerspring Qp ⅄   Y
IOM: 100-03, 4, 280.1; 100-03, 4, 280.7
DMEPOS Modifier(s): NU, RR, UE

⊛ **E0272** Mattress, foam rubber Qp ⅄   Y
IOM: 100-03, 4, 280.1; 100-03, 4, 280.7
DMEPOS Modifier(s): NU, RR, UE

◆ **E0273** Bed board   E
IOM: 100-03, 4, 280.1

◆ **E0274** Over-bed table   E
IOM: 100-03, 4, 280.1

⊛ **E0275** Bed pan, standard, metal or plastic Qp ⅄   Y
IOM: 100-03, 4, 280.1
DMEPOS Modifier(s): NU, RR, UE

⊛ **E0276** Bed pan, fracture, metal or plastic Qp ⅄   Y
IOM: 100-03, 4, 280.1
DMEPOS Modifier(s): NU, RR, UE

⊛ **E0277** Powered pressure-reducing air mattress Qp ⅄   Y
IOM: 100-03, 4, 280.1
DMEPOS Modifier(s): RR

✳ **E0280** Bed cradle, any type Qp ⅄   Y
DMEPOS Modifier(s): NU, RR, UE

⊛ **E0290** Hospital bed, fixed height, without side rails, with mattress Qp ⅄   Y
IOM: 100-02, 15, 110.1; 100-03, 4, 280.7
DMEPOS Modifier(s): RR

⊛ **E0291** Hospital bed, fixed height, without side rails, without mattress Qp ⅄   Y
IOM: 100-02, 15, 110.1; 100-03, 4, 280.7
DMEPOS Modifier(s): RR

⊛ **E0292** Hospital bed, variable height, hi-lo, without side rails, with mattress Qp ⅄   Y
IOM: 100-02, 15, 110.1; 100-03, 4, 280.7
DMEPOS Modifier(s): RR

⊛ **E0293** Hospital bed, variable height, hi-lo, without side rails, without mattress Qp ⅄   Y
IOM: 100-02, 15, 110.1; 100-03, 4, 280.7
DMEPOS Modifier(s): RR

⊛ **E0294** Hospital bed, semi-electric (head and foot adjustment), without side rails, with mattress Qp ⅄   Y
IOM: 100-02, 15, 110.1; 100-03, 4, 280.7
DMEPOS Modifier(s): RR

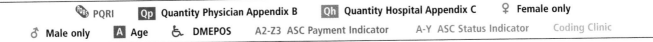

⊘ **E0295** Hospital bed, semi-electric (head and foot adjustment), without side rails, without mattress **Qp** ♿ Y

IOM: 100-02, 15, 110.1; 100-03, 4, 280.7

DMEPOS Modifier(s): RR

⊘ **E0296** Hospital bed, total electric (head, foot and height adjustments). Without side rails, with mattress **Qp** ♿ Y

IOM: 100-02, 15, 110.1; 100-03, 4, 280.7

DMEPOS Modifier(s): RR

⊘ **E0297** Hospital bed, total electric (head, foot and height adjustments), without side rails, without mattress **Qp** ♿ Y

IOM: 100-02, 15, 110.1; 100-03, 4, 280.7

DMEPOS Modifier(s): RR

✳ **E0300** Pediatric crib, hospital grade, fully enclosed **Qp** **A** ♿ Y

DMEPOS Modifier(s): NU, RR, UE

⊘ **E0301** Hospital bed, heavy duty, extra wide, with weight capacity greater than 350 pounds, but less than or equal to 600 pounds, with any type side rails, without mattress **Qp** ♿ Y

IOM: 100-03, 4, 280.7

DMEPOS Modifier(s): RR

⊘ **E0302** Hospital bed, extra heavy duty, extra wide, with weight capacity greater than 600 pounds, with any type side rails, without mattress **Qp** ♿ Y

IOM: 100-03, 4, 280.7

DMEPOS Modifier(s): RR

⊘ **E0303** Hospital bed, heavy duty, extra wide, with weight capacity greater than 350 pounds, but less than or equal to 600 pounds, with any type side rails, with mattress **Qp** ♿ Y

IOM: 100-03, 4, 280.7

DMEPOS Modifier(s): RR

⊘ **E0304** Hospital bed, extra heavy duty, extra wide, with weight capacity greater than 600 pounds, with any type side rails, with mattress **Qp** ♿ Y

IOM: 100-03, 4, 280.7

DMEPOS Modifier(s): RR

⊘ **E0305** Bed side rails, half length ♿ Y

IOM: 100-03, 4, 280.7

DMEPOS Modifier(s): RR

⊘ **E0310** Bed side rails, full length **Qp** ♿ Y

IOM: 100-03, 4, 280.7

DMEPOS Modifier(s): NU, RR, UE

◆ **E0315** Bed accessory: board, table, or support device, any type E

IOM: 100-03, 4, 280.1

✳ **E0316** Safety enclosure frame/canopy for use with hospital bed, any type **Qp** ♿ Y

DMEPOS Modifier(s): RR

⊘ **E0325** Urinal; male, jug-type, any material ♂ **Qp** ♿ Y

IOM: 100-03, 4, 280.1

DMEPOS Modifier(s): NU, RR, UE

⊘ **E0326** Urinal; female, jug-type, any material ♀ **Qp** ♿ Y

IOM: 100-03, 4, 280.1

DMEPOS Modifier(s): NU, RR, UE

✳ **E0328** Hospital bed, pediatric, manual, 360 degree side enclosures, top of headboard, footboard and side rails up to 24 inches above the spring, includes mattress **A** Y

✳ **E0329** Hospital bed, pediatric, electric or semi-electric, 360 degree side enclosures, top of headboard, footboard and side rails up to 24 inches above the spring, includes mattress **A** Y

✳ **E0350** Control unit for electronic bowel irrigation/evacuation system **Qp** E

Pulsed Irrigation Enhanced Evacuation (PIEE) is pulsed irrigation of severely impacted fecal material and may be necessary for patients who have not responded to traditional bowel program.

✳ **E0352** Disposable pack (water reservoir bag, speculum, valving mechanism and collection bag/box) for use with the electronic bowel irrigation/evacuation system E

Therapy kit includes 1 B-Valve circuit, 2 containment bags, 1 lubricating jelly, 1 bed pad, 1 tray liner-waste disposable bag, and 2 hose clamps

✳ **E0370** Air pressure elevator for heel E

✳ **E0371** Non powered advanced pressure reducing overlay for mattress, standard mattress length and width **Qp** ♿ Y

Patient has at least one large Stage III or Stage IV pressure sore (greater than 2 × 2 cm.) on trunk, with only two turning surfaces on which to lie

DMEPOS Modifier(s): RR

▶ New   → Revised   ✔ Reinstated   ~~deleted~~ Deleted

⊘ Special coverage instructions   ◆ Not covered or valid by Medicare   ✳ Carrier discretion

✳ **E0372**   Powered air overlay for mattress, standard mattress length and width Qp 占   Y

DMEPOS Modifier(s): RR

✳ **E0373**   Non powered advanced pressure reducing mattress Qp 占   Y

DMEPOS Modifier(s): RR

Oxygen and Related Respiratory Equipment

E0424-E0487:   Bill DME/MAC

✪ **E0424**   Stationary compressed gaseous oxygen system, rental; includes container, contents, regulator, flowmeter, humidifier, nebulizer, cannula or mask, and tubing Qp 占   Y

IOM: 100-03, 4, 280.1; 100-04, 20, 30.6

DMEPOS Modifier(s): RR

✪ **E0425**   Stationary compressed gas system, purchase; includes regulator, flowmeter, humidifier, nebulizer, cannula or mask, and tubing   E

IOM: 100-03, 4, 280.1; 100-04, 20, 30.6

✪ **E0430**   Portable gaseous oxygen system, purchase; includes regulator, flowmeter, humidifier, cannula or mask, and tubing   E

IOM: 100-03, 4, 280.1; 100-04, 20, 30.6

✪ **E0431**   Portable gaseous oxygen system, rental; includes portable container, regulator, flowmeter, humidifier, cannula or mask, and tubing Qp 占   Y

IOM: 100-03, 4, 280.1; 100-04, 20, 30.6

DMEPOS Modifier(s): RR

✳ **E0433**   Portable liquid oxygen system, rental; home liquefier used to fill portable liquid oxygen containers, includes portable containers, regulator, flowmeter, humidifier, cannula or mask and tubing, with or without supply reservoir and contents gauge Qh 占   Y

DMEPOS Modifier(s): RR

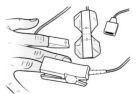

Figure 12   Oximeter device.

✪ **E0434**   Portable liquid oxygen system, rental; includes portable container, supply reservoir, humidifier, flowmeter, refill adaptor, contents gauge, cannula or mask, and tubing Qp 占   Y

Fee schedule payments for stationary oxygen system rentals are all-inclusive and represent monthly allowance for beneficiary. Non-Medicare payers may rent device to beneficiaries, or arrange for purchase of device

IOM: 100-03, 4, 280.1; 100-04, 20, 30.6

DMEPOS Modifier(s): RR

✪ **E0435**   Portable liquid oxygen system, purchase; includes portable container, supply reservoir, flowmeter, humidifier, contents gauge, cannula or mask, tubing and refill adaptor   E

IOM: 100-03, 4, 280.1; 100-04, 20, 30.6

✪ **E0439**   Stationary liquid oxygen system, rental; includes container, contents, regulator, flowmeter, humidifier, nebulizer, cannula or mask, & tubing Qp 占   Y

This allowance includes payment for equipment, contents, and accessories furnished during rental month

IOM: 100-03, 4, 280.1; 100-04, 20, 30.6

DMEPOS Modifier(s): RR

✪ **E0440**   Stationary liquid oxygen system, purchase; includes use of reservoir, contents indicator, regulator, flowmeter, humidifier, nebulizer, cannula or mask, and tubing   E

IOM: 100-03, 4, 280.1; 100-04, 20, 30.6

✳ **E0441**   Stationary oxygen contents, gaseous, 1 month's supply = 1 unit Qp 占   Y

IOM: 100-03, 4, 280.1; 100-04, 20, 30.6

✳ **E0442**   Stationary oxygen contents, liquid, 1 month's supply = 1 unit Qp 占   Y

IOM: 100-03, 4, 280.1; 100-04, 20, 30.6

✳ **E0443**   Portable oxygen contents, gaseous, 1 month's supply = 1 unit Qp 占   Y

IOM: 100-03, 4, 280.1; 100-04, 20, 30.6

✳ **E0444**   Portable oxygen contents, liquid, 1 month's supply = 1 unit Qp 占   Y

IOM: 100-03, 4, 280.1; 100-04, 20, 30.6

✳ **E0445**   Oximeter device for measuring blood oxygen levels non-invasively   N

◆ **E0446**   Topical oxygen delivery system, not otherwise specified, includes all supplies and accessories   E

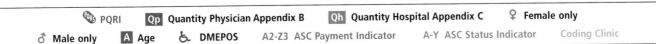

⊛ **E0450** Volume control ventilator, without pressure support mode, may include pressure control mode, used with invasive interface (e.g., tracheostomy tube) Qp ᪧ   Y

Patient confined to wheelchair during day may receive reimbursement for 2 ventilators. One ventilator is mounted to wheelchair and second used while in bed

IOM: 100-03, 4, 280.1

DMEPOS Modifier(s): RR

⊛ **E0455** Oxygen tent, excluding croup or pediatric tents Qp   Y

IOM: 100-03, 4, 280.1; 100-04, 20, 30.6

✻ **E0457** Chest shell (cuirass) Qp ᪧ   Y

DMEPOS Modifier(s): NU, RR, UE

✻ **E0459** Chest wrap Qp ᪧ   Y

DMEPOS Modifier(s): RR

⊛ **E0460** Negative pressure ventilator; portable or stationary Qp ᪧ   Y

Noninvasive device, generates airflow into lungs by creating negative pressure around chest by means of interface

IOM: 100-03, 4, 240.2

DMEPOS Modifier(s): RR

⊛ **E0461** Volume control ventilator, without pressure support mode, may include pressure control mode, used with non-invasive interface (e.g. mask) Qp ᪧ   Y

IOM: 100-03, 4, 240.2

DMEPOS Modifier(s): RR

✻ **E0462** Rocking bed with or without side rails Qp ᪧ   Y

DMEPOS Modifier(s): RR

✻ **E0463** Pressure support ventilator with volume control mode, may include pressure control mode, used with invasive interface (e.g., tracheostomy tube) Qp ᪧ   Y

DMEPOS Modifier(s): RR

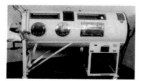

Figure 13 Pressure ventilator.

✻ **E0464** Pressure support ventilator with volume control mode, may include pressure control mode, used with non-invasive interface (e.g., mask) Qp ᪧ   Y

DMEPOS Modifier(s): RR

⊛ **E0470** Respiratory assist device, bi-level pressure capability, without backup rate feature, used with noninvasive interface, e.g., nasal or facial mask (intermittent assist device with continuous positive airway pressure device) Qp ᪧ   Y

IOM: 100-03, 4, 240.2

DMEPOS Modifier(s): RR

⊛ **E0471** Respiratory assist device, bi-level pressure capability, with back-up rate feature, used with noninvasive interface, e.g., nasal or facial mask (intermittent assist device with continuous positive airway pressure device) Qp ᪧ   Y

IOM: 100-03, 4, 240.2

DMEPOS Modifier(s): RR

⊛ **E0472** Respiratory assist device, bi-level pressure capability, with backup rate feature, used with invasive interface, e.g., tracheostomy tube (intermittent assist device with continuous positive airway pressure device) Qp ᪧ   Y

IOM: 100-03, 4, 240.2

DMEPOS Modifier(s): RR

⊛ **E0480** Percussor, electric or pneumatic, home model Qp ᪧ   Y

IOM: 100-03, 4, 240.2

DMEPOS Modifier(s): RR

◆ **E0481** Intrapulmonary percussive ventilation system and related accessories Qp   E

IOM: 100-03, 4, 240.2

✻ **E0482** Cough stimulating device, alternating positive and negative airway pressure Qp ᪧ   Y

DMEPOS Modifier(s): RR

✻ **E0483** High frequency chest wall oscillation air-pulse generator system, (includes hoses and vest), each Qp ᪧ   Y

DMEPOS Modifier(s): RR

✻ **E0484** Oscillatory positive expiratory pressure device, non-electric, any type, each Qp ᪧ   Y

DMEPOS Modifier(s): NU, RR, UE

▶ New   → Revised   ✔ Reinstated   ~~deleted~~ Deleted

⊛ Special coverage instructions   ◆ Not covered or valid by Medicare   ✻ Carrier discretion

✳ **E0485** Oral device/appliance used to reduce upper airway collapsibility, adjustable or non-adjustable, prefabricated, includes fitting and adjustment **Qp** 🚹   Y

    DMEPOS Modifier(s): NU, RR, UE

✳ **E0486** Oral device/appliance used to reduce upper airway collapsibility, adjustable or non-adjustable, custom fabricated, includes fitting and adjustment **Qp** 🚹   Y

    DMEPOS Modifier(s): NU, RR, UE

۞ **E0487** Spirometer, electronic, includes all accessories   N

IPPB Machines

۞ **E0500** IPPB machine, all types, with built-in nebulization; manual or automatic valves; internal or external power source **Qp** 🚹   Y

    Bill DME/MAC

    IOM: 100-03, 4, 240.2

    DMEPOS Modifier(s): RR

Humidifiers/Nebulizers/Compressors for Use with Oxygen IPPB Equipment

E0550-E0585:   Bill DME/MAC

۞ **E0550** Humidifier, durable for extensive supplemental humidification during IPPB treatments or oxygen delivery **Qp** 🚹   Y

    IOM: 100-03, 4, 240.2

    DMEPOS Modifier(s): RR

۞ **E0555** Humidifier, durable, glass or autoclavable plastic bottle type, for use with regulator or flowmeter **Qp**   Y

    IOM: 100-03, 4, 280.1; 100-04, 20, 30.6

۞ **E0560** Humidifier, durable for supplemental humidification during IPPB treatment or oxygen delivery **Qp** 🚹   Y

    IOM: 100-03, 4, 280.1

    DMEPOS Modifier(s): NU, RR, UE

✳ **E0561** Humidifier, non-heated, used with positive airway pressure device **Qp** 🚹   Y

    DMEPOS Modifier(s): NU, RR, UE

✳ **E0562** Humidifier, heated, used with positive airway pressure device **Qp** 🚹   Y

    DMEPOS Modifier(s): NU, RR, UE

✳ **E0565** Compressor, air power source for equipment which is not self-contained or cylinder driven **Qp** 🚹   Y

    DMEPOS Modifier(s): RR

۞ **E0570** Nebulizer, with compressor **Qp** 🚹   Y

    IOM: 100-03, 4, 240.2; 100-03, 4, 280.1

    DMEPOS Modifier(s): RR

~~E0571~~ ~~Aerosol compressor, battery powered, for use with small volume nebulizer~~   ✖

✳ **E0572** Aerosol compressor, adjustable pressure, light duty for intermittent use **Qp** 🚹   Y

    DMEPOS Modifier(s): RR

✳ **E0574** Ultrasonic/electronic aerosol generator with small volume nebulizer **Qp** 🚹   Y

    DMEPOS Modifier(s): RR

۞ **E0575** Nebulizer, ultrasonic, large volume **Qp** 🚹   Y

    IOM: 100-03, 4, 240.2

    DMEPOS Modifier(s): RR

۞ **E0580** Nebulizer, durable, glass or autoclavable plastic, bottle type, for use with regulator or flowmeter **Qp** 🚹   Y

    IOM: 100-03, 4, 240.2; 100-03, 4, 280.1

    DMEPOS Modifier(s): NU, RR, UE

۞ **E0585** Nebulizer, with compressor and heater **Qp** 🚹   Y

    IOM: 100-03, 4, 240.2; 100-03, 4, 280.1

    DMEPOS Modifier(s): RR

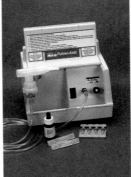

Figure 14 Nebulizer.

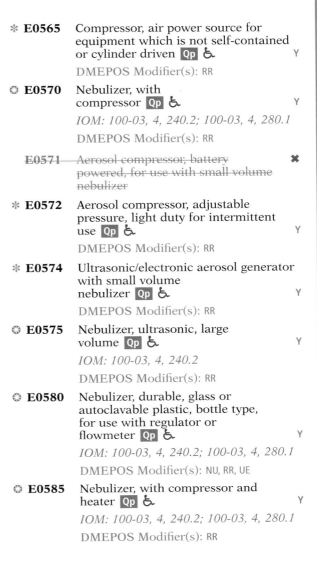

DURABLE MEDICAL EQUIPMENT   E0485 – E0585

Suction Pump/Room Vaporizers

E0600-E0606: Bill DME/MAC

✿ **E0600** Respiratory suction pump, home model, portable or stationary, electric Qp & Y

IOM: 100-03, 4, 240.2

DMEPOS Modifier(s): RR

✿ **E0601** Continuous airway pressure (CPAP) device Qp & Y

IOM: 100-03, 4, 240.4

DMEPOS Modifier(s): RR

∗ **E0602** Breast pump, manual, any type ♀ & Y

Bill either manual breast pump or breast pump kit

DMEPOS Modifier(s): NU, RR, UE

∗ **E0603** Breast pump, electric (AC and/or DC), any type ♀ N

∗ **E0604** Breast pump, hospital grade, electric (AC and/or DC), any type ♀ A

✿ **E0605** Vaporizer, room type Qp & Y

IOM: 100-03, 4, 240.2

DMEPOS Modifier(s): NU, RR, UE

✿ **E0606** Postural drainage board Qp & Y

IOM: 100-03, 4, 240.2

DMEPOS Modifier(s): RR

Monitoring Equipment

✿ **E0607** Home blood glucose monitor Qp & Y

Bill DME/MAC

Document recipient or caregiver is competent to monitor equipment and that device is designed for home rather than clinical use

IOM: 100-03, 4, 280.1; 100-03, 1, 40.2

DMEPOS Modifier(s): NU, RR, UE

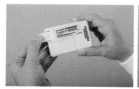 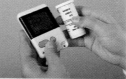

Figure 15 Glucose monitor.

Pacemaker Monitor

✿ **E0610** Pacemaker monitor, self-contained, (checks battery depletion, includes audible and visible check systems) Qp & Y

Bill DME/MAC

IOM: 100-03, 1, 20.8

DMEPOS Modifier(s): NU, RR, UE

✿ **E0615** Pacemaker monitor, self-contained, checks battery depletion and other pacemaker components, includes digital/visible check systems Qp & Y

Bill DME/MAC

IOM: 100-03, 1, 20.8

DMEPOS Modifier(s): NU, RR, UE

∗ **E0616** Implantable cardiac event recorder with memory, activator and programmer Qp Qh N1 N

Bill local carrier

Assign when two 30-day pre-symptom external loop recordings fail to establish a definitive diagnosis. Bill to local carrier.

∗ **E0617** External defibrillator with integrated electrocardiogram analysis Qp & Y

Bill DME/MAC

DMEPOS Modifier(s): RR, KF

∗ **E0618** Apnea monitor, without recording feature Qp Qh & Y

Bill DME/MAC

DMEPOS Modifier(s): RR

∗ **E0619** Apnea monitor, with recording feature Qp Qh & Y

Bill DME/MAC

DMEPOS Modifier(s): RR

∗ **E0620** Skin piercing device for collection of capillary blood, laser, each Qp & Y

Bill DME/MAC

DMEPOS Modifier(s): NU, RR, UE

Patient Lifts

E0621-E0642: Bill DME/MAC

✿ **E0621** Sling or seat, patient lift, canvas or nylon Qp & Y

IOM: 100-03, 4, 240.2, 280.4

DMEPOS Modifier(s): NU, RR, UE

▶ New → Revised ✔ Reinstated ~~deleted~~ Deleted

✿ Special coverage instructions ◆ Not covered or valid by Medicare ∗ Carrier discretion

◆ **E0625** Patient lift, bathroom or toilet, not otherwise classified E

IOM: 100-03, 4, 240.2

⊛ **E0627** Seat lift mechanism incorporated into a combination lift-chair mechanism Qp ♿ Y

IOM: 100-03, 4, 280.4; 100-04, 4, 20

Cross Reference Q0080

DMEPOS Modifier(s): NU, RR, UE

⊛ **E0628** Separate seat lift mechanism for use with patient owned furniture - electric Qp ♿ Y

IOM: 100-03, 4, 280.4; 100-04, 4, 20

Cross Reference Q0078

DMEPOS Modifier(s): NU, RR, UE

⊛ **E0629** Separate seat lift mechanism for use with patient owned furniture - non-electric Qp ♿ Y

IOM: 100-04, 4, 20

Cross Reference Q0079

DMEPOS Modifier(s): NU, RR, UE

⊛ **E0630** Patient lift, hydraulic or mechanical, includes any seat, sling, strap(s) or pad(s) Qp ♿ Y

IOM: 100-03, 4, 240.2

DMEPOS Modifier(s): RR

⊛ **E0635** Patient lift, electric, with seat or sling Qp ♿ Y

IOM: 100-03, 4, 240.2

DMEPOS Modifier(s): RR

✳ **E0636** Multipositional patient support system, with integrated lift, patient accessible controls Qp ♿ Y

DMEPOS Modifier(s): RR

→◆ **E0637** Combination sit to stand frame/table system, any size including pediatric, with seat lift feature, with or without wheels Qp E

IOM: 100-03, 4, 240.2

→◆ **E0638** Standing frame/table system, one position (e.g. upright, supine or prone stander), any size including pediatric, with or without wheels Qp E

IOM: 100-03, 4, 240.2

✳ **E0639** Patient lift, moveable from room to room with disassembly and reassembly, includes all components/accessories Qp E

✳ **E0640** Patient lift, fixed system, includes all components/accessories Qp E

→◆ **E0641** Standing frame/table system, multi-position (e.g. three-way stander), any size including pediatric, with or without wheels Qp E

IOM: 100-03, 4, 240.2

→◆ **E0642** Standing frame/table system, mobile (dynamic stander), any size including pediatric Qp E

IOM: 100-03, 4, 240.2

Pneumatic Compressor and Appliances

E0650-E0676: Bill DME/MAC

⊛ **E0650** Pneumatic compressor, non-segmental home model Qp ♿ Y

Lymphedema pumps are classified as segmented or nonsegmented, depending on whether distinct segments of devices can be inflated sequentially

IOM: 100-03, 4, 280.6

DMEPOS Modifier(s): NU, RR, UE

⊛ **E0651** Pneumatic compressor, segmental home model without calibrated gradient pressure Qp ♿ Y

IOM: 100-03, 4, 280.6

DMEPOS Modifier(s): NU, RR, UE

⊛ **E0652** Pneumatic compressor, segmental home model with calibrated gradient pressure Qp ♿ Y

IOM: 100-03, 4, 280.6

DMEPOS Modifier(s): NU, RR, UE

⊛ **E0655** Non-segmental pneumatic appliance for use with pneumatic compressor, half arm Qp ♿ Y

IOM: 100-03, 4, 280.6

DMEPOS Modifier(s): NU, RR, UE

⊛ **E0656** Segmental pneumatic appliance for use with pneumatic compressor, trunk Qp Qh ♿ Y

DMEPOS Modifier(s): NU, RR, UE

⊛ **E0657** Segmental pneumatic appliance for use with pneumatic compressor, chest Qp Qh ♿ Y

DMEPOS Modifier(s): NU, RR, UE

⊛ **E0660** Non-segmental pneumatic appliance for use with pneumatic compressor, full leg Qp ♿ Y

IOM: 100-03, 4, 280.6

DMEPOS Modifier(s): NU, RR, UE

| 🅟 PQRI | Qp Quantity Physician Appendix B | Qh Quantity Hospital Appendix C | ♀ Female only |
| ♂ Male only | A Age ♿ DMEPOS | A2-Z3 ASC Payment Indicator | A-Y ASC Status Indicator | Coding Clinic |

161

DURABLE MEDICAL EQUIPMENT E0625 – E0660

⊙ **E0665** Non-segmental pneumatic appliance for use with pneumatic compressor, full arm Qp ᕒ   Y

IOM: 100-03, 4, 280.6

DMEPOS Modifier(s): NU, RR, UE

⊙ **E0666** Non-segmental pneumatic appliance for use with pneumatic compressor, half leg Qp ᕒ   Y

IOM: 100-03, 4, 280.6

DMEPOS Modifier(s): NU, RR, UE

⊙ **E0667** Segmental pneumatic appliance for use with pneumatic compressor, full leg Qp ᕒ   Y

IOM: 100-03, 4, 280.6

DMEPOS Modifier(s): NU, RR, UE

⊙ **E0668** Segmental pneumatic appliance for use with pneumatic compressor, full arm Qp ᕒ   Y

IOM: 100-03, 4, 280.6

DMEPOS Modifier(s): NU, RR, UE

⊙ **E0669** Segmental pneumatic appliance for use with pneumatic compressor, half leg Qp ᕒ   Y

IOM: 100-03, 4, 280.6

DMEPOS Modifier(s): NU, RR, UE

⊙ **E0671** Segmental gradient pressure pneumatic appliance, full leg Qp ᕒ   Y

IOM: 100-03, 4, 280.6

DMEPOS Modifier(s): NU, RR, UE

⊙ **E0672** Segmental gradient pressure pneumatic appliance, full arm Qp ᕒ   Y

IOM: 100-03, 4, 280.6

DMEPOS Modifier(s): NU, RR, UE

⊙ **E0673** Segmental gradient pressure pneumatic appliance, half leg Qp ᕒ   Y

IOM: 100-03, 4, 280.6

DMEPOS Modifier(s): NU, RR, UE

✳ **E0675** Pneumatic compression device, high pressure, rapid inflation/deflation cycle, for arterial insufficiency (unilateral or bilateral system) Qp ᕒ   Y

DMEPOS Modifier(s): RR

✳ **E0676** Intermittent limb compression device (includes all accessories), not otherwise specified   Y

Ultraviolet Cabinet

E0691-E0694:   Bill DME/MAC

→ ✳ **E0691** Ultraviolet light therapy system, includes bulbs/lamps, timer and eye protection; treatment area 2 square feet or less Qp ᕒ   Y

DMEPOS Modifier(s): NU, RR, UE

✳ **E0692** Ultraviolet light therapy system panel, includes bulbs/lamps, timer and eye protection, 4 foot panel Qp ᕒ   Y

DMEPOS Modifier(s): NU, RR, UE

✳ **E0693** Ultraviolet light therapy system panel, includes bulbs/lamps, timer and eye protection, 6 foot panel Qp ᕒ   Y

DMEPOS Modifier(s): NU, RR, UE

✳ **E0694** Ultraviolet multidirectional light therapy system in 6 foot cabinet, includes bulbs/lamps, timer and eye protection Qp ᕒ   Y

DMEPOS Modifier(s): NU, RR, UE

Safety Equipment

E0700-E0705:   Bill DME/MAC

✳ **E0700** Safety equipment, device or accessory, any type   E

⊙ **E0705** Transfer device, any type, each Qp ᕒ   B

DMEPOS Modifier(s): NU, RR, UE

Restraints

✳ **E0710** Restraints, any type (body, chest, wrist or ankle)   E

Bill DME/MAC

Transcutaneous and/or Neuromuscular Electrical Nerve Stimulators (TENS)

⊙ **E0720** Transcutaneous electrical nerve stimulation (TENS) device, two lead, localized stimulation Qp ᕒ   Y

Bill DME/MAC

A Certificate of Medical Necessity (CMN) is not needed for a TENS rental, but is needed purchase.

IOM: 100-03, 2, 160.2; 100-03, 4, 280.1

DMEPOS Modifier(s): NU

▶ New   → Revised   ✔ Reinstated   ~~deleted~~ Deleted

⊙ Special coverage instructions   ◆ Not covered or valid by Medicare   ✳ Carrier discretion

⚙ **E0730** Transcutaneous electrical nerve stimulation (TENS) device, four or more leads, for multiple nerve stimulation Qp ♿ Y

Bill DME/MAC

IOM: 100-03, 2, 160.2; 100-03, 4, 280.1

DMEPOS Modifier(s): NU

⚙ **E0731** Form fitting conductive garment for delivery of TENS or NMES (with conductive fibers separated from the patient's skin by layers of fabric) Qp ♿ Y

Bill DME/MAC

IOM: 100-03, 2, 160.13

DMEPOS Modifier(s): NU

⚙ **E0740** Incontinence treatment system, pelvic floor stimulator, monitor, sensor and/or trainer Qp ♿ Y

Bill DME/MAC

IOM: 100-03, 4, 230.8

DMEPOS Modifier(s): NU, RR, UE

✳ **E0744** Neuromuscular stimulator for scoliosis Qp ♿ Y

Bill DME/MAC

DMEPOS Modifier(s): RR

⚙ **E0745** Neuromuscular stimulator, electronic shock unit Qp ♿ Y

Bill DME/MAC

IOM: 100-03, 2, 160.12

DMEPOS Modifier(s): RR

⚙ **E0746** Electromyography (EMG), biofeedback device Qp Qh N

Bill local carrier

IOM: 100-03, 1, 30.1

⚙ **E0747** Osteogenesis stimulator, electrical, non-invasive, other than spinal applications Qp ♿ Y

Bill DME/MAC

Devices are composed of two basic parts: Coils that wrap around cast and pulse generator that produces electric current

DMEPOS Modifier(s): NU, KF, RR, UE

⚙ **E0748** Osteogenesis stimulator, electrical, non-invasive, spinal applications Qp ♿ Y

Bill DME/MAC

Device should be applied within 30 days as adjunct to spinal fusion surgery

DMEPOS Modifier(s): NU, KF, RR, UE

⚙ **E0749** Osteogenesis stimulator, electrical, surgically implanted Qp Qh ♿ N1 N

Bill local carrier

DMEPOS Modifier(s): RR, KF

✳ **E0755** Electronic salivary reflex stimulator (intra-oral/non-invasive) Qp E

Bill DME/MAC

✳ **E0760** Osteogenesis stimulator, low intensity ultrasound, non-invasive Qp ♿ Y

Bill DME/MAC

Ultrasonic osteogenesis stimulator may not be used concurrently with other noninvasive stimulators

DMEPOS Modifier(s): NU, KF, RR, UE

⚙ **E0761** Non-thermal pulsed high frequency radiowaves, high peak power electromagnetic energy treatment device E

Bill DME/MAC

✳ **E0762** Transcutaneous electrical joint stimulation device system, includes all accessories Qp ♿ B

Bill DME/MAC

DMEPOS Modifier(s): NU, RR, UE

⚙ **E0764** Functional neuromuscular stimulator, transcutaneous stimulation of sequential muscle groups of ambulation with computer control, used for walking by spinal cord injured, entire system, after completion of training program Qp ♿ Y

Bill DME/MAC

IOM: 100-03, 2, 160.12

DMEPOS Modifier(s): NU, KF, RR, UE

➔ ✳ **E0765** FDA approved nerve stimulator, with replaceable batteries, for treatment of nausea and vomiting Qp ♿ Y

Bill DME/MAC

DMEPOS Modifier(s): NU, RR, UE

⚙ **E0769** Electrical stimulation or electromagnetic wound treatment device, not otherwise classified B

Bill DME/MAC

IOM: 100-04, 32, 11.1

⚙ **E0770** Functional electrical stimulator, transcutaneous stimulation of nerve and/or muscle groups, any type, complete system, not otherwise specified Y

Bill DME/MAC

PQRI	Qp Quantity Physician Appendix B	Qh Quantity Hospital Appendix C	♀ Female only
♂ Male only	A Age ♿ DMEPOS	A2-Z3 ASC Payment Indicator A-Y ASC Status Indicator	Coding Clinic

DURABLE MEDICAL EQUIPMENT E0730 – E0770

163

Infusion Supplies

* E0776 IV pole `Qp` ♿   Y

  Bill DME/MAC

  DMEPOS Modifier(s): NU, RR, UE

  PEN: On Fee Schedule,
  DMEPOS Modifier(s): BA, KE, NU, RR, UE

* E0779 Ambulatory infusion pump, mechanical, reusable, for infusion 8 hours or greater `Qp` ♿ Y

  Bill DME/MAC

  Requires prior authorization and copy of invoice

  DMEPOS Modifier(s): RR

  This is a capped rental infusion pump modifier. The correct monthly modifier (-KH, -KI, -KJ) is used to indicate which month the rental is for (i.e. -KH, month 1; -KI, months 2 and 3; -KJ, months 4 through 13).

* E0780 Ambulatory infusion pump, mechanical, reusable, for infusion less than 8 hours `Qp` ♿ Y

  Bill DME/MAC

  Requires prior authorization and copy of invoice

  DMEPOS Modifier(s): NU

☼ E0781 Ambulatory infusion pump, single or multiple channels, electric or battery operated with administrative equipment, worn by patient `Qp` ♿ Y

  Billable to both the local carrier and the DME/MAC. This item may be billed to the DME/MAC whenever the infusion is initiated in the physician's office but the patient does not return during the same business day.

  IOM: 100-03, 1, 50.3

  DMEPOS Modifier(s): RR

☼ E0782 Infusion pump, implantable, non-programmable (includes all components, e.g., pump, catheter, connectors, etc.) `Qp` `Qh` ♿ N1 N

  Bill local carrier

  IOM: 100-03, 1, 50.3

  DMEPOS Modifier(s): NU, KF, RR, UE

☼ E0783 Infusion pump system, implantable, programmable (includes all components, e.g., pump, catheter, connectors, etc.) `Qp` `Qh` ♿ N1 N

  Bill local carrier

  IOM: 100-03, 1, 50.3

  DMEPOS Modifier(s): NU, KF, RR, UE

☼ E0784 External ambulatory infusion pump, insulin `Qp` ♿ Y

  Bill DME/MAC

  IOM: 100-03, 4, 280.14

  DMEPOS Modifier(s): RR

☼ E0785 Implantable intraspinal (epidural/intrathecal) catheter used with implantable infusion pump, replacement `Qp` `Qh` ♿ N1 N

  Bill local carrier

  IOM: 100-03, 1, 50.3

  DMEPOS Modifier(s): KF

☼ E0786 Implantable programmable infusion pump, replacement (excludes implantable intraspinal catheter) `Qp` ♿ N1 N

  Bill local carrier

  IOM: 100-03, 1, 50.3

  DMEPOS Modifier(s): NU, KF, RR, UE

☼ E0791 Parenteral infusion pump, stationary, single or multi-channel `Qp` ♿ Y

  Bill DME/MAC

  IOM: 100-02, 15, 120; 100-03, 3, 180.2; 100-04, 20, 100.2.2

  DMEPOS Modifier(s): RR

Traction Equipment: All Types and Cervical

E0830-E0856: Bill DME/MAC

☼ E0830 Ambulatory traction device, all types, each N

  IOM: 100-03, 4, 280.1

  DMEPOS Modifier(s): NU

☼ E0840 Traction frame, attached to headboard, cervical traction `Qp` ♿ Y

  IOM: 100-03, 4, 280.1

  DMEPOS Modifier(s): NU, RR, UE

* E0849 Traction equipment, cervical, free-standing stand/frame, pneumatic, applying traction force to other than mandible `Qp` ♿ Y

  DMEPOS Modifier(s): NU, RR, UE

▶ **New**   → **Revised**   ✔ **Reinstated**   ~~deleted~~ **Deleted**

☼ **Special coverage instructions**   ◆ **Not covered or valid by Medicare**   * **Carrier discretion**

⊕ **E0850** Traction stand, free standing, cervical traction `Qp` ♿   Y

    IOM: 100-03, 4, 280.1

    DMEPOS Modifier(s): NU, RR, UE

✳ **E0855** Cervical traction equipment not requiring additional stand or frame `Qp` ♿   Y

    DMEPOS Modifier(s): NU, RR, UE

✳ **E0856** Cervical traction device, cervical collar with inflatable air bladder `Qp` `Qh` ♿   Y

    DMEPOS Modifier(s): NU, RR, UE

Traction: Overdoor

⊕ **E0860** Traction equipment, overdoor, cervical `Qp` ♿   Y

    Bill DME/MAC

    IOM: 100-03, 4, 280.1

    DMEPOS Modifier(s): NU, RR, UE

Traction: Extremity

E0870-E0880:   Bill DME/MAC

⊕ **E0870** Traction frame, attached to footboard, extremity traction, (e.g., Buck's) `Qp` ♿   Y

    IOM: 100-03, 4, 280.1

    DMEPOS Modifier(s): NU, RR, UE

⊕ **E0880** Traction stand, free standing, extremity traction, (e.g., Buck's) `Qp` ♿   Y

    IOM: 100-03, 4, 280.1

    DMEPOS Modifier(s): NU, RR, UE

Traction: Pelvic

E0890-E0900:   Bill DME/MAC

⊕ **E0890** Traction frame, attached to footboard, pelvic traction `Qp` ♿   Y

    IOM: 100-03, 4, 280.1

    DMEPOS Modifier(s): NU, RR, UE

⊕ **E0900** Traction stand, free standing, pelvic traction, (e.g., Buck's) `Qp` ♿   Y

    IOM: 100-03, 4, 280.1

    DMEPOS Modifier(s): NU, RR, UE

Trapeze Equipment, Fracture Frame, and Other Orthopedic Devices

E0910-E0948:   Bill DME/MAC

⊕ **E0910** Trapeze bars, A/K/A patient helper, attached to bed, with grab bar `Qp` ♿   Y

    IOM: 100-03, 4, 280.1

    DMEPOS Modifier(s): RR

⊕ **E0911** Trapeze bar, heavy duty, for patient weight capacity greater than 250 pounds, attached to bed, with grab bar `Qp` ♿   Y

    IOM: 100-03, 4, 280.1

    DMEPOS Modifier(s): RR

⊕ **E0912** Trapeze bar, heavy duty, for patient weight capacity greater than 250 pounds, free standing, complete with grab bar `Qp` ♿   Y

    IOM: 100-03, 4, 280.1

    DMEPOS Modifier(s): RR

⊕ **E0920** Fracture frame, attached to bed, includes weights `Qp` ♿   Y

    IOM: 100-03, 4, 280.1

    DMEPOS Modifier(s): RR

⊕ **E0930** Fracture frame, free standing, includes weights `Qp` ♿   Y

    IOM: 100-03, 4, 280.1

    DMEPOS Modifier(s): RR

⊕ **E0935** Continuous passive motion exercise device for use on knee only ♿   Y

    To qualify for coverage, use of device must commence within two days following surgery

    IOM: 100-03, 4, 280.1

    DMEPOS Modifier(s): RR

◆ **E0936** Continuous passive motion exercise device for use other than knee   E

⊕ **E0940** Trapeze bar, free standing, complete with grab bar `Qp` ♿   Y

    IOM: 100-03, 4, 280.1

    DMEPOS Modifier(s): RR

⊕ **E0941** Gravity assisted traction device, any type `Qp` ♿   Y

    IOM: 100-03, 4, 280.1

    DMEPOS Modifier(s): RR

✳ **E0942** Cervical head harness/halter `Qp` ♿   Y

    DMEPOS Modifier(s): NU, RR, UE

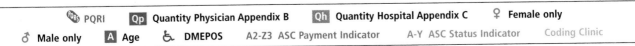

✳ **E0944** Pelvic belt/harness/boot Qp   Y
    DMEPOS Modifier(s): NU, RR, UE

✳ **E0945** Extremity belt/harness Qp   Y
    DMEPOS Modifier(s): NU, RR, UE

✪ **E0946** Fracture, frame, dual with cross bars, attached to bed, (e.g. Balken, 4 poster) Qp   Y
    IOM: 100-03, 4, 280.1
    DMEPOS Modifier(s): RR

✪ **E0947** Fracture frame, attachments for complex pelvic traction Qp   Y
    IOM: 100-03, 4, 280.1
    DMEPOS Modifier(s): NU, RR, UE

✪ **E0948** Fracture frame, attachments for complex cervical traction Qp   Y
    IOM: 100-03, 4, 280.1
    DMEPOS Modifier(s): NU, RR, UE

Wheelchair Accessories

E0950-E1030:   Bill DME/MAC

✪ **E0950** Wheelchair accessory, tray, each Qp Qh   Y
    IOM: 100-03, 4, 280.1
    DMEPOS Modifier(s): NU, KE, RR

✳ **E0951** Heel loop/holder, any type, with or without ankle strap, each Qp Qh   Y
    DMEPOS Modifier(s): NU, KE, RR

✪ **E0952** Toe loop/holder, any type, each Qp Qh   Y
    IOM: 100-03, 4, 280.1
    DMEPOS Modifier(s): NU, KE, RR

✳ **E0955** Wheelchair accessory, headrest, cushioned, any type, including fixed mounting hardware, each Qp   Y
    DMEPOS Modifier(s): NU, KE, RR

✳ **E0956** Wheelchair accessory, lateral trunk or hip support, any type, including fixed mounting hardware, each   Y
    DMEPOS Modifier(s): NU, KE, RR

✳ **E0957** Wheelchair accessory, medial thigh support, any type, including fixed mounting hardware, each Qp   Y
    DMEPOS Modifier(s): NU, KE, RR

✪ **E0958** Manual wheelchair accessory, one-arm drive attachment, each Qp Qh   Y
    IOM: 100-03, 4, 280.1
    DMEPOS Modifier(s): RR

✳ **E0959** Manual wheelchair accessory, adapter for amputee, each Qp   B
    IOM: 100-03, 4, 280.1
    DMEPOS Modifier(s): NU, RR, UE

✳ **E0960** Wheelchair accessory, shoulder harness/straps or chest strap, including any type mounting hardware Qp   Y
    DMEPOS Modifier(s): NU, KE, RR

✳ **E0961** Manual wheelchair accessory, wheel lock brake extension (handle), each Qp   B
    IOM: 100-03, 4, 280.1
    DMEPOS Modifier(s): NU, RR, UE

✳ **E0966** Manual wheelchair accessory, headrest extension, each Qp   B
    IOM: 100-03, 4, 280.1
    DMEPOS Modifier(s): NU, RR, UE

✪ **E0967** Manual wheelchair accessory, hand rim with projections, any type, each Qp   Y
    IOM: 100-03, 4, 280.1
    DMEPOS Modifier(s): NU, RR, UE

✪ **E0968** Commode seat, wheelchair Qp   Y
    IOM: 100-03, 4, 280.1
    DMEPOS Modifier(s): RR

✪ **E0969** Narrowing device, wheelchair   Y
    IOM: 100-03, 4, 280.1
    DMEPOS Modifier(s): NU, RR, UE

◆ **E0970** No.2 footplates, except for elevating leg rest Qp   E
    IOM: 100-03, 4, 280.1
    Cross Reference CPT K0037, K0042

✳ **E0971** Manual wheelchair accessory, anti-tipping device, each Qp   B
    IOM: 100-03, 4, 280.1
    Cross Reference CPT K0021
    DMEPOS Modifier(s): NU, RR, UE

✪ **E0973** Wheelchair accessory, adjustable height, detachable armrest, complete assembly, each Qp   B
    IOM: 100-03, 4, 280.1
    DMEPOS Modifier(s): NU, KE, RR

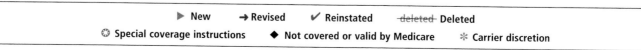

▶ New   → Revised   ✔ Reinstated   ~~deleted~~ Deleted
✪ Special coverage instructions   ◆ Not covered or valid by Medicare   ✳ Carrier discretion

⊘ **E0974** Manual wheelchair accessory, anti-rollback device, each Qp ♿ B

IOM: 100-03, 4, 280.1

DMEPOS Modifier(s): NU, RR, UE

→ ✳ **E0978** Wheelchair accessory, positioning belt/safety belt/pelvic strap, each Qp ♿ B

DMEPOS Modifier(s): NU, KE, RR

✳ **E0980** Safety vest, wheelchair ♿ Y

DMEPOS Modifier(s): NU, RR, UE

✳ **E0981** Wheelchair accessory, seat upholstery, replacement only, each Qp ♿ Y

DMEPOS Modifier(s): NU, KE, RR

✳ **E0982** Wheelchair accessory, back upholstery, replacement only, each Qp ♿ Y

DMEPOS Modifier(s): NU, KE, RR

✳ **E0983** Manual wheelchair accessory, power add-on to convert manual wheelchair to motorized wheelchair, joystick control Qp ♿ Y

DMEPOS Modifier(s): RR

✳ **E0984** Manual wheelchair accessory, power add-on to convert manual wheelchair to motorized wheelchair, tiller control Qp ♿ Y

DMEPOS Modifier(s): NU, RR, UE

✳ **E0985** Wheelchair accessory, seat lift mechanism Qp ♿ Y

DMEPOS Modifier(s): NU, RR, UE

✳ **E0986** Manual wheelchair accessory, push activated power assist, each Qp ♿ Y

DMEPOS Modifier(s): NU, RR, UE

▶ ✳ **E0988** Manual wheelchair accessory, lever-activated, wheel drive, pair Y

✳ **E0990** Wheelchair accessory, elevating leg rest, complete assembly, each Qp ♿ B

IOM: 100-03, 4, 280.1

DMEPOS Modifier(s): NU, KE, RR, UE

✳ **E0992** Manual wheelchair accessory, solid seat insert Qp ♿ B

DMEPOS Modifier(s): NU, RR, UE

⊘ **E0994** Arm rest, each Qp ♿ Y

IOM: 100-03, 4, 280.1

DMEPOS Modifier(s): NU, RR, UE

✳ **E0995** Wheelchair accessory, calf rest/pad, each Qp ♿ B

IOM: 100-03, 4, 280.1

DMEPOS Modifier(s): NU, KE, RR, UE

✳ **E1002** Wheelchair accessory, power seating system, tilt only Qp ♿ Y

DMEPOS Modifier(s): NU, KE, RR, UE

✳ **E1003** Wheelchair accessory, power seating system, recline only, without shear reduction Qp ♿ Y

DMEPOS Modifier(s): NU, KE, RR, UE

✳ **E1004** Wheelchair accessory, power seating system, recline only, with mechanical shear reduction Qp ♿ Y

DMEPOS Modifier(s): NU, KE, RR, UE

✳ **E1005** Wheelchair accessory, power seating system, recline only, with power shear reduction Qp ♿ Y

DMEPOS Modifier(s): NU, KE, RR, UE

✳ **E1006** Wheelchair accessory, power seating system, combination tilt and recline, without shear reduction Qp ♿ Y

DMEPOS Modifier(s): NU, KE, RR, UE

✳ **E1007** Wheelchair accessory, power seating system, combination tilt and recline, with mechanical shear reduction Qp ♿ Y

DMEPOS Modifier(s): NU, KE, RR, UE

✳ **E1008** Wheelchair accessory, power seating system, combination tilt and recline, with power shear reduction Qp ♿ Y

DMEPOS Modifier(s): NU, KE, RR, UE

✳ **E1009** Wheelchair accessory, addition to power seating system, mechanically linked leg elevation system, including pushrod and leg rest, each Qp ♿ Y

DMEPOS Modifier(s): NU, RR, UE

✳ **E1010** Wheelchair accessory, addition to power seating system, power leg elevation system, including leg rest, pair Qp ♿ Y

DMEPOS Modifier(s): NU, KE, RR, UE

⊘ **E1011** Modification to pediatric size wheelchair, width adjustment package (not to be dispensed with initial chair) Qp A ♿ Y

IOM: 100-03, 4, 280.1

DMEPOS Modifier(s): NU, RR, UE

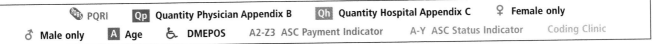

PQRI   Qp **Quantity Physician Appendix B**   Qh **Quantity Hospital Appendix C**   ♀ **Female only**
♂ **Male only**   A **Age**   ♿ **DMEPOS**   A2-Z3 **ASC Payment Indicator**   A-Y **ASC Status Indicator**   Coding Clinic

⚙ **E1014** Reclining back, addition to pediatric size wheelchair Qp A ♿   Y

IOM: 100-03, 4, 280.1

DMEPOS Modifier(s): NU, RR, UE

⚙ **E1015** Shock absorber for manual wheelchair, each Qp ♿   Y

IOM: 100-03, 4, 280.1

DMEPOS Modifier(s): NU, RR, UE

⚙ **E1016** Shock absorber for power wheelchair, each Qp ♿   Y

IOM: 100-03, 4, 280.1

DMEPOS Modifier(s): NU, KE, RR, UE

⚙ **E1017** Heavy duty shock absorber for heavy duty or extra heavy duty manual wheelchair, each Qp ♿   Y

IOM: 100-03, 4, 280.1

DMEPOS Modifier(s): NU, RR, UE

⚙ **E1018** Heavy duty shock absorber for heavy duty or extra heavy duty power wheelchair, each Qp ♿   Y

IOM: 100-03, 4, 280.1

DMEPOS Modifier(s): NU, RR, UE

⚙ **E1020** Residual limb support system for wheelchair Qp ♿   Y

IOM: 100-03, 3, 280.3

DMEPOS Modifier(s): NU, KE, RR, UE

✳ **E1028** Wheelchair accessory, manual swingaway, retractable or removable mounting hardware for joystick, other control interface or positioning accessory Qp ♿   Y

DMEPOS Modifier(s): NU, KE, RR, UE

✳ **E1029** Wheelchair accessory, ventilator tray, fixed Qp ♿   Y

DMEPOS Modifier(s): NU, KE, RR, UE

✳ **E1030** Wheelchair accessory, ventilator tray, gimbaled Qp ♿   Y

DMEPOS Modifier(s): NU, KE, RR, UE

Rollabout Chair and Transfer System

E1031-E1039: Bill DME/MAC

⚙ **E1031** Rollabout chair, any and all types with castors 5" or greater Qp ♿   Y

IOM: 100-03, 4, 280.1

DMEPOS Modifier(s): RR

✳ **E1035** Multi-positional patient transfer system, with integrated seat, operated by care giver, patient weight capacity up to and including 300 lbs Qp ♿   Y

IOM: 100-02, 15, 110

DMEPOS Modifier(s): RR

✳ **E1036** Multi-positional patient transfer system, extra-wide, with integrated seat, operated by caregiver, patient weight capacity greater than 300 lbs Qh ♿   Y

DMEPOS Modifier(s): RR

⚙ **E1037** Transport chair, pediatric size Qp A ♿   Y

IOM: 100-03, 4, 280.1

DMEPOS Modifier(s): RR

⚙ **E1038** Transport chair, adult size, patient weight capacity up to and including 300 pounds Qp A ♿   Y

IOM: 100-03, 4, 280.1

DMEPOS Modifier(s): RR

✳ **E1039** Transport chair, adult size, heavy duty, patient weight capacity greater than 300 pounds Qp A ♿   Y

DMEPOS Modifier(s): RR

Wheelchair: Fully Reclining

E1050-E1093: Bill DME/MAC

⚙ **E1050** Fully-reclining wheelchair, fixed full length arms, swing away detachable elevating leg rests Qp Qh ♿   Y

IOM: 100-03, 4, 280.1

DMEPOS Modifier(s): RR

⚙ **E1060** Fully-reclining wheelchair, detachable arms, desk or full length, swing away detachable elevating legrests Qp Qh ♿   Y

IOM: 100-03, 4, 280.1

DMEPOS Modifier(s): RR

⚙ **E1070** Fully-reclining wheelchair, detachable arms (desk or full length) swing away detachable footrests Qp Qh ♿   Y

IOM: 100-03, 4, 280.1

DMEPOS Modifier(s): RR

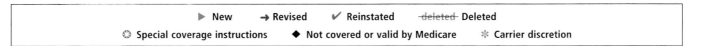

▶ New   → Revised   ✔ Reinstated   ~~deleted~~ Deleted

⚙ Special coverage instructions   ◆ Not covered or valid by Medicare   ✳ Carrier discretion

⊛ **E1083** Hemi-wheelchair, fixed full length arms, swing away detachable elevating leg rest `Qp` `Qh` ♿   Y

IOM: 100-03, 4, 280.1

DMEPOS Modifier(s): RR

⊛ **E1084** Hemi-wheelchair, detachable arms desk or full length arms, swing away detachable elevating leg rests `Qp` `Qh` ♿   Y

IOM: 100-03, 4, 280.1

DMEPOS Modifier(s): RR

◆ **E1085** Hemi-wheelchair, fixed full length arms, swing away detachable foot rests `Qp` `Qh`   E

IOM: 100-03, 4, 280.1

Cross Reference CPT K0002

◆ **E1086** Hemi-wheelchair, detachable arms desk or full length, swing away detachable footrests `Qp` `Qh`   E

IOM: 100-03, 4, 280.1

Cross Reference CPT K0002

⊛ **E1087** High strength lightweight wheelchair, fixed full length arms, swing away detachable elevating leg rests `Qp` `Qh` ♿   Y

IOM: 100-03, 4, 280.1

DMEPOS Modifier(s): RR

⊛ **E1088** High strength lightweight wheelchair, detachable arms desk or full length, swing away detachable elevating leg rests `Qp` `Qh` ♿   Y

IOM: 100-03, 4, 280.1

DMEPOS Modifier(s): RR

◆ **E1089** High strength lightweight wheelchair, fixed length arms, swing away detachable footrest `Qp` `Qh`   E

IOM: 100-03, 4, 280.1

Cross Reference CPT K0004

◆ **E1090** High strength lightweight wheelchair, detachable arms desk or full length, swing away detachable foot rests `Qp` `Qh`   E

IOM: 100-03, 4, 280.1

Cross Reference CPT K0004

⊛ **E1092** Wide heavy duty wheelchair, detachable arms (desk or full length) swing away detachable elevating leg rests `Qp` `Qh` ♿   Y

IOM: 100-03, 4, 280.1

DMEPOS Modifier(s): RR

⊛ **E1093** Wide heavy duty wheelchair, detachable arms (desk or full length arms), swing away detachable foot rests `Qp` `Qh` ♿   Y

IOM: 100-03, 4, 280.1

DMEPOS Modifier(s): RR

Wheelchair: Semi-reclining

E1100-E1110:   Bill DME/MAC

⊛ **E1100** Semi-reclining wheelchair, fixed full length arms, swing away detachable elevating leg rests `Qp` `Qh` ♿   Y

IOM: 100-03, 4, 280.1

DMEPOS Modifier(s): RR

⊛ **E1110** Semi-reclining wheelchair, detachable arms (desk or full length), elevating leg rest `Qp` `Qh` ♿   Y

IOM: 100-03, 4, 280.1

DMEPOS Modifier(s): RR

Wheelchair: Standard

E1130-E1161:   Bill DME/MAC

◆ **E1130** Standard wheelchair, fixed full length arms, fixed or swing away detachable footrests `Qp` `Qh`   E

IOM: 100-03, 4, 280.1

Cross Reference CPT K0001

◆ **E1140** Wheelchair, detachable arms, desk or full length, swing away detachable footrests `Qp` `Qh`   E

IOM: 100-03, 4, 280.1

Cross Reference CPT K0001

⊛ **E1150** Wheelchair, detachable arms, desk or full length, swing away detachable elevating legrests `Qp` ♿   Y

IOM: 100-03, 4, 280.1

DMEPOS Modifier(s): RR

⊛ **E1160** Wheelchair, fixed full length arms, swing away detachable elevating legrests `Qp` `Qh` ♿   Y

IOM: 100-03, 4, 280.1

DMEPOS Modifier(s): RR

→ ✳ **E1161** Manual adult size wheelchair, includes tilt in space `Qp` `Qh` `A` ♿   Y

DMEPOS Modifier(s): NU, RR, UE

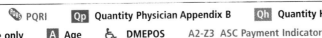
DURABLE MEDICAL EQUIPMENT   E1083 – E1161

Wheelchair: Amputee

E1170-E1200: Bill DME/MAC

⊛ **E1170** Amputee wheelchair, fixed full length arms, swing away detachable elevating legrests `Qp` `Qh` ♿   Y

IOM: 100-03, 4, 280.1

DMEPOS Modifier(s): RR

⊛ **E1171** Amputee wheelchair, fixed full length arms, without footrests or legrest `Qp` `Qh` ♿   Y

IOM: 100-03, 4, 280.1

DMEPOS Modifier(s): RR

⊛ **E1172** Amputee wheelchair, detachable arms (desk or full length) without footrests or legrest `Qp` `Qh` ♿   Y

IOM: 100-03, 4, 280.1

DMEPOS Modifier(s): RR

⊛ **E1180** Amputee wheelchair, detachable arms (desk or full length) swing away detachable footrests `Qp` `Qh` ♿   Y

IOM: 100-03, 4, 280.1

DMEPOS Modifier(s): RR

⊛ **E1190** Amputee wheelchair, detachable arms (desk or full length), swing away detachable elevating legrests `Qp` `Qh` ♿   Y

IOM: 100-03, 4, 280.1

DMEPOS Modifier(s): RR

⊛ **E1195** Heavy duty wheelchair, fixed full length arms, swing away detachable elevating legrests `Qp` `Qh` ♿   Y

IOM: 100-03, 4, 280.1

DMEPOS Modifier(s): RR

⊛ **E1200** Amputee wheelchair, fixed full length arms, swing away detachable footrest `Qp` `Qh` ♿   Y

IOM: 100-03, 4, 280.1

DMEPOS Modifier(s): RR

Wheelchair: Special Size

E1220-E1239: Bill DME/MAC

⊛ **E1220** Wheelchair; specially sized or constructed, (indicate brand name, model number, if any) and justification `Qp` `Qh`   Y

IOM: 100-03, 4, 280.3

⊛ **E1221** Wheelchair with fixed arm, footrests `Qp` `Qh` ♿   Y

IOM: 100-03, 4, 280.3

DMEPOS Modifier(s): RR

⊛ **E1222** Wheelchair with fixed arm, elevating legrests `Qp` `Qh` ♿   Y

IOM: 100-03, 4, 280.3

DMEPOS Modifier(s): RR

⊛ **E1223** Wheelchair with detachable arms, footrests `Qp` `Qh` ♿   Y

IOM: 100-03, 4, 280.3

DMEPOS Modifier(s): RR

⊛ **E1224** Wheelchair with detachable arms, elevating legrests `Qp` `Qh` ♿   Y

IOM: 100-03, 4, 280.3

DMEPOS Modifier(s): RR

⊛ **E1225** Wheelchair accessory, manual semi-reclining back, (recline greater than 15 degrees, but less than 80 degrees), each `Qp` ♿   Y

IOM: 100-03, 4, 280.3

DMEPOS Modifier(s): RR

⊛ **E1226** Wheelchair accessory, manual fully reclining back, (recline greater than 80 degrees), each `Qp` ♿   B

IOM: 100-03, 4, 280.1

DMEPOS Modifier(s): NU, RR, UE

⊛ **E1227** Special height arms for wheelchair ♿   Y

IOM: 100-03, 4, 280.3

DMEPOS Modifier(s): NU, RR, UE

⊛ **E1228** Special back height for wheelchair `Qp` ♿   Y

IOM: 100-03, 4, 280.3

DMEPOS Modifier(s): RR

✳ **E1229** Wheelchair, pediatric size, not otherwise specified `A`   Y

▶ New   → Revised   ✔ Reinstated   ~~deleted~~ Deleted

⊛ Special coverage instructions   ◆ Not covered or valid by Medicare   ✳ Carrier discretion

⊛ **E1230** Power operated vehicle (three or four wheel non-highway), specify brand name and model number Qp ♿   Y

Patient is unable to operate manual wheelchair; patient capable of safely operating controls for scooter; patient can transfer safely in and out of scooter

IOM: 100-08, 5, 5.2.3

DMEPOS Modifier(s): NU, RR, UE

⊛ **E1231** Wheelchair, pediatric size, tilt-in-space, rigid, adjustable, with seating system Qp A ♿   Y

IOM: 100-03, 4, 280.1

DMEPOS Modifier(s): NU, RR, UE

⊛ **E1232** Wheelchair, pediatric size, tilt-in-space, folding, adjustable, with seating system Qp A ♿   Y

IOM: 100-03, 4, 280.1

DMEPOS Modifier(s): NU, RR, UE

⊛ **E1233** Wheelchair, pediatric size, tilt-in-space, rigid, adjustable, without seating system Qp A ♿   Y

IOM: 100-03, 4, 280.1

DMEPOS Modifier(s): NU, RR, UE

⊛ **E1234** Wheelchair, pediatric size, tilt-in-space, folding, adjustable, without seating system Qp A ♿   Y

IOM: 100-03, 4, 280.1

DMEPOS Modifier(s): NU, RR, UE

⊛ **E1235** Wheelchair, pediatric size, rigid, adjustable, with seating system Qp A ♿   Y

IOM: 100-03, 4, 280.1

DMEPOS Modifier(s): NU, RR, UE

⊛ **E1236** Wheelchair, pediatric size, folding, adjustable, with seating system Qp A ♿   Y

IOM: 100-03, 4, 280.1

DMEPOS Modifier(s): NU, RR, UE

⊛ **E1237** Wheelchair, pediatric size, rigid, adjustable, without seating system Qp A ♿   Y

IOM: 100-03, 4, 280.1

DMEPOS Modifier(s): NU, RR, UE

⊛ **E1238** Wheelchair, pediatric size, folding, adjustable, without seating system Qp A ♿   Y

IOM: 100-03, 4, 280.1

DMEPOS Modifier(s): NU, RR, UE

＊ **E1239** Power wheelchair, pediatric size, not otherwise specified A   Y

Wheelchair: Lightweight

E1240-E1270:   Bill DME/MAC

⊛ **E1240** Lightweight wheelchair, detachable arms, (desk or full length) swing away detachable, elevating leg rests Qp Qh ♿   Y

IOM: 100-03, 4, 280.1

DMEPOS Modifier(s): RR

◆ **E1250** Lightweight wheelchair, fixed full length arms, swing away detachable footrest Qp Qh   E

IOM: 100-03, 4, 280.1

Cross Reference CPT K0003

◆ **E1260** Lightweight wheelchair, detachable arms (desk or full length) swing away detachable footrest Qp Qh   E

IOM: 100-03, 4, 280.1

Cross Reference CPT K0003

⊛ **E1270** Lightweight wheelchair, fixed full length arms, swing away detachable elevating legrests Qp Qh ♿   Y

IOM: 100-03, 4, 280.1

DMEPOS Modifier(s): RR

Wheelchair: Heavy Duty

E1280-E1298:   Bill DME/MAC

⊛ **E1280** Heavy duty wheelchair, detachable arms (desk or full length), elevating legrests Qp Qh ♿   Y

IOM: 100-03, 4, 280.1

DMEPOS Modifier(s): RR

◆ **E1285** Heavy duty wheelchair, fixed full length arms, swing away detachable footrest Qp Qh   E

IOM: 100-03, 4, 280.1

Cross Reference CPT K0006

◆ **E1290** Heavy duty wheelchair, detachable arms (desk or full length) swing away detachable footrest Qp Qh   E

IOM: 100-03, 4, 280.1

Cross Reference CPT K0006

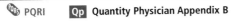 PQRI   **Qp** Quantity Physician Appendix B   **Qh** Quantity Hospital Appendix C   ♀ **Female only**

♂ **Male only**   **A** Age   ♿ **DMEPOS**   A2-Z3 **ASC Payment Indicator**   A-Y **ASC Status Indicator**   Coding Clinic

⊗ **E1295** Heavy duty wheelchair, fixed full length arms, elevating legrest `Qp` `Qh` ♿   Y

IOM: 100-03, 4, 280.1

DMEPOS Modifier(s): RR

⊗ **E1296** Special wheelchair seat height from floor ♿   Y

IOM: 100-03, 4, 280.3

DMEPOS Modifier(s): NU, RR, UE

⊗ **E1297** Special wheelchair seat depth, by upholstery ♿   Y

IOM: 100-03, 4, 280.3

DMEPOS Modifier(s): NU, RR, UE

⊗ **E1298** Special wheelchair seat depth and/or width, by construction ♿   Y

IOM: 100-03, 4, 280.3

DMEPOS Modifier(s): NU, RR, UE

Whirlpool Equipment

E1300-E1310: Bill DME/MAC

◆ **E1300** Whirlpool, portable (overtub type)   E

IOM: 100-03, 4, 280.1

⊗ **E1310** Whirlpool, non-portable (built-in type) `Qp` ♿   Y

IOM: 100-03, 4, 280.1

DMEPOS Modifier(s): NU, RR, UE

Additional Oxygen Related Equipment

⊗ **E1353** Regulator `Qp` ♿   Y

Bill DME/MAC

IOM: 100-03, 4, 240.2

✳ **E1354** Oxygen accessory, wheeled cart for portable cylinder or portable concentrator, any type, replacement only, each   Y

Bill DME/MAC

⊗ **E1355** Stand/rack `Qp` ♿   Y

Bill DME/MAC

IOM: 100-03, 4, 240.2

✳ **E1356** Oxygen accessory, battery pack/cartridge for portable concentrator, any type, replacement only, each   Y

Bill DME/MAC

✳ **E1357** Oxygen accessory, battery charger for portable concentrator, any type, replacement only, each   Y

Bill DME/MAC

◆ **E1358** Oxygen accessory, DC power adapter for portable concentrator, any type, replacement only, each   Y

Bill DME/MAC

⊗ **E1372** Immersion external heater for nebulizer `Qp` ♿   Y

Bill DME/MAC

IOM: 100-03, 4, 240.2

DMEPOS Modifier(s): NU, RR, UE

⊗ **E1390** Oxygen concentrator, single delivery port, capable of delivering 85 percent or greater oxygen concentration at the prescribed flow rate `Qp` ♿   Y

Bill DME/MAC

IOM: 100-03, 4, 240.2

DMEPOS Modifier(s): RR

⊗ **E1391** Oxygen concentrator, dual delivery port, capable of delivering 85 percent or greater oxygen concentration at the prescribed flow rate, each `Qp` ♿   Y

Bill DME/MAC

IOM: 100-03, 4, 240.2

DMEPOS Modifier(s): RR

⊗ **E1392** Portable oxygen concentrator, rental `Qp` ♿   Y

Bill DME/MAC

IOM: 100-03, 4, 240.2

DMEPOS Modifier(s): RR

✳ **E1399** Durable medical equipment, miscellaneous   Y

Local carrier if used with implanted DME. If other, bill DME/MAC.

Example: Therapeutic exercise putty; rubber exercise tubing; anti-vibration gloves

On DMEPOS fee schedule as a payable replacement for miscellaneous implanted or non-implanted items.

⊗ **E1405** Oxygen and water vapor enriching system with heated delivery `Qp` ♿   Y

Bill DME/MAC

IOM: 100-03, 4, 240.2

DMEPOS Modifier(s): RR

⊗ **E1406** Oxygen and water vapor enriching system without heated delivery `Qp` ♿   Y

Bill DME/MAC

IOM: 100-03, 4, 240.2

DMEPOS Modifier(s): RR

▶ New   → Revised   ✔ Reinstated   ~~deleted~~ Deleted

⊗ Special coverage instructions   ◆ Not covered or valid by Medicare   ✳ Carrier discretion

Artificial Kidney Machines and Accessories

E1500-E1699:   Bill DME/MAC

⚙ **E1500**   Centrifuge, for dialysis `Qp` `Qh`   A

⚙ **E1510**   Kidney, dialysate delivery syst. kidney machine, pump recirculating, air removal syst. flowrate meter, power off, heater and temperature control with alarm, I.V. poles, pressure gauge, concentrate container `Qp` `Qh`   A

⚙ **E1520**   Heparin infusion pump for hemodialysis `Qp` `Qh`   A

⚙ **E1530**   Air bubble detector for hemodialysis, each, replacement `Qp` `Qh`   A

⚙ **E1540**   Pressure alarm for hemodialysis, each, replacement `Qp` `Qh`   A

⚙ **E1550**   Bath conductivity meter for hemodialysis, each `Qp` `Qh`   A

⚙ **E1560**   Blood leak detector for hemodialysis, each, replacement `Qp` `Qh`   A

⚙ **E1570**   Adjustable chair, for ESRD patients `Qp` `Qh`   A

⚙ **E1575**   Transducer protectors/fluid barriers for hemodialysis, any size, per 10   A

⚙ **E1580**   Unipuncture control system for hemodialysis `Qp` `Qh`   A

⚙ **E1590**   Hemodialysis machine `Qp` `Qh`   A

⚙ **E1592**   Automatic intermittent peritoneal dialysis system `Qp` `Qh`   A

⚙ **E1594**   Cycler dialysis machine for peritoneal dialysis `Qp` `Qh`   A

⚙ **E1600**   Delivery and/or installation charges for hemodialysis equipment `Qp` `Qh`   A

⚙ **E1610**   Reverse osmosis water purification system, for hemodialysis `Qp` `Qh`   A

   IOM: 100-03, 4, 230.7

⚙ **E1615**   Deionizer water purification system, for hemodialysis `Qp` `Qh`   A

   IOM: 100-03, 4, 230.7

⚙ **E1620**   Blood pump for hemodialysis replacement `Qp` `Qh`   A

⚙ **E1625**   Water softening system, for hemodialysis `Qp` `Qh`   A

   IOM: 100-03, 4, 230.7

✳ **E1630**   Reciprocating peritoneal dialysis system `Qp` `Qh`   A

⚙ **E1632**   Wearable artificial kidney, each   A

⚙ **E1634**   Peritoneal dialysis clamps, each   B

   IOM: 100-04, 8, 60.4.2; 100-04, 8, 90.1; 100-04, 18, 80; 100-04, 18, 90

⚙ **E1635**   Compact (portable) travel hemodialyzer system `Qp` `Qh`   A

⚙ **E1636**   Sorbent cartridges, for hemodialysis, per 10   A

⚙ **E1637**   Hemostats, each   A

⚙ **E1639**   Scale, each `Qp` `Qh`   A

⚙ **E1699**   Dialysis equipment, not otherwise specified   A

Jaw Motion Rehabilitation System and Accessories

E1700-E1702:   Bill DME/MAC

✳ **E1700**   Jaw motion rehabilitation system `Qp` ♿   Y

   Must be prescribed by physician

   DMEPOS Modifier(s): NU, RR, UE

✳ **E1701**   Replacement cushions for jaw motion rehabilitation system, pkg. of 6 ♿   Y

✳ **E1702**   Replacement measuring scales for jaw motion rehabilitation system, pkg. of 200 ♿   Y

Other Orthopedic Devices

E1800-E1841:   Bill DME/MAC

✳ **E1800**   Dynamic adjustable elbow extension/flexion device, includes soft interface material `Qp` ♿   Y

   DMEPOS Modifier(s): RR

✳ **E1801**   Static progressive stretch elbow device, extension and/or flexion, with or without range of motion adjustment, includes all components and accessories `Qp` ♿   Y

   DMEPOS Modifier(s): RR

✳ **E1802**   Dynamic adjustable forearm pronation/supination device, includes soft interface material `Qp` ♿   Y

   DMEPOS Modifier(s): RR

✳ **E1805**   Dynamic adjustable wrist extension/flexion device, includes soft interface material `Qp` ♿   Y

   DMEPOS Modifier(s): RR

✳ **E1806**   Static progressive stretch wrist device, flexion and/or extension, with or without range of motion adjustment, includes all components and accessories `Qp` ♿   Y

   DMEPOS Modifier(s): RR

✳ **E1810** Dynamic adjustable knee extension/flexion device, includes soft interface material **Qp** ♿ Y

DMEPOS Modifier(s): RR

✳ **E1811** Static progressive stretch knee device, extension and/or flexion, with or without range of motion adjustment, includes all components and accessories **Qp** ♿ Y

DMEPOS Modifier(s): RR

✳ **E1812** Dynamic knee, extension/flexion device with active resistance control **Qp** ♿ Y

DMEPOS Modifier(s): RR

✳ **E1815** Dynamic adjustable ankle extension/flexion device, includes soft interface material **Qp** ♿ Y

DMEPOS Modifier(s): RR

✳ **E1816** Static progressive stretch ankle device, flexion and/or extension, with or without range of motion adjustment, includes all components and accessories **Qp** ♿ Y

DMEPOS Modifier(s): RR

✳ **E1818** Static progressive stretch forearm pronation/supination device with or without range of motion adjustment, includes all components and accessories **Qp** ♿ Y

DMEPOS Modifier(s): RR

✳ **E1820** Replacement soft interface material, dynamic adjustable extension/flexion device **Qp** ♿ Y

DMEPOS Modifier(s): NU, RR, UE

✳ **E1821** Replacement soft interface material/cuffs for bi-directional static progressive stretch device **Qp** ♿ Y

DMEPOS Modifier(s): NU, RR, UE

✳ **E1825** Dynamic adjustable finger extension/flexion device, includes soft interface material **Qp** ♿ Y

DMEPOS Modifier(s): RR

✳ **E1830** Dynamic adjustable toe extension/flexion device, includes soft interface material **Qp** ♿ Y

DMEPOS Modifier(s): RR

▶ ✳ **E1831** Static progressive stretch toe device, extension and/or flexion, with or without range of motion adjustment, includes all components and accessories **Qp** **Qh** ♿ Y

DMEPOS Modifier(s): RR

✳ **E1840** Dynamic adjustable shoulder flexion/abduction/rotation device, includes soft interface material **Qp** ♿ Y

DMEPOS Modifier(s): RR

✳ **E1841** Static progressive stretch shoulder device, with or without range of motion adjustment, includes all components and accessories **Qp** ♿ Y

DMEPOS Modifier(s): RR

MISCELLANEOUS (E1902-E2120)

✳ **E1902** Communication board, non-electronic augmentative or alternative communication device **Qp** **Qh** Y

✳ **E2000** Gastric suction pump, home model, portable or stationary, electric **Qp** ♿ Y

DMEPOS Modifier(s): RR

⊙ **E2100** Blood glucose monitor with integrated voice synthesizer **Qp** ♿ Y

IOM: 100-03, 4, 230.16

DMEPOS Modifier(s): NU, RR, UE

⊙ **E2101** Blood glucose monitor with integrated lancing/blood sample **Qp** ♿ Y

IOM: 100-03, 4, 230.16

DMEPOS Modifier(s): NU, RR, UE

✳ **E2120** Pulse generator system for tympanic treatment of inner ear endolymphatic fluid **Qp** ♿ Y

DMEPOS Modifier(s): RR

Wheelchair Assessories

E2201-E2397: Bill DME/MAC

✳ **E2201** Manual wheelchair accessory, nonstandard seat frame, width greater than or equal to 20 inches and less than 24 inches **Qp** ♿ Y

DMEPOS Modifier(s): NU, RR, UE

✳ **E2202** Manual wheelchair accessory, nonstandard seat frame width, 24-27 inches **Qp** ♿ Y

DMEPOS Modifier(s): NU, RR, UE

✳ **E2203** Manual wheelchair accessory, nonstandard seat frame depth, 20 to less than 22 inches **Qp** ♿ Y

DMEPOS Modifier(s): NU, RR, UE

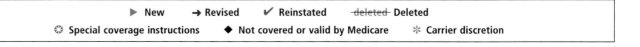

▶ New → Revised ✔ Reinstated deleted Deleted
⊙ Special coverage instructions ◆ Not covered or valid by Medicare ✳ Carrier discretion

✳ **E2204** Manual wheelchair accessory, nonstandard seat frame depth, 22 to 25 inches Qp   Y

   DMEPOS Modifier(s): NU, RR, UE

✳ **E2205** Manual wheelchair accessory, handrim without projections (includes ergonomic or contoured), any type, replacement only, each Qp   Y

   DMEPOS Modifier(s): NU, RR, UE

✳ **E2206** Manual wheelchair accessory, wheel lock assembly, complete, each Qp   Y

   DMEPOS Modifier(s): NU, RR, UE

✳ **E2207** Wheelchair accessory, crutch and cane holder, each Qp   Y

   DMEPOS Modifier(s): NU, RR, UE

✳ **E2208** Wheelchair accessory, cylinder tank carrier, each Qp   Y

   DMEPOS Modifier(s): NU, KE, RR, UE

✳ **E2209** Accessory arm trough, with or without hand support, each Qp   Y

   DMEPOS Modifier(s): NU, KE, RR, UE

✳ **E2210** Wheelchair accessory, bearings, any type, replacement only, each   Y

   DMEPOS Modifier(s): NU, KE, RR, UE

✳ **E2211** Manual wheelchair accessory, pneumatic propulsion tire, any size, each Qp   Y

   DMEPOS Modifier(s): NU, RR, UE

✳ **E2212** Manual wheelchair accessory, tube for pneumatic propulsion tire, any size, each Qp   Y

   DMEPOS Modifier(s): NU, RR, UE

✳ **E2213** Manual wheelchair accessory, insert for pneumatic propulsion tire (removable), any type, any size, each Qp   Y

   DMEPOS Modifier(s): NU, RR, UE

✳ **E2214** Manual wheelchair accessory, pneumatic caster tire, any size, each Qp   Y

   DMEPOS Modifier(s): NU, RR, UE

✳ **E2215** Manual wheelchair accessory, tube for pneumatic caster tire, any size, each Qp   Y

   DMEPOS Modifier(s): NU, RR, UE

✳ **E2216** Manual wheelchair accessory, foam filled propulsion tire, any size, each Qp   Y

   DMEPOS Modifier(s): NU, RR, UE

✳ **E2217** Manual wheelchair accessory, foam filled caster tire, any size, each Qp   Y

   DMEPOS Modifier(s): NU, RR, UE

✳ **E2218** Manual wheelchair accessory, foam propulsion tire, any size, each Qp   Y

   DMEPOS Modifier(s): NU, RR, UE

✳ **E2219** Manual wheelchair accessory, foam caster tire, any size, each Qp   Y

   DMEPOS Modifier(s): NU, RR, UE

✳ **E2220** Manual wheelchair accessory, solid (rubber/plastic) propulsion tire, any size, each Qp   Y

   DMEPOS Modifier(s): NU, RR, UE

✳ **E2221** Manual wheelchair accessory, solid (rubber/plastic) caster tire (removable), any size, each Qp   Y

   DMEPOS Modifier(s): NU, RR, UE

✳ **E2222** Manual wheelchair accessory, solid (rubber/plastic) caster tire with integrated wheel, any size, each Qp   Y

   DMEPOS Modifier(s): NU, RR, UE

✳ **E2224** Manual wheelchair accessory, propulsion wheel excludes tire, any size, each Qp   Y

   DMEPOS Modifier(s): NU, RR, UE

✳ **E2225** Manual wheelchair accessory, caster wheel excludes tire, any size, replacement only, each Qp   Y

   DMEPOS Modifier(s): NU, RR, UE

✳ **E2226** Manual wheelchair accessory, caster fork, any size, replacement only, each Qp   Y

   DMEPOS Modifier(s): NU, RR, UE

✳ **E2227** Manual wheelchair accessory, gear reduction drive wheel, each Qp   Y

   DMEPOS Modifier(s): NU, RR, UE

✳ **E2228** Manual wheelchair accessory, wheel braking system and lock, complete, each Qp   Y

   DMEPOS Modifier(s): NU, RR, UE

◆ **E2230** Manual wheelchair accessory, manual standing system   E

✳ **E2231** Manual wheelchair accessory, solid seat support base (replaces sling seat), includes any type mounting hardware Qp Qh   Y

   DMEPOS Modifier(s): NU, RR, UE

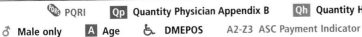

✳ **E2291**   Back, planar, for pediatric size wheelchair including fixed attaching hardware A   Y

✳ **E2292**   Seat, planar, for pediatric size wheelchair including fixed attaching hardware A   Y

✳ **E2293**   Back, contoured, for pediatric size wheelchair including fixed attaching hardware A   Y

✳ **E2294**   Seat, contoured, for pediatric size wheelchair including fixed attaching hardware A   Y

✳ **E2295**   Manual wheelchair accessory, for pediatric size wheelchair, dynamic seating frame, allows coordinated movement of multiple positioning features Qp Qh A   Y

✳ **E2300**   Power wheelchair accessory, power seat elevation system Qp   Y

✳ **E2301**   Power wheelchair accessory, power standing system Qp   Y

✳ **E2310**   Power wheelchair accessory, electronic connection between wheelchair controller and one power seating system motor, including all related electronics, indicator feature, mechanical function selection switch, and fixed mounting hardware Qp &   Y

DMEPOS Modifier(s): KE, NU, RR, UE

✳ **E2311**   Power wheelchair accessory, electronic connection between wheelchair controller and two or more power seating system motors, including all related electronics, indicator feature, mechanical function selection switch, and fixed mounting hardware Qp &   Y

DMEPOS Modifier(s): KE, NU, RR, UE

✳ **E2312**   Power wheelchair accessory, hand or chin control interface, mini-proportional remote joystick, proportional, including fixed mounting hardware Qp &   Y

DMEPOS Modifier(s): KC, NU, RR, UE

✳ **E2313**   Power wheelchair accessory, harness for upgrade to expandable controller, including all fasteners, connectors and mounting hardware, each Qp Qh &   Y

DMEPOS Modifier(s): NU, RR, UE

✳ **E2321**   Power wheelchair accessory, hand control interface, remote joystick, nonproportional, including all related electronics, mechanical stop switch, and fixed mounting hardware Qp &   Y

DMEPOS Modifier(s): KC, KE, NU, RR, UE

✳ **E2322**   Power wheelchair accessory, hand control interface, multiple mechanical switches, nonproportional, including all related electronics, mechanical stop switch, and fixed mounting hardware Qp &   Y

DMEPOS Modifier(s): KC, KE, NU, RR, UE

✳ **E2323**   Power wheelchair accessory, specialty joystick handle for hand control interface, prefabricated Qp   Y

DMEPOS Modifier(s): KE, NU, RR, UE

✳ **E2324**   Power wheelchair accessory, chin cup for chin control interface Qp &   Y

DMEPOS Modifier(s): KE, NU, RR, UE

✳ **E2325**   Power wheelchair accessory, sip and puff interface, nonproportional, including all related electronics, mechanical stop switch, and manual swingaway mounting hardware Qp &   Y

DMEPOS Modifier(s): KE, NU, RR, UE

✳ **E2326**   Power wheelchair accessory, breath tube kit for sip and puff interface Qp &   Y

DMEPOS Modifier(s): KE, NU, RR, UE

✳ **E2327**   Power wheelchair accessory, head control interface, mechanical, proportional, including all related electronics, mechanical direction change switch, and fixed mounting hardware Qp &   Y

DMEPOS Modifier(s): KC, KE, NU, RR, UE

✳ **E2328**   Power wheelchair accessory, head control or extremity control interface, electronic, proportional, including all related electronics and fixed mounting hardware Qp &   Y

DMEPOS Modifier(s): KE, NU, RR, UE

✳ **E2329**   Power wheelchair accessory, head control interface, contact switch mechanism, nonproportional, including all related electronics, mechanical stop switch, mechanical direction change switch, head array, and fixed mounting hardware Qp &   Y

DMEPOS Modifier(s): KE, NU, RR, UE

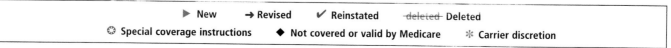

▶ New   → Revised   ✔ Reinstated   deleted Deleted

☼ Special coverage instructions   ◆ Not covered or valid by Medicare   ✳ Carrier discretion

✳ **E2330** Power wheelchair accessory, head control interface, proximity switch mechanism, nonproportional, including all related electronics, mechanical stop switch, mechanical direction change switch, head array, and fixed mounting hardware **Qp** ♿   Y

DMEPOS Modifier(s): KE, NU, RR, UE

✳ **E2331** Power wheelchair accessory, attendant control, proportional, including all related electronics and fixed mounting hardware **Qp**   Y

✳ **E2340** Power wheelchair accessory, nonstandard seat frame width, 20-23 inches **Qp** ♿   Y

DMEPOS Modifier(s): NU, RR, UE

✳ **E2341** Power wheelchair accessory, nonstandard seat frame width, 24-27 inches **Qp** ♿   Y

DMEPOS Modifier(s): NU, RR, UE

✳ **E2342** Power wheelchair accessory, nonstandard seat frame depth, 20 or 21 inches **Qp** ♿   Y

DMEPOS Modifier(s): NU, RR, UE

✳ **E2343** Power wheelchair accessory, nonstandard seat frame depth, 22-25 inches **Qp** ♿   Y

DMEPOS Modifier(s): NU, RR, UE

✳ **E2351** Power wheelchair accessory, electronic interface to operate speech generating device using power wheelchair control interface **Qp** ♿   Y

DMEPOS Modifier(s): KE, NU, RR, UE

▶ ✳ **E2358** Power wheelchair accessory, Group 34 non-sealed lead acid battery, each ♿   Y

▶ ✳ **E2359** Power wheelchair accessory, Group 34 sealed lead acid battery, each (e.g., gel cell, absorbed glassmat) ♿   Y

✳ **E2360** Power wheelchair accessory, 22 NF non-sealed lead acid battery, each ♿   Y

DMEPOS Modifier(s): KE, NU, RR, UE

✳ **E2361** Power wheelchair accessory, 22NF sealed lead acid battery, each, (e.g. gel cell, absorbed glassmat) **Qp** ♿   Y

DMEPOS Modifier(s): KE, NU, RR, UE

✳ **E2362** Power wheelchair accessory, group 24 non-sealed lead acid battery, each ♿   Y

DMEPOS Modifier(s): NU, RR, UE

✳ **E2363** Power wheelchair accessory, group 24 sealed lead acid battery, each (e.g. gel cell, absorbed glassmat) **Qp** ♿   Y

DMEPOS Modifier(s): KE, NU, RR, UE

✳ **E2364** Power wheelchair accessory, U-1 non-sealed lead acid battery, each ♿   Y

DMEPOS Modifier(s): NU, RR, UE

✳ **E2365** Power wheelchair accessory, U-1 sealed lead acid battery, each (e.g. gel cell, absorbed glassmat) **Qp** ♿   Y

DMEPOS Modifier(s): KE, NU, RR, UE

✳ **E2366** Power wheelchair accessory, battery charger, single mode, for use with only one battery type, sealed or non-sealed, each **Qp** ♿   Y

DMEPOS Modifier(s): KE, NU, RR, UE

✳ **E2367** Power wheelchair accessory, battery charger, dual mode, for use with either battery type, sealed or non-sealed, each **Qp** ♿   Y

DMEPOS Modifier(s): KE, NU, RR, UE

✳ **E2368** Power wheelchair component, motor, replacement only **Qp** ♿   Y

DMEPOS Modifier(s): KE, NU, RR, UE

✳ **E2369** Power wheelchair component, gear box, replacement only **Qp** ♿   Y

DMEPOS Modifier(s): KE, NU, RR, UE

✳ **E2370** Power wheelchair component, motor and gear box combination, replacement only **Qp** ♿   Y

DMEPOS Modifier(s): KE, NU, RR, UE

✳ **E2371** Power wheelchair accessory, group 27 sealed lead acid battery, (e.g. gel cell, absorbed glass mat), each **Qp** ♿   Y

DMEPOS Modifier(s): KE, NU, RR, UE

✳ **E2372** Power wheelchair accessory, group 27 non-sealed lead acid battery, each ♿   Y

DMEPOS Modifier(s): NU, RR, UE

✳ **E2373** Power wheelchair accessory, hand or chin control interface, compact remote joystick, proportional, including fixed mounting hardware ♿   Y

DMEPOS Modifier(s): KC, KE, NU, RR, UE

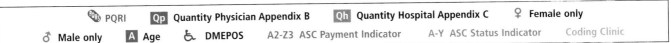

🅡 PQRI	**Qp** Quantity Physician Appendix B	**Qh** Quantity Hospital Appendix C	♀ Female only
♂ Male only	**A** Age ♿ DMEPOS	A2-Z3 ASC Payment Indicator A-Y ASC Status Indicator	Coding Clinic

⚙ **E2374** Power wheelchair accessory, hand or chin control interface, standard remote joystick (not including controller), proportional, including all related electronics and fixed mounting hardware, replacement only ♿   Y

DMEPOS Modifier(s): KE, NU, RR, UE

⚙ **E2375** Power wheelchair accessory, non-expandable controller, including all related electronics and mounting hardware, replacement only **Qp** ♿   Y

DMEPOS Modifier(s): KE, NU, RR, UE

⚙ **E2376** Power wheelchair accessory, expandable controller, including all related electronics and mounting hardware, replacement only ♿   Y

DMEPOS Modifier(s): KE, NU, RR, UE

⚙ **E2377** Power wheelchair accessory, expandable controller, including all related electronics and mounting hardware, upgrade provided at initial issue ♿   Y

DMEPOS Modifier(s): KE, NU, RR, UE

⚙ **E2381** Power wheelchair accessory, pneumatic drive wheel tire, any size, replacement only, each **Qp** ♿   Y

DMEPOS Modifier(s): KE, NU, RR, UE

⚙ **E2382** Power wheelchair accessory, tube for pneumatic drive wheel tire, any size, replacement only, each **Qp** ♿   Y

DMEPOS Modifier(s): KE, NU, RR, UE

⚙ **E2383** Power wheelchair accessory, insert for pneumatic drive wheel tire (removable), any type, any size, replacement only, each **Qp** ♿   Y

DMEPOS Modifier(s): KE, NU, RR, UE

⚙ **E2384** Power wheelchair accessory, pneumatic caster tire, any size, replacement only, each **Qp** ♿   Y

DMEPOS Modifier(s): KE, NU, RR, UE

⚙ **E2385** Power wheelchair accessory, tube for pneumatic caster tire, any size, replacement only, each **Qp** ♿   Y

DMEPOS Modifier(s): KE, NU, RR, UE

⚙ **E2386** Power wheelchair accessory, foam filled drive wheel tire, any size, replacement only, each ♿   Y

DMEPOS Modifier(s): KE, NU, RR, UE

⚙ **E2387** Power wheelchair accessory, foam filled caster tire, any size, replacement only, each **Qp** ♿   Y

DMEPOS Modifier(s): KE, NU, RR, UE

⚙ **E2388** Power wheelchair accessory, foam drive wheel tire, any size, replacement only, each ♿   Y

DMEPOS Modifier(s): KE, NU, RR, UE

⚙ **E2389** Power wheelchair accessory, foam caster tire, any size, replacement only, each **Qp** ♿   Y

DMEPOS Modifier(s): KE, NU, RR, UE

⚙ **E2390** Power wheelchair accessory, solid (rubber/plastic) drive wheel tire, any size, replacement only, each ♿   Y

DMEPOS Modifier(s): KE, NU, RR, UE

⚙ **E2391** Power wheelchair accessory, solid (rubber/plastic) caster tire (removable), any size, replacement only, each **Qp** ♿   Y

DMEPOS Modifier(s): KE, NU, RR, UE

⚙ **E2392** Power wheelchair accessory, solid (rubber/plastic) caster tire with integrated wheel, any size, replacement only, each **Qp** ♿   Y

DMEPOS Modifier(s): KE, NU, RR, UE

⚙ **E2394** Power wheelchair accessory, drive wheel excludes tire, any size, replacement only, each ♿   Y

DMEPOS Modifier(s): KE, NU, RR, UE

⚙ **E2395** Power wheelchair accessory, caster wheel excludes tire, any size, replacement only, each **Qp** ♿   Y

DMEPOS Modifier(s): KE, NU, RR, UE

⚙ **E2396** Power wheelchair accessory, caster fork, any size, replacement only, each **Qp** ♿   Y

DMEPOS Modifier(s): KE, NU, RR, UE

✳ **E2397** Power wheelchair accessory, lithium-based battery, each **Qp** **Qh** ♿   Y

DMEPOS Modifier(s): NU, RR, UE

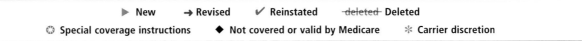

▶ New   → Revised   ✔ Reinstated   ~~deleted~~ Deleted

⚙ Special coverage instructions   ◆ Not covered or valid by Medicare   ✳ Carrier discretion

Negative Pressure

✻ **E2402** Negative pressure wound therapy electrical pump, stationary or portable Qp ♿ Y

Bill DME/MAC

Document at least every 30 calendar days the quantitative wound characteristics, including wound surface area (length, width and depth)

Medicare coverage up to a maximum of 15 dressing kits (A6550) per wound per month unless documentation states that the wound size requires more than one dressing kit for each dressing change.

DMEPOS Modifier(s): RR

Speech Device

E2500-E2599: Bill DME/MAC

✪ **E2500** Speech generating device, digitized speech, using pre-recorded messages, less than or equal to 8 minutes recording time Qp ♿ Y

IOM: 100-03, 1, 50.1

DMEPOS Modifier(s): NU, RR, UE

✪ **E2502** Speech generating device, digitized speech, using pre-recorded messages, greater than 8 minutes but less than or equal to 20 minutes recording time Qp ♿ Y

IOM: 100-03, 1, 50.1

DMEPOS Modifier(s): NU, RR, UE

✪ **E2504** Speech generating device, digitized speech, using pre-recorded messages, greater than 20 minutes but less than or equal to 40 minutes recording time Qp ♿ Y

IOM: 100-03, 1, 50.1

DMEPOS Modifier(s): NU, RR, UE

✪ **E2506** Speech generating device, digitized speech, using pre-recorded messages, greater than 40 minutes recording time Qp ♿ Y

IOM: 100-03, 1, 50.1

DMEPOS Modifier(s): NU, RR, UE

✪ **E2508** Speech generating device, synthesized speech, requiring message formulation by spelling and access by physical contact with the device Qp ♿ Y

IOM: 100-03, 1, 50.1

DMEPOS Modifier(s): NU, RR, UE

✪ **E2510** Speech generating device, synthesized speech, permitting multiple methods of message formulation and multiple methods of device access Qp ♿ Y

IOM: 100-03, 1, 50.1

DMEPOS Modifier(s): NU, RR, UE

✪ **E2511** Speech generating software program, for personal computer or personal digital assistant Qp ♿ Y

IOM: 100-03, 1, 50.1

DMEPOS Modifier(s): NU, RR, UE

✪ **E2512** Accessory for speech generating device, mounting system Qp ♿ Y

IOM: 100-03, 1, 50.1

DMEPOS Modifier(s): NU, RR, UE

✪ **E2599** Accessory for speech generating device, not otherwise classified Y

IOM: 100-03, 1, 50.1

Wheelchair, Cushion and Protection

E2601-E2621: Bill DME/MAC

✻ **E2601** General use wheelchair seat cushion, width less than 22 inches, any depth Qp ♿ Y

DMEPOS Modifier(s): NU, KE, RR, UE

✻ **E2602** General use wheelchair seat cushion, width 22 inches or greater, any depth Qp ♿ Y

DMEPOS Modifier(s): NU, KE, RR, UE

✻ **E2603** Skin protection wheelchair seat cushion, width less than 22 inches, any depth Qp ♿ Y

DMEPOS Modifier(s): NU, KE, RR, UE

✻ **E2604** Skin protection wheelchair seat cushion, width 22 inches or greater, any depth Qp ♿ Y

DMEPOS Modifier(s): NU, KE, RR, UE

✻ **E2605** Positioning wheelchair seat cushion, width less than 22 inches, any depth Qp ♿ Y

DMEPOS Modifier(s): NU, KE, RR, UE

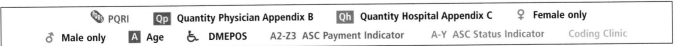

✳ **E2606** Positioning wheelchair seat cushion, width 22 inches or greater, any depth `Qp` ♿   Y

     DMEPOS Modifier(s): NU, KE, RR, UE

✳ **E2607** Skin protection and positioning wheelchair seat cushion, width less than 22 inches, any depth `Qp` ♿   Y

     DMEPOS Modifier(s): NU, KE, RR, UE

✳ **E2608** Skin protection and positioning wheelchair seat cushion, width 22 inches or greater, any depth `Qp` ♿   Y

     DMEPOS Modifier(s): NU, KE, RR, UE

✳ **E2609** Custom fabricated wheelchair seat cushion, any size `Qp` `Qh`   Y

✳ **E2610** Wheelchair seat cushion, powered   B

✳ **E2611** General use wheelchair back cushion, width less than 22 inches, any height, including any type mounting hardware `Qp` ♿   Y

     DMEPOS Modifier(s): NU, KE, RR, UE

✳ **E2612** General use wheelchair back cushion, width 22 inches or greater, any height, including any type mounting hardware `Qp` ♿   Y

     DMEPOS Modifier(s): NU, KE, RR, UE

✳ **E2613** Positioning wheelchair back cushion, posterior, width less than 22 inches, any height, including any type mounting hardware `Qp` ♿   Y

     DMEPOS Modifier(s): NU, KE, RR, UE

✳ **E2614** Positioning wheelchair back cushion, posterior, width 22 inches or greater, any height, including any type mounting hardware `Qp` ♿   Y

     DMEPOS Modifier(s): NU, KE, RR, UE

✳ **E2615** Positioning wheelchair back cushion, posterior-lateral, width less than 22 inches, any height, including any type mounting hardware `Qp` ♿   Y

     DMEPOS Modifier(s): NU, KE, RR, UE

✳ **E2616** Positioning wheelchair back cushion, posterior-lateral, width 22 inches or greater, any height, including any type mounting hardware `Qp` ♿   Y

     DMEPOS Modifier(s): NU, KE, RR, UE

✳ **E2617** Custom fabricated wheelchair back cushion, any size, including any type mounting hardware `Qp` `Qh`   Y

✳ **E2619** Replacement cover for wheelchair seat cushion or back cushion, each `Qp` ♿   Y

     DMEPOS Modifier(s): NU, KE, RR, UE

✳ **E2620** Positioning wheelchair back cushion, planar back with lateral supports, width less than 22 inches, any height, including any type mounting hardware `Qp` ♿   Y

     DMEPOS Modifier(s): NU, KE, RR, UE

✳ **E2621** Positioning wheelchair back cushion, planar back with lateral supports, width 22 inches or greater, any height, including any type mounting hardware `Qp` ♿   Y

     DMEPOS Modifier(s): NU, KE, RR, UE

SKIN PROTECTION, WHEELCHAIR (E2622-E2625)

▶ ✳ **E2622** Skin protection wheelchair seat cushion, adjustable, width less than 22 inches, any depth `Qp` `Qh` ♿   Y

     DMEPOS Modifier(s): NU, KE, RR, UE

▶ ✳ **E2623** Skin protection wheelchair seat cushion, adjustable, width 22 inches or greater, any depth `Qp` `Qh` ♿   Y

     DMEPOS Modifier(s): NU, KE, RR, UE

▶ ✳ **E2624** Skin protection and positioning wheelchair seat cushion, adjustable, width less than 22 inches, any depth `Qp` `Qh` ♿   Y

     DMEPOS Modifier(s): NU, KE, RR, UE

▶ ✳ **E2625** Skin protection and positioning wheelchair seat cushion, adjustable, width 22 inches or greater, any depth `Qp` `Qh` ♿   Y

     DMEPOS Modifier(s): NU, KE, RR, UE

▶ **New**   → **Revised**   ✔ **Reinstated**   ~~deleted~~ **Deleted**

✪ **Special coverage instructions**   ◆ **Not covered or valid by Medicare**   ✳ **Carrier discretion**

ARM SUPPORT
(E2626-E2633)

▶ ✳ **E2626** Wheelchair accessory, shoulder elbow, mobile arm support attached to wheelchair, balanced, adjustable   Y

▶ ✳ **E2627** Wheelchair accessory, shoulder elbow, mobile arm support attached to wheelchair, balanced, adjustable rancho type   Y

▶ ✳ **E2628** Wheelchair accessory, shoulder elbow, mobile arm support attached to wheelchair, balanced, reclining   Y

▶ ✳ **E2629** Wheelchair accessory, shoulder elbow, mobile arm support attached to wheelchair, balanced, friction arm support (friction dampening to proximal and distal joints)   Y

▶ ✳ **E2630** Wheelchair accessory, shoulder elbow, mobile arm support, monosuspension arm and hand support, overhead elbow forearm hand sling support, yoke type suspension support   Y

▶ ✳ **E2631** Wheelchair accessory, addition to mobile arm support, elevating proximal arm   Y

▶ ✳ **E2632** Wheelchair accessory, addition to mobile arm support, offset or lateral rocker arm with elastic balance control   Y

▶ ✳ **E2633** Wheelchair accessory, addition to mobile arm support, supinator   Y

Gait Trainer

E8000-E8002:   Bill DME/MAC

◆ **E8000** Gait trainer, pediatric size, posterior support, includes all accessories and components A   E

◆ **E8001** Gait trainer, pediatric size, upright support, includes all accessories and components A   E

◆ **E8002** Gait trainer, pediatric size, anterior support, includes all accessories and components A   E

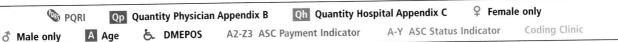

TEMPORARY PROCEDURES/PROFESSIONAL SERVICES (G0000-G9999)

NOTE: This section contains national codes assigned by CMS on a temporary basis to identify procedures/professional services.

Administration, Vaccine

G0008-G0010: Bill local carrier

✳ **G0008** Administration of influenza virus vaccine `Qp` `Qh`   S

Coinsurance and deductible do not apply. If provided, report significant, separately identifiable E/M for medically necessary services (V04.81)

✳ **G0009** Administration of pneumococcal vaccine `Qp` `Qh`   S

Reported once in a lifetime based on risk; Medicare covers cost of vaccine and administration (V03.82)

Copayment, coinsurance, and deductible waived. (https://www.cms. gov/MLNProducts/downloads/MPS_ QuickReferenceChart_1.pdf)

✳ **G0010** Administration of hepatitis B vaccine `Qp` `Qh`   S

Report for other than OPPs. Coinsurance and deductible apply; Medicare covers both cost of vaccine and administration (V05.3)

On or after January 1, 2011 the copayment/coinsurance and deductible are waived. (https://www.cms.gov/ MLNProducts/downloads/MPS_ QuickReferenceChart_1.pdf)

Semen Analysis

✳ **G0027** Semen analysis; presence and/or motility of sperm excluding Huhner `Qp` `Qh` ♂   A

Bill local carrier

Laboratory Certification: Hematology

Screening, Cervical

🄿 ☺ **G0101** Cervical or vaginal cancer screening; pelvic and clinical breast examination `Qp` `Qh` ♀   V

Bill local carrier

Covered once every two years and annually if high risk for cervical/vaginal cancer, or if childbearing age patient has had an abnormal Pap smear in preceding three years. High risk diagnosis, V15.89

Coding Clinic: 2002, Q4, P8

Screening, Prostate

G0102-G0103: Bill local carrier

☺ **G0102** Prostate cancer screening; digital rectal examination `Qp` `Qh` ♂   N

Covered annually by Medicare (V76.44). Not separately payable with an E/M code (99201-99499).

IOM: 100-02, 6, 10; 100-04, 4, 240
IOM: 100-04, 18, 50.1

☺ **G0103** Prostate cancer screening; prostate specific antigen test (PSA) `Qp` `Qh` ♂   Z3 A

Covered annually by Medicare (V76.44)

IOM: 100-02, 6, 10; 100-04, 4, 240
IOM: 100-04, 18, 50

Laboratory Certification: Routine chemistry

Screening, Colorectal

G0104-G0106: Bill local carrier

☺ **G0104** Colorectal cancer screening; flexible sigmoidoscopy `Qp` `Qh`   S

Covered once every 48 months for beneficiaries age 50+

Co-insurance waived under Section 4104.

Coding Clinic: 2011, Q2, P4

🄿 ☺ **G0105** Colorectal cancer screening; colonoscopy on individual at high risk `Qp` `Qh`   T

Screening colonoscopy covered once every 24 months for high risk for developing colorectal cancer. May use modifier 53 if appropriate (physician fee schedule)

Co-insurance waived under Section 4104.

Coding Clinic: 2011, Q2, P4

▶ New   → Revised   ✔ Reinstated   ~~deleted~~ Deleted

☺ Special coverage instructions   ◆ Not covered or valid by Medicare   ✳ Carrier discretion

🔵 ⊘ **G0106** Colorectal cancer screening; alternative to G0104, screening sigmoidoscopy, barium enema Qp Qh S

Barium enema (not high risk) (alternative to G0104). Covered once every 4 years for beneficiaries age 50+. Use modifier 26 for professional component only.

Coding Clinic: 2011, Q2, P4

Training Services, Diabetes

G0108-G0109: Bill local carrier

🔵 ✳ **G0108** Diabetes outpatient self-management training services, individual, per 30 minutes A

Report for beneficiaries diagnosed with diabetes

🔵 ✳ **G0109** Diabetes outpatient self-management training services, group session (2 or more) per 30 minutes A

Report for beneficiaries diagnosed with diabetes

Screening, Glaucoma

G0117-G0118: Bill local carrier

✳ **G0117** Glaucoma screening for high risk patients furnished by an optometrist or ophthalmologist Qp Qh S

Covered once per year (full 11 months between screenings). Bundled with all other ophthalmic services provided on same day. Diagnosis code V80.1

✳ **G0118** Glaucoma screening for high risk patient furnished under the direct supervision of an optometrist or ophthalmologist Qp Qh S

Covered once per year (full 11 months between screenings). Diagnosis code V80.1

Screening, Colorectal, Other

G0120-G0122: Bill local carrier

🔵 ⊘ **G0120** Colorectal cancer screening; alternative to G0105, screening colonoscopy, barium enema. Qp Qh S

Barium enema for patients with a high risk of developing colorectal. Covered once every 2 years. Used as an alternative to G0105. Use modifier 26 for professional component only

⊘ **G0121** Colorectal cancer screening; colonoscopy on individual not meeting criteria for high risk Qp Qh T

Screening colonoscopy for patients that are not high risk. Covered once every 10 years, but not within 48 months of a G0104. For non-Medicare patients report 45378.

Co-insurance waived under Section 4104.

◆ **G0122** Colorectal cancer screening; barium enema E

Medicare: this service is denied as noncovered, because it fails to meet the requirements of the benefit. The beneficiary is liable for payment.

Screening, Cytopathology

G0123-G0124: Bill local carrier

⊘ **G0123** Screening cytopathology, cervical or vaginal (any reporting system), collected in preservative fluid, automated thin layer preparation, screening by cytotechnologist under physician supervision Qp Qh ♀ A

Use G0123 or G0143 or G0144 or G0145 or G0147 or G0148 or P3000 for Pap smears NOT requiring physician interpretation (technical component)

IOM: 100-03, 3, 190.2; 100-04, 18, 30

Laboratory Certification: Cytology

⊘ **G0124** Screening cytopathology, cervical or vaginal (any reporting system), collected in preservative fluid, automated thin layer preparation, requiring interpretation by physician Qp Qh ♀ B

Report professional component for Pap smears requiring physician interpretation

IOM: 100-03, 3, 190.2; 100-04, 18, 30

Laboratory Certification: Cytology

Trimming, Nail

⊘ **G0127** Trimming of dystrophic nails, any number Qp Qh T

Bill local carrier

Must be used with a modifier (Q7, Q8, or Q9) to show that the foot care service is needed because the beneficiary has a systemic disease. Limit 1 unit of service

IOM: 100-02, 15, 290

🔵 PQRI	Qp **Quantity Physician Appendix B**	Qh **Quantity Hospital Appendix C**	♀ **Female only**
♂ **Male only** A **Age**	♿ **DMEPOS**	A2-Z3 **ASC Payment Indicator**	A-Y **ASC Status Indicator** Coding Clinic

Service, Nursing and OT

G0128-G0129: Bill local carrier

⊙ **G0128** Direct (face-to-face with patient) skilled nursing services of a registered nurse provided in a comprehensive outpatient rehabilitation facility, each 10 minutes beyond the first 5 minutes `Qp` `Qh`   B

A separate nursing service that is clearly identifiable in the Plan of Treatment and not part of other services. Documentation must support this service. Examples include: Insertion of a urinary catheter, intramuscular injections, bowel disimpaction, nursing assessment, and education. Restricted coverage by Medicare.

Medicare Statute 1833(a)

❋ **G0129** Occupational therapy services requiring the skills of a qualified occupational therapist, furnished as a component of a partial hospitalization treatment program, per session (45 minutes or more) `Qh`   P

Study, SEXA

⊙ **G0130** Single energy x-ray absorptiometry (SEXA) bone density study, one or more sites; appendicular skeleton (peripheral) (eg, radius, wrist, heel) `Qp` `Qh`   X

Bill local carrier

Covered every 24 months (more frequently if medically necessary). Use modifier 26 for professional component only

IOM: 100-03, 2, 150.3; 100-04, 13, 140.1

Screening, Cytopathology, Other

G0141-G0148: Bill local carrier

❋ **G0141** Screening cytopathology smears, cervical or vaginal, performed by automated system, with manual rescreening, requiring interpretation by physician `Qp` ♀   B

Co-insurance, copay, and deductible waived

Report professional component for Pap smears requiring physician interpretation. Refer to diagnosis of V15.89, V76.2, V76.47, or V76.49 to report appropriate risk level

Laboratory Certification: Cytology

❋ **G0143** Screening cytopathology, cervical or vaginal (any reporting system), collected in preservative fluid, automated thin layer preparation, with manual screening and rescreening by cytotechnologist under physician supervision `Qp` `Qh` ♀   A

Co-insurance, copay, and deductible waived

Laboratory Certification: Cytology

❋ **G0144** Screening cytopathology, cervical or vaginal (any reporting system), collected in preservative fluid, automated thin layer preparation, with screening by automated system, under physician supervision `Qp` `Qh` ♀   A

Co-insurance, copay, and deductible waived

Laboratory Certification: Cytology

❋ **G0145** Screening cytopathology, cervical or vaginal (any reporting system), collected in preservative fluid, automated thin layer preparation, with screening by automated system and manual rescreening under physician supervision `Qp` `Qh` ♀   A

Co-insurance, copay, and deductible waived

Laboratory Certification: Cytology

❋ **G0147** Screening cytopathology smears, cervical or vaginal; performed by automated system under physician supervision `Qp` `Qh` ♀   A

Co-insurance, copay, and deductible waived

Laboratory Certification: Cytology

❋ **G0148** Screening cytopathology smears, cervical or vaginal; performed by automated system with manual rescreening `Qp` `Qh` ♀   A

Co-insurance, copay, and deductible waived

Laboratory Certification: Cytology

Services, Allied Health

G0151-G0166: Bill local carrier

→ ❋ **G0151** Services performed by a qualified physical therapist in the home health or hospice setting, each 15 minutes   B

▶ New   → Revised   ✔ Reinstated   ~~deleted~~ Deleted
⊙ Special coverage instructions   ◆ Not covered or valid by Medicare   ❋ Carrier discretion

→ ✳ **G0152** Services performed by a qualified occupational therapist in the home health or hospice setting, each 15 minutes   B

→ ✳ **G0153** Services performed by a qualified speech-language pathologist in the home health or hospice setting, each 15 minutes   B

→ ✳ **G0154** Direct skilled nursing services of a licensed nurse (LPN or RN) in the home health or hospice setting, each 15 minutes   B

✳ **G0155** Services of clinical social worker in home health or hospice settings, each 15 minutes   B

✳ **G0156** Services of home health/health aide in home health or hospice settings, each 15 minutes   B

▶ ✳ **G0157** Services performed by a qualified physical therapist assistant in the home health or hospice setting, each 15 minutes   B

▶ ✳ **G0158** Services performed by a qualified occupational therapist assistant in the home health or hospice setting, each 15 minutes   B

▶ ✳ **G0159** Services performed by a qualified physical therapist, in the home health setting, in the establishment or delivery of a safe and effective physical therapy maintenance program, each 15 minutes   B

▶ ✳ **G0160** Services performed by a qualified occupational therapist, in the home health setting, in the establishment or delivery of a safe and effective occupational therapy maintenance program, each 15 minutes   B

▶ ✳ **G0161** Services performed by a qualified speech-language pathologist, in the home health setting, in the establishment or delivery of a safe and effective speech-language pathology maintenance program, each 15 minutes   B

▶ ✳ **G0162** Skilled services by a registered nurse (RN) for management and evaluation of the plan of care; each 15 minutes (the patient's underlying condition or complication requires an RN to ensure that essential non-skilled care achieves its purpose in the home health or hospice setting)   B

Transmittal No. 824 (CR7182)

▶ ✳ **G0163** Skilled services of a licensed nurse (LPN or RN) for the observation and assessment of the patient's condition, each 15 minutes (the of change in the patient's condition requires skilled nursing personnel to identify and evaluate the patient's need for possible modification of treatment in the home health or hospice setting)   B

Transmittal No. 824 (CR7182)

▶ ✳ **G0164** Skilled services of a licensed nurse (LPN or RN), in the training and/or education of a patient or family member, in the home health or hospice setting, each 15 minutes   B

Transmittal No. 824 (CR7182)

◎ **G0166** External counterpulsation, per treatment session Qp Qh   T

IOM: 100-03, 1, 20.20

Wound Closure

✳ **G0168** Wound closure utilizing tissue adhesive(s) only Qp Qh   B

Bill local carrier

Report for wound closure with only tissue adhesive. If a practitioner utilizes tissue adhesive in addition to staples or sutures to close a wound, HCPCS code G0168 is not separately reportable, but is included in the tissue repair.

The only closure material used for a simple repair, coverage based on payer.

Coding Clinic: 2005, Q1, P5; 2001, Q4, P12; Q3, P13

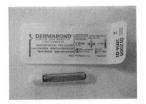

Figure 16 Tissue adhesive.

TEMPORARY PROCEDURES/PROFESSIONAL SERVICES   G0152 – G0168

Stereotactic Radiosurgery

⊙ **G0173** Linear accelerator based stereotactic radiosurgery, complete course of therapy in one session `Qp` `Qh` Z2 S

Bill local carrier

Do not bill with 77421

Team Conference

✳ **G0175** Scheduled interdisciplinary team conference (minimum of three exclusive of patient care nursing staff) with patient present `Qp` `Qh` V

Bill local carrier

Therapy, Activity

G0176-G0177: Bill local carrier

OPPS not separately payable

⊙ **G0176** Activity therapy, such as music, dance, art or play therapies not for recreation, related to the care and treatment of patient's disabling mental health problems, per session (45 minutes or more) `Qh` P

Paid in partial hospitalization

⊙ **G0177** Training and educational services related to the care and treatment of patient's disabling mental health problems per session (45 minutes or more) N

Paid in partial hospitalization

Physician Services

G0179-G0182: Bill local carrier

✳ **G0179** Physician re-certification for Medicare-covered home health services under a home health plan of care (patient not present), including contacts with home health agency and review of reports of patient status required by physicians to affirm the initial implementation of the plan of care that meets patient's needs, per re-certification period `Qp` M

The recertification code is used after a patient has received services for at least 60 days (or one certification period) when the physician signs the certification after the initial certification period.

✳ **G0180** Physician certification for Medicare-covered home health services under a home health plan of care (patient not present), including contacts with home health agency and review of reports of patient status required by physicians to affirm the initial implementation of the plan of care that meets patient's needs, per certification period `Qp` M

This code can be billed only when the patient has not received Medicare covered home health services for at least 60 days.

✳ **G0181** Physician supervision of a patient receiving Medicare-covered services provided by a participating home health agency (patient not present) requiring complex and multidisciplinary care modalities involving regular physician development and/or revision of care plans, review of subsequent reports of patient status, review of laboratory and other studies, communication (including telephone calls) with other health care professionals involved in the patient's care, integration of new information into the medical treatment plan and/or adjustment of medical therapy, within a calendar month, 30 minutes or more `Qp` M

✳ **G0182** Physician supervision of a patient under a Medicare-approved hospice (patient not present) requiring complex and multidisciplinary care modalities involving regular physician development and/or revision of care plans, review of subsequent reports of patient status, review of laboratory and other studies, communication (including telephone calls) with other health care professionals involved in the patient's care, integration of new information into the medical treatment plan and/or adjustment of medical therapy, within a calendar month, 30 minutes or more `Qp` M

Destruction

✳ **G0186** Destruction of localized lesion of choroid (for example, choroidal neovascularization); photocoagulation, feeder vessel technique (one or more sessions) `Qp` `Qh` T

Bill local carrier

▶ New   → Revised   ✔ Reinstated   ~~deleted~~ Deleted

⊙ Special coverage instructions   ◆ Not covered or valid by Medicare   ✳ Carrier discretion

Mammography

G0202-G0206: Bill local carrier

🅟🅠🅡🅢 ✳ **G0202** Screening mammography, producing direct digital image, bilateral, all views `Qp` `Qh` ♀   A

Screening mammogram reported based on technique, such as 76082, 76083, 76092, or G0202. Requires coinsurance, but no deductible. Diagnosis codes, V76.11 (high risk) or V76.12 (low risk). Use modifier 26 for professional component only

✳ **G0204** Diagnostic mammography, producing direct digital image, bilateral, all views `Qp` `Qh` ♀   A

Use modifier 26 for professional component only

✳ **G0206** Diagnostic mammography, producing direct digital image, unilateral, all views `Qp` `Qh` ♀   A

Use modifier 26 for professional component only

Coding Clinic: 2010, Q4, P5

Imaging, PET

G0219-G0235: Bill local carrier

◆ **G0219** PET imaging whole body; melanoma for non-covered indications   E

Example: Assessing regional lymph nodes in melanoma. Medicare non-covered.

IOM: 100-03, 4, 220.6

Coding Clinic: 2007, Q1, P6

◆ **G0235** PET imaging, any site, not otherwise specified   E

Example: Prostate cancer diagnosis and initial staging. Medicare non-covered.

IOM: 100-03, 4, 220.6

Coding Clinic: 2007, Q1, P6

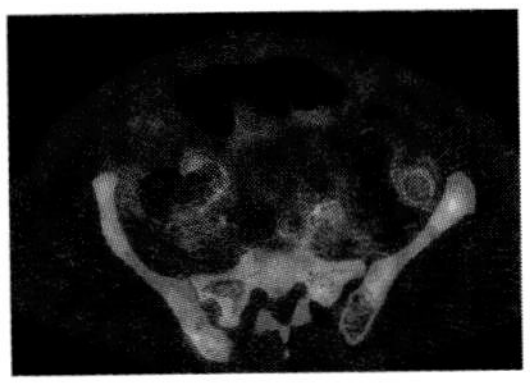

Figure 17   PET scan.

Therapeutic Procedures

G0237-G0239: Bill local carrier

✳ **G0237** Therapeutic procedures to increase strength or endurance of respiratory muscles, face to face, one on one, each 15 minutes (includes monitoring)   S

✳ **G0238** Therapeutic procedures to improve respiratory function, other than described by G0237, one on one, face to face, per 15 minutes (includes monitoring)   S

✳ **G0239** Therapeutic procedures to improve respiratory function or increase strength or endurance of respiratory muscles, two or more individuals (includes monitoring) `Qp` `Qh`   S

Physician Service, Diabetic

G0245-G0246: Bill local carrier

◎ **G0245** Initial physician evaluation and management of a diabetic patient with diabetic sensory neuropathy resulting in a loss of protective sensation (LOPS) which must include (1) the diagnosis of LOPS, (2) a patient history, (3) a physical examination that consist of at least the following elements: (A) visual inspection of the forefoot, hindfoot and toe web spaces, (B) evaluation of a protective sensation, (C) evaluation of foot structure and biomechanics, (D) evaluation of vascular status and skin integrity, and (E) evaluation and recommendation of footwear, and (4) patient education `Qp` `Qh`   V

Report one of the following diagnosis codes in conjunction with this code: 250.60, 250.61, 250.62, 250.63, or 357.2

IOM: 100-03, 1, 70.2.1

◎ **G0246** Follow-up physician evaluation and management of a diabetic patient with diabetic sensory neuropathy resulting in a loss of protective sensation (LOPS) to include at least the following: (1) a patient history, (2) a physical examination that includes: (A) visual inspection of the forefoot, hindfoot and toe web spaces, (B) evaluation of protective sensation, (C) evaluation of foot structure and biomechanics, (D) evaluation of vascular status and skin integrity, and (E) evaluation and recommendation of footwear, and (3) patient education `Qp` `Qh`   V

IOM: 100-03, 1, 70.2.1; 100-02, 15, 290

🅟🅠🅡🅢 PQRI	`Qp` Quantity Physician Appendix B	`Qh` Quantity Hospital Appendix C	♀ Female only
♂ Male only `A` Age ♿ DMEPOS	A2-Z3 ASC Payment Indicator	A-Y ASC Status Indicator	Coding Clinic

Foot Care

⊛ **G0247** Routine foot care by a physician of a diabetic patient with diabetic sensory neuropathy resulting in a loss of protective sensation (LOPS) to include, the local care of superficial wounds (i.e. superficial to muscle and fascia) and at least the following if present: (1) local care of superficial wounds, (2) debridement of corns and calluses, and (3) trimming and debridement of nails `Qp` `Qh`   T

Bill local carrier

IOM: 100-03, 1, 70.2.1

Demonstration, INR

G0248-G0250: Bill local carrier

⊛ **G0248** Demonstration, prior to initiation, of home INR monitoring for patient with either mechanical heart valve(s), chronic atrial fibrillation, or venous thromboembolism who meets Medicare coverage criteria, under the direction of a physician; includes: face-to-face demonstration of use and care of the INR monitor, obtaining at least one blood sample, provision of instructions for reporting home INR test results, and documentation of patient's ability to perform testing and report results `Qp` `Qh`   V

⊛ **G0249** Provision of test materials and equipment for home INR monitoring of patient with either mechanical heart valve(s), chronic atrial fibrillation, or venous thromboembolism who meets Medicare coverage criteria; includes provision of materials for use in the home and reporting of test results to physician; testing not occurring more frequently than once a week; testing materials, billing units of service include 4 tests `Qp` `Qh`   V

⊛ **G0250** Physician review, interpretation, and patient management of home INR testing for patient with either mechanical heart valve(s), chronic atrial fibrillation, or venous thromboembolism who meets Medicare coverage criteria; testing not occurring more frequently than once a week; billing units of service include 4 tests `Qp`   M

Stereotactic Radiosurgery

⊛ **G0251** Linear accelerator based stereotactic radiosurgery, delivery including collimator changes and custom plugging, fractionated treatment, all lesions, per session, maximum five sessions per course of treatment `Qp` `Qh`   Z2 S

Bill local carrier

Cannot bill with 77421. The indicator is "0" and the edit cannot be bypassed with a modifier. (https://www.cms.gov/NationalCorrectCodInitEd/NCCITrans/list.asp)

Imaging, PET

◆ **G0252** PET imaging, full and partial-ring PET scanners only, for initial diagnosis of breast cancer and/or surgical planning for breast cancer (e.g. initial staging of axillary lymph nodes)   E

Bill local carrier

IOM: 100-03, 4, 220.6

Coding Clinic: 2007, Q1, P6

SNCT

◆ **G0255** Current perception threshold/sensory nerve conduction test, (SNCT) per limb, any nerve   E

Bill local carrier

IOM: 100-03, 2, 160.23

Dialysis, Emergency

⊛ **G0257** Unscheduled or emergency dialysis treatment for an ESRD patient in a hospital outpatient department that is not certified as an ESRD facility `Qh`   S

Bill local carrier

Coding Clinic: 2003, Q1, P9

▶ New   → Revised   ✔ Reinstated   ~~deleted~~ Deleted
⊛ Special coverage instructions   ◆ Not covered or valid by Medicare   ✳ Carrier discretion

Injection, Arthrography

G0259-G0260: Bill local carrier

⚙ **G0259** Injection procedure for sacroiliac joint; arthrography [Qp] [Qh]   N

Replaces 27096 for reporting injections for Medicare beneficiaries

Used by Part A only (facility), not priced by Part B Medicare.

⚙ **G0260** Injection procedure for sacroiliac joint; provision of anesthetic, steroid and/or other therapeutic agent, with or without arthrography [Qp] [Qh]   T

ASCs report when a therapeutic sacroiliac joint injection is administered in ASC

Removal, Cerumen

✳ **G0268** Removal of impacted cerumen (one or both ears) by physician on same date of service as audiologic function testing [Qp] [Qh]   N

Bill local carrier

Report only when a physician, not an audiologist, performs the procedure.

Use with DX 380.4 when performed by physician.

Coding Clinic: 2003, Q1, P12

Placement, Occlusive Device

⚙ **G0269** Placement of occlusive device into either a venous or arterial access site, post surgical or interventional procedure (e.g. angioseal plug, vascular plug)   N

Bill local carrier

Report for replacement of vasoseal. Hospitals may report the closure device as a supply with C1760. Bundled status on Physician Fee Schedule.

Coding Clinic: 2010, Q4, P6

Therapy, Nutrition

G0270-G0271: Bill local carrier

⊕ ✳ **G0270** Medical nutrition therapy; reassessment and subsequent intervention(s) following second referral in same year for change in diagnosis, medical condition or treatment regimen (including additional hours needed for renal disease), individual, face to face with the patient, each 15 minutes   A

Requires physician referral for beneficiaries with diabetes or renal disease. Services must be provided by dietitian/nutritionist. Co-insurance and deductible waived.

⊕ ✳ **G0271** Medical nutrition therapy, reassessment and subsequent intervention(s) following second referral in same year for change in diagnosis, medical condition, or treatment regimen (including additional hours needed for renal disease), group (2 or more individuals), each 30 minutes   A

Requires physician referral for beneficiaries with diabetes or renal disease. Services must be provided by dietitian/nutritionist. Co-insurance and deductible waived.

Angiography

G0275-G0278: Bill local carrier

⊕ ✳ **G0275** Renal angiography, non-selective, one or both kidneys, performed at the same time as cardiac catheterization and/or coronary angiography, includes positioning or placement of any catheter in the abdominal aorta at or near the origins (OSTIA) of the renal arteries, injection of dye, flush aortogram, production of permanent images, and radiologic supervision and interpretation (list separately in addition to primary procedure) [Qp] [Qh]   N

Routine "drive-by angiography" at time of cardiac catheterization performed in the absence of accepted clinical indications that support medical necessity will be denied by Medicare

---

⊕ PQRI   [Qp] **Quantity Physician Appendix B**   [Qh] **Quantity Hospital Appendix C**   ♀ **Female only**
♂ **Male only**   [A] **Age**   & **DMEPOS**   A2-Z3 ASC Payment Indicator   A-Y ASC Status Indicator   Coding Clinic

(PQRS) * **G0278** Iliac and/or femoral artery angiography, non-selective, bilateral or ipsilateral to catheter insertion, performed at the same time as cardiac catheterization and/or coronary angiography, includes positioning or placement of the catheter in the distal aorta or ipsilateral femoral or iliac artery, injection of dye, production of permanent images, and radiologic supervision and interpretation (list separately in addition to primary procedure) **Qp** **Qh**   N

Medicare specific code not reported for iliac injection used as a guiding shot for a closure device

Coding Clinic: 2006, Q4, P7

Stimulation, Electrical

G0281-G0283:   Bill local carrier

* **G0281** Electrical stimulation, (unattended), to one or more areas, for chronic stage III and stage IV pressure ulcers, arterial ulcers, diabetic ulcers, and venous stasis ulcers not demonstrating measurable signs of healing after 30 days of conventional care, as part of a therapy plan of care **Qp** **Qh**   A

Reported by encounter/areas and not by site. Therapists report G0281 and G0283 rather than 97014

◆ **G0282** Electrical stimulation, (unattended), to one or more areas, for wound care other than described in G0281   E

IOM: 100-03, 4, 270.1

* **G0283** Electrical stimulation (unattended), to one or more areas for indication(s) other than wound care, as part of a therapy plan of care **Qp** **Qh**   A

Reported by encounter/areas and not by site. Therapists report G0281 and G0283 rather than 97014

Angiography, Arthroscopy

G0288-G0289:   Bill local carrier

* **G0288** Reconstruction, computed tomographic angiography of aorta for surgical planning for vascular surgery **Qp** **Qh**   N1   N

* **G0289** Arthroscopy, knee, surgical, for removal of loose body, foreign body, debridement/shaving of articular cartilage (chondroplasty) at the time of other surgical knee arthroscopy in a different compartment of the same knee **Qp** **Qh**   N

Add-on code reported with knee arthroscopy code for major procedure performed—reported once per extra compartment

"The code may be reported twice (or with a unit of two) if the physician performs these procedures in two compartments, in addition to the compartment where the main procedure was performed." (http://www.ama-assn.org/resources/doc/cpt/orthopaedics.pdf)

Placement, Transcatheter

G0290-G0291:   Bill local carrier

Includes angiography of same vessel.

☼ **G0290** Transcatheter placement of a drug eluting intracoronary stent(s), percutaneous, with or without other therapeutic intervention, any method; single vessel **Qp** **Qh**   T

Use site specific modifiers - LC, - LD, and - RC to designate artery. Part A claim.

Coding Clinic: 2007, Q1, P7; 2003, Q3, P11-12

☼ **G0291** Transcatheter placement of a drug eluting intracoronary stent(s), percutaneous, with or without other therapeutic intervention, any method; each additional vessel **Qp** **Qh**   T

Use site specific modifiers -LC, -LD, and -RC to designate artery. Part A claim.

Coding Clinic: 2003, Q3, P11-12

Procedure, Non-Covered

G0293-G0294:   Bill local carrier

☼ **G0293** Noncovered surgical procedure(s) using conscious sedation, regional, general or spinal anesthesia in a Medicare qualifying clinical trial, per day **Qp** **Qh**   X

☼ **G0294** Noncovered procedure(s) using either no anesthesia or local anesthesia only, in a Medicare qualifying clinical trial, per day **Qp** **Qh**   X

▶ New   → Revised   ✔ Reinstated   ~~deleted~~ Deleted

☼ Special coverage instructions   ◆ Not covered or valid by Medicare   * Carrier discretion

190

Therapy, Electromagnetic

◆ **G0295** Electromagnetic therapy, to one or more areas, for wound care other than described in G0329 or for other uses   E

Bill local carrier

IOM: 100-03, 4, 270.1

Services, Pulmonary Surgery

G0302-G0305:   Bill local carrier

✳ **G0302** Pre-operative pulmonary surgery services for preparation for LVRS, complete course of services, to include a minimum of 16 days of services **Qp** **Qh**   S

✳ **G0303** Pre-operative pulmonary surgery services for preparation for LVRS, 10 to 15 days of services **Qp** **Qh**   S

✳ **G0304** Pre-operative pulmonary surgery services for preparation for LVRS, 1 to 9 days of services **Qp** **Qh**   S

✳ **G0305** Post-discharge pulmonary surgery services after LVRS, minimum of 6 days of services **Qp** **Qh**   S

Laboratory

G0306-G0328:   Bill local carrier

→ ✳ **G0306** Complete CBC, automated (HgB, HCT, RBC, WBC, without platelet count) and automated WBC differential count **Qp** **Qh**   A

Laboratory Certification: Hematology

→ ✳ **G0307** Complete CBC, automated (HgB, HCT, RBC, WBC; without platelet count) **Qp** **Qh**   A

Laboratory Certification: Hematology

☉ **G0328** Colorectal cancer screening; fecal occult blood test, immunoassay, 1-3 simultaneous **Qp** **Qh**   A

Co-insurance and deductible waived

Reported for Medicare patients 50+; one FOBT per year, with either G0107 (guaiac-based) or G0328 (immunoassay-based)

Laboratory Certification: Routine Chemistry, Hematology

US machine

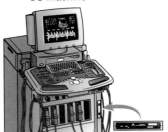

Electromagnetic device

Figure 18 Electromagnetic device.

Therapy, Electromagnetic

✳ **G0329** Electromagnetic therapy, to one or more areas for chronic stage III and stage IV pressure ulcers, arterial ulcers, and diabetic ulcers and venous stasis ulcers not demonstrating measurable signs of healing after 30 days of conventional care as part of a therapy plan of care **Qp** **Qh**   A

Bill local carrier

Fee, Pharmacy

☉ **G0333** Pharmacy dispensing fee for inhalation drug(s); initial 30-day supply as a beneficiary **Qp**   M

Bill DME/MAC

Medicare will reimburse an initial dispensing fee to a pharmacy for initial 30-day period of inhalation drugs furnished through DME

Hospice

✳ **G0337** Hospice evaluation and counseling services, pre-election **Qp** **Qh**   B

Bill local carrier

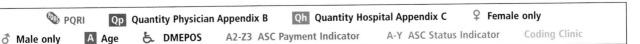

PQRI	**Qp** Quantity Physician Appendix B	**Qh** Quantity Hospital Appendix C	♀ Female only
♂ Male only **A** Age ♿ DMEPOS	A2-Z3 ASC Payment Indicator	A-Y ASC Status Indicator	Coding Clinic

Radiosurgery, Robotic

G0339-G0340: Bill local carrier

→ ✳ **G0339** Image-guided robotic linear accelerator-based stereotactic radiosurgery, complete course of therapy in one session or first session of fractionated treatment `Qp` `Qh` Z2 S

Do not report with 77421

→ ✳ **G0340** Image-guided robotic linear accelerator-based stereotactic radiosurgery, delivery including collimator changes and custom plugging, fractionated treatment, all lesions, per session, second through fifth sessions, maximum five sessions per course of treatment `Qp` `Qh` Z2 S

Do not report with 77421

Islet Cell

G0341-G0343: Bill local carrier

⊙ **G0341** Percutaneous islet cell transplant, includes portal vein catheterization and infusion `Qp` C

IOM: 100-03, 4, 260.3; 100-04, 32, 70

⊙ **G0342** Laparoscopy for islet cell transplant, includes portal vein catheterization and infusion `Qp` C

IOM: 100-03, 4, 260.3

⊙ **G0343** Laparotomy for islet cell transplant, includes portal vein catheterization and infusion `Qp` C

IOM: 100-03, 4, 260.3

Aspiration, Bone Marrow

✳ **G0364** Bone marrow aspiration performed with bone marrow biopsy through the same incision on the same date of service `Qp` `Qh` X

Bill local carrier

For Medicare patients, reported rather than 38220

Mapping, Vessel

G0365-G0372: Bill local carrier

✳ **G0365** Vessel mapping of vessels for hemodialysis access (services for preoperative vessel mapping prior to creation of hemodialysis access using an autogenous hemodialysis conduit, including arterial inflow and venous outflow) `Qp` `Qh` S

Includes evaluation of the relevant arterial and venous vessels. Use modifier 26 for professional component only

⊙ **G0372** Physician service required to establish and document the need for a power mobility device `Qp` M

Providers should bill the E/M code and G0372 on the same claim.

Services, Observation and ED

G0378-G0384: Bill local carrier

⊙ **G0378** Hospital observation service, per hour N

Report all related services in addition to G0378. Report units of hours spent in observation (rounded to the nearest hour). Hospitals report the ED or clinic visit with a CPT code or, if applicable, G0379 (direct admit to observation) and G0378 (hospital observation services, per hour)

Coding Clinic: 2007, Q1, P10; 2006, Q3, P7-8

⊙ **G0379** Direct admission of patient for hospital observation care `Qh` Q3

Report all related services in addition to G0379. Report units of hours spent in observation (rounded to the nearest hour). Hospitals report the ED or clinic visit with a CPT code or, if applicable, G0379 (direct admit to observation) and G0378 (hospital observation services, per hour)

Coding Clinic: 2007, Q1, P7

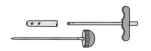

Figure 19 Bone aspiration needles.

| ▶ New | → Revised | ✔ Reinstated | ~~deleted~~ Deleted |
| ⊙ Special coverage instructions | ◆ Not covered or valid by Medicare | ✳ Carrier discretion |

✳ **G0380** Level 1 hospital emergency department visit provided in a type B emergency department; (the ED must meet at least one of the following requirements: (1) it is licensed by the state in which it is located under applicable state law as an emergency room or emergency department; (2) it is held out to the public (by name, posted signs, advertising, or other means) as a place that provides care for emergency medical conditions on an urgent basis without requiring a previously scheduled appointment; or (3) during the calendar year immediately preceding the calendar year in which a determination under 42 CFR 489.24 is being made, based on a representative sample of patient visits that occurred during that calendar year, it provides at least one-third of all of its outpatient visits for the treatment of emergency medical conditions on an urgent basis without requiring a previously scheduled appointment) **Qh** V

Coding Clinic: 2009, Q1, P4; 2007, Q2, P1

✳ **G0381** Level 2 hospital emergency department visit provided in a type B emergency department; (the ED must meet at least one of the following requirements: (1) it is licensed by the state in which it is located under applicable state law as an emergency room or emergency department; (2) it is held out to the public (by name, posted signs, advertising, or other means) as a place that provides care for emergency medical conditions on an urgent basis without requiring a previously scheduled appointment; or (3) during the calendar year immediately preceding the calendar year in which a determination under 42 CFR 489.24 is being made, based on a representative sample of patient visits that occurred during that calendar year, it provides at least one-third of all of its outpatient visits for the treatment of emergency medical conditions on an urgent basis without requiring a previously scheduled appointment) **Qh** V

Coding Clinic: 2009, Q1, P4; 2007, Q2, P1

✳ **G0382** Level 3 hospital emergency department visit provided in a type B emergency department; (the ED must meet at least one of the following requirements: (1) it is licensed by the state in which it is located under applicable state law as an emergency room or emergency department; (2) it is held out to the public (by name, posted signs, advertising, or other means) as a place that provides care for emergency medical conditions on an urgent basis without requiring a previously scheduled appointment; or (3) during the calendar year immediately preceding the calendar year in which a determination under 42 CFR 489.24 is being made, based on a representative sample of patient visits that occurred during that calendar year, it provides at least one-third of all of its outpatient visits for the treatment of emergency medical conditions on an urgent basis without requiring a previously scheduled appointment) **Qh** V

Coding Clinic: 2009, Q1, P4; 2007, Q2, P1

✳ **G0383** Level 4 hospital emergency department visit provided in a type B emergency department; (the ED must meet at least one of the following requirements: (1) it is licensed by the state in which it is located under applicable state law as an emergency room or emergency department; (2) it is held out to the public (by name, posted signs, advertising, or other means) as a place that provides care for emergency medical conditions on an urgent basis without requiring a previously scheduled appointment; or (3) during the calendar year immediately preceding the calendar year in which a determination under 42 CFR 489.24 is being made, based on a representative sample of patient visits that occurred during that calendar year, it provides at least one-third of all of its outpatient visits for the treatment of emergency medical conditions on an urgent basis without requiring a previously scheduled appointment) **Qh** V

Coding Clinic: 2009, Q1, P4; 2007, Q2, P1

(PQRS) PQRI	**Qp** Quantity Physician Appendix B	**Qh** Quantity Hospital Appendix C	♀ Female only	
♂ Male only	**A** Age	🦽 DMEPOS	A2-Z3 ASC Payment Indicator	A-Y ASC Status Indicator Coding Clinic

✻ **G0384** Level 5 hospital emergency department visit provided in a type B emergency department; (the ED must meet at least one of the following requirements: (1) it is licensed by the state in which it is located under applicable state law as an emergency room or emergency department; (2) it is held out to the public (by name, posted signs, advertising, or other means) as a place that provides care for emergency medical conditions on an urgent basis without requiring a previously scheduled appointment; or (3) during the calendar year immediately preceding the calendar year in which a determination under 42 CFR § 489.24 is being made, based on a representative sample of patient visits that occurred during that calendar year, it provides at least one-third of all of its outpatient visits for the treatment of emergency medical conditions on an urgent basis without requiring a previously scheduled appointment) `Qh`   Q3

Coding Clinic: 2009, Q1, P4; 2007, Q2, P1

Ultrasound, AAA

⊚ **G0389** Ultrasound B-scan and/or real time with image documentation; for abdominal aortic aneurysm (AAA) screening `Qp` `Qh`   S

Bill local carrier

Use modifier 26 for professional component only

Eligible beneficiaries must receive a referral for an AAA ultrasound screening as a result of an IPPE (initial preventative physical examination). This is a once in a lifetime benefit per eligible beneficiary. (http://www.cms.gov/MLNProducts/downloads/MPS_QuickReferenceChart_1.pdf)

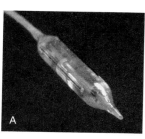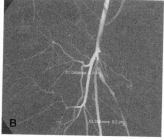

Figure 20 Angioplasty balloon.

Team, Trauma Response

⊚ **G0390** Trauma response team associated with hospital critical care service `Qh`   S

Bill local carrier

Coding Clinic: 2007, Q2, P5

Assessment/Intervention

G0396-G0397:   Bill local carrier

✻ **G0396** Alcohol and/or substance (other than tobacco) abuse structured assessment (e.g., AUDIT, DAST), and brief intervention 15 to 30 minutes `Qp` `Qh`   S

Bill instead of 99408 and 99409

✻ **G0397** Alcohol and/or substance (other than tobacco) abuse structured assessment (e.g., AUDIT, DAST), and intervention, greater than 30 minutes `Qp` `Qh`   S

Bill instead of 99408 and 99409

Home Sleep Study Test

✻ **G0398** Home sleep study test (HST) with type II portable monitor, unattended; minimum of 7 channels: EEG, EOG, EMG, ECG/heart rate, airflow, respiratory effort and oxygen saturation `Qp` `Qh`   S

Bill local carrier

✻ **G0399** Home sleep test (HST) with type III portable monitor, unattended; minimum of 4 channels: 2 respiratory movement/airflow, 1 ECG/heart rate and 1 oxygen saturation `Qp` `Qh`   S

✻ **G0400** Home sleep test (HST) with type IV portable monitor, unattended; minimum of 3 channels `Qp` `Qh`   S

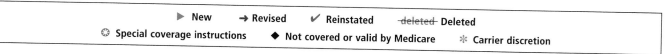

▶ New   → Revised   ✔ Reinstated   ~~deleted~~ Deleted
⊚ Special coverage instructions   ◆ Not covered or valid by Medicare   ✻ Carrier discretion

Examination, Initial Medicare

✳ **G0402**   Initial preventive physical examination; face-to-face visit, services limited to new beneficiary during the first 12 months of Medicare enrollment   V

Depending on circumstances, 99201-99215 may be assigned with modifier 25 to report an E/M service as a significant, separately identifiable service in addition to the Initial Preventive Physical Examination (IPPE), G0402.

Copayment and coinsurance waived, deductible waived after 01/01/11. (http://www.cms.gov/MLNProducts/downloads/MPS_QuickReferenceChart_1.pdf)

Coding Clinic: 2009, Q4, P8

Electrocardiogram

G0403-G0405:   Bill local carrier

✳ **G0403**   Electrocardiogram, routine ECG with 12 leads; performed as a screening for the initial preventive physical examination with interpretation and report   M

Optional service may be ordered or performed at discretion of physician. Once in a life-time screening, stemming from a referral from Initial Preventive Physical Examination (IPPE). Both deductible and co-payment apply.

✳ **G0404**   Electrocardiogram, routine ECG with 12 leads; tracing only, without interpretation and report, performed as a screening for the initial preventive physical examination   S

✳ **G0405**   Electrocardiogram, routine ECG with 12 leads; interpretation and report only, performed as a screening for the initial preventive physical examination   B

Telehealth

G0406-G0408:   Bill local carrier

→ ✳ **G0406**   Follow-up inpatient consultation, limited, physicians typically spend 15 minutes communicating with the patient via telehealth **Qp**   B

These telehealth modifers are required when billing for telehealth services with codes G0406-G0408 and G0425-G0427:
- GT, via interactive audio and video telecommunications system
- GQ, via asynchronous telecommunications system

→ ✳ **G0407**   Follow-up inpatient consultation, intermediate, physicians typically spend 25 minutes communicating with the patient via telehealth **Qp**   B

→ ✳ **G0408**   Follow-up inpatient consultation, complex, physicians typically spend 35 minutes communicating with the patient via telehealth **Qp**   B

Services, Social, Psychological

G0409-G0411:   Bill local carrier

✳ **G0409**   Social work and psychological services, directly relating to and/or furthering the patient's rehabilitation goals, each 15 minutes, face-to-face; individual (services provided by a CORF-qualified social worker or psychologist in a CORF)   M

✳ **G0410**   Group psychotherapy other than of a multiple-family group, in a partial hospitalization setting, approximately 45 to 50 minutes   P

Coding Clinic: 2009, Q4, P9, 10

✳ **G0411**   Interactive group psychotherapy, in a partial hospitalization setting, approximately 45 to 50 minutes   P

Coding Clinic: 2009, Q4, P9, 10

Treatment, Bone

G0412-G0415:   Bill local carrier

✳ **G0412**   Open treatment of iliac spine(s), tuberosity avulsion, or iliac wing fracture(s), unilateral or bilateral for pelvic bone fracture patterns which do not disrupt the pelvic ring includes internal fixation, when performed   C

* **G0413** Percutaneous skeletal fixation of posterior pelvic bone fracture and/or dislocation, for fracture patterns which disrupt the pelvic ring, unilateral or bilateral, (includes ilium, sacroiliac joint and/or sacrum)   T

* **G0414** Open treatment of anterior pelvic bone fracture and/or dislocation for fracture patterns which disrupt the pelvic ring, unilateral or bilateral, includes internal fixation when performed (includes pubic symphysis and/or superior/inferior rami)   C

* **G0415** Open treatment of posterior pelvic bone fracture and/or dislocation, for fracture patterns which disrupt the pelvic ring, unilateral or bilateral, includes internal fixation, when performed (includes ilium, sacroiliac joint and/or sacrum)   C

Pathology, Surgical

G0416-G0419: Bill local carrier

* **G0416** Surgical pathology, gross and microscopic examination for prostate needle saturation biopsy sampling, 1-20 specimens `Qp` `Qh` ♂   X

    This testing requires a facility to have either a CLIA certificate of registration (certificate type code 9), a CLIA certificate of compliance (certificate type code 1), or a CLIA certificate of accreditation (certificate type code 3). A facility without a valid, current, CLIA certificate, with a current CLIA certificate of waiver (certificate type code 2) or with a current CLIA certificate for provider-performed microscopy procedures (certificate type code 4), must not be permitted to be paid for these tests. This code has a -TC, -26 (physician), or gobal component.

    Laboratory Certification: Histopathology

* **G0417** Surgical pathology, gross and microscopic examination for prostate needle saturation biopsy sampling, 21-40 specimens `Qp` `Qh` ♂   S

    Laboratory Certification: Histopathology

* **G0418** Surgical pathology, gross and microscopic examination for prostate needle saturation biopsy sampling, 41-60 specimens `Qp` `Qh` ♂   S

    Use modifier 26 for professional component only

    Laboratory Certification: Histopathology

* **G0419** Surgical pathology, gross and microscopic examination for prostate needle saturation biopsy sampling, greater than 60 specimens `Qp` `Qh` ♂   S

    Use modifier 26 for professional component only

    Laboratory Certification: Histopathology

Educational Services, Rehabilitation, Telehealth, and Drug Screening

G0420-G0441: Bill local carrier

* **G0420** Face-to-face educational services related to the care of chronic kidney disease; individual, per session, per one hour   A

    CKD is kidney damage of 3 months or longer, regardless of the cause of kidney damage. Sessions billed in increments of one hour (if session is less than 1 hour, it must last at least 31 minutes to be billable. Sessions less than one hour and longer than 31 minutes is billable as one session. No more than 6 sessions of KDE services in a beneficiary's lifetime

* **G0421** Face-to-face educational services related to the care of chronic kidney disease; group, per session, per one hour   A

    Group setting: 2 to 20, report codes G0420 and G0421 with diagnosis code 585.4.

* **G0422** Intensive cardiac rehabilitation; with or without continuous ECG monitoring with exercise, per session   S

    Includes the same service as 93798 but at a greater frequency; may be reported with as many as six hourly sessions on a single date of service. Includes medical nutrition services to reduce cardiac disease risk factors.

▶ **New**   → **Revised**   ✔ **Reinstated**   ~~deleted~~ **Deleted**

⊙ **Special coverage instructions**   ◆ **Not covered or valid by Medicare**   * **Carrier discretion**

✳ **G0423** Intensive cardiac rehabilitation; with or without continuous ECG monitoring; without exercise, per session　S

Includes the same service as 93797 but at a greater frequency; may be reported with as many as six hourly sessions on a single date of service. Includes medical nutrition services to reduce cardiac disease risk factors.

✳ **G0424** Pulmonary rehabilitation, including exercise (includes monitoring), one hour, per session, up to two sessions per day　S

Includes therapeutic services and all related monitoring services to inprove respiratory function. Do not report with G0237, G0238, or G0239.

→ ✳ **G0425** Telehealth consultation, emergency department or initial inpatient, typically 30 minutes communicating with the patient via telehealth **Qp**　B

Problem Focused: Problem focused history and examination, with straightforward medical decision making complexity. Typically 30 minutes communicating with patient via telehealth

→ ✳ **G0426** Initial inpatient telehealth consultation, emergency department or initial inpatient, typically 50 minutes communicating with the patient via telehealth **Qp**　B

Detailed: Detailed history and examination, with moderate medical decision making complexity. Typically 50 minutes communicating with patient via telehealth

→ ✳ **G0427** Initial inpatient telehealth consultation, emergency department or initial inpatient, typically 70 minutes or more communicating with the patient via telehealth **Qp**　B

Comprehensive: Comprehensive history and examination, with high medical decision making complexity. Typically 70 minutes or more communicating with patient via telehealth.

▶ ◆ **G0428** Collagen meniscus implant procedure for filling meniscal defects (e.g., CMI, collagen scaffold, menaflex)　E

▶ ✳ **G0429** Dermal filler injection(s) for the treatment of facial lipodystrophy syndrome (LDS) (e.g., as a result of highly active antiretroviral therapy) **Qp Qh**　B

Designated for dermal fillers Sculptra® and Radiesse (Medicare). (https://www.cms.gov/ContractorLearningResources/downloads/JA6953.pdf)

Coding Clinic: 2010, Q3, P8

→ ✳ **G0431** Drug screen, qualitative; multiple drug classes by high complexity test method (e.g., immunoassay, enzyme assay), per patient encounter **Qp Qh**　A

http://www.cms.hhs.gov/mlnmattersarticles/downloads/se1001.pdf.

Laboratory Certification: Toxicology

→ ✳ **G0432** Infectious agent antibody detection by enzyme immunoassay (EIA) technique, HIV-1 and/or HIV-2, screening **Qp Qh**　A

Laboratory Certification: Virology, General immunology

Coding Clinic: 2010, Q2, P10

→ ✳ **G0433** Infectious agent antibody detection by enzyme-linked immunosorbent assay (ELISA) technique, HIV-1 and/or HIV-2, screening **Qp Qh**　A

Coding Clinic: 2010, Q2, P10

▶ ✳ **G0434** Drug screen, other than chromatographic; any number of drug classes, by CLIA waived test or moderate complexity test, per patient encounter **Qp Qh**　A

Laboratory Certification: Virology, General immunology

→ ✳ **G0435** Infectious agent antibody detection by rapid antibody test, HIV-1 and/or HIV-2, screening **Qp Qh**　A

Coding Clinic: 2010, Q2, P10

▶ ✳ **G0436** Smoking and tobacco cessation counseling visit for the asymptomatic patient; intermediate, greater than 3 minutes, up to 10 minutes **Qp Qh**　X

Coding Clinic: 2011, Q1, P5

▶ ✳ **G0437** Smoking and tobacco cessation counseling visit for the asymptomatic patient; intensive, greater than 10 minutes **Qp Qh**　X

Coding Clinic: 2011, Q1, P5

▶ ✳ **G0438** Annual wellness visit; includes a personalized prevention plan of service (PPS), initial visit Qp Qh A

▶ ✳ **G0439** Annual wellness visit, includes a personalized prevention plan of service (PPS), subsequent visit Qp Qh A

~~G0440~~ ~~Application of tissue cultured allogeneic skin substitute or dermal substitute; for use on lower limb, includes the site preparation and debridement if performed; first 25 sq cm or less~~ ✖

~~G0441~~ ~~Application of tissue cultured allogeneic skin substitute or dermal substitute; for use on lower limb, includes the site preparation and debridement if performed; each additional 25 sq cm~~ ✖

▶ ✳ **G0442** Annual alcohol misuse screening, 15 minutes

▶ ✳ **G0443** Brief face-to-face behavioral counseling for alcohol misuse, 15 minutes

▶ ✳ **G0444** Annual depression screening, 15 minutes

▶ ✳ **G0445** High intensity behavioral counseling to prevent sexually transmitted infection; face-to-face, individual, includes: education, skills training and guidance on how to change sexual behavior; performed semi-annually, 30 minutes

▶ ✳ **G0446** Intensive behavioral therapy to reduce cardiovascular disease risk, individual, face-to-face, bi-annual, 15 minutes

▶ ✳ **G0447** Face-to-face behavioral counseling for obesity, 15 minutes

▶ ✳ **G0448** Insertion or replacement of a permanent pacing cardioverter-defibrillator system with transvenous lead(s), single or dual chamber with insertion of pacing electrode, cardiac venous system, for left ventricular pacing B

▶ ✳ **G0449** Annual face-to-face obesity screening, 15 minutes

▶ ✳ **G0450** Screening for sexually transmitted infections, includes laboratory tests for chlamydia, gonorrhea, syphilis and hepatitis B

▶ ✳ **G0451** Development testing, with interpretation and report, per standardized instrument form S

▶ ✳ **G0908** Most recent hemoglobin (HGB) level >12.0 g/dl M

▶ ✳ **G0909** Hemoglobin level measurement not documented, reason not otherwise specified M

▶ ✳ **G0910** Most recent hemoglobin level <= 12.0 g/dl M

▶ ✳ **G0911** Assessed level of activity and symptoms M

▶ ✳ **G0912** Level of activity and symptoms not assessed M

▶ ✳ **G0913** Improvement in visual function achieved within 90 days following cataract surgery M

▶ ✳ **G0914** Patient care survey was not completed by patient M

▶ ✳ **G0915** Improvement in visual function not achieved within 90 days following cataract surgery M

▶ ✳ **G0916** Satisfaction with care achieved within 90 days following cataract surgery M

▶ ✳ **G0917** Patient satisfaction survey was not completed by patient M

▶ ✳ **G0918** Satisfaction with care not achieved within 90 days following cataract surgery M

▶ ✳ **G0919** Influenza immunization ordered or recommended (to be given at alternate location or alternate provider); vaccine not available at time of visit M

▶ ✳ **G0920** Type, anatomic location, and activity all documented M

▶ ✳ **G0921** Documentation of patient reason(s) for not being able to assess M

▶ ✳ **G0922** No documentation of disease type, anatomic location, and activity, reason not otherwise specified M

Tositumomab

✳ **G3001** Administration and supply of tositumomab, 450 mg S

Bill local carrier

The therapeutic regimen consists of a dosimetric step of tositumomab infusion followed 7–14 days later by a therapeutic step of iodine I-131 tositumomab infusion.

▶ New ➔ Revised ✔ Reinstated ~~deleted~~ Deleted
◎ Special coverage instructions ◆ Not covered or valid by Medicare ✳ Carrier discretion

Documentation

G8126-G9140: Bill local carrier

⊛ **G8126** Patient documented as being treated with antidepressant medication during the entire 12 week acute treatment phase   M

⊛ **G8127** Patient not documented as being treated with antidepressant medication during the entire 12 weeks acute treatment phase   M

⊛ **G8128** Clinician documented that patient was not an eligible candidate for antidepressant medication during the entire 12 week acute treatment phase measure   M

⊛ **G8395** Left ventricular ejection fraction (LVEF) > = 40% or documentation as normal or mildly depressed left ventricular systolic function   M

⊛ **G8396** Left ventricular ejection fraction (LVEF) not performed or documented   M

⊛ **G8397** Dilated macular or fundus exam performed, including documentation of the presence or absence of macular edema and level of severity of retinopathy   M

⊛ **G8398** Dilated macular or fundus exam not performed   M

⊛ **G8399** Patient with central dual-energy x-ray absorptiometry (DXA) results documented or ordered or pharmacologic therapy (other than minerals/vitamins) for osteoporosis prescribed)   M

⊛ **G8400** Patient with central dual-energy x-ray absorptiometry (DXA) results not documented or not ordered or pharmacologic therapy (other than minerals/vitamins) for osteoporosis not prescribed   M

⊛ **G8401** Clinician documented that patient was not an eligible candidate for screening or therapy for osteoporosis for women measure ♀   M

⊛ **G8404** Lower extremity neurological exam performed and documented   M

⊛ **G8405** Lower extremity neurological exam not performed   M

⊛ **G8406** Clinician documented that patient was not an eligible candidate for lower extremity neurological exam measure   M

⊛ **G8410** Footwear evaluation performed and documented   M

⊛ **G8415** Footwear evaluation was not performed   M

⊛ **G8416** Clinician documented that patient was not an eligible candidate for footwear evaluation measure   M

⊛ **G8417** Calculated BMI above the upper parameter and a follow-up plan was documented in the medical record   M

⊛ **G8418** Calculated BMI below the lower parameter and a follow-up plan was documented in the medical record   M

⊛ **G8419** Calculated BMI outside normal parameters, no follow-up plan was documented in the medical record   M

⊛ **G8420** Calculated BMI within normal parameters and documented   M

⊛ **G8421** BMI not calculated   M

⊛ **G8422** Patient not eligible for BMI calculation   M

→ ⊛ **G8427** List of current medications (includes prescription, over-the-counter, herbals, vitamin/mineral/dietary [nutritional] supplements) documented by the provider, including drug name, dosage, frequency and route   M

→ ⊛ **G8428** Current medications (includes prescription, over-the-counter, herbals, vitamin/mineral/dietary [nutritional] supplements) with drug name, dosage, frequency and route not documented by the provider, reason not specified   M

⊛ **G8430** Provider documentation that patient is not eligible for medication assessment   M

→ ⊛ **G8431** Positive screen for clinical depression using an age-appropriate standardized tool and a follow-up plan documented   M

→ ⊛ **G8432** No documentation of clinical depression screening using an age-appropriate standardized tool   M

→ ⊛ **G8433** Screening for clinical depression using an age-appropriate standardized tool not documented, patient not eligible/ appropriate   M

~~G8440~~ ~~Documentation of pain assessment (including location, intensity and description) prior to initiation of therapy or documentation of the absence of pain as a result of assessment through discussion with the patient including the use of a standardized tool and a follow-up plan is documented~~ ✖

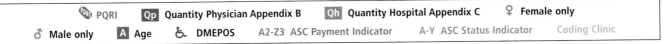

~~G8441~~ ~~No documentation of pain assessment (including location, intensity and description) prior to initiation of therapy~~ ✖

(PQRS) ✳ **G8442** Documentation that patient is not eligible for pain assessment   M

(PQRS) → ✳ **G8447** Patient encounter was documented using an EHR system that has been certified by an authorized testing and certification body (ATCB)   M

(PQRS) → ✳ **G8448** Patient encounter was documented using a PQRI qualified EHR or other acceptable systems   M

(PQRS) ✳ **G8450** Beta-blocker therapy prescribed for patients with left ventricular ejection fraction (LVEF) <40% or documentation as moderately or severely depressed left ventricular systolic function   M

(PQRS) ✳ **G8451** Clinician documented patient with left ventricular ejection fraction (LVEF) <40% or documentation as moderately or severely depressed left ventricular systolic function was not eligible candidate for beta-blocker therapy   M

(PQRS) ✳ **G8452** Beta-blocker therapy not prescribed for patients with left ventricular ejection fraction (LVEF) <40% or documentation as moderately or severely depressed left ventricular systolic function   M

(PQRS) ✳ **G8458** Clinician documented that patient is not an eligible candidate for genotype testing; patient not receiving antiviral treatment for hepatitis C   M

(PQRS) ✳ **G8459** Clinician documented that patient is receiving antiviral treatment for hepatitis C   M

(PQRS) ✳ **G8460** Clinician documented that patient is not an eligible candidate for quantitative RNA testing at week 12; patient not receiving antiviral treatment for hepatitis C   M

(PQRS) ✳ **G8461** Patient receiving antiviral treatment for hepatitis C   M

(PQRS) ✳ **G8462** Clinician documented that patient is not an eligible candidate for counseling regarding contraception prior to antiviral treatment; patient not receiving antiviral treatment for hepatitis C   M

(PQRS) ✳ **G8463** Patient receiving antiviral treatment for hepatitis C documented   M

(PQRS) ✳ **G8464** Clinician documented that prostate cancer patient is not an eligible candidate for adjuvant hormonal therapy; low or intermediate risk of recurrence or risk of recurrence not determined   M

(PQRS) ✳ **G8465** High risk of recurrence of prostate cancer ♂   M

(PQRS) ✳ **G8468** Angiotensin converting enzyme (ACE) inhibitor or angiotensin receptor blocker (ARB) therapy prescribed for patients with a left ventricular ejection fraction (LVEF) <40% or documentation of moderately or severely depressed left ventricular systolic function   M

(PQRS) ✳ **G8469** Clinician documented that patient with a left ventricular ejection fraction (LVEF) <40% or documentation of moderately or severely depressed left ventricular systolic function was not an eligible candidate for angiotensin converting enzyme (ACE) inhibitor or angiotensin receptor blocker (ARB) therapy   M

(PQRS) ✳ **G8470** Patient with left ventricular ejection fraction (LVEF) > =40% or documentation as normal or mildly depressed left ventricular systolic function   M

(PQRS) ✳ **G8471** Left ventricular ejection fraction (LVEF) was not performed or documented   M

(PQRS) ✳ **G8472** Angiotensin converting enzyme (ACE) inhibitor or angiotensin receptor blocker (ARB) therapy not prescribed for patients with a left ventricular ejection fraction (LVEF) <40% or documentation of moderately or severely depressed left ventricular systolic function, reason not specified   M

(PQRS) ✳ **G8473** Angiotensin converting enzyme (ACE) inhibitor or angiotensin receptor blocker (ARB) therapy prescribed   M

(PQRS) ✳ **G8474** Angiotensin converting enzyme (ACE) inhibitor or angiotensin receptor blocker (ARB) therapy not prescribed for reasons documented by the clinician   M

(PQRS) ✳ **G8475** Angiotensin converting enzyme (ACE) inhibitor or angiotensin receptor blocker (ARB) therapy not prescribed, reason not specified   M

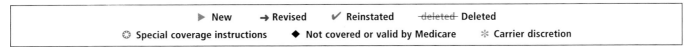

▶ New   → Revised   ✔ Reinstated   ~~deleted~~ Deleted
◎ Special coverage instructions   ◆ Not covered or valid by Medicare   ✳ Carrier discretion

(PQRI) * **G8476** Most recent blood pressure has a systolic measurement of <130 mm/Hg and a diastolic measurement of <80 mm/Hg — M

(PQRI) * **G8477** Most recent blood pressure has a systolic measurement of > =130 mm/Hg and/or a diastolic measurement of > =80 mm/Hg — M

(PQRI) * **G8478** Blood pressure measurement not performed or documented, reason not specified — M

(PQRI) → * **G8482** Influenza immunization administered or previously received — M

(PQRI) * **G8483** Influenza immunization was not ordered or administered for reasons documented by clinician — M

(PQRI) * **G8484** Influenza immunization was not ordered or administered, reason not specified — M

* **G8485** I intend to report the diabetes mellitus measures group — M

* **G8486** I intend to report the preventive care measures group — M

* **G8487** I intend to report the chronic kidney disease (CKD) measures group — M

* **G8489** I intend to report the Coronary Artery Disease (CAD) measures group — M

* **G8490** I intend to report the Rheumatoid Arthritis measures group — M

* **G8491** I intend to report the HIV/AIDS measures group — M

* **G8492** I intend to report the Perioperative Care measures group — M

* **G8493** I intend to report the Back Pain measures group — M

* **G8494** All quality actions for the applicable measures in the Diabetes Mellitus measures group have been performed for this patient — M
Composite code, do not report with G8485

* **G8495** All quality actions for the applicable measures in the CKD measures group have been performed for this patient — M
Composite code, do not report with G8487

* **G8496** All quality actions for the applicable measures in the Preventive Care measures group have been performed for this patient — M
Composite code, do not report with G8486

* **G8497** All quality actions for the applicable measures in the Coronary Artery Bypass Graft (CABG) measures group have been performed for this patient — M
Composite code.

* **G8498** All quality actions for the applicable measures in the Coronary Artery Disease (CAD) measures group have been performed for this patient — M
Composite code.

* **G8499** All quality actions for the applicable measures in the Rheumatoid Arthritis measures group have been performed for this patient — M
Composite code, do not report with G8490

* **G8500** All quality actions for the applicable measures in the HIV/AIDS measures group have been performed for this patient — M
Composite code.

* **G8501** All quality actions for the applicable measures in the Perioperative Care measures group have been performed for this patient — M
Composite code, do not report with G8492

* **G8502** All quality actions for the applicable measures in the Back Pain measures group have been performed for this patient — M
Composite code, do not report with G8493

(PQRI) * **G8506** Patient receiving angiotensin converting enzyme (ACE) inhibitor or angiotensin receptor blocker (ARB) therapy — M

~~**G8508** Documentation of pain assessment (including location, intensity and description) prior to initiation of therapy or documentation of the absence of pain as a result of assessment through discussion with the patient including the use of a standardized tool; no documentation of a follow up plan, patient not eligible~~ ✖

(PQRI) → * **G8509** Documentation of positive pain assessment; no documentation of a follow-up plan, reason not specified — M

(PQRI) → * **G8510** Negative screen for clinical depression using an age-appropriate standardized tool, follow-up not required — M

→ * **G8511** Positive screen for clinical depression using an age-appropriate standardized tool documented, follow up plan not documented, reason not specified   M

* **G8524** Patch closure used for patient undergoing conventional CEA   M

* **G8525** Clinician documented that patient did not receive conventional CEA   M

* **G8526** Patch closure not used for patient undergoing conventional CEA, reason not specified   M

* **G8530** Autogenous AV fistula received   M

* **G8531** Clinician documented that patient was not an eligible candidate for autogenous AV fistula   M

* **G8532** Clinician documented that patient received vascular access other than autogenous AV fistula, reason not specified   M

~~G8534   Documentation of an elder maltreatment screen and follow-up plan~~   ✖

* **G8535** No documentation of an elder maltreatment screen, patient not eligible ▪A   M

* **G8536** No documentation of an elder maltreatment screen, reason not specified ▪A   M

~~G8537   Elder maltreatment screen documented, follow up plan not documented, patient not eligible~~   ✖

~~G8538   Elder maltreatment screen documented, follow up plan not documented, reason not specified~~   ✖

→ * **G8539** Documentation of a current functional outcome assessment using a standardized tool and documentation of a care plan based on identified deficiencies   M

* **G8540** Documentation that the patient is not eligible for a functional outcome assessment using a standardized tool   M

* **G8541** No documentation of a current functional outcome assessment using a standardized tool, reason not specified   M

→ * **G8542** Documentation of a current functional outcome assessment using a standardized tool; no functional deficiencies identified, care plan not required   M

* **G8543** Documentation of a current functional outcome assessment using a standardized tool; no documentation of a care plan, reason not specified   M

* **G8544** I intend to report the coronary artery bypass graft (CABG) measures group   M

* **G8545** I intend to report the Hepatitis C measures group   M

* **G8546** I intend to report the Community-Acquired Pneumonia (CAP) measures group   M

* **G8547** I intend to report the Ischemic Vascular Disease (IVD) measures group   M

* **G8548** I intend to report the Heart Failure (HF) measures group   M

* **G8549** All quality actions for the applicable measures in the Hepatitis C measures group have been performed for this patient   M

Composite code, do not report with G8545

* **G8550** All quality actions for the applicable measures in the Community-Acquired Pneumonia (CAP) measures group have been performed for this patient   M

Composite code, do not report with G8546

* **G8551** All quality actions for the applicable measures in the Heart Failure (HF) measures group have been performed for this patient   M

Composite code.

* **G8552** All quality actions for the applicable measures in the Ischemic Vascular Disease (IVD) measures group have been performed for this patient   M

Composite code, do not report with G8547

→ * **G8553** Prescription generated and transmitted via a qualified ERX system or a certified EHR system   M

* **G8556** Referred to a physician (preferably a physician with training in disorders of the ear) for an otologic evaluation   M

* **G8557** Patient is not eligible for the referral for otologic evaluation measure   M

* **G8558** Not referred to a physician (preferably a physician with training in disorders of the ear) for an otologic evaluation, reason not specified   M

* **G8559** Patient referred to a physician (preferably a physician with training in disorders of the ear) for an otologic evaluation   M

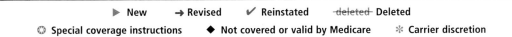

▶ New   → Revised   ✔ Reinstated   ~~deleted~~ Deleted
✪ Special coverage instructions   ◆ Not covered or valid by Medicare   * Carrier discretion

(PQRS)	* **G8560**	Patient has a history of active drainage from the ear within the previous 90 days	M
(PQRS)	* **G8561**	Patient is not eligible for the referral for otologic evaluation for patients with a history of active drainage measure	M
(PQRS)	* **G8562**	Patient does not have a history of active drainage from the ear within the previous 90 days	M
(PQRS)	* **G8563**	Patient not referred to a physician (preferably a physician with training in disorders of the ear) for an otologic evaluation, reason not specified	M
(PQRS)	* **G8564**	Patient was referred to a physician (preferably a physician with training in disorders of the ear) for an otologic evaluation, reason not specified)	M
(PQRS)	* **G8565**	Verification and documentation of sudden or rapidly progressive hearing loss	M
(PQRS)	* **G8566**	Patient is not eligible for the "referral for otologic evaluation for sudden or rapidly progressive hearing loss" measure	M
(PQRS)	* **G8567**	Patient does not have verification and documentation of sudden or rapidly progressive hearing loss	M
(PQRS)	* **G8568**	Patient was not referred to a physician (preferably a physician with training in disorders of the ear) for an otologic evaluation, reason not specified	M
	* **G8569**	Prolonged intubation (>24 hrs) required	M
	* **G8570**	Prolonged intubation (>24 hrs) not required	M
(PQRS)	* **G8571**	Development of deep sternal wound infection within 30 days postoperatively	M
(PQRS)	* **G8572**	No deep sternal wound infection	M
(PQRS)	→ * **G8573**	Stroke following isolated CABG surgery	M
(PQRS)	→ * **G8574**	No stroke following isolated CABG surgery	M
(PQRS)	→ * **G8575**	Developed postoperative renal failure or required dialysis	M
(PQRS)	→ * **G8576**	No postoperative renal failure/ dialysis not required	M
(PQRS)	→ * **G8577**	Reexploration required due to mediastinal bleeding with or without tamponade, graft occlusion, valve disfunction, or other cardiac reason	M

(PQRS)	→ * **G8578**	Reexploration not required due to mediastinal bleeding with or without tamponade, graft occlusion, valve dysfunction, or other cardiac reason	M
(PQRS)	* **G8579**	Antiplatelet medication at discharge	M
(PQRS)	→ * **G8580**	Antiplatelet medication contraindicated	M
(PQRS)	* **G8581**	No antiplatelet medication at discharge	M
(PQRS)	* **G8582**	Beta-blocker at discharge	M
(PQRS)	→ * **G8583**	Beta-blocker contraindicated	M
(PQRS)	* **G8584**	No beta-blocker at discharge	M
(PQRS)	* **G8585**	Anti-lipid treatment at discharge	M
(PQRS)	→ * **G8586**	Anti-lipid treatment contraindicated	M
(PQRS)	* **G8587**	No anti-lipid treatment at discharge	M
(PQRS)	* **G8588**	Most recent systolic blood pressure < 140 mmhg	M
(PQRS)	* **G8589**	Most recent systolic blood pressure >= 140 mmhg	M
(PQRS)	* **G8590**	Most recent diastolic blood pressure < 90 mmhg	M
(PQRS)	* **G8591**	Most recent diastolic blood pressure >= 90 mmhg	M
(PQRS)	* **G8592**	No documentation of blood pressure measurement	M
(PQRS)	* **G8593**	Lipid profile results documented and reviewed (must include total cholesterol, HDL-C, triglycerides and calculated LDL-C)	M
(PQRS)	* **G8594**	Lipid profile not performed, reason not otherwise specified	M
(PQRS)	* **G8595**	Most recent LDL-C < 100 mg/dl	M
(PQRS)	* **G8596**	LDL-C was not performed	M
(PQRS)	* **G8597**	Most recent LDL-C >= 100 mg/dl	M
(PQRS)	* **G8598**	Aspirin or another antithrombotic therapy used	M
(PQRS)	* **G8599**	Aspirin or another antithrombotic therapy not used, reason not otherwise specified	M
(PQRS)	* **G8600**	IV T-PA initiated within three hours (<= 180 minutes) of time last known well	M
(PQRS)	* **G8601**	IV T-PA not initiated within three hours (<= 180 minutes) of time last known well for reasons documented by clinician	M

Ⓟ   ✳ **G8602**   IV T-PA not initiated within three hours (<= 180 minutes) of time last known well, reason not specified   M

Ⓟ   ✳ **G8603**   Score on the spoken language comprehension functional communication measure at discharge was higher than at admission   M

Ⓟ   ✳ **G8604**   Score on the spoken language comprehension functional communication measure at discharge was not higher than at admission, reason not specified   M

Ⓟ → ✳ **G8605**   Patient treated for spoken langue comprehension but not scored on the spoken language comprehension functional communication measure either at admission or at discharge   M

Ⓟ   ✳ **G8606**   Score on the attention functional communication measure at discharge was higher than at admission   M

Ⓟ   ✳ **G8607**   Score on the attention functional communication measure at discharge was not higher than at admission, reason not specified   M

Ⓟ → ✳ **G8608**   Patient treated for attention but not scored on the attention functional communication measure either at admission or at discharge   M

Ⓟ   ✳ **G8609**   Score on the memory functional communication measure at discharge was higher than at admission   M

Ⓟ   ✳ **G8610**   Score on the memory functional communication measure at discharge was not higher than at admission, reason not specified   M

Ⓟ → ✳ **G8611**   Patient treated for memory but not scored on the memory functional communication measure either at admission or at discharge   M

Ⓟ   ✳ **G8612**   Score on the motor speech functional communication measure at discharge was higher than at admission   M

Ⓟ   ✳ **G8613**   Score on the motor speech functional communication measure at discharge was not higher than at admission, reason not specified   M

Ⓟ → ✳ **G8614**   Patient treated for motor speech but not scored on the motor speech comprehension functional communication measure either at admission or at discharge   M

Ⓟ   ✳ **G8615**   Score on the reading functional communication measure at discharge was higher than at admission   M

Ⓟ   ✳ **G8616**   Score on the reading functional communication measure at discharge was not higher than at admission, reason not specified   M

Ⓟ → ✳ **G8617**   Patient treated for reading but not scored on the reading functional communication measure either at admission or at discharge   M

Ⓟ   ✳ **G8618**   Score on the spoken language expression functional communication measure at discharge was higher than at admission   M

Ⓟ   ✳ **G8619**   Score on the spoken language expression functional communication measure at discharge was not higher than at admission, reason not specified   M

Ⓟ → ✳ **G8620**   Patient treated for spoken language expression but not scored on the spoken language expression functional communication measure either at admission or at discharge   M

Ⓟ   ✳ **G8621**   Score on the writing functional communication measure at discharge was higher than at admission   M

Ⓟ   ✳ **G8622**   Score on the writing functional communication measure at discharge was not higher than at admission, reason not specified   M

Ⓟ → ✳ **G8623**   Patient treated for writing but not scored on the writing functional communication measure either at admission or at discharge   M

Ⓟ   ✳ **G8624**   Score on the swallowing functional communication measure at discharge was higher than at admission   M

Ⓟ   ✳ **G8625**   Score on the swallowing functional communication measure at discharge was not higher than at admission, reason not specified   M

Ⓟ → ✳ **G8626**   Patient treated for swallowing but not scored on the swallowing functional communication measure at admission or at discharge   M

Ⓟ   ✳ **G8627**   Surgical procedure performed within 30 days following cataract surgery for major complications (e.g. retained nuclear fragments, endophthalmitis, dislocated or wrong power IOL, retinal detachment, or wound dehiscence)   M

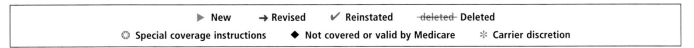

▶ New   → Revised   ✔ Reinstated   ~~deleted~~ Deleted

⊙ Special coverage instructions   ◆ Not covered or valid by Medicare   ✳ Carrier discretion

G8602 – G8627   TEMPORARY PROCEDURES/PROFESSIONAL SERVICES

G8628 Surgical procedure not performed within 30 days following cataract surgery for major complications (e.g. retained nuclear fragments, endophthalmitis, dislocated or wrong power IOL, retinal detachment, or wound dehiscence) M

G8629 Documentation of order for prophylactic parenteral antibiotic to be given within one hour (if fluoroquinolone or vancomycin, two hours) prior to surgical incision (or start of procedure when no incision is required) M

G8630 Documentation that administration of prophylactic parenteral antibiotics was initiated within one hour (if fluoroquinolone or vancomycin, two hours) prior to surgical incision (or start of procedure when no incision is required), as ordered M

G8631 Clinician documented that patient was not an eligible candidate for ordering prophylactic parenteral antibiotics to be given within one hour (if fluoroquinolone or vancomycin, two hours) prior to surgical incision (or start of procedure when no incision is required) M

G8632 Prophylactic parenteral antibiotics were not ordered to be given or given within one hour (if fluoroquinolone or vancomycin, two hours) prior to the surgical incision (or start of procedure when no incision is required), reason not otherwise specified) M

G8633 Pharmacologic therapy (other than minierals/vitamins) for osteoporosis prescribed M

G8634 Clinician documented patient not an eligible candidate to receive pharmacologic therapy for osteoporosis M

G8635 Pharmacologic therapy for osteoporosis was not prescribed, reason not otherwise specified M

G8636 Influenza immunization administered or previously received ✖

G8637 Clinician documented that patient is not eligible to receive the influenza immunization ✖

G8638 Influenza immunization not administered or previously received, reason not otherwise specified ✖

G8639 Influenza immunization was administered or previously received ✖

G8640 Clinician has documented that patient is not eligible to receive the influenza immunization ✖

G8641 Influenza immunization was not administered or previously received, reason not otherwise specified ✖

G8642 The eligible professional practices in a rural area without sufficient high speed internet access and requests a hardship exemption from the application of the payment adjustment under Section 1848(a)(5)(a) of the Social Security Act M

G8643 The eligible professional practices in an area without sufficient available pharmacies for electronic prescribing and requests a hardship exemption for the application of the payment adjustment under Section 1848(a)(5)(a) of the Social Security Act M

G8644 Eligible professional does not have prescribing privileges M

G8645 I intend to report the asthma measures group M

G8646 All quality actions for the applicable measures in the asthma measures group have been performed for this patient M

G8647 Risk-adjusted functional status change residual score for the knee successfully calculated and the score was equal to zero (0) or greater than zero (>0) M

G8648 Risk-adjusted functional status change residual score for the knee successfully calculated and the score was less than zero (<0) M

G8649 Risk-adjusted functional status change residual scores for the knee not measured because the patient did not complete FOTO'S functional intake on admission and/or follow up status survey near discharge, patient not eligible/not appropriate M

G8650 Risk-adjusted functional status change residual scores for the knee not measured because the patient did not complete FOTO'S functional intake on admission and/or follow up status survey near discharge, reason not specified M

G8651 Risk-adjusted functional status change residual score for the hip successfully calculated and the score was equal to zero (0) or greater than zero (>0) M

PQRI | Qp Quantity Physician Appendix B | Qh Quantity Hospital Appendix C | ♀ Female only
♂ Male only | A Age | DMEPOS | A2-Z3 ASC Payment Indicator | A-Y ASC Status Indicator | Coding Clinic

(PQRS) ▶ ✳ **G8652**   Risk-adjusted functional status change residual score for the hip successfully calculated and the score was less than zero (<0)   M

(PQRS) ▶ ✳ **G8653**   Risk-adjusted functional status change residual scores for the hip not measured because the patient did not complete FOTO'S functional intake on admission and/or follow up status survey near discharge, patient not eligible/not appropriate   M

(PQRS) ▶ ✳ **G8654**   Risk-adjusted functional status change residual scores for the hip not measured because the patient did not complete FOTO'S functional intake on admission and/or follow up status survey near discharge, reason not specified   M

(PQRS) ▶ ✳ **G8655**   Risk-adjusted functional status change residual score for the lower leg, foot or ankle successfully calculated and the score was equal to zero (0) or greater than zero (>0)   M

(PQRS) ▶ ✳ **G8656**   Risk-adjusted functional status change residual score for the lower leg, foot or ankle successfully calculated and the score was less than zero (<0)   M

(PQRS) ▶ ✳ **G8657**   Risk-adjusted functional status change residual scores for the lower leg, foot or ankle not measured because the patient did not complete FOTO'S functional intake on admission and/or follow up status survey near discharge, patient not eligible/not appropriate   M

(PQRS) ▶ ✳ **G8658**   Risk-adjusted functional status change residual scores for the lower leg, foot or ankle not measured because the patient did not complete FOTO'S functional intake on admission and/or follow up status survey near discharge, reason not specified   M

(PQRS) ▶ ✳ **G8659**   Risk-adjusted functional status change residual score for the lumbar spine successfully calculated and the score was equal to zero (0) or greater than zero (>0)   M

(PQRS) ▶ ✳ **G8660**   Risk-adjusted functional status change residual score for the lumbar spine successfully calculated and the score was less than zero (<0)   M

(PQRS) ▶ ✳ **G8661**   Risk-adjusted functional status change residual scores for the lumbar spine not measured because the patient did not complete FOTO'S functional intake on admission and/or follow up status survey near discharge, patient not eligible/not appropriate   M

(PQRS) ▶ ✳ **G8662**   Risk-adjusted functional status change residual scores for the lumbar spine not measured because the patient did not complete FOTO'S functional intake on admission and/or follow up status survey near discharge, reason not specified   M

(PQRS) ▶ ✳ **G8663**   Risk-adjusted functional status change residual score for the shoulder successfully calculated and the score was equal to zero (0) or greater than zero (>0)   M

(PQRS) ▶ ✳ **G8664**   Risk-adjusted functional status change residual score for the shoulder successfully calculated and the score was less than zero (<0)   M

(PQRS) ▶ ✳ **G8665**   Risk-adjusted functional status change residual scores for the shoulder not measured because the patient did not complete FOTO'S functional intake on admission and/or follow up status survey near discharge, patient not eligible/not appropriate   M

(PQRS) ▶ ✳ **G8666**   Risk-adjusted functional status change residual scores for the shoulder not measured because the patient did not complete FOTO'S functional intake on admission and/or follow up status survey near discharge, reason not specified   M

(PQRS) ▶ ✳ **G8667**   Risk-adjusted functional status change residual score for the elbow, wrist or hand successfully calculated and the score was equal to zero (0) or greater than zero (>0)   M

(PQRS) ▶ ✳ **G8668**   Risk-adjusted functional status change residual score for the elbow, wrist or hand successfully calculated and the score was less than zero (<0)   M

(PQRS) ▶ ✳ **G8669**   Risk-adjusted functional status change residual scores for the elbow, wrist or hand not measured because the patient did not complete FOTO'S functional intake on admission and/or follow up status survey near discharge, patient not eligible/not appropriate   M

(PQRS) ▶ ✳ **G8670**   Risk-adjusted functional status change residual scores for the elbow, wrist or hand not measured because the patient did not complete FOTO'S functional intake on admission and/or follow up status survey near discharge, reason not specified   M

▶ New   → Revised   ✔ Reinstated   ~~deleted~~ Deleted

⊙ Special coverage instructions   ◆ Not covered or valid by Medicare   ✳ Carrier discretion

⊘ ▶ ✳ **G8671** Risk-adjusted functional status change residual score for the neck, cranium, mandible, thoracic spine, ribs, or other general orthopedic impairment successfully calculated and the score was equal to zero (0) or greater than zero (>0)   M

⊘ ▶ ✳ **G8672** Risk-adjusted functional status change residual score for the neck, cranium, mandible, thoracic spine, ribs, or other general orthopedic impairment successfully calculated and the score was less than zero (<0)   M

⊘ ▶ ✳ **G8673** Risk-adjusted functional status change residual scores for the neck, cranium, mandible, thoracic spine, ribs, or other general orthopedic impairment not measured because the patient did not complete FOTO'S functional intake on admission and/or follow up status survey near discharge, patient not eligible/not appropriate   M

⊘ ▶ ✳ **G8674** Risk-adjusted functional status change residual scores for the neck, cranium, mandible, thoracic spine, ribs, or other general orthopedic impairment not measured because the patient did not complete FOTO'S functional intake on admission and/or follow up status survey near discharge, reason not specified   M

~~G8675~~ ~~Most recent systolic blood pressure ≥ 140 mm hg~~   ✖

~~G8676~~ ~~Most recent diastolic blood pressure ≥ 90 mm hg~~   ✖

~~G8677~~ ~~Most recent systolic blood pressure < 130 mm hg~~   ✖

~~G8678~~ ~~Most recent systolic blood pressure 130 to 139 mm hg~~   ✖

~~G8679~~ ~~Most recent diastolic blood pressure < 80 mm hg~~   ✖

~~G8680~~ ~~Most recent diastolic blood pressure 80-89 mm hg~~   ✖

~~G8681~~ ~~Patient hospitalized with principal diagnosis of heart failure during the measurement period~~   ✖

⊘ ▶ ✳ **G8682** Left ventricular function testing performed during the measurement period   M

⊘ ▶ ✳ **G8683** Clinician documented that patient is not an eligible candidate for left ventricular function testing during the measurement period   M

~~G8684~~ ~~Patient not hospitalized with principal diagnosis of heart failure during the measurement period~~   ✖

⊘ ▶ ✳ **G8685** Left ventricular function testing not performed during the measurement period, reason not specified

~~G8686~~ ~~Currently a tobacco smoker or current exposure to secondhand smoke~~   ✖

~~G8687~~ ~~Currently a tobacco non-user and no exposure to secondhand smoke~~   ✖

~~G8688~~ ~~Currently a smokeless tobacco user (eg, chew, snuff) and no exposure to secondhand smoke~~   ✖

~~G8689~~ ~~Tobacco use not assessed, reason not otherwise specified~~   ✖

~~G8690~~ ~~Current tobacco smoker or current exposure to secondhand smoke~~   ✖

~~G8691~~ ~~Current tobacco non-user and no exposure to secondhand smoke~~   ✖

~~G8692~~ ~~Current smokeless tobacco user (eg, chew, snuff) and no exposure to secondhand smoke~~   ✖

~~G8693~~ ~~Tobacco use not assessed, reason not specified~~   ✖

▶ ✳ **G8694** Left ventriucular ejection fraction (LVEF) <40%   M

▶ ✳ **G8695** Left ventricular ejection fraction (LVEF) >= 40% or documentation as mildly depressed left ventricular systolic function or normal   M

▶ ✳ **G8696** Antithrombotic therapy prescribed at discharge   M

▶ ✳ **G8697** Antithrombotic therapy not prescribed for documented reasons   M

▶ ✳ **G8698** Antithrombotic therapy was not prescribed at discharge, reason not otherwise specified   M

▶ ✳ **G8699** Rehabilitation services (occupational, physical or speech) ordered at or prior to discharge   M

▶ ✳ **G8700** Rehabilitation services (occupational, physical or speech) not indicated at or prior to discharge   M

▶ ✳ **G8701** Rehabilitation services were not ordered, reason not otherwise specified   M

▶ ✳ **G8702** Documentation that prophylactic antibiotics were given within 4 hours prior to surgical incision or intraoperatively   M

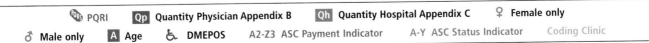

⊘ PQRI   **Qp** Quantity Physician Appendix B   **Qh** Quantity Hospital Appendix C   ♀ Female only

♂ Male only   **A** Age   ♿ DMEPOS   A2-Z3 ASC Payment Indicator   A-Y ASC Status Indicator   Coding Clinic

▶ ✳ **G8703** Documentation that prophylactic antibiotics were neither given within 4 hours prior to surgical incision nor intraoperatively   M

▶ ✳ **G8704** 12-lead electrocardiogram (ECG) performed   M

▶ ✳ **G8705** Documentation of medical reason(s) for not performing a 12-lead electrocardiogram (ECG)   M

▶ ✳ **G8706** Documentation of patient reason(s) for not performing a 12-lead electrocardiogram (ECG)   M

▶ ✳ **G8707** 12-lead electrocardiogram (ECG) not performed, reason not otherwise specified   M

▶ ✳ **G8708** Patient not prescribed or dispensed antibiotic   M

▶ ✳ **G8709** Patient prescribed or dispensed antibiotic for documented medical reason(s)   M

▶ ✳ **G8710** Patient prescribed or dispensed antibiotic   M

▶ ✳ **G8711** Prescribed or dispensed antibiotic   M

▶ ✳ **G8712** Antibiotic not prescribed or dispensed   M

▶ ✳ **G8713** SPKT/V greater than or equal to 1.2 (single-pool clearance of urea [KT] / volume [V])   M

▶ ✳ **G8714** Hemodialysis treatment performed exactly three times per week   M

▶ ✳ **G8715** Hemodialysis treatment performed less than three times per week or greater than three times per week   M

▶ ✳ **G8716** Documentation of reason(s) for patient not having greater than or equal to 1.2 (single-pool clearance of urea [KT] / volume [V])   M

▶ ✳ **G8717** SPKT/V less than 1.2 (single-pool clearance of urea [KT] / volume [V]), reason not specified   M

▶ ✳ **G8718** Total KT/V greater than or equal to 1.7 per week (total clearance of urea [KT] / volume [V])   M

▶ ✳ **G8720** Total KT/V less than 1.7 per week (total clearance of urea [KT] / volume [V]), reason not specified   M

▶ ✳ **G8721** PT category (primary tumor), PN category (regional lymph nodes), and histologic grade were documented in pathology report   M

▶ ✳ **G8722** Medical reason(s) documented for not including PT category, PN category and histologic grade in the pathology report   M

▶ ✳ **G8723** Specimen site is other than anatomic location of primary tumor   M

▶ ✳ **G8724** PT category, PN category and histologic grade were not documented in the pathology report, reason not otherwise specified   M

▶ ✳ **G8725** Fasting lipid profile performed (triglycerides, LDL-C, HDL-C and total cholesterol)   M

▶ ✳ **G8726** Clinician has documented reason for not performing fasting lipid profile   M

▶ ✳ **G8727** Patient receiving hemodialysis, peritoneal dialysis or kidney transplantation   M

▶ ✳ **G8728** Fasting lipid profile not performed, reason not otherwise specified   M

▶ ✳ **G8730** Pain assessment documented as positive utilizing a standardized tool and a follow-up plan is documented   M

▶ ✳ **G8731** Pain assessment documented as negative, no follow-up plan is required   M

▶ ✳ **G8732** No documentation of pain assessment   M

▶ ✳ **G8733** Documentation of a positive elder maltreatment screen and documented follow-up plan **A**   M

▶ ✳ **G8734** Elder maltreatment screen documented as negative, no follow-up required **A**   M

▶ ✳ **G8735** Elder maltreatment screen documented as positive, follow-up plan not documented, reason not specified **A**   M

▶ ✳ **G8736** Most current LDL-C <100 mg/dl   M

▶ ✳ **G8737** Most current LDL-C >=100 mg/dl   M

▶ ✳ **G8738** Left ventricular ejection fraction (LVEF) <40% or documentation of severely or moderately depressed left ventricular systolic function   M

▶ ✳ **G8739** Left ventricular ejection fraction (LVEF) >= 40% or documentation as normal or mildly depressed left ventricular systolic function   M

▶ New   → Revised   ✔ Reinstated   ~~deleted~~ Deleted

☼ Special coverage instructions   ◆ Not covered or valid by Medicare   ✳ Carrier discretion

▶ ✳ **G8740** Left ventricular ejection fraction (LVEF) not performed or assessed, reason not specified M

▶ ✳ **G8741** Patient not treated for spoken language comprehension disorder M

▶ ✳ **G8742** Patient not treated for attention disorder M

▶ ✳ **G8743** Patient not treated for memory disorder M

▶ ✳ **G8744** Patient not treated for motor speech disorder M

▶ ✳ **G8745** Patient not treated for reading disorder M

▶ ✳ **G8746** Patient not treated for spoken language expression disorder M

▶ ✳ **G8747** Patient not treated for writing disorder M

▶ ✳ **G8748** Patient not treated for swallowing disorder M

▶ ✳ **G8749** Absence of signs of melanoma (cough, dyspnea, tenderness, localized neurologic signs such as weakness, jaundice or any other sign suggesting systemic spread) or absence of symptoms of melanoma (pain, paresthesia, or any other symptom suggesting the possibility of systemic spread of melanoma) M

▶ ✳ **G8750** Presence of signs of melanoma (cough, dyspnea, tenderness, localized neurologic signs such as weakness, jaundice or any other sign suggesting systemic spread) or presence of symptoms of melanoma (pain, paresthesia, or any other symptom suggesting the possibility of systemic spread of melanoma) M

▶ ✳ **G8751** Smoking status and exposure to secondhand smoke in the home not assessed, reason not specified M

▶ ✳ **G8752** Most recent systolic blood pressure <140 mm hg M

▶ ✳ **G8753** Most recent systolic blood pressure >= 140 mm hg M

▶ ✳ **G8754** Most recent diastolic blood pressure <90 mm hg M

▶ ✳ **G8755** Most recent diastolic blood pressure >= 90 mm hg M

▶ ✳ **G8756** No documentation of blood pressure measurement, reason not otherwise specified M

▶ ✳ **G8757** All quality actions for the applicable measures in the chronic obstructive pulmonary disease measures group have been performed for this patient M

▶ ✳ **G8758** All quality actions for the applicable measures in the inflammatory bowel disease measures group have been performed for this patient M

▶ ✳ **G8759** All quality actions for the applicable measures in the obstructive sleep apnea measures group have been performed for this patient M

▶ ✳ **G8760** All quality actions for the applicable measures in the epilepsy measures group have been performed for this patient M

▶ ✳ **G8761** All quality actions for the applicable measures in the dementia measures group have been performed for this patient M

▶ ✳ **G8762** All quality actions for the applicable measures in the Parkinson's disease measures group have been performed for this patient M

▶ ✳ **G8763** All quality actions for the applicable measures in the hypertension measures group have been performed for this patient M

▶ ✳ **G8764** All quality actions for the applicable measures in the cardiovascular prevention measures group have been performed for this patient M

▶ ✳ **G8765** All quality actions for the applicable measures in the cataract measures group have been performed for this patient M

▶ ✳ **G8767** Lipid panel results documented and reviewed (must include total cholesterol, HDL-C, triglycerides and calculated LDL-C) M

▶ ✳ **G8768** Documentation of medical reason(s) for not performing lipid profile (e.g., patients who have a terminal illness or for whom treatment of hypertension with standard treatment goals is not clinically appropriate) M

▶ ✳ **G8769** Lipid profile not performed, reason not otherwise specified M

▶ ✳ **G8770** Urine protein test result documented and reviewed M

▶ ✳ **G8771** Documentation of diagnosis of chronic kidney disease M

▶ ✳ **G8772** Documentation of medical reason(s) for not performing urine protein test (e.g., patients who have a terminal illness or for whom treatment of hypertension with standard treatment goals is not clinically appropriate)   M

▶ ✳ **G8773** Urine protein test was not performed, reason not otherwise specified   M

▶ ✳ **G8774** Serum creatinine test result documented and reviewed   M

▶ ✳ **G8775** Documentation of medical reason(s) for not performing serum creatinine test (e.g., patients who have a terminal illness or for whom treatment of hypertension with standard treatment goals is not clinically appropriate)   M

▶ ✳ **G8776** Serum creatinine test not performed, reason not otherwise specified   M

▶ ✳ **G8777** Diabetes screening test performed   M

▶ ✳ **G8778** Documentation of medical reason(s) for not performing diabetes screening test(e.g., patients who have a terminal illness or for whom treatment of hypertension with standard treatment goals is not clinically appropriate, or patients with a diagnosis of diabetes)   M

▶ ✳ **G8779** Diabetes screening test not performed, reason not otherwise specified   M

▶ ✳ **G8780** Counseling for diet and physical activity performed   M

▶ ✳ **G8781** Documentation of medical reason(s) for patient not receiving counseling for diet and physical activity (e.g., patients who have a terminal illness or for whom treatment of hypertension with standard treatment goals is not clinically appropriate)   M

▶ ✳ **G8782** Counseling for diet and physical activity not performed, reason not otherwise specified   M

▶ ✳ **G8783** Blood pressure screening performed as recommended by the defined screening interval   M

▶ ✳ **G8784** Blood pressure not assessed, patient not eligible   M

▶ ✳ **G8785** Blood pressure screening not performed as recommended by screening interval, reason not otherwise specified   M

▶ ✳ **G8786** Severity of angina assessed according to level of activity   M

▶ ✳ **G8787** Angina assessed as present   M

▶ ✳ **G8788** Angina assessed as absent   M

▶ ✳ **G8789** Severity of angina not assessed according to level of activity   M

▶ ✳ **G8790** Most recent office visit systolic blood pressure <130 mm hg   M

▶ ✳ **G8791** Most recent office visit systolic blood pressure, 130-139 mm hg   M

▶ ✳ **G8792** Most recent office visit systolic blood pressure >=140 mm hg   M

▶ ✳ **G8793** Most recent office visit diastolic blood pressure, <80 mm hg   M

▶ ✳ **G8794** Most recent office visit diastolic blood pressure, 80-89 mm hg   M

▶ ✳ **G8795** Most recent office visit diastolic blood pressure >=90 mm hg   M

▶ ✳ **G8796** Blood pressure measurement not documented, reason not otherwise specified   M

▶ ✳ **G8797** Specimen site other than anatomic location of esophagus   M

▶ ✳ **G8798** Specimen site other than anatomic location of prostate   M

▶ ✳ **G8799** Anticoagulation ordered   M

▶ ✳ **G8800** Anticoagulation not ordered for reasons documented by clinician   M

▶ ✳ **G8801** Anticoagulation was not ordered, reason not specified   M

▶ ✳ **G8802** Pregnancy test (urine or serum) ordered   M

▶ ✳ **G8803** Pregnancy test (urine or serum) not ordered for reasons documented by clinician   M

▶ ✳ **G8805** Pregnancy test (urine or serum) was not ordered, reason not specified   M

▶ ✳ **G8806** Performance of trans-abdominal or trans-vaginal ultrasound   M

▶ ✳ **G8807** Trans-abdominal or trans-vaginal ultrasound not performed for reasons documented by clinician   M

▶ ✳ **G8808** Performance of trans-abdominal or trans-vaginal ultrasound not ordered, reason not specified   M

▶ ✳ **G8809** Rh-immunoglobulin (RhoGAM) ordered   M

▶ ✳ **G8810** R-immunoglobulin (RhoGAM) not ordered for reasons documented by clinician   M

▶ New   → Revised   ✔ Reinstated   ~~deleted~~ Deleted

⊘ Special coverage instructions   ◆ Not covered or valid by Medicare   ✳ Carrier discretion

▶ ✳ **G8811** Documentation RH-immunoglobulin (RhoGAM) was not ordered, reason not specified M

▶ ✳ **G8812** Patient is not eligible for follow-up CTA, duplex, or MRA M

▶ ✳ **G8813** Follow-up CTA, duplex, or MRA of the abdomen and pelvis performed M

▶ ✳ **G8814** Follow-up CTA, duplex, or MRA of the abdomen and pelvis not performed M

▶ ✳ **G8815** Statin therapy not prescribed for documented reasons M

▶ ✳ **G8816** Statin medication prescribed at discharge M

▶ ✳ **G8817** Statin therapy not prescribed at discharge, reason not specified M

▶ ✳ **G8818** Patient discharge to home no later than post-operative day #7 M

▶ ✳ **G8819** Aneurysm minor diameter <= 5.5 cm M

▶ ✳ **G8820** Aneurysm minor diameter 5.6-6.0 cm M

▶ ✳ **G8821** Abdominal aortic aneurysm is not infareral M

▶ ✳ **G8822** Male patients with aneurysms minor diameter >6 cm ♂ M

▶ ✳ **G8823** Female patients with aneurysm minor diameter >6 cm ♀ M

▶ ✳ **G8824** Female patients with aneurysm minor diameter 5.6-6.0 cm ♀ M

▶ ✳ **G8825** Patient not discharged to home by post-operative day #7 M

▶ ✳ **G8826** Patient discharge to home no later than post-operative day #2 following EVAR M

▶ ✳ **G8827** Aneurysm minor diameter <= 5.5 cm for women ♀ M

▶ ✳ **G8828** Aneurysm minor diameter <= 5.5 cm for men ♂ M

▶ ✳ **G8829** Aneurysm minor diameter 5.6-6.0 cm for men ♂ M

▶ ✳ **G8830** Aneurysm minor diameter >6 cm for men ♂ M

▶ ✳ **G8831** Aneurysm minor diameter >6 cm for women ♀ M

▶ ✳ **G8832** Aneurysm minor diameter 5.6-6.0 cm for women ♀ M

▶ ✳ **G8833** Patient not discharged to home by post-operative day #2 following EVAR M

▶ ✳ **G8834** Patient discharged to home no later than post-operative day #2 following CEA M

▶ ✳ **G8835** Asymptomatic patient with no history of any transient ischemic attack or stroke in any carotid or vertebrobasilar territory M

▶ ✳ **G8836** Symptomatic patient with ipsilateral stroke or TIA within 120 days prior to CEA M

▶ ✳ **G8837** Other symptomatic patient with ipsilateral carotid territory TIA or stroke >120 days prior to CEA, or contralateral carotid territory TIA or stroke or vertebrobasilar TIA or stroke M

▶ ✳ **G8838** Patient not discharged to home by post-operative day #2 M

▶ ✳ **G8839** Sleep apnea symptoms assessed, including presence or absence of snoring and daytime sleepiness M

▶ ✳ **G8840** Documentation of reason(s) for not performing an assessment of sleep symptoms (e.g., patient didn't have initial daytime sleepiness, patient visits between initial testing and initiation of therapy) M

▶ ✳ **G8841** Sleep apnea symptoms not assessed, reason not otherwise specified M

▶ ✳ **G8842** Apnea Hypopnea Index (AHI) or Respiratory Disturbance Index (RDI) measured at the time of initial diagnosis M

▶ ✳ **G8843** Documentation of reason(s) for not measuring an Apnea Hypopnea Index (AHI) or a Respiratory Disturbance Index (RDI) at the time of initial diagnosis M

▶ ✳ **G8844** Apnea Hypopnea Index (AHI) or Respiratory Disturbance Index (RDI) not measured at the time of initial diagnosis, reason not specified M

▶ ✳ **G8845** Positive airway pressure therapy prescribed M

▶ ✳ **G8846** Moderate or severe obstructive sleep apnea (Apnea Hypopnea Index (AHI) or Respiratory Disturbance Index (RDI) of 15 or greater) M

▶ ✳ **G8847** Positive airway pressure therapy not prescribed M

▶ ✳ **G8848** Mild obstructive sleep apnea (Apnea Hypopnea Index (AHI) or Respiratory Disturbance Index (RDI) of less than 15)   M

▶ ✳ **G8849** Documentation of reason(s) for not prescribing positive airway pressure therapy   M

▶ ✳ **G8850** Positive airway pressure therapy not prescribed, reason not otherwise specified   M

▶ ✳ **G8851** Objective measurement of adherence to positive airway pressure therapy, documented   M

▶ ✳ **G8852** Positive airway pressure therapy prescribed   M

▶ ✳ **G8853** Positive airway pressure therapy not prescribed   M

▶ ✳ **G8854** Documentation of reason(s) for not objectively measuring adherence to positive airway pressure therapy   M

▶ ✳ **G8855** Objective measurement of adherence to positive airway pressure therapy not performed, reason not otherwise specified   M

▶ ✳ **G8856** Referral to a physician for an otologic evaluation performed   M

▶ ✳ **G8857** Patient is not eligible for the referral for otologic evaluation measure (e.g., patients who are already under the care of a physician for acute or chronic dizziness)   M

▶ ✳ **G8858** Referral to a physician for an otologic evaluation not performed, reason not specified   M

▶ ✳ **G8859** Patient receiving corticosteroids greater than or equal to 10 mg/day for 60 or greater consecutive days   M

▶ ✳ **G8860** Patients who have received dose of corticosteroids greater than or equal to10 mg/day for 60 or greater consecutive days   M

▶ ✳ **G8861** Central dual-energy x-ray absorptiometry (DXA) ordered or documented, review of systems and medication history or pharmacologic therapy (other than minerals/vitamins) for osteoporosis prescribed   M

▶ ✳ **G8862** Patients not receiving corticosteroids greater than or equal to 10 mg/day for 60 or greater consecutive days   M

▶ ✳ **G8863** Patients not assessed for risk of bone loss, reason not otherwise specified   M

▶ ✳ **G8864** Pneumococcal vaccine administered or previously received   M

▶ ✳ **G8865** Documentation of medical reason(s) for not administering or previously receiving pneumococcal vaccine (e.g., patient allergic reaction, potential adverse drug reaction)   M

▶ ✳ **G8866** Documentation of patient reason(s) for not administering or previously receiving pneumococcal vaccine (e.g., patient refusal)   M

▶ ✳ **G8867** Pneumococcal vaccine not administered or previously received, reason not otherwise specified   M

▶ ✳ **G8868** Patients receiving a first course of anti-TNF therapy   M

▶ ✳ **G8869** Patient has documented immunity to hepatitis B and is receiving a first course of anti-TNF therapy   M

▶ ✳ **G8870** Hepatitis B vaccine injection administered or previously received and is receiving a first course of anti-TNF therapy   M

▶ ✳ **G8871** Patient not receiving a first course of anti-TNF therapy   M

▶ ✳ **G8872** Excised tissue evaluated by imaging intraoperatively to confirm successful inclusion of targeted lesion   M

▶ ✳ **G8873** Patients with needle localization specimens which are not amenable to intraoperative imaging such as MRI needle wire localization, or targets which are tentatively identified on mammogram or ultrasound which do not contain a biopsy marker but which can be verified on intraoperative inspection or pathology   M

▶ ✳ **G8874** Excised tissue not evaluated by imaging intraoperatively to confirm successful inclusion of targeted lesion   M

▶ ✳ **G8875** Clinician diagnosed breast cancer preoperatively by a minimally invasive biopsy method   M

▶ ✳ **G8876** Documentation of reason(s) for not performing minimally invasive biopsy to diagnose breast cancer properatively   M

▶ ✳ **G8877** Clinician did not attempt to achieve the diagnosis of breast cancer preoperatively by a minimally invasive biopsy method, reason not otherwise specified   M

▶ ✳ **G8878** Sentinel lymph node biopsy procedure performed   M

▶ **New**   → **Revised**   ✔ **Reinstated**   ~~deleted~~ **Deleted**
◎ **Special coverage instructions**   ◆ **Not covered or valid by Medicare**   ✳ **Carrier discretion**

▶ ✳ **G8879** Clinically node negative (T1N0M0 or T2N0M0) invasive breast cancer M

▶ ✳ **G8880** Documentation of reason(s) sentinel lymph node biopsy not performed M

▶ ✳ **G8881** Stage of breast cancer is greater than T1N0M0 or T2N0M0 M

▶ ✳ **G8882** Sentinel lymph node biopsy procedure not performed M

▶ ✳ **G8883** Biopsy results reviewed, communicated, tracked and documented M

▶ ✳ **G8884** Clinician documented reason that patient's biopsy results were not reviewed M

▶ ✳ **G8885** Biopsy results not reviewed, communicated, tracked or documented M

▶ ✳ **G8886** Most recent blood pressure under control M

▶ ✳ **G8887** Documentation of medical reason(s) for most recent blood pressure not being under control (e.g., patients with comorbid conditions that cause an increase in blood pressure or require treatment with medications that cause an increase in blood pressure, or patients who had a terminal illness or for whom treatment of hypertension with standard treatment goals is not clinically appropriate) M

▶ ✳ **G8888** Most recent blood pressure not under control, results documented and reviewed M

▶ ✳ **G8889** No documentation of blood pressure measurement, reason not otherwise specified M

▶ ✳ **G8890** Most recent LDL-C under control, results documented and reviewed M

▶ ✳ **G8891** Documentation of medical reason(s) for most recent LSL-C not under control (e.g., patients who had a terminal illness or for whom treatment of hypertension with standard treatment goals is not clinically appropriate) M

▶ ✳ **G8892** Documentation of medical reason(s) for not performing LDL-C test (e.g., patients who had a terminal illness or for whom treatment of hypertension with standard treatment goals is not clinically appropriate) M

▶ ✳ **G8893** Most recent LDL-C not under control, results documented and reviewed M

▶ ✳ **G8894** LDL-C not performed, reason not specified M

▶ ✳ **G8895** Oral aspirin or other anticoagulant/ antiplatelet therapy prescribed M

▶ ✳ **G8896** Documentation of medical reason(s) for not prescribing oral aspirin or other anticoagulant/antiplatelet therapy (e.g., under age 30, patient documented to be low risk, patient with terminal illness or treatment of hypertension with standard treatment goals is not clinically appropriate) M

▶ ✳ **G8897** Oral aspirin or other anticoagulant/ antiplatelet therapy was not prescribed, reason not otherwise specified M

▶ ✳ **G8898** I intend to report the chronic obstructive pulmonary disease measures group M

▶ ✳ **G8899** I intend to report the inflammatory bowel disease measures group M

▶ ✳ **G8900** I intend to report the obstructive sleep apnea measures group M

▶ ✳ **G8901** I intend to report the epilepsy measures group M

▶ ✳ **G8902** I intend to report the dementia measures group M

▶ ✳ **G8903** I intend to report the Parkinson's disease measures group M

▶ ✳ **G8904** I intend to report the hypertension measures group M

▶ ✳ **G8905** I intend to report the cardiovascular prevention measures group M

▶ ✳ **G8906** I intend to report the cataract measures group M

✺ **G9001** Coordinated care fee, initial rate B

✺ **G9002** Coordinated care fee, maintenance rate B

✺ **G9003** Coordinated care fee, risk adjusted high, initial B

✺ **G9004** Coordinated care fee, risk adjusted low, initial B

✺ **G9005** Coordinated care fee, risk adjusted maintenance B

✺ **G9006** Coordinated care fee, home monitoring B

✺ **G9007** Coordinated care fee, scheduled team conference B

✺ **G9008** Coordinated care fee, physician coordinated care oversight services B

🅟 PQRI	**Qp** Quantity Physician Appendix B	**Qh** Quantity Hospital Appendix C	♀ **Female only**	
♂ **Male only**	🄐 **Age**	& **DMEPOS**	A2-Z3 ASC Payment Indicator	A-Y ASC Status Indicator	Coding Clinic

⊛ **G9009** Coordinated care fee, risk adjusted maintenance, level 3   B

⊛ **G9010** Coordinated care fee, risk adjusted maintenance, level 4   B

⊛ **G9011** Coordinated care fee, risk adjusted maintenance, level 5   B

⊛ **G9012** Other specified case management services not elsewhere classified   B

◆ **G9013** ESRD demo basic bundle Level I   E

     Medicare non-covered.

◆ **G9014** ESRD demo expanded bundle, including venous access and related services   E

     Medicare non-covered.

◆ **G9016** Smoking cessation counseling, individual, in the absence of or in addition to any other evaluation and management service, per session (6-10 minutes) [demo project code only]   E

     Medicare non-covered.

✳ **G9017** Amantadine hydrochloride, oral, per 100 mg (for use in a Medicare-approved demonstration project)   A

✳ **G9018** Zanamivir, inhalation powder, administered through inhaler, per 10 mg (for use in a Medicare-approved demonstration project)   A

✳ **G9019** Oseltamivir phosphate, oral, per 75 mg (for use in a Medicare-approved demonstration project)   A

✳ **G9020** Rimantadine hydrochloride, oral, per 100 mg (for use in a Medicare-approved demonstration project)   A

✳ **G9033** Amantadine hydrochloride, oral brand, per 100 mg (for use in a Medicare-approved demonstration project)   A

✳ **G9034** Zanamivir, inhalation powder, administered through inhaler, brand, per 10 mg (for use in a Medicare-approved demonstration project)   A

✳ **G9035** Oseltamivir phosphate, oral, brand, per 75 mg (for use in a Medicare-approved demonstration project)   A

✳ **G9036** Rimantadine hydrochloride, oral, brand, per 100 mg (for use in a Medicare-approved demonstration project)   A

~~G9041~~ ~~Rehabilitation services for low vision by qualified occupational therapist, direct one on one contact, each 15 minutes~~ ✖

~~G9042~~ ~~Rehabilitation services for low vision by certified orientation and mobility specialists, direct one-on-one contact, each 15 minutes~~ ✖

~~G9043~~ ~~Rehabilitation services for low vision by certified low vision rehabilitation therapist, direct one-on-one contact, each 15 minutes~~ ✖

~~G9044~~ ~~Rehabilitation services for low vision by certified low vision rehabilitation teacher, direct one-on-one contact, each 15 minutes~~ ✖

◆ **G9050** Oncology; primary focus of visit; work-up, evaluation, or staging at the time of cancer diagnosis or recurrence (for use in a Medicare-approved demonstration project)   E

◆ **G9051** Oncology; primary focus of visit; treatment decision-making after disease is staged or restaged, discussion of treatment options, supervising/ coordinating active cancer directed therapy or managing consequences of cancer directed therapy (for use in a Medicare-approved demonstration project)   E

◆ **G9052** Oncology; primary focus of visit; surveillance for disease recurrence for patient who has completed definitive cancer-directed therapy and currently lacks evidence of recurrent disease; cancer directed therapy might be considered in the future (for use in a Medicare-approved demonstration project)   E

◆ **G9053** Oncology; primary focus of visit; expectant management of patient with evidence of cancer for whom no cancer directed therapy is being administered or arranged at present; cancer directed therapy might be considered in the future (for use in a Medicare-approved demonstration project)   E

◆ **G9054** Oncology; primary focus of visit; supervising, coordinating or managing care of patient with terminal cancer or for whom other medical illness prevents further cancer treatment; includes symptom management, end-of-life care planning, management of palliative therapies (for use in a Medicare-approved demonstration project)   E

▶ New   → Revised   ✔ Reinstated   ~~deleted~~ Deleted

⊛ Special coverage instructions   ◆ Not covered or valid by Medicare   ✳ Carrier discretion

◆ **G9055** Oncology; primary focus of visit; other, unspecified service not otherwise listed (for use in a Medicare-approved demonstration project)   E

◆ **G9056** Oncology; practice guidelines; management adheres to guidelines (for use in a Medicare-approved demonstration project)   E

◆ **G9057** Oncology; practice guidelines; management differs from guidelines as a result of patient enrollment in an institutional review board approved clinical trial (for use in a Medicare-approved demonstration project)   E

◆ **G9058** Oncology; practice guidelines; management differs from guidelines because the treating physician disagrees with guideline recommendations (for use in a Medicare-approved demonstration project)   E

◆ **G9059** Oncology; practice guidelines; management differs from guidelines because the patient, after being offered treatment consistent with guidelines, has opted for alternative treatment or management, including no treatment (for use in a Medicare-approved demonstration project)   E

◆ **G9060** Oncology; practice guidelines; management differs from guidelines for reason(s) associated with patient comorbid illness or performance status not factored into guidelines (for use in a Medicare-approved demonstration project)   E

◆ **G9061** Oncology; practice guidelines; patient's condition not addressed by available guidelines (for use in a Medicare-approved demonstration project)   E

◆ **G9062** Oncology; practice guidelines; management differs from guidelines for other reason(s) not listed (for use in a Medicare-approved demonstration project)   E

✳ **G9063** Oncology; disease status; limited to non-small cell lung cancer; extent of disease initially established as stage I (prior to neo-adjuvant therapy, if any) with no evidence of disease progression, recurrence, or metastases (for use in a Medicare-approved demonstration project)   M

✳ **G9064** Oncology; disease status; limited to non-small cell lung cancer; extent of disease initially established as stage II (prior to neo-adjuvant therapy, if any) with no evidence of disease progression, recurrence, or metastases (for use in a Medicare-approved demonstration project)   M

✳ **G9065** Oncology; disease status; limited to non-small cell lung cancer; extent of disease initially established as stage IIIA (prior to neo-adjuvant therapy, if any) with no evidence of disease progression, recurrence, or metastases (for use in a Medicare-approved demonstration project)   M

✳ **G9066** Oncology; disease status; limited to non-small cell lung cancer; stage IIIB-IV at diagnosis, metastatic, locally recurrent, or progressive (for use in a Medicare-approved demonstration project)   M

✳ **G9067** Oncology; disease status; limited to non-small cell lung cancer; extent of disease unknown, staging in progress, or not listed (for use in a Medicare-approved demonstration project)   M

✳ **G9068** Oncology; disease status; limited to small cell and combined small cell/non-small cell; extent of disease initially established as limited with no evidence of disease progression, recurrence, or metastases (for use in a Medicare-approved demonstration project)   M

✳ **G9069** Oncology; disease status; small cell lung cancer, limited to small cell and combined small cell/non-small cell; extensive stage at diagnosis, metastatic, locally recurrent, or progressive (for use in a Medicare-approved demonstration project)   M

✳ **G9070** Oncology; disease status; small cell lung cancer, limited to small cell and combined small cell/non-small cell; extent of disease unknown, staging in progress, or not listed (for use in a Medicare-approved demonstration project)   M

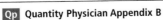 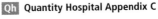

✳ **G9071** Oncology; disease status; invasive female breast cancer (does not include ductal carcinoma in situ); adenocarcinoma as predominant cell type; stage I or stage IIA-IIB; or T3, N1, M0; and ER and/or PR positive; with no evidence of disease progression, recurrence, or metastases (for use in a Medicare-approved demonstration project) ♀   M

✳ **G9072** Oncology; disease status; invasive female breast cancer (does not include ductal carcinoma in situ); adenocarcinoma as predominant cell type; stage I, or stage IIA-IIB; or T3, N1, M0; and ER and PR negative; with no evidence of disease progression, recurrence, or metastases (for use in a Medicare-approved demonstration project) ♀   M

✳ **G9073** Oncology; disease status; invasive female breast cancer (does not include ductal carcinoma in situ); adenocarcinoma as predominant cell type; stage IIIA-IIIB; and not T3, N1, M0; and ER and/or PR positive; with no evidence of disease progression, recurrence, or metastases (for use in a Medicare-approved demonstration project) ♀   M

✳ **G9074** Oncology; disease status; invasive female breast cancer (does not include ductal carcinoma in situ); adenocarcinoma as predominant cell type; stage IIIA-IIIB; and not T3, N1, M0; and ER and PR negative; with no evidence of disease progression, recurrence, or metastases (for use in a Medicare-approved demonstration project) ♀   M

✳ **G9075** Oncology; disease status; invasive female breast cancer (does not include ductal carcinoma in situ); adenocarcinoma as predominant cell type; M1 at diagnosis, metastatic, locally recurrent, or progressive (for use in a Medicare-approved demonstration project) ♀   M

✳ **G9077** Oncology; disease status; prostate cancer, limited to adenocarcinoma as predominant cell type; T1-T2c and Gleason 2-7 and PSA < or equal to 20 at diagnosis with no evidence of disease progression, recurrence, or metastases (for use in a Medicare-approved demonstration project) ♂   M

✳ **G9078** Oncology; disease status; prostate cancer, limited to adenocarcinoma as predominant cell type; T2 or T3a Gleason 8-10 or PSA > 20 at diagnosis with no evidence of disease progression, recurrence, or metastases (for use in a Medicare-approved demonstration project) ♂   M

✳ **G9079** Oncology; disease status; prostate cancer, limited to adenocarcinoma as predominant cell type; T3b-T4, any N; any T, N1 at diagnosis with no evidence of disease progression, recurrence, or metastases (for use in a Medicare-approved demonstration project) ♂   M

✳ **G9080** Oncology; disease status; prostate cancer, limited to adenocarcinoma; after initial treatment with rising PSA or failure of PSA decline (for use in a Medicare-approved demonstration project) ♂   M

✳ **G9083** Oncology; disease status; prostate cancer, limited to adenocarcinoma; extent of disease unknown, staging in progress, or not listed (for use in a Medicare-approved demonstration project) ♂   M

✳ **G9084** Oncology; disease status; colon cancer, limited to invasive cancer, adenocarcinoma as predominant cell type; extent of disease initially established as T1-3, N0, M0 with no evidence of disease progression, recurrence, or metastases (for use in a Medicare-approved demonstration project)   M

✳ **G9085** Oncology; disease status; colon cancer, limited to invasive cancer, adenocarcinoma as predominant cell type; extent of disease initially established as T4, N0, M0 with no evidence of disease progression, recurrence, or metastases (for use in a Medicare-approved demonstration project)   M

✳ **G9086** Oncology; disease status; colon cancer, limited to invasive cancer, adenocarcinoma as predominant cell type; extent of disease initially established as T1-4, N1-2, M0 with no evidence of disease progression, recurrence, or metastases (for use in a Medicare-approved demonstration project)   M

▶ New   → Revised   ✔ Reinstated   ~~deleted~~ Deleted
✪ Special coverage instructions   ◆ Not covered or valid by Medicare   ✳ Carrier discretion

✳ **G9087** Oncology; disease status; colon cancer, limited to invasive cancer, adenocarcinoma as predominant cell type; M1 at diagnosis, metastatic, locally recurrent, or progressive with current clinical, radiologic, or biochemical evidence of disease (for use in a Medicare-approved demonstration project) M

✳ **G9088** Oncology; disease status; colon cancer, limited to invasive cancer, adenocarcinoma as predominant cell type; M1 at diagnosis, metastatic, locally recurrent, or progressive without current clinical, radiologic, or biochemical evidence of disease (for use in a Medicare-approved demonstration project) M

✳ **G9089** Oncology; disease status; colon cancer, limited to invasive cancer, adenocarcinoma as predominant cell type; extent of disease unknown, staging in progress, or not listed (for use in a Medicare-approved demonstration project) M

✳ **G9090** Oncology; disease status; rectal cancer, limited to invasive cancer, adenocarcinoma as predominant cell type; extent of disease initially established as T1-2, N0, M0 (prior to neo-adjuvant therapy, if any) with no evidence of disease progression, recurrence, or metastases (for use in a Medicare-approved demonstration project) M

✳ **G9091** Oncology; disease status; rectal cancer, limited to invasive cancer, adenocarcinoma as predominant cell type; extent of disease initially established as T3, N0, M0 (prior to neo-adjuvant therapy, if any) with no evidence of disease progression, recurrence, or metastases (for use in a Medicare-approved demonstration project) M

✳ **G9092** Oncology; disease status; rectal cancer, limited to invasive cancer, adenocarcinoma as predominant cell type; extent of disease initially established as T1-3, N1-2, M0 (prior to neo-adjuvant therapy, if any) with no evidence of disease progression, recurrence or metastases (for use in a Medicare-approved demonstration project) M

✳ **G9093** Oncology; disease status; rectal cancer, limited to invasive cancer, adenocarcinoma as predominant cell type; extent of disease initially established as T4, any N, M0 (prior to neo-adjuvant therapy, if any) with no evidence of disease progression, recurrence, or metastases (for use in a Medicare-approved demonstration project) M

✳ **G9094** Oncology; disease status; rectal cancer, limited to invasive cancer, adenocarcinoma as predominant cell type; M1 at diagnosis, metastatic, locally recurrent, or progressive (for use in a Medicare-approved demonstration project) M

✳ **G9095** Oncology; disease status; rectal cancer, limited to invasive cancer, adenocarcinoma as predominant cell type; extent of disease unknown, staging in progress, or not listed (for use in a Medicare-approved demonstration project) M

✳ **G9096** Oncology; disease status; esophageal cancer, limited to adenocarcinoma or squamous cell carcinoma as predominant cell type; extent of disease initially established as T1-T3, N0-N1 or NX (prior to neo-adjuvant therapy, if any) with no evidence of disease progression, recurrence, or metastases (for use in a Medicare-approved demonstration project) M

✳ **G9097** Oncology; disease status; esophageal cancer, limited to adenocarcinoma or squamous cell carcinoma as predominant cell type; extent of disease initially established as T4, any N, M0 (prior to neo-adjuvant therapy, if any) with no evidence of disease progression, recurrence, or metastases (for use in a Medicare-approved demonstration project) M

✳ **G9098** Oncology; disease status; esophageal cancer, limited to adenocarcinoma or squamous cell carcinoma as predominant cell type; M1 at diagnosis, meta-static, locally recurrent, or progressive (for use in a Medicare-approved demonstration project) M

✳ **G9099** Oncology; disease status; esophageal cancer, limited to adenocarcinoma or squamous cell carcinoma as predominant cell type; extent of disease unknown, staging in progress, or not listed (for use in a Medicare-approved demonstration project) M

🔬 PQRI	**Qp** Quantity Physician Appendix B	**Qh** Quantity Hospital Appendix C	♀ Female only
♂ Male only	**A** Age	♿ DMEPOS	A2-Z3 ASC Payment Indicator	A-Y ASC Status Indicator	Coding Clinic

✳ **G9100**   Oncology; disease status; gastric cancer, limited to adenocarcinoma as predominant cell type; post R0 resection (with or without neoadjuvant therapy) with no evidence of disease recurrence, progression, or metastases (for use in a Medicare-approved demonstration project)   M

✳ **G9101**   Oncology; disease status; gastric cancer, limited to adenocarcinoma as predominant cell type; post R1 or R2 resection (with or without neoadjuvant therapy) with no evidence of disease progression, or metastases (for use in a Medicare-approved demonstration project)   M

✳ **G9102**   Oncology; disease status; gastric cancer, limited to adenocarcinoma as predominant cell type; clinical or pathologic M0, unresectable with no evidence of disease progression, or metastases (for use in a Medicare-approved demonstration project)   M

✳ **G9103**   Oncology; disease status; gastric cancer, limited to adenocarcinoma as predominant cell type; clinical or pathologic M1 at diagnosis, metastatic, locally recurrent, or progressive (for use in a Medicare-approved demonstration project)   M

✳ **G9104**   Oncology; disease status; gastric cancer, limited to adenocarcinoma as predominant cell type; extent of disease unknown, staging in progress, or not listed (for use in a Medicare-approved demonstration project)   M

✳ **G9105**   Oncology; disease status; pancreatic cancer, limited to adenocarcinoma as predominant cell type; post R0 resection without evidence of disease progression, recurrence, or metastases (for use in a Medicare-approved demonstration project)   M

✳ **G9106**   Oncology; disease status; pancreatic cancer, limited to adenocarcinoma; post R1 or R2 resection with no evidence of disease progression or metastases (for use in a Medicare-approved demonstration project)   M

✳ **G9107**   Oncology; disease status; pancreatic cancer, limited to adenocarcinoma; unresectable at diagnosis, M1 at diagnosis, metastatic, locally recurrent, or progressive (for use in a Medicare-approved demonstration project)   M

✳ **G9108**   Oncology; disease status; pancreatic cancer, limited to adenocarcinoma; extent of disease unknown, staging in progress, or not listed (for use in a Medicare-approved demonstration project)   M

✳ **G9109**   Oncology; disease status; head and neck cancer, limited to cancers of oral cavity, pharynx and larynx with squamous cell as predominant cell type; extent of disease initially established as T1-T2 and N0, M0 (prior to neo-adjuvant therapy, if any) with no evidence of disease progression, recurrence, or metastases (for use in a Medicare-approved demonstration project)   M

✳ **G9110**   Oncology; disease status; head and neck cancer, limited to cancers of oral cavity, pharynx, and larynx with squamous cell as predominant cell type; extent of disease initially established as T3-4 and/ or N1-3, M0 (prior to neo-adjuvant therapy, if any) with no evidence of disease progression, recurrence, or metastases (for use in a Medicare-approved demonstration project)   M

✳ **G9111**   Oncology; disease status; head and neck cancer, limited to cancers of oral cavity, pharynx and larynx with squamous cell as predominant cell type; M1 at diagnosis, metastatic, locally recurrent, or progressive (for use in a Medicare-approved demonstration project)   M

✳ **G9112**   Oncology; disease status; head and neck cancer, limited to cancers of oral cavity, pharynx and larynx with squamous cell as predominant cell type; extent of disease unknown, staging in progress, or not listed (for use in a Medicare-approved demonstration project)   M

✳ **G9113**   Oncology; disease status; ovarian cancer, limited to epithelial cancer; pathologic stage IA-B (grade 1) without evidence of disease progression, recurrence, or metastases (for use in a Medicare-approved demonstration project) ♀   M

✳ **G9114**   Oncology; disease status; ovarian cancer, limited to epithelial cancer; pathologic stage IA-B (grade 2-3); or stage IC (all grades); or stage II; without evidence of disease progression, recurrence, or metastases (for use in a Medicare-approved demonstration project) ♀   M

▶ New   → Revised   ✔ Reinstated   deleted Deleted

☉ Special coverage instructions   ◆ Not covered or valid by Medicare   ✳ Carrier discretion

✳ **G9115** Oncology; disease status; ovarian cancer, limited to epithelial cancer; pathologic stage III-IV; without evidence of progression, recurrence, or metastases (for use in a Medicare-approved demonstration project) ♀   M

✳ **G9116** Oncology; disease status; ovarian cancer, limited to epithelial cancer; evidence of disease progression, or recurrence and/or platinum resistance (for use in a Medicare-approved demonstration project) ♀   M

✳ **G9117** Oncology; disease status; ovarian cancer, limited to epithelial cancer; extent of disease unknown, staging in progress, or not listed (for use in a Medicare-approved demonstration project) ♀   M

✳ **G9123** Oncology; disease status; chronic myelogenous leukemia, limited to Philadelphia chromosome positive and/or BCR-ABL positive; chronic phase not in hematologic, cytogenetic, or molecular remission (for use in a Medicare-approved demonstration project)   M

✳ **G9124** Oncology; disease status; chronic myelogenous leukemia, limited to Philadelphia chromosome positive and/or BCR-ABL positive; accelerated phase not in hematologic cytogenetic, or molecular remission (for use in a Medicare-approved demonstration project)   M

✳ **G9125** Oncology; disease status; chronic myelogenous leukemia, limited to Philadelphia chromosome positive and/or BCR-ABL positive; blast phase not in hematologic, cytogenetic, or molecular remission (for use in a Medicare-approved demonstration project)   M

✳ **G9126** Oncology; disease status; chronic myelogenous leukemia, limited to Philadelphia chromosome positive and/or BCR-ABL positive; in hematologic, cytogenetic, or molecular remission (for use in a Medicare-approved demonstration project)   M

G9128 Oncology: disease status; limited to multiple myeloma, systemic disease; smouldering, stage I (for use in a Medicare-approved demonstration project)   M

✳ **G9129** Oncology; disease status; limited to multiple myeloma, systemic disease; stage II or higher (for use in a Medicare-approved demonstration project)   M

✳ **G9130** Oncology; disease status; limited to multiple myeloma, systemic disease; extent of disease unknown, staging in progress, or not listed (for use in a Medicare-approved demonstration project)   M

✳ **G9131** Oncology; disease status; invasive female breast cancer (does not include ductal carcinoma in situ); adenocarcinoma as predominant cell type; extent of disease unknown, staging in progress, or not listed (for use in a Medicare-approved demonstration project) ♀   M

✳ **G9132** Oncology; disease status; prostate cancer, limited to adenocarcinoma; hormone-refractory/androgen-independent (e.g., rising PSA on anti-androgen therapy or post-orchiectomy); clinical metastases (for use in a Medicare-approved demonstration project) ♂   M

✳ **G9133** Oncology; disease status; prostate cancer, limited to adenocarcinoma; hormone-responsive; clinical metastases or M1 at diagnosis (for use in a Medicare-approved demonstration project) ♂   M

✳ **G9134** Oncology; disease status; non-Hodgkin's lymphoma, any cellular classification; stage I, II at diagnosis, not relapsed, not refractory (for use in a Medicare-approved demonstration project)   M

✳ **G9135** Oncology; disease status; non-Hodgkin's lymphoma, any cellular classification; stage III, IV, not relapsed, not refractory (for use in a Medicare-approved demonstration project)   M

✳ **G9136** Oncology; disease status; non-Hodgkin's lymphoma, transformed from original cellular diagnosis to a second cellular classification (for use in a Medicare-approved demonstration project)   M

✳ **G9137** Oncology; disease status; non-Hodgkin's lymphoma, any cellular classification; relapsed/refractory (for use in a Medicare-approved demonstration project)   M

 PQRI   **Qp** Quantity Physician Appendix B   **Qh** Quantity Hospital Appendix C   ♀ **Female only**

♂ **Male only**   **A** Age   � **DMEPOS**   A2-Z3 ASC Payment Indicator   A-Y ASC Status Indicator   Coding Clinic

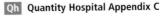

* **G9138** Oncology; disease status; non-Hodgkin's lymphoma, any cellular classification; diagnostic evaluation, stage not determined, evaluation of possible relapse or non-response to therapy, or not listed (for use in a Medicare-approved demonstration project)   M

* **G9139** Oncology; disease status; chronic myelogenous leukemia, limited to Philadelphia chromosome positive and/or BCR-ABL positive; extent of disease unknown, staging in progress, not listed (for use in a Medicare-approved demonstration project)   M

* **G9140** Frontier extended stay clinic demonstration; for a patient stay in a clinic approved for the CMS demonstration project; the following measures should be present: the stay must be equal to or greater than 4 hours; weather or other conditions must prevent transfer or the case falls into a category of monitoring and observation cases that are permitted by the rules of the demonstration; there is a maximum frontier extended stay clinic (FESC) visit of 48 hours, except in the case when weather or other conditions prevent transfer; payment is made on each period up to 4 hours, after the first 4 hours   A

Influenza A (H1N1) and Warfarin Responsiveness Testing

* **G9141** Influenza A (H1N1) immunization administration (includes the physician counseling the patient/family)   S

Payment for G9141 will be the same as that for G0008 and G0009, which is currently based on 90471. Beneficiary copayment and deductible do not apply. Bill the H1N1 flu administration with V04.81

Coding Clinic: 2010, Q3, P9; 2009, Q3, P10

* **G9142** Influenza A (H1N1) vaccine, any route of administration   E

http://www.cdc.gov/h1n1flu/

Under OPPS, G9142 will be assigned status indicator "E," indicating that payment will not be made by Medicare when this code is submitted for an outpatient service. (Transmittal 1803, October 1, 2009)

Coding Clinic: 2010, Q3, P9; 2009, Q3, P10

* **G9143** Warfarin responsiveness testing by genetic technique using any method, any number of specimen(s)   A

This would be a once-in-a-lifetime test unless there is a reason to believe that the patient's personal genetic characteristics would change over time. (https://www.cms.gov/ContractorLearningResources/downloads/JA6715.pdf)

Coding Clinic: 2010, Q2, P10

▶ ◆ **G9147** Outpatient intravenous insulin treatment (OIVIT) either pulsatile or continuous, by any means, guided by the results of measurements for: respiratory quotient; and/or, urine urea nitrogen (UUN); and/or, arterial, venous or capillary glucose; and/or potassium concentration   E

On December 23, 2009, CMS issued a national non-coverage decision on the use of OIVIT. CR 6775.

Not covered on Physician Fee Schedule

Coding Clinic: 2010, Q2, P10

▶ * **G9156** Evaluation for wheelchair requiring face to face visit with physician   M

▶ New   → Revised   ✔ Reinstated   ~~deleted~~ Deleted

☺ Special coverage instructions   ◆ Not covered or valid by Medicare   * Carrier discretion

BEHAVIORAL HEALTH AND/OR SUBSTANCE ABUSE TREATMENT SERVICES (H0001-H9999)

Used by Medicaid state agencies because no national code exists to meet the reporting needs of these agencies.

◆ **H0001** Alcohol and/or drug assessment

◆ **H0002** Behavioral health screening to determine eligibility for admission to treatment program

◆ **H0003** Alcohol and/or drug screening; laboratory analysis of specimens for presence of alcohol and/or drugs

◆ **H0004** Behavioral health counseling and therapy, per 15 minutes

◆ **H0005** Alcohol and/or drug services; group counseling by a clinician

◆ **H0006** Alcohol and/or drug services; case management

◆ **H0007** Alcohol and/or drug services; crisis intervention (outpatient)

◆ **H0008** Alcohol and/or drug services; sub-acute detoxification (hospital inpatient)

◆ **H0009** Alcohol and/or drug services; acute detoxification (hospital inpatient)

◆ **H0010** Alcohol and/or drug services; sub-acute detoxification (residential addiction program inpatient)

◆ **H0011** Alcohol and/or drug services; acute detoxification (residential addiction program inpatient)

◆ **H0012** Alcohol and/or drug services; sub-acute detoxification (residential addiction program outpatient)

◆ **H0013** Alcohol and/or drug services; acute detoxification (residential addiction program outpatient)

◆ **H0014** Alcohol and/or drug services; ambulatory detoxification

◆ **H0015** Alcohol and/or drug services; intensive outpatient (treatment program that operates at least 3 hours/day and at least 3 days/week and is based on an individualized treatment plan), including assessment, counseling; crisis intervention, and activity therapies or education

◆ **H0016** Alcohol and/or drug services; medical/somatic (medical intervention in ambulatory setting)

◆ **H0017** Behavioral health; residential (hospital residential treatment program), without room and board, per diem

◆ **H0018** Behavioral health; short-term residential (non-hospital residential treatment program), without room and board, per diem

◆ **H0019** Behavioral health; long-term residential (non-medical, non-acute care in a residential treatment program where stay is typically longer than 30 days), without room and board, per diem

◆ **H0020** Alcohol and/or drug services; methadone administration and/or service (provision of the drug by a licensed program)

◆ **H0021** Alcohol and/or drug training service (for staff and personnel not employed by providers)

◆ **H0022** Alcohol and/or drug intervention service (planned facilitation)

◆ **H0023** Behavioral health outreach service (planned approach to reach a targeted population)

◆ **H0024** Behavioral health prevention information dissemination service (one-way direct or non-direct contact with service audiences to affect knowledge and attitude)

◆ **H0025** Behavioral health prevention education service (delivery of services with target population to affect knowledge, attitude and/or behavior)

◆ **H0026** Alcohol and/or drug prevention process service, community-based (delivery of services to develop skills of impactors)

◆ **H0027** Alcohol and/or drug prevention environmental service (broad range of external activities geared toward modifying systems in order to mainstream prevention through policy and law)

◆ **H0028** Alcohol and/or drug prevention problem identification and referral service (e.g. student assistance and employee assistance programs), does not include assessment

◆ **H0029** Alcohol and/or drug prevention alternatives service (services for populations that exclude alcohol and other drug use e.g. alcohol-free social events)

◆ **H0030** Behavioral health hotline service

◆ **H0031** Mental health assessment, by non-physician

◆ **H0032** Mental health service plan development by non-physician

◆ **H0033** Oral medication administration, direct observation

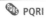 PQRI	**Qp** Quantity Physician Appendix B	**Qh** Quantity Hospital Appendix C	♀ Female only
♂ Male only	**A** Age	🦽 DMEPOS	A2-Z3 ASC Payment Indicator	A-Y ASC Status Indicator	Coding Clinic

221

◆ **H0034** Medication training and support, per 15 minutes

◆ **H0035** Mental health partial hospitalization, treatment, less than 24 hours

◆ **H0036** Community psychiatric supportive treatment, face-to-face, per 15 minutes

◆ **H0037** Community psychiatric supportive treatment program, per diem

◆ **H0038** Self-help/peer services, per 15 minutes

◆ **H0039** Assertive community treatment, face-to-face, per 15 minutes

◆ **H0040** Assertive community treatment program, per diem

◆ **H0041** Foster care, child, non-therapeutic, per diem **A**

◆ **H0042** Foster care, child, non-therapeutic, per month **A**

◆ **H0043** Supported housing, per diem

◆ **H0044** Supported housing, per month

◆ **H0045** Respite care services, not in the home, per diem

◆ **H0046** Mental health services, not otherwise specified

◆ **H0047** Alcohol and/or other drug abuse services, not otherwise specified

◆ **H0048** Alcohol and/or other drug testing: collection and handling only, specimens other than blood

◆ **H0049** Alcohol and/or drug screening

◆ **H0050** Alcohol and/or drug services, brief intervention, per 15 minutes

◆ **H1000** Prenatal care, at-risk assessment ♀

◆ **H1001** Prenatal care, at-risk enhanced service; antepartum management ♀

◆ **H1002** Prenatal care, at-risk enhanced service; care coordination ♀

◆ **H1003** Prenatal care, at-risk enhanced service; education ♀

◆ **H1004** Prenatal care, at-risk enhanced service; follow-up home visit ♀

◆ **H1005** Prenatal care, at-risk enhanced service package (includes H1001-H1004) ♀

◆ **H1010** Non-medical family planning education, per session

◆ **H1011** Family assessment by licensed behavioral health professional for state defined purposes

◆ **H2000** Comprehensive multidisciplinary evaluation

◆ **H2001** Rehabilitation program, per 1/2 day

◆ **H2010** Comprehensive medication services, per 15 minutes

◆ **H2011** Crisis intervention service, per 15 minutes

◆ **H2012** Behavioral health day treatment, per hour

◆ **H2013** Psychiatric health facility service, per diem

◆ **H2014** Skills training and development, per 15 minutes

◆ **H2015** Comprehensive community support services, per 15 minutes

◆ **H2016** Comprehensive community support services, per diem

◆ **H2017** Psychosocial rehabilitation services, per 15 minutes

◆ **H2018** Psychosocial rehabilitation services, per diem

◆ **H2019** Therapeutic behavioral services, per 15 minutes

◆ **H2020** Therapeutic behavioral services, per diem

◆ **H2021** Community-based wrap-around services, per 15 minutes

◆ **H2022** Community-based wrap-around services, per diem

◆ **H2023** Supported employment, per 15 minutes

◆ **H2024** Supported employment, per diem

◆ **H2025** Ongoing support to maintain employment, per 15 minutes

◆ **H2026** Ongoing support to maintain employment, per diem

◆ **H2027** Psychoeducational service, per 15 minutes

◆ **H2028** Sexual offender treatment service, per 15 minutes

◆ **H2029** Sexual offender treatment service, per diem

◆ **H2030** Mental health clubhouse services, per 15 minutes

◆ **H2031** Mental health clubhouse services, per diem

◆ **H2032** Activity therapy, per 15 minutes

◆ **H2033** Multisystemic therapy for juveniles, per 15 minutes

◆ **H2034** Alcohol and/or drug abuse halfway house services, per diem

◆ **H2035** Alcohol and/or other drug treatment program, per hour

◆ **H2036** Alcohol and/or other drug treatment program, per diem

◆ **H2037** Developmental delay prevention activities, dependent child of client, per 15 minutes **A**

▶ New   → Revised   ✔ Reinstated   ~~deleted~~ Deleted

◎ Special coverage instructions   ◆ Not covered or valid by Medicare   ✳ Carrier discretion

DRUGS OTHER THAN CHEMOTHERAPY
(J0100-J9999)

J0120-J3570: Bill local carrier if incident to a physician's service or used in an implanted infusion pump. If other, bill DME/MAC.

✪ **J0120** Injection, tetracycline, **up to 250 mg**   N1   N

Other: Achromycin

IOM: 100-02, 15, 50

→ ✳ **J0129** Injection, abatacept, **10 mg**   K2   K

Other: Orencia

✪ **J0130** Injection, abciximab, **10 mg** (Code may be used for Medicare when drug administered under the direct supervision of a physician; not for use when drug is self-administered)   K2   K

NDC: ReoPro

IOM: 100-02, 15, 50

▶ ✳ **J0131** Injection, acetaminophen, **10 mg**   K2   G

✳ **J0132** Injection, acetylcysteine, **100 mg**   K2   K

✳ **J0133** Injection, acyclovir, **5 mg**   N1   N

✳ **J0135** Injection, adalimumab, **20 mg**   K2   K

NDC: Humira

IOM: 100-02, 15, 50

✪ **J0150** Injection, adenosine, for therapeutic use, **6 mg** (not to be used to report any adenosine phosphate compounds, instead use A9270)   N1   N

NDC: Adenocard

IOM: 100-02, 15, 50

Coding Clinic: 2002, Q2, P10

✳ **J0152** Injection, adenosine, for diagnostic use, **30 mg** (not to be used to report any adenosine phosphate compounds; instead use A9270)   K2   K

NDC: Adenoscan

▶ ✪ **J0171** Injection, adrenalin, epinephrine, **0.1 mg**   N1   N

IOM: 100-02, 15, 50

Coding Clinic: 2011, Q1, P8

✳ **J0180** Injection, agalsidase beta, **1 mg**   K2   K

NDC: Fabrazyme

IOM: 100-02, 15, 50

✪ **J0190** Injection, biperiden lactate, **per 5 mg**   E

Other: Akineton

IOM: 100-02, 15, 50

✪ **J0200** Injection, alatrofloxacin mesylate, **100 mg**   N1   N

Other: Trovan

IOM: 100-02, 15, 50

✪ **J0205** Injection, alglucerase, **per 10 units**   K2   K

NDC: Ceredase

IOM: 100-02, 15, 50

✪ **J0207** Injection, amifostine, **500 mg**   K2   K

NDC: Ethyol

IOM: 100-02, 15, 50

✪ **J0210** Injection, methyldopa HCL, **up to 250 mg**   K2   K

Other: Aldomet

IOM: 100-02, 15, 50

✳ **J0215** Injection, alefacept, **0.5 mg**   K2   K

NDC: Amevive

→ ✳ **J0220** Injection, alglucosidase alfa, not otherwise specified, **10 mg**   K2   K

▶ ✳ **J0221** Injection, alglucosidase alfa, (lumizyme), **10 mg**   K2   G

NDC: Myozyme

→ ✪ **J0256** Injection, alpha 1 - proteinase inhibitor (human), not otherwise specified, **10 mg**   K2   K

NDC: Aralast, Aralast NP, Prolastin, Prolastin-C, Zemaira

IOM: 100-02, 15, 50

▶ ✪ **J0257** Injection, alpha 1 proteinase inhibitor (human), (glassia), **10 mg**   K2   K

IOM: 100-02, 15, 50

✪ **J0270** Injection, alprostadil, **per 1.25 mcg** (Code may be used for Medicare when drug administered under the direct supervision of a physician, not for use when drug is self administered)   B

NDC: Caverject, Caverject Impulse, Edex, Prostin VR

Other: Prostaglandin E1

IOM: 100-02, 15, 50

✪ **J0275** Alprostadil urethral suppository (Code may be used for Medicare when drug administered under the direct supervision of a physician, not for use when drug is self administered)   B

Other: Muse

IOM: 100-02, 15, 50

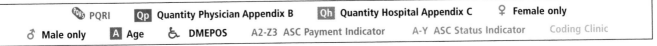

PQRI	**Qp** Quantity Physician Appendix B	**Qh** Quantity Hospital Appendix C	♀ Female only
♂ Male only **A** Age ⚕ DMEPOS	A2-Z3 ASC Payment Indicator	A-Y ASC Status Indicator	Coding Clinic

✳ **J0278** Injection, amikacin sulfate, **100 mg** N1 N

Other: Amikin

⊛ **J0280** Injection, aminophylline, **up to 250 mg** N1 N

IOM: 100-02, 15, 50

⊛ **J0282** Injection, amiodarone hydrochloride, **30 mg** N1 N

Other: Cordarone

IOM: 100-02, 15, 50

⊛ **J0285** Injection, amphotericin B, **50 mg** N1 N

Other: ABLC, Amphocin, Fungizone

IOM: 100-02, 15, 50

⊛ **J0287** Injection, amphotericin B lipid complex, **10 mg** K2 K

NDC: Abelcet

IOM: 100-02, 15, 50

⊛ **J0288** Injection, amphotericin B cholesteryl sulfate complex, **10 mg** K2 K

NDC: Amphotec

Other: Abelcet

IOM: 100-02, 15, 50

⊛ **J0289** Injection, amphotericin B liposome, **10 mg** K2 K

NDC: AmBisome

Other: Abelcet

IOM: 100-02, 15, 50

⊛ **J0290** Injection, ampicillin sodium, **500 mg** N1 N

Other: Omnipen-N, Polycillin-N, Totacillin-N

IOM: 100-02, 15, 50

⊛ **J0295** Injection, ampicillin sodium/sulbactam sodium, **per 1.5 gm** N1 N

NDC: Unasyn

Other: Omnipen-N, Polycillin-N, Totacillin-N

IOM: 100-02, 15, 50

⊛ **J0300** Injection, amobarbital, **up to 125 mg** K2 K

Other: Amytal

IOM: 100-02, 15, 50

⊛ **J0330** Injection, succinylcholine chloride, **up to 20 mg** N1 N

Other: Anectine, Quelicin

IOM: 100-02, 15, 50

✳ **J0348** Injection, anidulafungin, **1 mg** K2 K

NDC: Eraxis

⊛ **J0350** Injection, anistreplase, **per 30 units** E

Other: Eminase

IOM: 100-02, 15, 50

⊛ **J0360** Injection, hydralazine hydrochloride, **up to 20 mg** N1 N

Other: Apresoline

IOM: 100-02, 15, 50

✳ **J0364** Injection, apomorphine hydrochloride, **1 mg** K2 K

NDC: Apokyn

⊛ **J0365** Injection, aprotinin, **10,000 KIU** N1 N

NDC: Trasylol

IOM: 100-02, 15, 50

⊛ **J0380** Injection, metaraminol bitartrate, **per 10 mg** N1 N

Other: Aramine

IOM: 100-02, 15, 50

⊛ **J0390** Injection, chloroquine hydrochloride, **up to 250 mg** N1 N

Benefit only for diagnosed malaria or amebiasis

Other: Aralen

IOM: 100-02, 15, 50

⊛ **J0395** Injection, arbutamine HCL, **1 mg** E

IOM: 100-02, 15, 50

✳ **J0400** Injection, aripiprazole, intramuscular, **0.25 mg** N1 N

Other: Abilify

⊛ **J0456** Injection, azithromycin, **500 mg** N1 N

NDC: Zithromax

IOM: 100-02, 15, 50

⊛ **J0461** Injection, atropine sulfate, **0.01 mg** N1 N

IOM: 100-02, 15, 50

⊛ **J0470** Injection, dimercaprol, per 100 mg N1 N

NDC: BAL In Oil

IOM: 100-02, 15, 50

⊛ **J0475** Injection, baclofen, **10 mg** K2 K

NDC: Gablofen, Lioresal

IOM: 100-02, 15, 50

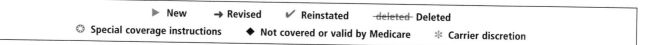

▶ **New** → **Revised** ✔ **Reinstated** ~~deleted~~ **Deleted**
⊛ **Special coverage instructions** ◆ **Not covered or valid by Medicare** ✳ **Carrier discretion**

✿ **J0476** Injection, baclofen **50 mcg** for intrathecal trial K2 K

NDC: Gablofen, Lioresal

IOM: 100-02, 15, 50

✿ **J0480** Injection, basiliximab, **20 mg** K2 K

NDC: Simulect

IOM: 100-02, 15, 50

▶ ✳ **J0490** Injection, belimumab, **10 mg** K2 G

✿ **J0500** Injection, dicyclomine HCL, **up to 20 mg** N1 N

NDC: Bentyl

Other: Antispas, Dibent, Dicyclocot, Dilomine, Di-Spa, Neoquess, Or-Tyl, Spasmoject

IOM: 100-02, 15, 50

✿ **J0515** Injection, benztropine mesylate, **per 1 mg** N1 N

NDC: Cogentin

IOM: 100-02, 15, 50

✿ **J0520** Injection, bethanechol chloride, myotonachol or urecholine, **up to 5 mg** N1 N

IOM: 100-02, 15, 50

▶ ✳ **J0558** Injection, penicillin G benzathine and penicillin G procaine, **100,000 units** N1 N

NDC: Bicillin C-R

Coding Clinic: 2011, Q1, P8

▶ ✿ **J0561** Injection, penicillin G benzathine, **100,000 units** N1 N

NDC: Bicillin L-A

IOM: 100-02, 15, 50

Coding Clinic: 2011, Q1, P8

✳ **J0583** Injection, bivalirudin, **1 mg** K2 K

NDC: Angiomax

✳ **J0585** Injection, onabotulinumtoxinaA, **1 unit** K2 K

NDC: Botox, Botox Cosmetic

Other: Oculinum

IOM: 100-02, 15, 50

✳ **J0586** Injection, abobotulinumtoxinaA, **5 units** K2 K

NDC: Dysport

✳ **J0587** Injection, rimabotulinumtoxinB, **100 units** K2 K

NDC: Myobloc

IOM: 100-02, 15, 50

▶ ✳ **J0588** Injection, incobotulinumtoxin A, **1 unit** K2 G

✿ **J0592** Injection, buprenorphine hydrochloride, **0.1 mg** N1 N

NDC: Buprenex

IOM: 100-02, 15, 50

✳ **J0594** Injection, busulfan, **1 mg** K2 K

✳ **J0595** Injection, butorphanol tartrate, **1 mg** N1 N

NDC: Stadol

▶ ✳ **J0597** Injection, C-1 esterase inhibitor (human), Berinet, **10 units** K2 G

Coding Clinic: 2011, Q1, P7

➔ ✳ **J0598** Injection, C1 esterase inhibitor (human), cinryze, **10 units** K2 K

✿ **J0600** Injection, edetate calcium disodium, **up to 1000 mg** K2 K

NDC: Calcium Disodium Versenate

IOM: 100-02, 15, 50

✿ **J0610** Injection, calcium gluconate, **per 10 ml** N1 N

Other: Kaleinate

IOM: 100-02, 15, 50

✿ **J0620** Injection, calcium glycerophosphate and calcium lactate, **per 10 ml** N1 N

Other: Calphosan

MCM 2049

IOM: 100-02, 15, 50

✿ **J0630** Injection, calcitonin (salmon), **up to 400 units** N1 N

NDC: Miacalcin

Other: Calcimar, Calcitonin-salmon

IOM: 100-02, 15, 50

✿ **J0636** Injection, calcitriol, **0.1 mcg** N1 N

Non-dialysis use

NDC: Calcijex

Other: Calcitriol in almond oil

IOM: 100-02, 15, 50

✳ **J0637** Injection, caspofungin acetate, **5 mg** K2 K

NDC: Cancidas

▶ ✳ **J0638** Injection, canakinumab, **1 mg** K2 G

NDC: Ilaris

✿ **J0640** Injection, leucovorin calcium, **per 50 mg** N1 N

Other: Wellcovorin

IOM: 100-02, 15, 50

Coding Clinic: 2009, Q1, P10

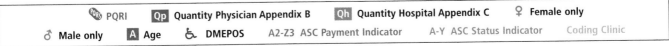

⊛ **J0641** Injection, levoleucovorin calcium, **0.5 mg** K2 K

Part of treatment regimen for osteosarcoma

⊛ **J0670** Injection, mepivacaine HCL, **per 10 ml** N1 N

NDC: Carbocaine, Polocaine, Polocaine-MPF

Other: Isocaine HCl

IOM: 100-02, 15, 50

⊛ **J0690** Injection, cefezolin sodium, **500 mg** N1 N

NDC: Ancef, Kefzol

IOM: 100-02, 15, 50

✳ **J0692** Injection, cefepime HCL, **500 mg** N1 N

NDC: Maxipime

⊛ **J0694** Injection, cefoxitin sodium, **1 gm** N1 N

NDC: Mefoxin

IOM: 100-02, 15, 50,

Cross Reference Q0090

⊛ **J0696** Injection, ceftriaxone sodium, **per 250 mg** N1 N

NDC: Rocephin

IOM: 100-02, 15, 50

⊛ **J0697** Injection, sterile cefuroxime sodium, **per 750 mg** N1 N

NDC: Zinacef

Other: Kefurox

IOM: 100-02, 15, 50

⊛ **J0698** Injection, cefotaxime sodium, **per g** N1 N

NDC: Claforan

IOM: 100-02, 15, 50

⊛ **J0702** Injection, betamethasone acetate **3 mg** and betamethasone sodium phosphate **3 mg** N1 N

NDC: Celestone Soluspan

IOM: 100-02, 15, 50

✳ **J0706** Injection, caffeine citrate, **5 mg** N1 N

Other: Cafcit, Cipro IV, Ciprofloxacin

⊛ **J0710** Injection, cephapirin sodium, **up to 1 gm** N1 N

Other: Cefadyl

IOM: 100-02, 15, 50

▶ ✳ **J0712** Injection, ceftaroline fosamil, **10 mg** K2 G

⊛ **J0713** Injection, ceftazidime, **per 500 mg** N1 N

NDC: Fortaz, Tazicef

IOM: 100-02, 15, 50

⊛ **J0715** Injection, ceftizoxime sodium, **per 500 mg** N1 N

Other: Cefizox

IOM: 100-02, 15, 50

✳ **J0718** Injection, certolizumab pegol, **1 mg** K2 K

NDC: Cimzia

⊛ **J0720** Injection, chloramphenicol sodium succinate, **up to 1 gm** N1 N

IOM: 100-02, 15, 50

⊛ **J0725** Injection, chorionic gonadotropin, **per 1,000 USP units** N1 N

NDC: Pregnyl, Novarel

Other: A.P.L., Chorex-5, Chorex-10, Chorignon, Choron-10, Corgonject-5, Follutein, Glukor, Gonic, Profasi HP

IOM: 100-02, 15, 50

⊛ **J0735** Injection, clonidine hydrochloride (HCL), **1 mg** N1 N

NDC: Duraclon

IOM: 100-02, 15, 50

⊛ **J0740** Injection, cidofovir, **375 mg** K2 K

NDC: Vistide

IOM: 100-02, 15, 50

⊛ **J0743** Injection, cilastatin sodium; imipenem, **per 250 mg** N1 N

NDC: Primaxin

IOM: 100-02, 15, 50

✳ **J0744** Injection, ciprofloxacin for intravenous infusion, **200 mg** N1 N

Other: Cipro IV

⊛ **J0745** Injection, codeine phosphate, **per 30 mg** N1 N

IOM: 100-02, 15, 50

⊛ **J0760** Injection, colchicine, **per 1 mg** N1 N

IOM: 100-02, 15, 50

⊛ **J0770** Injection, colistimethate sodium, **up to 150 mg** N1 N

NDC: Coly-Mycin M

IOM: 100-02, 15, 50

▶ ✳ **J0775** Injection, collagenase, clostridium histolyticum, **0.01 mg** K2 G

NDC: Xiaflex

Coding Clinic: 2011, Q1, P7

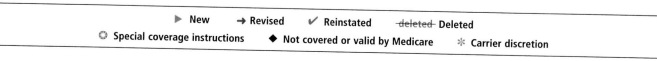

▶ New   → Revised   ✔ Reinstated   ~~deleted~~ Deleted
⊛ Special coverage instructions   ◆ Not covered or valid by Medicare   ✳ Carrier discretion

⊛ **J0780** Injection, prochlorperazine, **up to 10 mg** N1 N

Other: Compa-Z, Compazine, Cotranzine, Ultrazine-10

IOM: 100-02, 15, 50

⊛ **J0795** Injection, corticorelin ovine triflutate, **1 microgram** K2 K

NDC: Acthrel

IOM: 100-02, 15, 50

⊛ **J0800** Injection, corticotropin, **up to 40 units** K2 K

NDC: Acthar H.P.

Other: H.P. Acthar, ACTH

IOM: 100-02, 15, 50

✳ **J0833** Injection, cosyntropin, not otherwise specified, **0.25 mg** K2 K

✳ **J0834** Injection, cosyntropin (Cortrosyn), **0.25 mg** N1 N

▶ ✳ **J0840** Injection, crotalidae polyvalent immune fab (ovine), **up to 1 gram** K2 G

⊛ **J0850** Injection, cytomegalovirus immune globulin intravenous (human), **per vial** K2 K

Prophylaxis to prevent cytomegalovirus disease associated with transplantation of kidney, lung, liver, pancreas, and heart.

NDC: CytoGam

IOM: 100-02, 15, 50

✳ **J0878** Injection, daptomycin, **1 mg** K2 K

NDC: Cubicin

⊛ **J0881** Injection, darbepoetin alfa, **1 microgram** (non-ESRD use) K2 K

NDC: Aranesp

⊛ **J0882** Injection, darbepoetin alfa, **1 microgram** (for ESRD on dialysis) A

NDC: Aranesp

IOM: 100-02, 6, 10; 100-04, 4, 240

⊛ **J0885** Injection, epoetin alfa, (for non-ESRD use), **1000 units** K2 K

NDC: Epogen, Procrit

IOM: 100-02, 15, 50

Coding Clinic: 2006, Q2, P5

⊛ **J0886** Injection, epoetin alfa, **1000 units** (for ESRD on dialysis) A

NDC: Epogen, Procrit

IOM: 100-02, 6, 10; 100-04, 4, 240

Coding Clinic: 2006, Q2, P5

✳ **J0894** Injection, decitabine, **1 mg** K2 K

Indicated for treatment of myelodysplastic syndromes (MDS)

⊛ **J0895** Injection, deferoxamine mesylate, **500 mg** N1 N

NDC: Desferal

Other: Desferal mesylate

IOM: 100-02, 15, 50,

Cross Reference Q0087

▶ ✳ **J0897** Injection, denosumab, **1 mg** K2 G

⊛ **J0900** Injection, testosterone enanthate and estradiol valerate, **up to 1 cc** N1 N

Other: Andrest 90-4, Andro-Estro 90-4, Androgyn L.A., Deladumone, Deladumone OB, Delatest, Delatestadiol, Ditate-DS, Dua-Gen LA, Duoval PA, Estra-Testrin, TEEV, Testadiate, Testradiol 90/4, Valertest

IOM: 100-02, 15, 50

⊛ **J0945** Injection, brompheniramine maleate, **per 10 mg** N1 N

Other: Codimal-A, Cophene-B, Dehist, Histaject, Nasahist B, ND Stat, Oraminic II, Sinusol-B

IOM: 100-02, 15, 50

⊛ **J1000** Injection, depo-estradiol cypionate, **up to 5 mg** N1 N

Other: Depogen, DepGynogen, Dura-Estrin, Estra-D, Estro-Cyp, Estroject LA, Estronol-LA

IOM: 100-02, 15, 50

⊛ **J1020** Injection, methylprednisolone acetate, **20 mg** N1 N

NDC: Depo-Medrol, Methylpred

Other: DepMedalone, Depoject, Depopred, D-Med 80, Duralone, Medralone, M-Prednisol, Rep-Pred

IOM: 100-02, 15, 50

Coding Clinic: 2005, Q3, P10

 PQRI   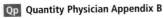 **Qp** Quantity Physician Appendix B   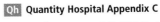 **Qh** Quantity Hospital Appendix C   ♀ **Female only**

♂ **Male only**   **A** Age   ♿ **DMEPOS**   A2-Z3 **ASC Payment Indicator**   A-Y **ASC Status Indicator**   Coding Clinic

⊛ **J1030** Injection, methylprednisolone acetate,
40 mg   N1 N

NDC: Depo-Medrol

*Other: DepMedalone, Depoject,
Depropred, D-Med 80, Duralone,
Medralone, M-Prednisol, Rep-Pred*

IOM: 100-02, 15, 50

Coding Clinic: 2005, Q3, P10

⊛ **J1040** Injection, methylprednisolone acetate,
80 mg   N1 N

NDC: Depo-Medrol

*Other: DepMedalone, Depoject,
Depropred, D-Med 80, Duralone,
Medralone, M-Prednisol, Rep-Pred*

IOM: 100-02, 15, 50

⊛ **J1051** Injection, medroxyprogesterone
acetate, **50 mg** ♀   N1 N

NDC: Depo-Provera

IOM: 100-02, 15, 50

◆ **J1055** Injection, medroxyprogesterone acetate
for contraceptive use, **150 mg** ♀   E

Other: Depo Provera

Medicare Statute 1862a1

✳ **J1056** Injection, medroxyprogesterone acetate/
estradiol cypionate, **5 mg/25 mg** ♀   E

Other: Lunelle

⊛ **J1060** Injection, testosterone cypionate and
estradiol cypionate, **up to 1 ml**   N1 N

*Other: Andro/Fem, De-Comberol,
DepAndrogyn, Depo-Testadiol,
Depotestogen, Duratestrin, Estradiol
cypionate, Test-Estro-C, Test-Estro
Cypionates, Valertest No. 1*

IOM: 100-02, 15, 50

⊛ **J1070** Injection, testosterone cypionate, **up to
100 mg**   N1 N

NDC: Depo-Testosterone

*Other: Andro-Cyp, Andronaq-LA,
Andronate, DepAndro, Depotest,
Duratest, Testa-C, Testadiate-Depo,
Testaject-LA, Testoject-LA,*

IOM: 100-02, 15, 50

⊛ **J1080** Injection, testosterone cypionate, **1 cc,
200 mg**   N1 N

NDC: Depo-Testosterone

*Other: Andro-Cyp, Andronaq-LA,
Andronate, DepAndro, Depotest,
Duratest, Testa-C, Testadiate-Depo,
Testaject-LA, Testoject-LA*

IOM: 100-02, 15, 50

⊛ **J1094** Injection, dexamethasone acetate,
1 mg   N1 N

*Other: Cortastat LA, Dalalone LA,
Decadrone LA, Decaject LA,
Dexacen-LA-8, Dexamethasone
Micronized, Dexasone L.A., Dexone-LA*

IOM: 100-02, 15, 50

⊛ **J1100** Injection, dexamethasone sodium
phosphate, **1 mg**   N1 N

*Other: Cortastat 10, Dalalone, Decadron
Phosphate, Decaject, Dexacen-4, Dexone,
Hexadrol Phosphate, Solurex*

IOM: 100-02, 15, 50

⊛ **J1110** Injection, dihydroergotamine mesylate,
per 1 mg   N1 N

NDC: D.H.E. 45

IOM: 100-02, 15, 50

⊛ **J1120** Injection, acetazolamide sodium, **up to
500 mg**   N1 N

Other: Diamox

IOM: 100-02, 15, 50

⊛ **J1160** Injection, digoxin, **up to
0.5 mg**   N1 N

NDC: Lanoxin

IOM: 100-02, 15, 50

⊛ **J1162** Injection, digoxin immune Fab (ovine),
per vial   K2 K

NDC: Digibind, DigiFab

IOM: 100-02, 15, 50

⊛ **J1165** Injection, phenytoin sodium, **per
50 mg**   N1 N

Other: Dilantin

IOM: 100-02, 15, 50

⊛ **J1170** Injection, hydromorphone, **up to
4 mg**   N1 N

NDC: Dilaudid, Dilaudid-HP

IOM: 100-02, 15, 50

⊛ **J1180** Injection, dyphylline, **up to
500 mg**   N1 N

Other: Dilor, Lufyllin

IOM: 100-02, 15, 50

⊛ **J1190** Injection, dexrazoxane hydrochloride,
per 250 mg   K2 K

NDC: Totect, Zinecard

IOM: 100-02, 15, 50

▶ **New**   → **Revised**   ✔ **Reinstated**   ~~deleted~~ **Deleted**

⊛ **Special coverage instructions**   ◆ **Not covered or valid by Medicare**   ✳ **Carrier discretion**

⊕ **J1200**   Injection, diphenhydramine HCL, **up to 50 mg**   N1   N

NDC: Benadryl

Other: Bena-D, Truxadryl

IOM: 100-02, 15, 50

⊕ **J1205**   Injection, chlorothiazide sodium, **per 500 mg**   K2   K

NDC: Diuril

IOM: 100-02, 15, 50

⊕ **J1212**   Injection, DMSO, dimethyl sulfoxide, 50%, **50 ml**   K2   K

NDC: Rimso-50

IOM: 100-02, 15, 50; 100-03, 4, 230.12

⊕ **J1230**   Injection, methadone HCL, **up to 10 mg**   N1   N

MCM 2049

IOM: 100-02, 15, 50

⊕ **J1240**   Injection, dimenhydrinate, **up to 50 mg**   N1   N

Other: Dinate, Dommanate, Dramamine, Dramanate, Dramilin, Dramocen, Dramoject, Dymenate, Hydrate, Marmine, Wehamine

IOM: 100-02, 15, 50

⊕ **J1245**   Injection, dipyridamole, **per 10 mg**   N1   N

Other: Persantine

IOM: 100-04, 15, 50; 100-04, 12, 30.6

⊕ **J1250**   Injection, dobutamine HCL, **per 250 mg**   N1   N

Other: Dobutrex

IOM: 100-02, 15, 50

⊕ **J1260**   Injection, dolasetron mesylate, **10 mg**   N1   N

NDC: Anzemet

IOM: 100-02, 15, 50

✳ **J1265**   Injection, dopamine HCL, **40 mg**   N1   N

✳ **J1267**   Injection, doripenem, **10 mg**   N1   N

NDC: Doribax

✳ **J1270**   Injection, doxercalciferol, **1 mcg**   N1   N

NDC: Hectorol

▶ ✳ **J1290**   Injection, ecallantide, **1 mg**   K2   G

NDC: Kalbitor

Coding Clinic: 2011, Q1, P7

✳ **J1300**   Injection, eculizumab, **10 mg**   K2   K

NDC: Soliris

⊕ **J1320**   Injection, amitriptyline HCL, **up to 20 mg**   N1   N

Other: Elavil, Enovil

IOM: 100-02, 15, 50

✳ **J1324**   Injection, enfuvirtide, **1 mg**   K2   K

Other: Fuzeon

⊕ **J1325**   Injection, epoprostenol, **0.5 mg**   N1   N

NDC: Flolan

IOM: 100-02, 15, 50

⊕ **J1327**   Injection, eptifibatide, **5 mg**   K2   K

NDC: Integrilin

IOM: 100-02, 15, 50

⊕ **J1330**   Injection, ergonovine maleate, **up to 0.2 mg**   N1   N

Benefit limited to obstetrical diagnosis

IOM: 100-02, 15, 50

✳ **J1335**   Injection, ertapenem sodium, **500 mg**   N1   N

NDC: Invanz

⊕ **J1364**   Injection, erythromycin lactobionate, **per 500 mg**   N1   N

IOM: 100-02, 15, 50

⊕ **J1380**   Injection, estradiol valerate, **up to 10 mg**   N1   N

NDC: Delestrogen

Other: Dioval, Duragen, Estra-L, Gynogen L.A., L.A.E. 20, Valergen

IOM: 100-02, 15, 50

Coding Clinic: 2011, Q1, P8

⊕ **J1410**   Injection, estrogen conjugated, **per 25 mg**   K2   K

NDC: Premarin

IOM: 100-02, 15, 50

⊕ **J1430**   Injection, ethanolamine oleate, **100 mg**   K2   K

Other: Ethamolin

IOM: 100-02, 15, 50

⊕ **J1435**   Injection, estrone, **per 1 mg**   E

Other: Estragyn, Estronol, Kestrone 5, Theelin Aqueous

IOM: 100-02, 15, 50

⊕ **J1436**   Injection, etidronate disodium, **per 300 mg**   N1   N

Other: Didronel

IOM: 100-02, 15, 50

⊙ **J1438** Injection, etanercept, **25 mg** (Code may be used for Medicare when drug administered under the direct supervision of a physician, not for use when drug is self-administered.) K2 K

NDC: Enbrel

IOM: 100-02, 15, 50

⊙ **J1440** Injection, filgrastim (G-CSF), **300 mcg** K2 K

NDC: Neupogen

IOM: 100-02, 15, 50

⊙ **J1441** Injection, filgrastim (G-CSF), **480 mcg** K2 K

Other: Neupogen

IOM: 100-02, 15, 50

⊙ **J1450** Injection, fluconazole, **200 mg** N1 N

NDC: Diflucan

IOM: 100-02, 15, 50

⊙ **J1451** Injection, fomepizole, **15 mg** K2 K

NDC: Antizol

IOM: 100-02, 15, 50

⊙ **J1452** Injection, fomivirsen sodium, intraocular, **1.65 mg** E

IOM: 100-02, 15, 50

✳ **J1453** Injection, fosaprepitant, **1 mg** K2 K

Prevents chemotherapy-induced nausea and vomiting

NDC: Emend

⊙ **J1455** Injection, foscarnet sodium, **per 1000 mg** K2 K

NDC: Foscavir

IOM: 100-02, 15, 50

✳ **J1457** Injection, gallium nitrate, **1 mg** N1 N

NDC: Ganite

✳ **J1458** Injection, galsulfase, **1 mg** K2 K

NDC: Naglazyme

✳ **J1459** Injection, immune globulin (Privigen), intravenous, non-lyophilized (e.g., liquid), **500 mg** K2 K

⊙ **J1460** Injection, gamma globulin, intramuscular, **1 cc** K2 K

NDC: GamaSTAN, Immune Globulin (Human)

Other: Gammar

IOM: 100-02, 15, 50

Coding Clinic: 2011, Q1, P8

▶ ✳ **J1557** Injection, immune globulin, (gammaplex), intravenous, non-lyophilized (e.g., liquid), **500 mg** K2 G

▶ ✳ **J1559** Injection, immune globulin, (hizentra), **100 mg** K2 K

Coding Clinic: 2011, Q1, P6

⊙ **J1560** Injection, gamma globulin, intramuscular, **over 10 cc** K2 K

NDC: GamaSTAN, Immune Globin (Human)

Other: Gammar

IOM: 100-02, 15, 50

→ ⊙ **J1561** Injection, immune globulin, (Gamunex/ Gamunex-C-Gammaked), non-lyophilized (e.g. liquid), **500 mg** K2 K

NDC: Gamunex

IOM: 100-02, 15, 50

✳ **J1562** Injection, immune globulin (Vivaglobin), **100 mg** K2 K

⊙ **J1566** Injection, immune globulin, intravenous, lyophilized (e.g., powder), not otherwise specified, **500 mg** K2 K

NDC: Carimune, Gammagard S/D, Panglobulin NF

Other: Polygam

IOM: 100-02, 15, 50

✳ **J1568** Injection, immune globulin, (Octagam), intravenous, non-lyophilized (e.g., liquid), **500 mg** K2 K

⊙ **J1569** Injection, immune globulin, (Gammagard Liquid), intravenous, non-lyophilized, (e.g. liquid), **500 mg** K2 K

IOM: 100-02, 15, 50

⊙ **J1570** Injection, ganciclovir sodium, **500 mg** K2 K

NDC: Cytovene

IOM: 100-02, 15, 50

⊙ **J1571** Injection, hepatitis B immune globulin (HepaGam B), intramuscular, **0.5 ml** K2 K

IOM: 100-02, 15, 50

Coding Clinic: 2008, Q3, P7-8

⊙ **J1572** Injection, immune globulin, (flebogamma/flebogamma DIF) intravenous, non-lyophilized (e.g. liquid), **500 mg** K2 G

IOM: 100-02, 15, 50

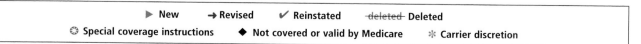

▶ New → Revised ✔ Reinstated ~~deleted~~ Deleted
⊙ Special coverage instructions ◆ Not covered or valid by Medicare ✳ Carrier discretion

✳ **J1573** Injection, hepatitis B immune globulin (HepaGam B), intravenous, **0.5 ml** K2 K

Coding Clinic: 2008, Q3, P8

⚙ **J1580** Injection, Garamycin, gentamicin, **up to 80 mg** N1 N

NDC: Gentamicin Sulfate

Other: Jenamicin

IOM: 100-02, 15, 50

✳ **J1590** Injection, gatifloxacin, **10 mg** N1 N

Other: Tequin

⚙ **J1595** Injection, glatiramer acetate, **20 mg** K2 K

Other: Copaxone

IOM: 100-02, 15, 50

▶ ✳ **J1599** Injection, immune globulin, intravenous, non-lyophilized (e.g., liquid), not otherwise specified, **500 mg** N1 N

Coding Clinic: 2011, P1, Q6

⚙ **J1600** Injection, gold sodium thiomalate, **up to 50 mg** N1 N

NDC: Myochrysine

IOM: 100-02, 15, 50

⚙ **J1610** Injection, glucagon hydrochloride, **per 1 mg** K2 K

NDC: GlucaGen, Glucagon Emergency

IOM: 100-02, 15, 50

⚙ **J1620** Injection, gonadorelin hydrochloride, **per 100 mcg** K2 K

Other: Factrel

IOM: 100-02, 15, 50

⚙ **J1626** Injection, granisetron hydrochloride, **100 mcg** N1 N

NDC: Kytril

IOM: 100-02, 15, 50

⚙ **J1630** Injection, haloperidol, **up to 5 mg** N1 N

NDC: Haldol, Haloperidol Lactate

IOM: 100-02, 15, 50

⚙ **J1631** Injection, haloperidol decanoate, **per 50 mg** N1 N

NDC: Haldol Decanoate

IOM: 100-02, 15, 50

⚙ **J1640** Injection, hemin, **1 mg** K2 K

NDC: Panhematin

IOM: 100-02, 15, 50

⚙ **J1642** Injection, heparin sodium, (heparin lock flush), **per 10 units** K2 K

NDC: Heparine Combination, Heparine (Porcine) In Nacl, Heparin (Porcine) Lock Flush, Heparin Sodium Flush, Heparin Sodium Lock Flush, Hep Flush-10, Hep-Lock, Hep-Lock Flush, Vasceze

Other: Hep-Lock U/P

IOM: 100-02, 15, 50

⚙ **J1644** Injection, heparin sodium, **per 1000 units** K2 K

NDC: Heparin (Porcine), Heparin Sodium (Porcine)

Other: Liquaemin Sodium

IOM: 100-02, 15, 50

⚙ **J1645** Injection, dalteparin sodium, **per 2500 IU** N1 N

NDC: Fragmin

IOM: 100-02, 15, 50

✳ **J1650** Injection, enoxaparin sodium, **10 mg** N1 N

NDC: Lovenox

⚙ **J1652** Injection, fondaparinux sodium, **0.5 mg** N1 N

NDC: Arixtra

IOM: 100-02, 15, 50

✳ **J1655** Injection, tinzaparin sodium, **1000 IU** N1 N

NDC: Innohep

⚙ **J1670** Injection, tetanus immune globulin, human, **up to 250 units** K2 K

Indicated for transient protection against tetanus post-exposure to tetanus (V03.7).

NDC: Hypertet S/D

Other: Hyper-tet

IOM: 100-02, 15, 50

⚙ **J1675** Injection, histrelin acetate, **10 micrograms** B

IOM: 100-02, 15, 50

✳ **J1680** Injection, human fibrinogen concentrate, **100 mg** K2 K

⚙ **J1700** Injection, hydrocortisone acetate, **up to 25 mg** N1 N

Other: Hydrocortone Acetate

IOM: 100-02, 15, 50

🐷 PQRI	**Qp** Quantity Physician Appendix B	**Qh** Quantity Hospital Appendix C	♀ **Female only**
♂ **Male only**	**A** **Age**	♿ **DMEPOS**	A2-Z3 **ASC Payment Indicator** A-Y **ASC Status Indicator** Coding Clinic

⚙ **J1710** Injection, hydrocortisone sodium phosphate, **up to 50 mg**　　N1　N

Other: A-hydroCort, Hydrocortone phosphate, Solu-Cortef

IOM: 100-02, 15, 50

⚙ **J1720** Injection, hydrocortisone sodium succinate, **up to 100 mg**　　N1　N

NDC: A-Hydrocort, Solu-Cortef

IOM: 100-02, 15, 50

▶ ✳ **J1725** Injection, hydroxyprogesterone caproate, **1 mg**　　K2　K

⚙ **J1730** Injection, diazoxide, **up to 300 mg**　　N1　K

Other: Hyperstat

IOM: 100-02, 15, 50

✳ **J1740** Injection, ibandronate sodium, **1 mg**　　K2　K

Other: Boniva

⚙ **J1742** Injection, ibutilide fumarate, **1 mg**　　K2　K

NDC: Corvert

IOM: 100-02, 15, 50

✳ **J1743** Injection, idursulfase, **1 mg**　　K2　K

Other: Elaprase

⚙ **J1745** Injection, infliximab, **10 mg**　　K2　K

Report total number of 10 mg increments administered; medical record must document failed or incomplete control of arthritis with use of other antirheumatic modalities

NDC: Remicade

IOM: 100-02, 15, 50

⚙ **J1750** Injection, iron dextran, **50 mg**　　K2　K

IOM: 100-02, 15, 50

NDC: Dexferrum, Infed

✳ **J1756** Injection, iron sucrose, **1 mg**　　K2　K

NDC: Venofer

▶ ⚙ **J1786** Injection, imiglucerase, **10 units**　　K2　K

NDC: Cerezyme

IOM: 100-02, 15, 50

Coding Clinic: 2011, Q1, P8

⚙ **J1790** Injection, droperidol, **up to 5 mg**　　N1　N

NDC: Inapsine

IOM: 100-02, 15, 50

⚙ **J1800** Injection, propranolol HCL, **up to 1 mg**　　N1　N

NDC: Inderal

IOM: 100-02, 15, 50

⚙ **J1810** Injection, droperidol and fentanyl citrate, **up to 2 ml ampule**　　E

Other: Innovar

IOM: 100-02, 15, 50

⚙ **J1815** Injection, insulin, **per 5 units**　　N1　N

NDC: Apidra, Humalog, Humulin, Iletin-I, Lantus, Novolin, Novolog, Relion

Other: Lispro-PFC

IOM: 100-02, 15, 50; 100-03, 4, 280.14

✳ **J1817** Insulin for administration through DME (i.e., insulin pump) **per 50 units**　　N1　N

NDC: Apidra, Humalog, Humulin, Iletin, Lantus, Novolin, Novolog, Relion

Other: Apidra Solostar, Insulin-Humalog, Insulin Lispro

▶ ◆ **J1826** Injection, interferon beta-1a, **30 mcg**　　E

Coding Clinic: 2011, Q2, P9; Q1, P8

⚙ **J1830** Injection interferon beta-1b, **0.25 mg** (Code may be used for Medicare when drug administered under the direct supervision of a physician, not for use when drug is self administered)　　K2　K

Other: Betaseron

IOM: 100-02, 15, 50

✳ **J1835** Injection, itraconazole, **50 mg**　　K2　K

Other: Sporanox

⚙ **J1840** Injection, kanamycin sulfate, **up to 500 mg**　　N1　N

Other: Kantrex, Klebcil

IOM: 100-02, 15, 50

⚙ **J1850** Injection, kanamycin sulfate, **up to 75 mg**　　N1　N

Other: Kantrex, Klebcil

IOM: 100-02, 15, 50

⚙ **J1885** Injection, ketorolac tromethamine, **per 15 mg**　　N1　N

Other: Toradol

IOM: 100-02, 15, 50

⚙ **J1890** Injection, cephalothin sodium, **up to 1 gram**　　N1　N

Other: Keflin

IOM: 100-02, 15, 50

▶ New　　→ Revised　　✔ Reinstated　　~~deleted~~ Deleted

⚙ Special coverage instructions　　◆ Not covered or valid by Medicare　　✳ Carrier discretion

✳ **J1930** Injection, lanreotide, **1 mg** K2 K

Treats acromegaly and symptoms caused by neuroendocrine tumors

NDC: Somatuline Depot

✳ **J1931** Injection, laronidase, **0.1 mg** K2 K

NDC: Aldurazyme

❂ **J1940** Injection, furosemide, **up to 20 mg** N1 N

Other: Lasix

MCM 2049

IOM: 100-02, 15, 50

❂ **J1945** Injection, lepirudin, **50 mg** K2 K

NDC: Refludan

IOM: 100-02, 15, 50

❂ **J1950** Injection, leuprolide acetate (for depot suspension), **per 3.75 mg** K2 K

NDC: Lupron Depot, Lupron Depot-Ped

IOM: 100-02, 15, 50

✳ **J1953** Injection, levetiracetam, **10 mg** N1 N

❂ **J1955** Injection, levocarnitine, **per 1 gm** B

NDC: Carnitor

Other: L-Carnitine

IOM: 100-02, 15, 50

❂ **J1956** Injection, levofloxacin, **250 mg** N1 N

NDC: Levaquin

IOM: 100-02, 15, 50

❂ **J1960** Injection, levorphanol tartrate, **up to 2 mg** N1 N

Other: Levo-Dromoran

MCM 2049

IOM: 100-02, 15, 50

❂ **J1980** Injection, hyoscyamine sulfate, **up to 0.25 mg** N1 N

NDC: Levsin

IOM: 100-02, 15, 50

❂ **J1990** Injection, chlordiazepoxide HCL, **up to 100 mg** N1 N

Other: Librium

IOM: 100-02, 15, 50

❂ **J2001** Injection, lidocaine HCL for intravenous infusion, **10 mg** N1 N

NDC: Lidocaine in D5W, Xylocaine (Cardiac)

Other: Anestacaine, Caine-1, Dilocaine, L-Caine, Lidoject, Nervocaine, Nulicaine, Xylocaine

IOM: 100-02, 15, 50

❂ **J2010** Injection, lincomycin HCL, **up to 300 mg** N1 N

NDC: Lincocin

IOM: 100-02, 15, 50

✳ **J2020** Injection, linezolid, **200 mg** K2 K

NDC: Zyvox

❂ **J2060** Injection, lorazepam, **2 mg** N1 N

NDC: Ativan

IOM: 100-02, 15, 50

❂ **J2150** Injection, mannitol, **25% in 50 ml** N1 N

MCM 2049

IOM: 100-02, 15, 50

✳ **J2170** Injection, mecasermin, **1 mg** K2 K

Other: Increlex

❂ **J2175** Injection, meperidine hydrochloride, **per 100 mg** N1 N

NDC: Demerol

IOM: 100-02, 15, 50

❂ **J2180** Injection, meperidine and promethazine HCL, **up to 50 mg** N1 N

Other: Mepergan

IOM: 100-02, 15, 50

✳ **J2185** Injection, meropenem, **100 mg** N1 N

NDC: Merrem

❂ **J2210** Injection, methylergonovine maleate, **up to 0.2 mg** N1 N

Benefit limited to obstetrical diagnoses for prevention and control of post-partum hemorrhage

NDC: Methergine

IOM: 100-02, 15, 50

✳ **J2248** Injection, micafungin sodium, **1 mg** K2 K

Other: Mycamine

❂ **J2250** Injection, midazolam hydrochloride, **per 1 mg** N1 N

Other: Versed

IOM: 100-02, 15, 50

❂ **J2260** Injection, milrinone lactate, **5 mg** N1 N

NDC: Primacor

IOM: 100-02, 15, 50

▶ ✳ **J2265** Injection, minocycline hydrochloride, **1 mg**

🅟 PQRI	**Qp** Quantity Physician Appendix B	**Qh** Quantity Hospital Appendix C	♀ Female only	
♂ Male only	🅐 Age	�ɕ DMEPOS	A2-Z3 ASC Payment Indicator	A-Y ASC Status Indicator Coding Clinic

⊙ **J2270**   Injection, morphine sulfate,
up to 10 mg   N1 N

Other: Astromorph PF, Duramorph

IOM: 100-02, 15, 50

⊙ **J2271**   Injection, morphine sulfate,
100 mg   N1 N

Other: Astramorph PF, Duramorph

IOM: 100-02, 15, 50; 100-03, 4, 280.1

⊙ **J2275**   Injection, morphine sulfate
(preservative-free sterile solution),
per 10 mg   N1 N

*NDC: Astramorph, Duramorph,
Infumorph*

IOM: 100-02, 15, 50; 100-03, 4, 280.1

⊙ **J2278**   Injection, ziconotide,
1 microgram   K2 K

NDC: Prialt

✳ **J2280**   Injection, moxifloxacin,
100 mg   N1 N

NDC: Avelox

⊙ **J2300**   Injection, nalbuphine hydrochloride,
per 10 mg   N1 N

NDC: Nubain

IOM: 100-02, 15, 50

⊙ **J2310**   Injection, naloxone hydrochloride,
per 1 mg   N1 N

Other: Narcan

IOM: 100-02, 15, 50

✳ **J2315**   Injection, naltrexone, depot form,
1 mg   K2 K

NDC: Vivitrol

⊙ **J2320**   Injection, nandrolone decanoate, **up to
50 mg**   N1 N

*Other: Anabolin LA 100, Androlone,
Deca-Durabolin, Decolone, Hybolin
Decanoate, Nandrobolic LA,
Neo-Durabolic*

IOM: 100-02, 15, 50

Coding Clinic: 2011, Q1, P8

✳ **J2323**   Injection, natalizumab, **1 mg**   K2 K

Other: Tysabri

⊙ **J2325**   Injection, nesiritide, **0.1 mg**   K2 K

NDC: Natrecor

IOM: 100-02, 15, 50

✳ **J2353**   Injection, octreotide, depot form for
intramuscular injection, **1 mg**   K2 K

NDC: Sandostatin LAR Depot

✳ **J2354**   Injection, octreotide, non-depot form
for subcutaneous or intravenous
injection, **25 mcg**   N1 N

Other: Sandostatin LAR Depot

⊙ **J2355**   Injection, oprelvekin, **5 mg**   K2 K

NDC: Neumega

IOM: 100-02, 15, 50

✳ **J2357**   Injection, omalizumab, **5 mg**   K2 K

NDC: Xolair

▶ ✳ **J2358**   Injection, olanzapine, long-acting,
1 mg   K2 K

NDC: Zyprexa, Relprevv

Coding Clinic: 2011, Q1, P6

⊙ **J2360**   Injection, orphenadrine citrate, **up to
60 mg**   N1 N

NDC: Norflex

*Other: Antiflex, Banflex, Flexoject,
Flexon, K-Flex, Mio-Rel, Neocyten,
O-Flex, Orfro, Orphenate*

IOM: 100-02, 15, 50

⊙ **J2370**   Injection, phenylephrine HCL,
up to 1 ml   N1 N

NDC: Neo-Synephrine

IOM: 100-02, 15, 50

⊙ **J2400**   Injection, chloroprocaine
hydrochloride, **per 30 ml**   N1 N

NDC: Nesacaine, Nesacaine-MPF

IOM: 100-02, 15, 50

⊙ **J2405**   Injection, ondansetron hydrochloride,
per 1 mg   N1 N

NDC: Zofran

IOM: 100-02, 15, 50

⊙ **J2410**   Injection, oxymorphone HCL, **up to
1 mg**   N1 N

NDC: Numorphan, Opana

IOM: 100-02, 15, 50

✳ **J2425**   Injection, palifermin,
50 micrograms   K2 K

NDC: Kepivance

▶ ✳ **J2426**   Injection, paliperidone palmitate
extended release, **1 mg**   K2 K

NDC: Invega Sustenna

Coding Clinic: 2011, Q1, P7

⊙ **J2430**   Injection, pamidronate disodium,
per 30 mg   N1 N

NDC: Aredia

IOM: 100-02, 15, 50

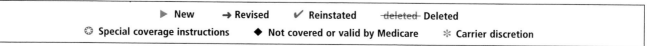

▶ **New**   → **Revised**   ✔ **Reinstated**   ~~deleted~~ **Deleted**
⊙ **Special coverage instructions**   ◆ **Not covered or valid by Medicare**   ✳ **Carrier discretion**

⚙ **J2440** Injection, papaverine HCL, **up to 60 mg**   N1 N

IOM: 100-02, 15, 50

⚙ **J2460** Injection, oxytetracycline HCL, **up to 50 mg**   E

Other: Terramycin IM

IOM: 100-02, 15, 50

✳ **J2469** Injection, palonosetron HCL, **25 mcg**   K2 K

Example: 0.25 mgm dose = 10 units. Example of use is acute, delayed, nausea and vomiting due to chemotherapy

NDC: Aloxi

⚙ **J2501** Injection, paricalcitol, **1 mcg**   N1 N

NDC: Zemplar

IOM: 100-02, 15, 50

✳ **J2503** Injection, pegaptanib sodium, **0.3 mg**   K2 K

NDC: Macugen

⚙ **J2504** Injection, pegademase bovine, **25 IU**   K2 K

NDC: Adagen

IOM: 100-02, 15, 50

✳ **J2505** Injection, pegfilgrastim, **6 mg**   K2 K

Report 1 unit per 6 mg.

NDC: Neulasta

▶✳ **J2507** Injection, pegloticase, **1 mg**   K2 G

⚙ **J2510** Injection, penicillin G procaine, aqueous, **up to 600,000 units**   N1 N

NDC: Wycillin

Other: Crysticillin, Duracillin AS, Pfizerpen AS

IOM: 100-02, 15, 50

⚙ **J2513** Injection, pentastarch, 10% solution, **100 ml**   K2 K

IOM: 100-02, 15, 50

⚙ **J2515** Injection, pentobarbital sodium, **per 50 mg**   N1 N

NDC: Nembutal

IOM: 100-02, 15, 50

⚙ **J2540** Injection, penicillin G potassium, **up to 600,000 units**   N1 N

NDC: Pfizerpen-G

IOM: 100-02, 15, 50

⚙ **J2543** Injection, piperacillin sodium/ tazobactam sodium, **1 gram/ 0.125 grams (1.125 grams)**   N1 N

NDC: Zosyn

IOM: 100-02, 15, 50

⚙ **J2545** Pentamidine isethionate, inhalation solution, FDA-approved final product, non-compounded, administered through DME, unit dose form, **per 300 mg**   B

NDC: Nebupent

⚙ **J2550** Injection, promethazine HCL, **up to 50 mg**   N1 N

Administration of phenergan suppository considered part of E/M encounter

NDC: Phenergan

Other: Anergan, Phenazine, Prorex, Prothazine

IOM: 100-02, 15, 50

⚙ **J2560** Injection, phenobarbital sodium, **up to 120 mg**   N1 N

NDC: Luminal

IOM: 100-02, 15, 50

✳ **J2562** Injection, plerixafor, **1 mg**   K2 K

FDA approved for non-Hodgkin lymphoma and multiple myeloma in 2008.

NDC: Mozobil

⚙ **J2590** Injection, oxytocin, **up to 10 units**   N1 N

NDC: Pitocin

Other: Syntocinon

IOM: 100-02, 15, 50

⚙ **J2597** Injection, desmopressin acetate, **per 1 mcg**   N1 N

NDC: DDAVP

IOM: 100-02, 15, 50

⚙ **J2650** Injection, prednisolone acetate, **up to 1 ml**   N1 N

Other: Cotolone, Key-Pred, Predalone, Predcor, Predicort

IOM: 100-02, 15, 50

⚙ **J2670** Injection, tolazoline HCL, **up to 25 mg**   N1 N

Other: Priscoline Hydrochloride

IOM: 100-02, 15, 50

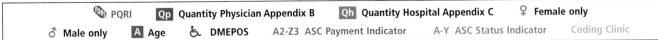

PQRI   **Qp** Quantity Physician Appendix B   **Qh** Quantity Hospital Appendix C   ♀ Female only   ♂ Male only   **A** Age   ♿ DMEPOS   A2-Z3 ASC Payment Indicator   A-Y ASC Status Indicator   Coding Clinic

⚙ **J2675** Injection, progesterone, **per 50 mg** N1 N

Other: Gesterol 50, Progestaject

IOM: 100-02, 15, 50

⚙ **J2680** Injection, fluphenazine decanoate, **up to 25 mg** N1 N

Other: Prolixin Decanoate

MCM 2049

IOM: 100-02, 15, 50

⚙ **J2690** Injection, procainamide HCL, **up to 1 gm** ♀ N1 N

Benefit limited to obstetrical diagnoses

Other: Pronestyl, Prostaphlin

IOM: 100-02, 15, 50

⚙ **J2700** Injection, oxacillin sodium, **up to 250 mg** K2 K

NDC: Bactocill

IOM: 100-02, 15, 50

⚙ **J2710** Injection, neostigmine methylsulfate, **up to 0.5 mg** N1 N

Other: Prostigmin

IOM: 100-02, 15, 50

⚙ **J2720** Injection, protamine sulfate, **per 10 mg** N1 N

IOM: 100-02, 15, 50

✻ **J2724** Injection, protein C concentrate, intravenous, human, **10 IU** K2 K

NDC: Ceprotin

⚙ **J2725** Injection, protirelin, **per 250 mcg** N1 K

Other: Relefact TRH, Thypinone

IOM: 100-02, 15, 50

⚙ **J2730** Injection, pralidoxime chloride, **up to 1 gm** K2 K

NDC: Protopam Chloride

IOM: 100-02, 15, 50

⚙ **J2760** Injection, phentolamine mesylate, **up to 5 mg** K2 K

Other: Regitine

IOM: 100-02, 15, 50

⚙ **J2765** Injection, metoclopramide HCL, **up to 10 mg** N1 N

NDC: Reglan

IOM: 100-02, 15, 50

⚙ **J2770** Injection, quinupristin/dalfopristin, **500 mg (150/350)** K2 K

NDC: Synercid

IOM: 100-02, 15, 50

✻ **J2778** Injection, ranibizumab, **0.1 mg** K2 K

May be reported for exudative senile macular degeneration (wet AMD) with 67028 (RT or LT)

Other: Lucentis

⚙ **J2780** Injection, ranitidine hydrochloride, **25 mg** N1 N

NDC: Zantac

IOM: 100-02, 15, 50

✻ **J2783** Injection, rasburicase, **0.5 mg** K2 K

NDC: Elitek

✻ **J2785** Injection, regadenoson, **0.1 mg** K2 K

One billing unit equal to 0.1 mg of regadenoson

⚙ **J2788** Injection, Rho D immune globulin, human, minidose, **50 mcg (250 IU)** K2 K

NDC: Bay Rho-D, MicRhoGAM

Other: HypRho-D, RhoGam

IOM: 100-02, 15, 50

⚙ **J2790** Injection, Rho D immune globulin, human, full dose, **300 mcg (1500 IU)** K2 K

Administered to pregnant female to prevent hemolistic disease of newborn. Report 90384 to private payer

NDC: Hyperrho S/D, RhoGAM

Other: Gamulin Rh, HypRho-D, Rhesonativ

IOM: 100-02, 15, 50

⚙ **J2791** Injection, Rho(D) immune globulin (human), (Rhophylac), intramuscular or intravenous, **100 IU** K2 K

Agent must be billed per 100 IU in both physician office and hospital outpatient settings

IOM: 100-02, 15, 50

⚙ **J2792** Injection, Rho D immune globulin intravenous, human, solvent detergent, **100 IU** K2 K

NDC: WinRHo-SDF

Other: Gamulin RH, Hyperrho S/D

IOM: 100-02, 15, 50

⚙ **J2793** Injection, rilonacept, **1 mg** K2 K

IOM: 100-02, 15, 50

✻ **J2794** Injection, risperidone, long acting, **0.5 mg** K2 K

NDC: Risperdal Costa

▶ **New** → **Revised** ✔ **Reinstated** ~~deleted~~ **Deleted**

⚙ **Special coverage instructions** ◆ **Not covered or valid by Medicare** ✻ **Carrier discretion**

✳ **J2795** Injection, ropivacaine hydrochloride, **1 mg** N1 N

NDC: Naropin

✳ **J2796** Injection, romiplostim, **10 micrograms** K2 K

Stimulates bone marrow megakarocytes to produce platelets (i.e., ITP).

NDC: Nplate

✿ **J2800** Injection, methocarbamol, **up to 10 ml** N1 N

NDC: Robaxin

IOM: 100-02, 15, 50

✳ **J2805** Injection, sincalide, **5 micrograms** N1 N

✿ **J2810** Injection, theophylline, **per 40 mg** N1 N

IOM: 100-02, 15, 50

✿ **J2820** Injection, sargramostim (GM-CSF), **50 mcg** K2 K

NDC: Leukine

Other: Prokine

IOM: 100-02, 15, 50

✿ **J2850** Injection, secretin, synthetic, human, **1 microgram** K2 K

NDC: Chirhostim

IOM: 100-02, 15, 50

✿ **J2910** Injection, aurothioglucose, **up to 50 mg** N1 N

Other: Solganal

IOM: 100-02, 15, 50

✿ **J2916** Injection, sodium ferric gluconate complex in sucrose injection, **12.5 mg** N1 N

NDC: Ferrlecit

IOM: 100-02, 15, 50

✿ **J2920** Injection, methylprednisolone sodium succinate, **up to 40 mg** N1 N

NDC: A-MethaPred, Solu-Medrol

IOM: 100-02, 15, 50

✿ **J2930** Injection, methylprednisolone sodium succinate, **up to 125 mg** N1 N

NDC: A-MethaPred, Solu-Medrol

IOM: 100-02, 15, 50

✿ **J2940** Injection, somatrem, **1 mg** E

IOM: 100-02, 15, 50,

Medicare Statute 1861s2b

✿ **J2941** Injection, somatropin, **1 mg** K2 K

Other: Genotropin, Humatrope, Nutropin, Omnitrope, Saizen, Serostim, Zorbtive

IOM: 100-02, 15, 50,

Medicare Statute 1861s2b

✿ **J2950** Injection, promazine HCL, **up to 25 mg** N1 N

Other: Prozine-50, Sparine

IOM: 100-02, 15, 50

✿ **J2993** Injection, reteplase, **18.1 mg** K2 K

NDC: Retavase

IOM: 100-02, 15, 50

✿ **J2995** Injection, streptokinase, **per 250,000 IU** K2 K

Bill 1 unit for each 250,000 IU

Other: Kabikinase, Streptase

IOM: 100-02, 15, 50

✿ **J2997** Injection, alteplase recombinant, **1 mg** K2 K

Thrombolytic agent, treatment of occluded catheters. Bill units of 1 mg administered

NDC: Activase, Cathflo Activase

IOM: 100-02, 15, 50

✿ **J3000** Injection, streptomycin, **up to 1 gm** N1 N

IOM: 100-02, 15, 50

✿ **J3010** Injection, fentanyl citrate, **0.1 mg** N1 N

NDC: Sublimaze

IOM: 100-02, 15, 50

✿ **J3030** Injection, sumatriptan succinate, **6 mg** (Code may be used for Medicare when drug administered under the direct supervision of a physician, not for use when drug is self administered) N1 K

NDC: Imitrex, Sumavel Dosepro

IOM: 100-02, 15, 150

✿ **J3070** Injection, pentazocine, **30 mg** N1 N

NDC: Talwin

IOM: 100-02, 15, 50

 PQRI 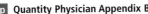 **Qp** Quantity Physician Appendix B 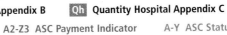 **Qh** Quantity Hospital Appendix C ♀ Female only

♂ Male only **A** Age ♿ DMEPOS A2-Z3 ASC Payment Indicator A-Y ASC Status Indicator Coding Clinic

▶ ✳ **J3095** Injection, televancin, **10 mg**   K2 G

Prescribed for the treatment of adults with complicated skin and skin structure infections (cSSSI) of the following Gram-positive microorganisms: *Staphylococcus aureus*; *Streptococcus* pyogenes, *Streptococcus* agalactiae, *Streptococcus* anginosus group. Separately payable under the ASC payment system.

NDC: Vibativ

Coding Clinic: 2011, Q1, P7

✳ **J3101** Injection, tenecteplase, **1 mg**   K2 K

NDC: TNKase

☼ **J3105** Injection, terbutaline sulfate, **up to 1 mg**   N1 N

Other: Brethine

IOM: 100-02, 15, 50

☼ **J3110** Injection, teriparatide, **10 mcg**   B

Other: Forteo

☼ **J3120** Injection, testosterone enanthate, **up to 100 mg**   N1 N

NDC: Delatestryl

Other: Andro LA 200, Andropository 100, Andryl 200, Delatest, Durathate-200, Everone, Testone LA, Testrin PA

IOM: 100-02, 15, 50

☼ **J3130** Injection, testosterone enanthate, **up to 200 mg**   N1 N

NDC: Delatestryl

Other: Andro LA 200, Andropository 100, Andryl 200, Delatest, Durathate-200, Everone, Testone LA, Testrin PA

IOM: 100-02, 15, 50

☼ **J3140** Injection, testosterone suspension, **up to 50 mg**   N1 N

Other: Adronaq-50, Histerone, Testaqua, Testro AQ, Testoject-50

IOM: 100-02, 15, 50

☼ **J3150** Injection, testosterone propionate, **up to 100 mg**   N1 N

Other: DepAndro 100, Testex

IOM: 100-02, 15, 50

☼ **J3230** Injection, chlorpromazine HCL, **up to 50 mg**   N1 N

Other: Ormazine, Thorazine

IOM: 100-02, 15, 50

☼ **J3240** Injection, thyrotropin alfa, **0.9 mg provided in 1.1 mg vial**   K2 K

NDC: Thyrogen

IOM: 100-02, 15, 50

✳ **J3243** Injection, tigecycline, **1 mg**   K2 K

✳ **J3246** Injection, tirofiban HCL, **0.25 mg**   K2 K

NDC: Aggrastat

☼ **J3250** Injection, trimethobenzamide HCL, **up to 200 mg**   N1 N

NDC: Benzacot, Tigan

Other: Arrestin, Tiject 20

IOM: 100-02, 15, 50

☼ **J3260** Injection, tobramycin sulfate, **up to 80 mg**   N1 N

Other: Nebcin

IOM: 100-02, 15, 50

▶ ✳ **J3262** Injection, tocilizumab, **1 mg**   K2 G

Indicated for the treatment of adult patients with moderately to severely active rheumatoid arthritis (RA) who have had an inadequate response to one or more tumor necrosis factor (TNF) antagonist therapies.

NDC: Actemra

Coding Clinic: 2011, Q1, P7

☼ **J3265** Injection, torsemide, **10 mg/ml**   N1 N

Other: Demadex

IOM: 100-02, 15, 50

☼ **J3280** Injection, thiethylperazine maleate, **up to 10 mg**   N1 N

Other: Norzine, Torecan

IOM: 100-02, 15, 50

✳ **J3285** Injection, treprostinil, **1 mg**   K2 K

NDC: Remodulin

☼ **J3300** Injection, triamcinolone acetonide, preservative free, **1 mg**   K2 K

☼ **J3301** Injection, triamcinolone acetonide, not otherwise specified, **10 mg**   N1 N

NDC: Kenalog

Other: Cenacort A-40, Kenaject-40, Triam A, Triesence, Tri-Kort, Trilog

IOM: 100-02, 15, 50

☼ **J3302** Injection, triamcinolone diacetate, **per 5 mg**   N1 N

NDC: Clincacort

Other: Amcort, Aristocort, Cenacort Forte, Triamcot, Trilone

IOM: 100-02, 15, 50

▶ New   → Revised   ✔ Reinstated   ~~deleted~~ Deleted
☼ Special coverage instructions   ◆ Not covered or valid by Medicare   ✳ Carrier discretion

⊙ **J3303** Injection, triamcinolone hexacetonide, **per 5 mg**   N1 N

NDC: Aristospan

IOM: 100-02, 15, 50

⊙ **J3305** Injection, trimetrexate glucuronate, **per 25 mg**   E

Other: NeuTrexin

IOM: 100-02, 15, 50

⊙ **J3310** Injection, perphenazine, **up to 5 mg**   K2 K

Other: Trilafon

IOM: 100-02, 15, 50

⊙ **J3315** Injection, triptorelin pamoate, **3.75 mg**   K2 K

NDC: Trelstar

IOM: 100-02, 15, 50

⊙ **J3320** Injection, spectinomycin dihydrochloride, **up to 2 gm**   E

Other: Trobicin

IOM: 100-02, 15, 50

⊙ **J3350** Injection, urea, **up to 40 gm**   K2 K

Other: Ureaphil

IOM: 100-02, 15, 50

⊙ **J3355** Injection, urofollitropin, **75 IU**   K2 K

NDC: Bravelle

Other: Metrodin

IOM: 100-02, 15, 50

▶ ✳ **J3357** Injection, ustekinumab, **1 mg**   K2 G

NDC: Stelara

Coding Clinic: 2011, Q1, P7

⊙ **J3360** Injection, diazepam, **up to 5 mg**   N1 N

Other: Valium, Zetran

IOM: 100-02, 15, 50

Coding Clinic: 2007, Q2, P6-7

⊙ **J3364** Injection, urokinase, **5000 IU vial**   N1 N

NDC: Abbokinase

IOM: 100-02, 15, 50

⊙ **J3365** Injection, IV, urokinase, **250,000 IU vial**   K2 K

Other: Kinlytic

IOM: 100-02, 15, 50,

Cross Reference Q0089

⊙ **J3370** Injection, vancomycin HCL, **500 mg**   N1 N

NDC: Vancocin

Other: Vancoled

IOM: 100-02, 15, 50; 100-03, 4, 280.14

▶ ✳ **J3385** Injection, velaglucerase alfa, **100 units**   K2 G

Enzyme replacement therapy in Gaucher Disease that results from a specific enzyme deficiency in the body, caused by a genetic mutation received from both parents. Type 1 is the most prevalent Ashkenazi Jewish genetic disease, occurring in one in every 1,000.

NDC: VPRIV

Coding Clinic: 2011, Q1, P7

⊙ **J3396** Injection, verteporfin, **0.1 mg**   K2 K

NDC: Visudyne

IOM: 100-03, 1, 80.2; 100-03, 1, 80.3

⊙ **J3400** Injection, triflupromazine HCL, **up to 20 mg**   E

Other: Vesprin

IOM: 100-02, 15, 50

⊙ **J3410** Injection, hydroxyzine HCL, **up to 25 mg**   N1 N

NDC: Restall

Other: Hyzine-50, Vistacot, Vistaject 25

IOM: 100-02, 15, 50

✳ **J3411** Injection, thiamine HCL, **100 mg**   N1 N

✳ **J3415** Injection, pyridoxine HCL, **100 mg**   N1 N

Other: Rodex

⊙ **J3420** Injection, vitamin B-12 cyanocobalamin, **up to 1000 mcg**   N1 N

Medicare carriers may have local coverage decisions regarding vitamin B_{12} injections that provide reimbursement only for patients with certain types of anemia and other conditions

NDC: Cobal-1000, Nervidox-6 S

Other: Cobolin-M, Hydroxocobalamin, Neuroforte-R, Redisol, Rubramin PC, Sytobex, Vita #12

IOM: 100-02, 15, 50; 100-03, 2, 150.6

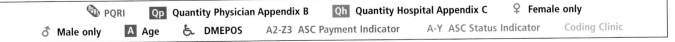

⊛ **J3430** Injection, phytonadione (vitamin K), **per 1 mg**   N1 N

NDC: Vitamin K1

Other: Aqua-Mephyton, Konakion, Menadione, Synkavite

IOM: 100-02, 15, 50

⊛ **J3465** Injection, voriconazole, **10 mg**   K2 K

NDC: VFEND

IOM: 100-02, 15, 50

⊛ **J3470** Injection, hyaluronidase, **up to 150 units**   N1 N

NDC: Amphadase

Other: Vitrase, Wydase

IOM: 100-02, 15, 50

⊛ **J3471** Injection, hyaluronidase, ovine, preservative free, **per 1 USP unit (up to 999 USP units)**   N1 N

NDC: Vitrase

⊛ **J3472** Injection, hyaluronidase, ovine, preservative free, **per 1000 USP units**   N1 N

NDC: Vitrase

⊛ **J3473** Injection, hyaluronidase, recombinant, **1 USP unit**   N1 N

Other: Hylenex

IOM: 100-02, 15, 50

⊛ **J3475** Injection, magnesium sulfate, **per 500 mg**   N1 N

IOM: 100-02, 15, 50

⊛ **J3480** Injection, potassium chloride, **per 2 meq**   N1 N

IOM: 100-02, 15, 50

⊛ **J3485** Injection, zidovudine, **10 mg**   N1 N

NDC: Retrovir

IOM: 100-02, 15, 50

⁑ **J3486** Injection, ziprasidone mesylate, **10 mg**   N1 N

NDC: Geodon

⁑ **J3487** Injection, zoledronic acid (Zometa), **1 mg**   K2 K

NDC: Zometa

⊛ **J3488** Injection, zoledronic acid (Reclast), **1 mg**   K2 K

Physician to specify 5 units for approved 5 mg dosing of Reclast

NDC: Reclast

⊛ **J3490** Unclassified drugs   N1 N

Bill on paper. Bill one unit. Identify drug and total dosage in "Remarks" field.

Other: Acthib, Aminocaproic Acid, Baciim, Bacitracin, Benzocaine, Betamethasone Acetate, Brevital Sodium, Bumetanide, Bupivacaine, Cefotetan, Cimetidine, Ciprofloxacin, Cleocin Phosphate, Clindamycin, Cortisone Acetate, Definity, Diprivan, Engerix-B, Ethanolamine, Famotidine, Ganirelix, Gonal-F, Hyaluronic Acid, Kineret, Marcaine, Metronidazole, Nafcillin, Naltrexone, Ovidrel, Pegasys, Peg-Intron, Penicillin G Sodium, Prodrox, Propofol, Protonix, Recombivax, Rifadin, Rifampin, Sensorcaine-MPF, Smz-TMP, Sodium Hyaluronate, Sufenta, Sufentanil Citrate, Timentin, Treanda, Twinrix, Valcyte, Veritas Collagen Matrix

IOM: 100-02, 15, 50

◆ **J3520** Edetate disodium, **per 150 mg**   E

Other: Chealamide, Disotate, Endrate ethylenediamine-tetra-acetic

IOM: 100-03, 1, 20.21; 100-03, 1, 20.22

⊛ **J3530** Nasal vaccine inhalation   N1 N

IOM: 100-02, 15, 50

◆ **J3535** Drug administered through a metered dose inhaler   E

Other: Ipratropium bromide

IOM: 100-02, 15, 50

◆ **J3570** Laetrile, amygdalin, vitamin B-17   E

IOM: 100-03, 1, 30.7

⁑ **J3590** Unclassified biologics   N1 N

Bill local carrier

Bill on paper. Bill one unit. Identify drug and total dosage in "Remarks" field.

Other: Bayhep B, Hyperhep-B, NABI-HB

Miscellaneous Drugs and Solutions

⊛ **J7030** Infusion, normal saline solution, **1000 cc**   N1 N

Bill local carrier if incident to a physician's service or used in an implanted infusion pump. If other, bill DME/MAC

NDC: Sodium Chloride

IOM: 100-02, 15, 50

▶ New   → Revised   ✔ Reinstated   ~~deleted~~ Deleted

⊛ Special coverage instructions   ◆ Not covered or valid by Medicare   ⁑ Carrier discretion

❂ **J7040** Infusion, normal saline solution, sterile **(500 ml=1 unit)** N1 N

Bill local carrier if incident to a physician's service or used in an implanted infusion pump. If other, bill DME/MAC

NDC: Sodium Chloride

IOM: 100-02, 15, 50

❂ **J7042** 5% dextrose/normal saline **(500 ml = 1 unit)** N1 N

Bill local carrier if incident to a physician's service or used in an implanted infusion pump. If other, bill DME/MAC

NDC: Dextrose-Nacl

IOM: 100-02, 15, 50

❂ **J7050** Infusion, normal saline solution, **250 cc** N1 N

Bill local carrier if incident to a physician's service or used in an implanted infusion pump. If other, bill DME/MAC

NDC: Sodium Chloride

IOM: 100-02, 15, 50

❂ **J7060** 5% dextrose/water **(500 ml = 1 unit)** N1 N

Bill local carrier if incident to a physician's service or used in an implanted infusion pump. If other, bill DME/MAC

IOM: 100-02, 15, 50

❂ **J7070** Infusion, D 5 W, **1000 cc** N1 N

Bill local carrier if incident to a physician's service or used in an implanted infusion pump. If other, bill DME/MAC

NDC: Dextrose

IOM: 100-02, 15, 50

❂ **J7100** Infusion, dextran 40, **500 ml** N1 N

Bill local carrier if incident to a physician's service or used in an implanted infusion pump. If other, bill DME/MAC

Other: Gentran, LMD, LMD in Dextrose, Rheomacrodex

IOM: 100-02, 15, 50

❂ **J7110** Infusion, dextran 75, **500 ml** N1 N

Bill local carrier if incident to a physician's service or used in an implanted infusion pump. If other, bill DME/MAC

NDC: Dextran 70 w/NACL, Dextran 75 in D5W

Other: Gentran

IOM: 100-02, 15, 50

❂ **J7120** Ringer's lactate infusion, **up to 1000 cc** N1 N

Bill local carrier if incident to a physician's service or used in an implanted infusion pump. If other, bill DME/MAC

Replacement fluid or electrolytes.

NDC: Lactated Ringers

IOM: 100-02, 15, 50

~~J7130~~ ~~Hypertonic saline solution, 50 or 100 meq, 20 cc vial~~ ✖

▶ ❂ **J7131** Hypertonic saline solution, **1 ml** N1 N

IOM: 100-02, 15, 50

▶ ✳ **J7180** Injection, factor XIII (antihemophilic factor, human), 1 i.u. K2 G

▶ ❂ **J7183** Injection, von Willebrand factor complex (human), wilate, **1 i.u. vwf:rco** K2 G

~~J7184~~ ~~Injection, von Willebrand factor complex (human), Wilate, per 100 IU VWF:RCO~~ ✖

IOM: 100-02, 15, 50 K2 G

✳ **J7185** Injection, Factor VIII (antihemophilic factor, recombinant) (Xyntha), **per IU** K2 K

Reported in place of temporary code Q2023.

❂ **J7186** Injection, anti-hemophilic factor VIII/ von Willebrand factor complex (human), **per factor VIII IU** K2 K

Bill local carrier

NDC: Alphanate

IOM: 100-02, 15, 50

❂ **J7187** Injection, von Willebrand factor complex (HUMATE-P), **per IU VWF: RCO** K2 K

Bill local carrier

NDC: Humate-P Low Dilutent

Other: Wilate

IOM: 100-02, 15, 50

ⓟ PQRI	**Qp** Quantity Physician Appendix B	**Qh** Quantity Hospital Appendix C	♀ Female only
♂ Male only	**A** Age ♿ DMEPOS A2-Z3 ASC Payment Indicator	A-Y ASC Status Indicator	Coding Clinic

⚙ **J7189** Factor VIIa (anti-hemophilic factor, recombinant), **per 1 microgram** K2 K

Bill local carrier

NDC: NovoSeven

IOM: 100-02, 15, 50

⚙ **J7190** Factor VIII anti-hemophilic factor, human, **per IU** K2 K

Bill local carrier

NDC: Alphanate, Alphanate/von Willebrand factor complex, Hemofil M, Koate DVI, Monarc-M, Monoclate-P

Other: Koate-HP, Kogenate, Recombinate

IOM: 100-02, 15, 50

⚙ **J7191** Factor VIII, anti-hemophilic factor (porcine), **per IU** K2 K

Bill local carrier

Other: Hyate C, Koate-HP, Recombinate

IOM: 100-02, 15, 50

＊ **J7192** Factor VIII (anti-hemophilic factor, recombinant) **per IU,** not otherwise specified K2 K

Bill local carrier

NDC: Advate, Helixate FS, Kogenate FS, Poly Bio-Set, Recombinate

Other: Refacto

IOM: 100-02, 15, 50

⚙ **J7193** Factor IX (anti-hemophilic factor, purified, non-recombinant) **per IU** K2 K

Bill local carrier

NDC: AlphaNine SD, Mononine

IOM: 100-02, 15, 50

⚙ **J7194** Factor IX, complex, **per IU** K2 K

Bill local carrier

NDC: Bebulin VH, Profilnine SD

Other: Konyne-80, Profilnine Heat-treated, Proplex SX-T, Proplex T

IOM: 100-02, 15, 50

⚙ **J7195** Factor IX (anti-hemophilic factor, recombinant) **per IU** K2 K

Bill local carrier

NDC: Benefix

Other: Konyne 80, Proplex T

IOM: 100-02, 15, 50

▶ ＊ **J7196** Injection, antithrombin recombinant, **50 i.u.** K2 K

Other: ATryn

Coding Clinic: 2011, Q1, P6

⚙ **J7197** Anti-thrombin III (human), **per IU** K2 K

Bill local carrier

NDC: Thrombate III

IOM: 100-02, 15, 50

⚙ **J7198** Anti-inhibitor, **per IU** K2 K

Bill local carrier

Diagnosis examples: 286.0 Congenital Factor VIII disorder; 286.1 Congenital Factor IX disorder; 286.4 VonWillebrand's disease

NDC: Feiba VH Immuno

Other: Autoplex T, Hemophilia clotting factors

IOM: 100-02, 15, 50; 100-03, 2, 110.3

⚙ **J7199** Hemophilia clotting factor, not otherwise classified B

Bill local carrier

Other: Autoplex T

IOM: 100-02, 15, 50; 100-03, 2, 110.3

◆ **J7300** Intrauterine copper contraceptive E

Bill local carrier

Report IVD insertion with 58300. Bill usual and customary charge.

Other: Paragard T 380 A

Medicare Statute 1862a1

◆ **J7302** Levonorgestrel-releasing intrauterine contraceptive system, **52 mg** ♀ E

Bill local carrier

Other: Mirena

Medicare Statute 1862a1

◆ **J7303** Contraceptive supply, hormone containing vaginal ring, each ♀ E

Bill local carrier

Medicare Statute 1862.1

◆ **J7304** Contraceptive supply, hormone containing patch, each ♀ E

Bill local carrier

Only billed by Family Planning Clinics

Medicare Statute 1862.1

◆ **J7306** Levonorgestrel (contraceptive) implant system, including implants and supplies E

Bill local carrier

◆ **J7307** Etonogestrel (contraceptive) implant system, including implant and supplies E

Bill local carrier

▶ New → Revised ✔ Reinstated deleted Deleted
⚙ Special coverage instructions ◆ Not covered or valid by Medicare ＊ Carrier discretion

* **J7308** Aminolevulinic acid HCL for topical administration, 20%, single unit dosage form **(354 mg)** K2 K

Bill local carrier

NDC: Levulan Kerastick

▶ ⊛ **J7309** Methyl aminolevulinate (MAL) for topical administration, 16.8%, **1 gram** K2 K

Coding Clinic: 2011, Q1, P6

⊛ **J7310** Ganciclovir, **4.5 mg,** long-acting implant K2 K

Bill local carrier

NDC: Vitrasert

IOM: 100-02, 15, 50

* **J7311** Fluocinolone acetonide, intravitreal implant K2 K

Bill local carrier

Treatment of chronic noninfectious posterior segment uveitis

Other: Retisert

▶ * **J7312** Injection, dexamethasone, intravitreal implant, **0.1 mg** K2 K

To bill for Ozurdex services submit the following codes: J7312 and 67028 with the modifier -22 (for the increased work difficulty and increased risk). Indicated for the treatment of macular edema occurring after branch retinal vein occlusion (BRVO) or central retinal vein occlusion (CRVO) and non-infectious uveitis affecting the posterior segment of the eye.

MDC: Ozurdex

Coding Clinic: 2011, Q1, P7

* **J7321** Hyaluronan or derivative, Hyalgan or Supartz, for intra-articular injection, **per dose** K2 K

Bill local carrier

Therapeutic goal is to restore visco-elasticity of synovial hyaluronan, thereby decreasing pain, improving mobility and restoring natural protective functions of hyaluronan in joint

* **J7323** Hyaluronan or derivative, Euflexxa, for intra-articular injection, **per dose** K2 K

Bill local carrier

* **J7324** Hyaluronan or derivative, Orthovisc, for intra-articular injection, **per dose** K2 K

Bill local carrier

* **J7325** Hyaluronan or derivative, Synvisc or Synvisc-One, for intra-articular injection, **1 mg** K2 K

▶ * **J7326** Hyaluronan or derivative, Gel-One, for intra-articular injection, **per dose** K2 K

* **J7330** Autologous cultured chondrocytes, **implant** B

Bill local carrier

NDC: Carticel

Coding Clinic: 2010, Q4, P3

▶ * **J7335** Capsaicin 8% patch, **per 10 square centimeters** K2 G

NDC: Qutenza

Coding Clinic: 2011, Q1, P7

Immunosuppressive Drugs (Includes Non-injectibles)

J7500-J7599: Bill local carrier if incident to a physician's service or used in an implanted infusion pump. If other, bill DME/MAC

⊛ **J7500** Azathioprine, oral, **50 mg** N1 N

NDC: Azasan, Imuran

IOM: 100-02, 15, 50

⊛ **J7501** Azathioprine, parenteral, **100 mg** K2 K

Other: Imuran

IOM: 100-02, 15, 50

⊛ **J7502** Cyclosporine, oral, **100 mg** N1 N

NDC: Gengraf, Neoral, Sandimmune

IOM: 100-02, 15, 50

⊛ **J7504** Lymphocyte immune globulin, antithymocyte globulin, equine, parenteral, **250 mg** K2 K

NDC: Atgam

IOM: 100-02, 15, 50; 100-03, 2, 110.3

⊛ **J7505** Muromonab-CD3, parenteral, **5 mg** K2 K

NDC: Orthoclone OKT3

Other: Monoclonal antibodies (parenteral)

IOM: 100-02, 15, 50

⊛ **J7506** Prednisone, oral, **per 5 mg** N1 N

Unit billing example, fifty 10 mg prednisone tablets dispensed, report J7506, 100 units (1 unit of J7506 = 5 mg)

NDC: Deltasone, Liquid Pred, Sterapred

Other: Prednicot

IOM: 100-02, 15, 50

PQRI | Qp Quantity Physician Appendix B | Qh Quantity Hospital Appendix C | ♀ Female only | ♂ Male only | A Age | & DMEPOS | A2-Z3 ASC Payment Indicator | A-Y ASC Status Indicator | Coding Clinic

◎ **J7507** Tacrolimus, oral, **per 1 mg** N1 N
NDC: Prograf
IOM: 100-02, 15, 50

◎ **J7509** Methylprednisolone oral, **per 4 mg** N1 N
NDC: Medrol
Other: Methylpred DP
IOM: 100-02, 15, 50

◎ **J7510** Prednisolone oral, **per 5 mg** N1 N
Other: Cotolone, Delta-Cortef, Prelone
IOM: 100-02, 15, 50

✳ **J7511** Lymphocyte immune globulin, antithymocyte globulin, rabbit, parenteral, **25 mg** K2 K
NDC: Thymoglobulin

◎ **J7513** Daclizumab, parenteral, **25 mg** K2 K
NDC: Zenapax
IOM: 100-02, 15, 50

✳ **J7515** Cyclosporine, oral, **25 mg** N1 N
NDC: Gengraf, Neoral, Sandimmune

✳ **J7516** Cyclosporin, parenteral, **250 mg** N1 N
NDC: Sandimmune

✳ **J7517** Mycophenolate mofetil, oral, **250 mg** N1 N
NDC: CellCept

◎ **J7518** Mycophenolic acid, oral, **180 mg** N1 N
NDC: Myfortic
IOM: 100-04, 4, 240; 100-4, 17, 80.3.1

◎ **J7520** Sirolimus, oral, **1 mg** N1 N
NDC: Rapamune
IOM: 100-02, 15, 50

◎ **J7525** Tacrolimus, parenteral, **5 mg** K2 K
NDC: Prograf
IOM: 100-02, 15, 50

◎ **J7599** Immunosuppressive drug, not otherwise classified N1 N
Bill on paper. Bill one unit. Identify drug and total dosage in "Remarks" field.
IOM: 100-02, 15, 50

Inhalation Solutions

J7604-J7799: If "incident to" a physician's service, do not bill; otherwise, bill DME/MAC.

✳ **J7604** Acetylcysteine, inhalation solution, compounded product, administered through DME, unit dose form, **per gram** M
Other: Mucomyst (unit dose form), N-acetyl-L-cysteine

✳ **J7605** Arformoterol, inhalation solution, FDA approved final product, non-compounded, administered through DME, unit dose form, **15 micrograms** M
Maintenance treatment of bronchoconstriction in patients with chronic obstructive pulmonary disease (COPD)
Other: Brovana

✳ **J7606** Formoterol fumarate, inhalation solution, FDA approved final product, non-compounded, administered through DME, unit dose form, **20 micrograms** M
NDC: Perforomist

✳ **J7607** Levalbuterol, inhalation solution, compounded product, administered through DME, concentrated form, **0.5 mg** M

◎ **J7608** Acetylcysteine, inhalation solution, FDA-approved final product, non-compounded, administered through DME, unit dose form, **per gram** M
Other: Mucomyst

✳ **J7609** Albuterol, inhalation solution, compounded product, administered through DME, unit dose, **1 mg** M
Patient's home, medications—such as albuterol when administered through a nebulizer—are considered DME and are payable under Part B.
Other: Xopenex

✳ **J7610** Albuterol, inhalation solution, compounded product, administered through DME, concentrated form, **1 mg** M
Other: Xopenex

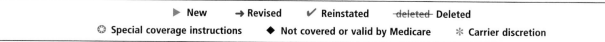

▶ **New**   → **Revised**   ✔ **Reinstated**   ~~deleted~~ **Deleted**
◎ **Special coverage instructions**   ◆ **Not covered or valid by Medicare**   ✳ **Carrier discretion**

⊕ **J7611** Albuterol, inhalation solution, FDA-approved final product, non-compounded, administered through DME, concentrated form, **1 mg** M

Report once for each milligram administered. For example, 2 mg of concentrated albuterol (usually diluted with saline), reported with J7611×2

NDC: Proventil, Ventolin

Other: Xopenex

⊕ **J7612** Levalbuterol, inhalation solution, FDA-approved final product, non-compounded, administered through DME, concentrated form, **0.5 mg** M

NDC: Xopenex

⊕ **J7613** Albuterol, inhalation solution, FDA-approved final product, non-compounded, administered through DME, unit dose, **1 mg** M

NDC: Accuneb

⊕ **J7614** Levalbuterol, inhalation solution, FDA-approved final product, non-compounded, administered through DME, unit dose, **0.5 mg** M

NDC: Xopenex

✳ **J7615** Levalbuterol, inhalation solution, compounded product, administered through DME, unit dose, **0.5 mg** M

⊕ **J7620** Albuterol, **up to 2.5 mg** and ipratropium bromide, **up to 0.5 mg,** FDA-approved final product, non-compounded, administered through DME M

NDC: DuoNeb

✳ **J7622** Beclomethasone, inhalation solution, compounded product, administered through DME, unit dose form, **per milligram** M

✳ **J7624** Betamethasone, inhalation solution, compounded product, administered through DME, unit dose form, **per mg** M

Other: Celestone Soluspan

✳ **J7626** Budesonide inhalation solution, FDA-approved final product, non-compounded, administered through DME, unit dose form, **up to 0.5 mg** M

NDC: Pulmicort

✳ **J7627** Budesonide, inhalation solution, compounded product, administered through DME, unit dose form, **up to 0.5 mg** M

Other: Pulmicort Respulses

⊕ **J7628** Bitolterol mesylate, inhalation solution, compounded product, administered through DME, concentrated form, **per milligram** M

Other: Tornalate

⊕ **J7629** Bitolterol mesylate, inhalation solution, compounded product, administered through DME, unit dose form, **per milligram** M

Other: Tornalate

⊕ **J7631** Cromolyn sodium, inhalation solution, FDA-approved final product, non-compounded, administered through DME, unit dose form, **per 10 milligrams** M

NDC: Intal

✳ **J7632** Cromolyn sodium, inhalation solution, compounded product, administered through DME, unit dose form, **per 10 milligrams** M

✳ **J7633** Budesonide, inhalation solution, FDA-approved final product, non-compounded, administered through DME, concentrated form, **per 0.25 milligram** M

Other: Pulmicort Respules

✳ **J7634** Budesonide, inhalation solution, compounded product, administered through DME, concentrated form, **per 0.25 milligram** M

⊕ **J7635** Atropine, inhalation solution, compounded product, administered through DME, concentrated form, **per milligram** M

⊕ **J7636** Atropine, inhalation solution, compounded product, administered through DME, unit dose form, **per milligram** M

⊕ **J7637** Dexamethasone, inhalation solution, compounded product, administered through DME, concentrated form, **per milligram** M

⊕ **J7638** Dexamethasone, inhalation solution, compounded product, administered through DME, unit dose form, **per milligram** M

⊕ **J7639** Dornase alfa, inhalation solution, FDA-approved final product, non-compounded, administered through DME, unit dose form, **per milligram** M

NDC: Pulmozyme

✳ **J7640** Formoterol, inhalation solution, compounded product, administered through DME, unit dose form, **12 micrograms** E

PQRI PQRI	**Qp** Quantity Physician Appendix B		**Qh** Quantity Hospital Appendix C	♀ **Female only**
♂ **Male only**	**A** Age	﴾ **DMEPOS**	A2-Z3 ASC Payment Indicator	A-Y ASC Status Indicator Coding Clinic

✳ **J7641** Flunisolide, inhalation solution, compounded product, administered through DME, unit dose, **per milligram** M

✿ **J7642** Glycopyrrolate, inhalation solution, compounded product, administered through DME, concentrated form, **per milligram** M

✿ **J7643** Glycopyrrolate, inhalation solution, compounded product, administered through DME, unit dose form, **per milligram** M

Other: Robinul

✿ **J7644** Ipratropium bromide, inhalation solution, FDA-approved final product, non-compounded, administered through DME, unit dose form, **per milligram** M

NDC: Atrovent

✳ **J7645** Ipratropium bromide, inhalation solution, compounded product, administered through DME, unit dose form, **per milligram** M

✳ **J7647** Isoetharine HCL, inhalation solution, compounded product, administered through DME, concentrated form, **per milligram** M

Other: Bronkosol

✿ **J7648** Isoetharine HCL, inhalation solution, FDA-approved final product, non-compounded, administered through DME, concentrated form, **per milligram** M

Other: Bronkosol

✿ **J7649** Isoetharine HCL, inhalation solution, FDA-approved final product, non-compounded, administered through DME, unit dose form, **per milligram** M

Other: Bronkosol

✳ **J7650** Isoetharine HCL, inhalation solution, compounded product, administered through DME, unit dose form, **per milligram** M

Other: Bronkosol

✳ **J7657** Isoproterenol HCL, inhalation solution, compounded product, administered through DME, concentrated form, **per milligram** M

Other: Isuprel

✿ **J7658** Isoproterenol HCL inhalation solution, FDA-approved final product, non-compounded, administered through DME, concentrated form, **per milligram** M

Other: Isuprel

✿ **J7659** Isoproterenol HCL, inhalation solution, FDA-approved final product, non-compounded, administered through DME, unit dose form, **per milligram** M

Other: Isuprel

✳ **J7660** Isoproterenol HCL, inhalation solution, compounded product, administered through DME, unit dose form, **per milligram** M

Other: Isuprel

▶ ✳ **J7665** Mannitol, administered through an inhaler, **5 mg** M

✳ **J7667** Metaproterenol sulfate, inhalation solution, compounded product, concentrated form, **per 10 milligrams** M

Other: Metaprel

✿ **J7668** Metaproterenol sulfate, inhalation solution, FDA-approved final product, non-compounded, administered through DME, concentrated form, **per 10 milligrams** M

Other: Metaprel

✿ **J7669** Metaproterenol sulfate, inhalation solution, FDA-approved final product, non-compounded, administered through DME, unit dose form, **per 10 milligrams** M

NDC: Alupent

Other: Metaprel

✳ **J7670** Metaproterenol sulfate, inhalation solution, compounded product, administered through DME, unit dose form, **per 10 milligrams** M

Other: Metaprel

✳ **J7674** Methacholine chloride administered as inhalation solution through a nebulizer, **per 1 mg** N1 N

NDC: Provocholine

✳ **J7676** Pentamidine isethionate, inhalation solution, compounded product, administered through DME, unit dose form, **per 300 mg** M

Other: Pentam

✿ **J7680** Terbutaline sulfate, inhalation solution, compounded product, administered through DME, concentrated form, **per milligram** M

Other: Brethine

▶ **New** → **Revised** ✔ **Reinstated** ~~deleted~~ **Deleted**
✿ **Special coverage instructions** ◆ **Not covered or valid by Medicare** ✳ **Carrier discretion**

⊕ **J7681** Terbutaline sulfate, inhalation solution, compounded product, administered through DME, unit dose form, **per milligram** M

Other: Brethine

⊕ **J7682** Tobramycin, inhalation solution, FDA-approved final product, non-compounded unit dose form, administered through DME, **per 300 milligrams** M

NDC: Tobi

Other: Nebcin

⊕ **J7683** Triamcinolone, inhalation solution, compounded product, administered through DME, concentrated form, **per milligram** M

⊕ **J7684** Triamcinolone, inhalation solution, compounded product, administered through DME, unit dose form, **per milligram** M

Other: Triamcinolone acetonide

✳ **J7685** Tobramycin, inhalation solution, compounded product, administered through DME, unit dose form, **per 300 milligrams** M

▶ ✳ **J7686** Treprostinil, inhalation solution, FDA-approved final product, non-compounded, administered through DME, unit dose form, **1.74 mg** M

NDC: Tyvaso

⊕ **J7699** NOC drugs, inhalation solution administered through DME M

Other: Gentamicin Sulfate, Sodium chloride, Tyvaso

⊕ **J7799** NOC drugs, other than inhalation drugs, administered through DME N1 N

Bill on paper. Bill one unit and identify drug and total dosage in the "Remark" field.

Other: Dextrose, Epinephrine, Mannitol, Osmitrol, Phenylephrine, Resectisol, Sodium chloride

IOM: 100-02, 15, 110.3

Other

⊕ **J8498** Antiemetic drug, rectal/suppository, not otherwise specified B

Bill DME/MAC

Other: Compazine, Compro, Phenadoz, Phenergan, Prochlorperazine, Promethazine, Promethegan, Thorazine

Medicare Statute 1861(s)2t

◆ **J8499** Prescription drug, oral, non chemotherapeutic, NOS E

If "incident to" a physician's service, do not bill; otherwise, bill DME/MAC

Other: Acyclovir, Millipred, Zovirax

IOM: 100-02, 15, 50

⊕ **J8501** Aprepitant, oral, **5 mg** K2 K

Bill DME/MAC

NDC: Emend

⊕ **J8510** Busulfan; oral, **2 mg** K2 K

Bill DME/MAC

NDC: Myleran

IOM 100-02, 15, 50; 100-04, 4, 240; 100-04, 17, 80.1.1

◆ **J8515** Cabergoline, oral, **0.25 mg** E

Bill DME/MAC

IOM: 100-02, 15, 50; 100-04, 4, 240

⊕ **J8520** Capecitabine, oral, **150 mg** K2 K

Bill DME/MAC

NDC: Xeloda

IOM: 100-02, 15, 50; 100-04, 4, 240; 100-04, 17, 80.1.1

⊕ **J8521** Capecitabine, oral, **500 mg** K2 K

Bill DME/MAC

NDC: Xeloda

IOM: 100-02, 15, 50; 100-04, 4, 240; 100-04, 17, 80.1.1

⊕ **J8530** Cyclophosphamide; oral, **25 mg** N1 N

Bill DME/MAC

NDC: Cytoxan

IOM: 100-02, 15, 50; 100-04, 4, 240; 100-04, 17, 80.1.1

⊕ **J8540** Dexamethasone, oral, **0.25 mg** N1 N

Bill DME/MAC

Other: Decadron, Dexone, Dexpak

Medicare Statute 1861(s)2t

⊕ **J8560** Etoposide; oral, **50 mg** K2 K

Bill DME/MAC

NDC: VePesid

IOM: 100-02, 15, 50; 100-04, 4, 230.1; 100-04, 4, 240; 100-04, 17, 80.1.1

▶ ⊕ **J8561** Everolimus, oral, **0.25 mg** K2 K

IOM: 100-02, 15, 50

PQRI | **Qp** Quantity Physician Appendix B | **Qh** Quantity Hospital Appendix C | ♀ Female only | ♂ Male only | **A** Age | DMEPOS | A2-Z3 ASC Payment Indicator | A-Y ASC Status Indicator | Coding Clinic

▶ ✳ **J8562** Fludarabine phosphate, oral, **10 mg**   K2   G

Bill DME/MAC

NDC: Oforta

Coding Clinic: 2011, Q1, P9

◆ **J8565** Gefitinib, oral, **250 mg**   E

Bill DME/MAC

Other: Iressa

⊕ **J8597** Antiemetic drug, oral, not otherwise specified   N1   N

Bill DME/MAC

Medicare Statute 1861(s)2t

⊕ **J8600** Melphalan; oral, **2 mg**   N1   N

Bill DME/MAC

NDC: Alkeran

IOM: 100-02, 15, 50; 100-04, 4, 240; 100-04, 17, 80.1.1

⊕ **J8610** Methotrexate; oral, **2.5 mg**   N1   N

Bill DME/MAC

NDC: Rheumatrex, Trexall

IOM: 100-02, 15, 50; 100-04, 4, 240; 100-04, 17, 80.1.1

✳ **J8650** Nabilone, oral, **1 mg**   E

Bill DME/MAC

⊕ **J8700** Temozolomide, oral, **5 mg**   K2   K

Bill DME/MAC

NDC: Temodar

IOM: 100-02, 15, 50; 100-04, 4, 240

✳ **J8705** Topotecan, oral, **0.25 mg**   K2   K

Bill DME/MAC

Treatment for ovarian and lung cancers, etc. Report J9350 (Topotecan, 4 mg) for intravenous version

⊕ **J8999** Prescription drug, oral, chemotherapeutic, NOS   B

Bill DME/MAC

Other: Arimidex, Aromasin, Ceenu, Droxia, Flutamide, Hydrea, Hydroxyurea, Leukeran, Malulane, Megace, Megestrol Acetate, Mercaptopurine, Nolvadex, Purinethol, Tamoxifen Citrate

IOM: 100-02, 15, 50; 100-04, 4, 250; 100-04, 17, 80.1.1; 100-04, 17, 80.1.2

CHEMOTHERAPY DRUGS (J9000-J9999)

NOTE: These codes cover the cost of the chemotherapy drug only, not to include the administration

J9000-J9999: Bill local carrier if incident to a physician's service or used in an implanted infusion pump. If other, bill DME/MAC

⊕ **J9000** Injection, doxorubicin hydrochloride, **10 mg**   N1   N

NDC: Adriamycin

Other: Rubex

IOM: 100-02, 15, 50

Coding Clinic: 2007, Q4, P5

⊕ **J9001** Injection, doxorubicin hydrochloride, all lipid formulations, **10 mg**   K2   K

NDC: Doxil

IOM: 100-02, 15, 50

⊕ **J9010** Injection, alemtuzumab, **10 mg**   K2   K

NDC: Campath

Medicare Statute 1833(t)

⊕ **J9015** Injection, aldesleukin, **per single use vial**   K2   K

NDC: Proleukin

IOM: 100-02, 15, 50

✳ **J9017** Injection, arsenic trioxide, **1 mg**   K2   K

NDC: Trisenox

⊕ **J9020** Injection, asparaginase, **10,000 units**   K2   K

NDC: Elspar

IOM: 100-02, 15, 50

✳ **J9025** Injection, azacitidine, **1 mg**   K2   K

NDC: Vidaza

✳ **J9027** Injection, clofarabine, **1 mg**   K2   K

NDC: Clolar

⊕ **J9031** BCG (intravesical), **per instillation**   K2   K

NDC: TheraCys, Tice BCG

IOM: 100-02, 15, 50

✳ **J9033** Injection, bendamustine HCL, **1 mg**   K2   K

Treatment for form of non-Hodgkin's lymphoma; standard administration time is as an intravenous infusion over 30 minutes

NDC: Treanda

▶ New   → Revised   ✔ Reinstated   ~~deleted~~ Deleted

⊕ Special coverage instructions   ◆ Not covered or valid by Medicare   ✳ Carrier discretion

✳ **J9035** Injection, bevacizumab, **10 mg**   K2 K

For malignant neoplasm of breast, considered J9207.

NDC: Avastin

⊙ **J9040** Injection, bleomycin sulfate, **15 units**   N1 N

NDC: Blenoxane

IOM: 100-02, 15, 50

✳ **J9041** Injection, bortezomib, **0.1 mg**   K2 K

NDC: Velcade

▶ ✳ **J9043** Injection, cabazitaxel, **1 mg**   K2 G

⊙ **J9045** Injection, carboplatin, **50 mg**   N1 N

NDC: Paraplatin

IOM: 100-02, 15, 50

⊙ **J9050** Injection, carmustine, **100 mg**   K2 K

NDC: BiCNU

IOM: 100-02, 15, 50

✳ **J9055** Injection, cetuximab, **10 mg**   K2 K

NDC: Erbitux

→ ⊙ **J9060** Injection, cisplatin, powder or solution, **10 mg**   N1 N

NDC: Plantinol AQ

IOM: 100-02, 15, 50

Coding Clinic: 2011, Q1, P8

⊙ **J9065** Injection, cladribine, **per 1 mg**   K2 K

NDC: Leustatin

IOM: 100-02, 15, 50

⊙ **J9070** Cyclophosphamide, **100 mg**   K2 K

NDC: Cytoxan

Other: Neosar

IOM: 100-02, 15, 50

Coding Clinic: 2011, Q1, P8-9

✳ **J9098** Injection, cytarabine liposome, **10 mg**   K2 K

NDC: DepoCyt

⊙ **J9100** Injection, cytarabine, **100 mg**   N1 N

Other: Cytosar-U

IOM: 100-02, 15, 50

Coding Clinic: 2011, Q1, P9

⊙ **J9120** Injection, dactinomycin, **0.5 mg**   K2 K

NDC: Cosmegen

IOM: 100-02, 15, 50

⊙ **J9130** Dacarbazine, **100 mg**   N1 N

Other: DTIC-Dome

IOM: 100-02, 15, 50

Coding Clinic: 2011, Q1, P9

⊙ **J9150** Injection, daunorubicin, **10 mg**   K2 K

NDC: Cerubidine

IOM: 100-02, 15, 50

⊙ **J9151** Injection, daunorubicin citrate, liposomal formulation, **10 mg**   K2 K

NDC: Daunoxome

IOM: 100-02, 15, 50

✳ **J9155** Injection, degarelix, **1 mg**   K2 K

Report 1 unit for every 1 mg.

NDC: Firmagon

✳ **J9160** Injection, denileukin diftitox, **300 micrograms**   K2 K

NDC: Ontak

⊙ **J9165** Injection, diethylstilbestrol diphosphate, **250 mg**   E

Other: Stilphostrol

IOM: 100-02, 15, 50

⊙ **J9171** Injection, docetaxel, **1 mg**   K2 K

Report 1 unit for every 1 mg.

NDC: Taxotere

IOM: 100-02, 15, 50

⊙ **J9175** Injection, Elliott's B solution, **1 ml**   N1 N

NDC: Elliott's b

IOM: 100-02, 15, 50

✳ **J9178** Injection, epirubicin HCL, **2 mg**   K2 K

NDC: Ellence

▶ ✳ **J9179** Injection, eribulin mesylate, **0.1 mg**   K2 G

⊙ **J9181** Injection, etoposide, **10 mg**   N1 N

NDC: Etopophos, VePesid

IOM: 100-02, 15, 50

⊙ **J9185** Injection, fludarabine phosphate, **50 mg**   K2 K

NDC: Fludara

IOM: 100-02, 15, 50

⊙ **J9190** Injection, fluorouracil, **500 mg**   N1 N

NDC: Adrucil

IOM: 100-02, 15, 50

⊙ **J9200** Injection, floxuridine, **500 mg**   K2 K

Other: FUDR

IOM: 100-02, 15, 50

⊙ **J9201** Injection, gemcitabine hydrochloride, **200 mg**   K2 K

NDC: Gemzar

IOM: 100-02, 15, 50

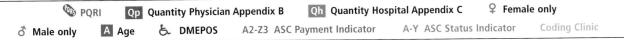

PQRI   Qp **Quantity Physician Appendix B**   Qh **Quantity Hospital Appendix C**   ♀ **Female only**

♂ **Male only**   A **Age**   & **DMEPOS**   A2-Z3 **ASC Payment Indicator**   A-Y **ASC Status Indicator**   Coding Clinic

⊘ **J9202**   Goserelin acetate implant, **per 3.6 mg**   K2   K
NDC: Zoladex
IOM: 100-02, 15, 50

⊘ **J9206**   Injection, irinotecan, **20 mg**   K2   K
NDC: Camptosar
IOM: 100-02, 15, 50

✳ **J9207**   Injection, ixabepilone, **1 mg**   K2   K

➜ ⊘ **J9208**   Injection, ifosfamide, **1 gm**   K2   K
NDC: Ifex
IOM: 100-02, 15, 50

⊘ **J9209**   Injection, mesna, **200 mg**   N1   N
NDC: Mesnex
IOM: 100-02, 15, 50

⊘ **J9211**   Injection, idarubicin hydrochloride, **5 mg**   K2   K
NDC: Idamycin PFS
IOM: 100-02, 15, 50

⊘ **J9212**   Injection, interferon alfacon-1, recombinant, **1 mcg**   N1   N
Other: Infergen
IOM: 100-02, 15, 50

⊘ **J9213**   Injection, interferon, alfa-2a, recombinant, **3 million units**   N1   N
IOM: 100-02, 15, 50

⊘ **J9214**   Injection, interferon, alfa-2b, recombinant, **1 million units**   K2   K
NDC: Intron-A
IOM: 100-02, 15, 50

⊘ **J9215**   Injection, interferon, alfa-n3 (human leukocyte derived), **250,000 IU**   K2   K
Other: Alferon N
IOM: 100-02, 15, 50

⊘ **J9216**   Injection, interferon, gamma-1B, **3 million units**   K2   K
Other: Actimmune
IOM: 100-02, 15, 50

⊘ **J9217**   Leuprolide acetate (for depot suspension), **7.5 mg**   K2   K
NDC: Eligard, Lupron Depot
IOM: 100-02, 15, 50

⊘ **J9218**   Leuprolide acetate, **per 1 mg**   K2   K
NDC: Lupron
IOM: 100-02, 15, 50

⊘ **J9219**   Leuprolide acetate implant, **65 mg**   K2   K
NDC: Viadur
IOM: 100-02, 15, 50

⊘ **J9225**   Histrelin implant (Vantas), **50 mg**   K2   K
IOM: 100-02, 15, 50

⊘ **J9226**   Histrelin implant (Supprelin LA), **50 mg**   K2   K
Other: Vantas
IOM: 100-02, 15, 50

▶ ✳ **J9228**   Injection, ipilimumab, **1 mg**   K2   G

⊘ **J9230**   Injection, mechlorethamine hydrochloride, (nitrogen mustard), **10 mg**   K2   K
NDC: Mustargen
IOM: 100-02, 15, 50

⊘ **J9245**   Injection, melphalan hydrochloride, **50 mg**   K2   K
NDC: Alkeran
IOM: 100-02, 15, 50

⊘ **J9250**   Methotrexate sodium, **5 mg**   N1   N
Other: Folex
IOM: 100-02, 15, 50

⊘ **J9260**   Methotrexate sodium, **50 mg**   N1   N
Other: Folex
IOM: 100-02, 15, 50

✳ **J9261**   Injection, nelarabine, **50 mg**   K2   K
NDC: Arranon

✳ **J9263**   Injection, oxaliplatin, **0.5 mg**   K2   K
Eloxatin, platinum-based anticancer drug that destroys cancer cells
NDC: Eloxatin
Coding Clinic: 2009, Q1, P10

✳ **J9264**   Injection, paclitaxel protein-bound particles, **1 mg**   K2   K
NDC: Abraxane

⊘ **J9265**   Injection, paclitaxel, **30 mg**   N1   N
NDC: Onxol, Taxol
IOM: 100-02, 15, 50

⊘ **J9266**   Injection, pegaspargase, **per single dose vial**   K2   K
NDC: Oncaspar
IOM: 100-02, 15, 50

⊘ **J9268**   Injection, pentostatin, **10 mg**   K2   K
NDC: Nipent
IOM: 100-02, 15, 50

▶ **New**   ➜ **Revised**   ✔ **Reinstated**   ~~deleted~~ **Deleted**
⊘ **Special coverage instructions**   ◆ **Not covered or valid by Medicare**   ✳ **Carrier discretion**

⊛ **J9270** Injection, plicamycin, **2.5 mg** N1 N

Other: Mithracin

IOM: 100-02, 15, 50

⊛ **J9280** Mitomycin, **5 mg** K2 K

NDC: Mutamycin

IOM: 100-02, 15, 50

Coding Clinic: 2011, Q1, P9

⊛ **J9293** Injection, mitoxantrone hydrochloride, **per 5 mg** K2 K

Other: Novantrone

IOM: 100-02, 15, 50

✳ **J9300** Injection, gemtuzumab ozogamicin, **5 mg** K2 K

NDC: Mylotarg

▶ ✳ **J9302** Injection, ofatumumab, **10 mg** K2 G

NDC: Arzerra

Other: Doulinum

Coding Clinic: 2011, Q1, P7

✳ **J9303** Injection, panitumumab, **10 mg** K2 K

Other: Vectibix

✳ **J9305** Injection, pemetrexed, **10 mg** K2 K

NDC: Alimta

▶ ✳ **J9307** Injection, pralatrexate, **1 mg** K2 G

NDC: Folotyn

Coding Clinic: 2011, Q1, P7

⊛ **J9310** Injection, rituximab, **100 mg** K2 K

NDC: RituXan

IOM: 100-02, 15, 50

▶ ✳ **J9315** Injection, romidepsin, **1 mg** K2 G

NDC: Istodax

Coding Clinic: 2011, Q1, P7

⊛ **J9320** Injection, streptozocin, **1 gram** K2 K

NDC: Zanosar

IOM: 100-02, 15, 50

✳ **J9328** Injection, temozolomide, **1 mg** K2 K

Intravenous formulation, not for oral administration

NDC: Temodar

✳ **J9330** Injection, temsirolimus, **1 mg** K2 K

Treatment for advanced renal cell carcinoma; standard administration is intravenous infusion greater than 30-60 minutes

Other: Torisel

⊛ **J9340** Injection, thiotepa, **15 mg** K2 K

Other: Thiethylenethiophosphoramide/T

IOM: 100-02, 15, 50

▶ ✳ **J9351** Injection, topotecan, **0.1 mg** K2 K

NDC: Hycamtin

Coding Clinic: 2011, Q1, P9

✳ **J9355** Injection, trastuzumab, **10 mg** K2 K

NDC: Herceptin

⊛ **J9357** Injection, valrubicin, intravesical, **200 mg** K2 K

NDC: Valstar

IOM: 100-02, 15, 50

⊛ **J9360** Injection, vinblastine sulfate, **1 mg** N1 N

Other: Alkaban-AQ, Velban, Velsar

IOM: 100-02, 15, 50

⊛ **J9370** Vincristine sulfate, **1 mg** N1 N

NDC: Vincasar PFS

Other: Oncovin

IOM: 100-02, 15, 50

Coding Clinic: 2011, Q1, P9

⊛ **J9390** Injection, vinorelbine tartrate, **10 mg** K2 K

NDC: Navelbine

IOM: 100-02, 15, 50

✳ **J9395** Injection, fulvestrant, **25 mg** K2 K

NDC: Faslodex

⊛ **J9600** Injection, porfimer sodium, **75 mg** K2 K

NDC: Photofrin

IOM: 100-02, 15, 50

⊛ **J9999** Not otherwise classified, antineoplastic drugs N1 N

Bill on paper, bill one unit, and identify drug and total dosage in "Remarks" field. Include invoice of cost or NDC number in "Remarks" field.

Other: Allopurinol Sodium, Ifosfamide/Mesna

IOM: 100-02, 15, 50; 100-03, 2, 110.2

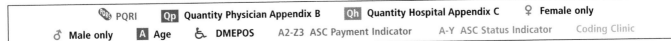

PQRS PQRI   **Qp** Quantity Physician Appendix B   **Qh** Quantity Hospital Appendix C   ♀ Female only

♂ Male only   **A** Age   ♿ DMEPOS   A2-Z3 ASC Payment Indicator   A-Y ASC Status Indicator   Coding Clinic

TEMPORARY CODES ASSIGNED TO DME REGIONAL CARRIERS (K0000-K9999)

Wheelchairs and Accessories

NOTE: This section contains national codes assigned by CMS on a temporary basis and for the exclusive use of the durable medical equipment regional carriers (DMERC).

✳ **K0001**   Standard wheelchair `Qp` ♿   Y

     Bill DME/MAC

     Capped rental

     DMEPOS Modifier(s): RR

✳ **K0002**   Standard hemi (low seat) wheelchair `Qp` ♿   Y

     Bill DME/MAC

     Capped rental

     DMEPOS Modifier(s): RR

✳ **K0003**   Lightweight wheelchair `Qp` ♿   Y

     Bill DME/MAC

     Capped rental

     DMEPOS Modifier(s): RR

✳ **K0004**   High strength, lightweight wheelchair `Qp` ♿   Y

     Bill DME/MAC

     Capped rental

     DMEPOS Modifier(s): RR

✳ **K0005**   Ultralightweight wheelchair `Qp` ♿   Y

     Bill DME/MAC

     Capped rental. Inexpensive and routinely purchased DME

     DMEPOS Modifier(s): NU, RR, UE

✳ **K0006**   Heavy duty wheelchair `Qp` ♿   Y

     Bill DME/MAC

     Capped rental

     DMEPOS Modifier(s): RR

✳ **K0007**   Extra heavy duty wheelchair `Qp` ♿   Y

     Bill DME/MAC

     Capped rental

     DMEPOS Modifier(s): RR

✳ **K0009**   Other manual wheelchair/base `Qp`   Y

     Not Otherwise Classified.

✳ **K0010**   Standard - weight frame motorized/power wheelchair ♿   Y

     Capped rental. Codes K0010-K0014 are not for manual wheelchairs with add-on power packs. Use the appropriate code for the manual wheelchair base provided (K0001-K0009) and code K0460

     DMEPOS Modifier(s): RR

✳ **K0011**   Standard - weight frame motorized/power wheelchair with programmable control parameters for speed adjustment, tremor dampening, acceleration control and braking ♿   Y

     Capped rental. A patient who requires a power wheelchair usually is totally nonambulatory and has severe weakness of the upper extremities due to a neurologic or muscular disease/condition

     DMEPOS Modifier(s): KF, RR

✳ **K0012**   Lightweight portable motorized/power wheelchair ♿   Y

     Capped rental

     DMEPOS Modifier(s): RR

✳ **K0014**   Other motorized/power wheelchair base   Y

     Capped rental

✳ **K0015**   Detachable, non-adjustable height armrest, each `Qp` ♿   Y

     Inexpensive and routinely purchased DME

     DMEPOS Modifier(s): KE, NU, RR, UE

✳ **K0017**   Detachable, adjustable height armrest, base, each `Qp` ♿   Y

     Inexpensive and routinely purchased DME

     DMEPOS Modifier(s): KE, NU, RR, UE

✳ **K0018**   Detachable, adjustable height armrest, upper portion, each `Qp` ♿   Y

     Inexpensive and routinely purchased DME

     DMEPOS Modifier(s): KE, NU, RR, UE

✳ **K0019**   Arm pad, each `Qp` ♿   Y

     Inexpensive and routinely purchased DME

     DMEPOS Modifier(s): KE, NU, RR, UE

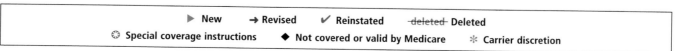

▶ New   → Revised   ✔ Reinstated   deleted Deleted

✪ Special coverage instructions   ◆ Not covered or valid by Medicare   ✳ Carrier discretion

✳ **K0020** Fixed, adjustable height armrest, pair Qp ♿   Y

Inexpensive and routinely purchased DME

DMEPOS Modifier(s): KE, NU, RR, UE

✳ **K0037** High mount flip-up footrest, each Qp ♿   Y

Inexpensive and routinely purchased DME

DMEPOS Modifier(s): KE, NU, RR, UE

✳ **K0038** Leg strap, each Qp ♿   Y

Inexpensive and routinely purchased DME

DMEPOS Modifier(s): KE, NU, RR, UE

✳ **K0039** Leg strap, H style, each Qp ♿   Y

Inexpensive and routinely purchased DME

DMEPOS Modifier(s): KE, NU, RR, UE

✳ **K0040** Adjustable angle footplate, each Qp ♿   Y

Inexpensive and routinely purchased DME

DMEPOS Modifier(s): KE, NU, RR, UE

✳ **K0041** Large size footplate, each Qp ♿   Y

Inexpensive and routinely purchased DME

DMEPOS Modifier(s): KE, NU, RR, UE

✳ **K0042** Standard size footplate, each Qp ♿   Y

Inexpensive and routinely purchased DME

DMEPOS Modifier(s): KE, NU, RR, UE

✳ **K0043** Footrest, lower extension tube, each Qp ♿   Y

Inexpensive and routinely purchased DME

DMEPOS Modifier(s): KE, NU, RR, UE

✳ **K0044** Footrest, upper hanger bracket, each Qp ♿   Y

Inexpensive and routinely purchased DME

DMEPOS Modifier(s): KE, NU, RR, UE

✳ **K0045** Footrest, complete assembly Qp ♿   Y

Inexpensive and routinely purchased DME

DMEPOS Modifier(s): KE, NU, RR, UE

✳ **K0046** Elevating legrest, lower extension tube, each Qp ♿   Y

Inexpensive and routinely purchased DME

DMEPOS Modifier(s): KE, NU, RR, UE

✳ **K0047** Elevating legrest, upper hanger bracket, each Qp ♿   Y

Inexpensive and routinely purchased DME

DMEPOS Modifier(s): KE, NU, RR, UE

✳ **K0050** Ratchet assembly Qp ♿   Y

Inexpensive and routinely purchased DME

DMEPOS Modifier(s): KE, NU, RR, UE

✳ **K0051** Cam release assembly, footrest or legrests, each Qp ♿   Y

Inexpensive and routinely purchased DME

DMEPOS Modifier(s): KE, NU, RR, UE

✳ **K0052** Swing-away, detachable footrests, each Qp ♿   Y

Inexpensive and routinely purchased DME

DMEPOS Modifier(s): KE, NU, RR, UE

✳ **K0053** Elevating footrests, articulating (telescoping), each Qp ♿   Y

Inexpensive and routinely purchased DME

DMEPOS Modifier(s): KE, NU, RR, UE

✳ **K0056** Seat height less than 17″ or equal to or greater than 21″ for a high strength, lightweight, or ultralightweight wheelchair Qp ♿   Y

Inexpensive and routinely purchased DME

DMEPOS Modifier(s): NU, RR, UE

✳ **K0065** Spoke protectors, each Qp ♿   Y

Inexpensive and routinely purchased DME

DMEPOS Modifier(s): NU, RR, UE

✳ **K0069** Rear wheel assembly, complete, with solid tire, spokes or molded, each Qp ♿   Y

Inexpensive and routinely purchased DME

DMEPOS Modifier(s): NU, RR, UE

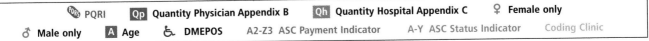

🄿 PQRI   **Qp** Quantity Physician Appendix B   **Qh** Quantity Hospital Appendix C   ♀ **Female only**
♂ **Male only**   **A** Age   ♿ **DMEPOS**   A2-Z3 ASC Payment Indicator   A-Y ASC Status Indicator   Coding Clinic

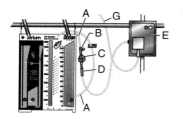

Figure 21 Infusion pump.

✳ **K0070** Rear wheel assembly, complete, with pneumatic tire, spokes or molded, each [Qp] [&] Y

Inexpensive and routinely purchased DME

DMEPOS Modifier(s): NU, RR, UE

✳ **K0071** Front caster assembly, complete, with pneumatic tire, each [Qp] [&] Y

Caster assembly includes a caster fork (E2396), wheel rim, and tire. Inexpensive and routinely purchased DME

DMEPOS Modifier(s): NU, RR, UE

✳ **K0072** Front caster assembly, complete, with semi-pneumatic tire, each [Qp] [&] Y

Inexpensive and routinely purchased DME

DMEPOS Modifier(s): NU, RR, UE

✳ **K0073** Caster pin lock, each [Qp] [&] Y

Inexpensive and routinely purchased DME

DMEPOS Modifier(s): NU, RR, UE

✳ **K0077** Front caster assembly, complete, with solid tire, each [Qp] [&] Y

DMEPOS Modifier(s): NU, RR, UE

✳ **K0098** Drive belt for power wheelchair [&] Y

Inexpensive and routinely purchased DME

DMEPOS Modifier(s): KE, NU, RR, UE

✳ **K0105** IV hanger, each [Qp] [&] Y

Inexpensive and routinely purchased DME

DMEPOS Modifier(s): NU, RR, UE

✳ **K0108** Wheelchair component or accessory, not otherwise specified Y

⊛ **K0195** Elevating leg rests, pair (for use with capped rental wheelchair base) [Qp] [&] Y

Bill DME/MAC

Medically necessary replacement items are covered if rollabout chair or transport chair covered

IOM: 100-03, 4, 280.1

DMEPOS Modifier(s): KE, RR

⊛ **K0455** Infusion pump used for uninterrupted parenteral administration of medication (e.g., epoprostenol or treprostinol) [Qp] [&] Y

Bill DME/MAC

An EIP may also be referred to as an external insulin pump, ambulatory pump, or mini-infuser. CMN/DIF required. Frequent and substantial service DME

IOM: 100-03, 1, 50.3

DMEPOS Modifier(s): RR

⊛ **K0462** Temporary replacement for patient owned equipment being repaired, any type [Qp] Y

Bill DME/MAC

Only report for maintenance and service for an item for which initial claim was paid. The term power mobility device (PMD) includes power operated vehicles (POVs) and power wheelchairs (PWCs). Not Otherwise Classified.

IOM: 100-04, 20, 40.1

⊛ **K0552** Supplies for external drug infusion pump, syringe type cartridge, sterile, each [&] Y

Bill DME/MAC

Supplies.

IOM: 100-03, 1, 50.3

✳ **K0601** Replacement battery for external infusion pump owned by patient, silver oxide, 1.5 volt, each [&] Y

Bill DME/MAC

Inexpensive and routinely purchased DME

DMEPOS Modifier(s): NU

✳ **K0602** Replacement battery for external infusion pump owned by patient, silver oxide, 3 volt, each [&] Y

Bill DME/MAC

Inexpensive and routinely purchased DME

DMEPOS Modifier(s): NU

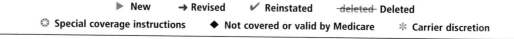

▶ New → Revised ✔ Reinstated ~~deleted~~ Deleted
⊛ Special coverage instructions ◆ Not covered or valid by Medicare ✳ Carrier discretion

✳ **K0603** Replacement battery for external infusion pump owned by patient, alkaline, 1.5 volt, each ♿   Y

Bill DME/MAC

Inexpensive and routinely purchased DME

DMEPOS Modifier(s): NU

✳ **K0604** Replacement battery for external infusion pump owned by patient, lithium, 3.6 volt, each ♿   Y

Bill DME/MAC

Inexpensive and routinely purchased DME

DMEPOS Modifier(s): NU

✳ **K0605** Replacement battery for external infusion pump owned by patient, lithium, 4.5 volt, each ♿   Y

Bill DME/MAC

Inexpensive and routinely purchased DME

DMEPOS Modifier(s): NU

✳ **K0606** Automatic external defibrillator, with integrated electrocardiogram analysis, garment type Qp ♿   Y

Bill DME/MAC

Capped rental

DMEPOS Modifier(s): KE, RR

✳ **K0607** Replacement battery for automated external defibrillator, garment type only, each Qp ♿   Y

Bill DME/MAC

Inexpensive and routinely purchased DME

DMEPOS Modifier(s): KF, NU, RR, UE

✳ **K0608** Replacement garment for use with automated external defibrillator, each Qp ♿   Y

Bill DME/MAC

Inexpensive and routinely purchased DME

DMEPOS Modifier(s): KF, NU, RR, UE

✳ **K0609** Replacement electrodes for use with automated external defibrillator, garment type only, each Qp ♿   Y

Bill DME/MAC

Supplies.

DMEPOS Modifier(s): KF

→ ✳ **K0669** Wheelchair accessory, wheelchair seat or back cushion, does not meet specific code criteria or no written coding verification from DME PDAC   Y

Bill DME/MAC

Inexpensive and routinely purchased DME

✳ **K0672** Addition to lower extremity orthosis, removable soft interface, all components, replacement only, each ♿   A

Bill DME/MAC

Prosthetics/Orthotics

→ ✳ **K0730** Controlled dose inhalation drug delivery system Qp ♿   Y

Bill DME/MAC

Inexpensive and routinely purchased DME

DMEPOS Modifier(s): NU, RR, UE

✳ **K0733** Power wheelchair accessory, 12 to 24 amp hour sealed lead acid battery, each (e.g., gel cell, absorbed glassmat) Qp ♿   Y

Bill DME/MAC

Inexpensive and routinely purchased DME

DMEPOS Modifier(s): KF, NU, RR, UE

✳ **K0738** Portable gaseous oxygen system, rental; home compressor used to fill portable oxygen cylinders; includes portable containers, regulator, flowmeter, humidifier, cannula or mask, and tubing Qp ♿   Y

Bill DME/MAC

Oxygen and oxygen equipment

DMEPOS Modifier(s): RR

✳ **K0739** Repair or nonroutine service for durable medical equipment other than oxygen equipment requiring the skill of a technician, labor component, per 15 minutes   Y

Local carrier if used with implanted DME. If other, bill DME/MAC.

◆ **K0740** Repair or nonroutine service for oxygen equipment requiring the skill of a technician, labor component, per 15 minutes   E

Bill DME/MAC

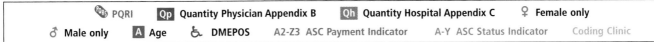

▶ ☼ **K0741** Portable gaseous oxygen system, rental, includes portable container, regulator, flowmeter, humidifier, cannula or mask, and tubing, for cluster headaches   Y

▶ ☼ **K0742** Portable oxygen contents, gaseous, 1 month's supply = 1 unit, for cluster headaches, for initial months supply or to replace used contents   Y

▶ ✳ **K0743** Suction pump, home model, portable, for use on wounds   Y

Bill DME/MAC

▶ ✳ **K0744** Absorptive wound dressing for use with suction pump, home model, portable, pad size 16 square inches or less   A

Bill DME/MAC

▶ ✳ **K0745** Absorptive wound dressing for use with suction pump, home model, portable, pad size more than 16 square inches but less than or equal to 48 square inches   A

Bill DME/MAC

▶ ✳ **K0746** Absorptive wound dressing for use with suction pump, home model, portable, pad size greater than 48 square inches   A

Bill DME/MAC

✳ **K0800** Power operated vehicle, group 1 standard, patient weight capacity up to and including 300 pounds **Qp** ♿   Y

Bill DME/MAC

Power mobility device (PMD) includes power operated vehicles (POVs) and power wheelchairs (PWCs). Inexpensive and routinely purchased DME

DMEPOS Modifier(s): NU, RR, UE

✳ **K0801** Power operated vehicle, group 1 heavy duty, patient weight capacity 301 to 450 pounds **Qp** ♿   Y

Bill DME/MAC

Inexpensive and routinely purchased DME

DMEPOS Modifier(s): NU, RR, UE

✳ **K0802** Power operated vehicle, group 1 very heavy duty, patient weight capacity 451 to 600 pounds **Qp** ♿   Y

Bill DME/MAC

Inexpensive and routinely purchased DME

DMEPOS Modifier(s): NU, RR, UE

✳ **K0806** Power operated vehicle, group 2 standard, patient weight capacity up to and including 300 pounds **Qp** ♿   Y

Bill DME/MAC

Inexpensive and routinely purchased DME

DMEPOS Modifier(s): NU, RR, UE

✳ **K0807** Power operated vehicle, group 2 heavy duty, patient weight capacity 301 to 450 pounds **Qp** ♿   Y

Bill DME/MAC

Inexpensive and routinely purchased DME

DMEPOS Modifier(s): NU, RR, UE

✳ **K0808** Power operated vehicle, group 2 very heavy duty, patient weight capacity 451 to 600 pounds **Qp** ♿   Y

Bill DME/MAC

Inexpensive and routinely purchased DME

DMEPOS Modifier(s): NU, RR, UE

✳ **K0812** Power operated vehicle, not otherwise classified   Y

Bill DME/MAC

Not Otherwise Classified.

✳ **K0813** Power wheelchair, group 1 standard, portable, sling/solid seat and back, patient weight capacity up to and including 300 pounds **Qp** ♿   Y

Bill DME/MAC

Capped rental

DMEPOS Modifier(s): RR

✳ **K0814** Power wheelchair, group 1 standard, portable, captains chair, patient weight capacity up to and including 300 pounds **Qp** ♿   Y

Bill DME/MAC

Capped rental

DMEPOS Modifier(s): RR

✳ **K0815** Power wheelchair, group 1 standard, sling/solid seat and back, patient weight capacity up to and including 300 pounds **Qp** ♿   Y

Bill DME/MAC

Capped rental

DMEPOS Modifier(s): RR

▶ New   → Revised   ✔ Reinstated   ~~deleted~~ Deleted

☼ Special coverage instructions   ◆ Not covered or valid by Medicare   ✳ Carrier discretion

✻ **K0816** Power wheelchair, group 1 standard, captains chair, patient weight capacity up to and including 300 pounds **Qp** ♿   Y

Bill DME/MAC

Capped rental

DMEPOS Modifier(s): RR

✻ **K0820** Power wheelchair, group 2 standard, portable, sling/solid seat/back, patient weight capacity up to and including 300 pounds **Qp** ♿   Y

Bill DME/MAC

Capped rental

DMEPOS Modifier(s): RR

✻ **K0821** Power wheelchair, group 2 standard, portable, captains chair, patient weight capacity up to and including 300 pounds **Qp** ♿   Y

Bill DME/MAC

Capped rental

DMEPOS Modifier(s): RR

✻ **K0822** Power wheelchair, group 2 standard, sling/solid seat/back, patient weight capacity up to and including 300 pounds **Qp** ♿   Y

Bill DME/MAC

Capped rental

DMEPOS Modifier(s): RR

✻ **K0823** Power wheelchair, group 2 standard, captains chair, patient weight capacity up to and including 300 pounds **Qp** ♿   Y

Bill DME/MAC

Capped rental

DMEPOS Modifier(s): RR

✻ **K0824** Power wheelchair, group 2 heavy duty, sling/solid seat/back, patient weight capacity 301 to 450 pounds **Qp** ♿   Y

Bill DME/MAC

Capped rental

DMEPOS Modifier(s): RR

✻ **K0825** Power wheelchair, group 2 heavy duty, captains chair, patient weight capacity 301 to 450 pounds **Qp** ♿   Y

Bill DME/MAC

Capped rental

DMEPOS Modifier(s): RR

✻ **K0826** Power wheelchair, group 2 very heavy duty, sling/solid seat/back, patient weight capacity 451 to 600 pounds **Qp** ♿   Y

Bill DME/MAC

Capped rental

DMEPOS Modifier(s): RR

✻ **K0827** Power wheelchair, group 2 very heavy duty, captains chair, patient weight capacity 451 to 600 pounds **Qp** ♿   Y

Bill DME/MAC

Capped rental

DMEPOS Modifier(s): RR

✻ **K0828** Power wheelchair, group 2 extra heavy duty, sling/solid seat/back, patient weight capacity 601 pounds or more **Qp** ♿   Y

Bill DME/MAC

Capped rental

DMEPOS Modifier(s): RR

✻ **K0829** Power wheelchair, group 2 extra heavy duty, captains chair, patient weight 601 pounds or more **Qp** ♿   Y

Bill DME/MAC

Capped rental

DMEPOS Modifier(s): RR

✻ **K0830** Power wheelchair, group 2 standard, seat elevator, sling/solid seat/back, patient weight capacity up to and including 300 pounds **Qp**   Y

Bill DME/MAC

Capped rental

DMEPOS Modifier(s): NU, RR, UE

✻ **K0831** Power wheelchair, group 2 standard, seat elevator, captains chair, patient weight capacity up to and including 300 pounds **Qp**   Y

Bill DME/MAC

DMEPOS Modifier(s): NU, RR, UE

✻ **K0835** Power wheelchair, group 2 standard, single power option, sling/solid seat/back, patient weight capacity up to and including 300 pounds **Qp** ♿   Y

Bill DME/MAC

Capped rental

DMEPOS Modifier(s): RR

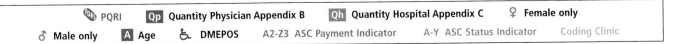

PQRI   **Qp** Quantity Physician Appendix B   **Qh** Quantity Hospital Appendix C   ♀ Female only

♂ Male only   **A** Age   ♿ DMEPOS   A2-Z3 ASC Payment Indicator   A-Y ASC Status Indicator   Coding Clinic

✳ **K0836** Power wheelchair, group 2 standard, single power option, captains chair, patient weight capacity up to and including 300 pounds Qp ♿ Y

Bill DME/MAC

Capped rental

DMEPOS Modifier(s): RR

✳ **K0837** Power wheelchair, group 2 heavy duty, single power option, sling/solid seat/back, patient weight capacity 301 to 450 pounds Qp ♿ Y

Bill DME/MAC

Capped rental

DMEPOS Modifier(s): RR

✳ **K0838** Power wheelchair, group 2 heavy duty, single power option, captains chair, patient weight capacity 301 to 450 pounds Qp ♿ Y

Bill DME/MAC

Capped rental

DMEPOS Modifier(s): RR

✳ **K0839** Power wheelchair, group 2 very heavy duty, single power option sling/solid seat/back, patient weight capacity 451 to 600 pounds Qp ♿ Y

Bill DME/MAC

Capped rental

DMEPOS Modifier(s): RR

✳ **K0840** Power wheelchair, group 2 extra heavy duty, single power option, sling/solid seat/back, patient weight capacity 601 pounds or more Qp ♿ Y

Bill DME/MAC

Capped rental

DMEPOS Modifier(s): RR

✳ **K0841** Power wheelchair, group 2 standard, multiple power option, sling/solid seat/back, patient weight capacity up to and including 300 pounds Qp ♿ Y

Bill DME/MAC

Capped rental

DMEPOS Modifier(s): RR

✳ **K0842** Power wheelchair, group 2 standard, multiple power option, captains chair, patient weight capacity up to and including 300 pounds Qp ♿ Y

Bill DME/MAC

Capped rental

DMEPOS Modifier(s): RR

✳ **K0843** Power wheelchair, group 2 heavy duty, multiple power option, sling/solid seat/back, patient weight capacity 301 to 450 pounds Qp ♿ Y

Bill DME/MAC

Capped rental

DMEPOS Modifier(s): RR

✳ **K0848** Power wheelchair, group 3 standard, sling/solid seat/back, patient weight capacity up to and including 300 pounds Qp ♿ Y

Bill DME/MAC

Capped rental

DMEPOS Modifier(s): RR

✳ **K0849** Power wheelchair, group 3 standard, captains chair, patient weight capacity up to and including 300 pounds Qp ♿ Y

Bill DME/MAC

Capped rental

DMEPOS Modifier(s): RR

✳ **K0850** Power wheelchair, group 3 heavy duty, sling/solid seat/back, patient weight capacity 301 to 450 pounds Qp ♿ Y

Bill DME/MAC

Capped rental

DMEPOS Modifier(s): RR

✳ **K0851** Power wheelchair, group 3 heavy duty, captains chair, patient weight capacity 301 to 450 pounds Qp ♿ Y

Bill DME/MAC

Capped rental

DMEPOS Modifier(s): RR

✳ **K0852** Power wheelchair, group 3 very heavy duty, sling/solid seat/back, patient weight capacity 451 to 600 pounds Qp ♿ Y

Bill DME/MAC

Capped rental

DMEPOS Modifier(s): RR

✳ **K0853** Power wheelchair, group 3 very heavy duty, captains chair, patient weight capacity 451 to 600 pounds ♿ Y

Bill DME/MAC

Capped rental

DMEPOS Modifier(s): RR

▶ New   → Revised   ✔ Reinstated   ~~deleted~~ Deleted

☺ Special coverage instructions   ◆ Not covered or valid by Medicare   ✳ Carrier discretion

* **K0854** Power wheelchair, group 3 extra heavy duty, sling/solid seat/back, patient weight capacity 601 pounds or more Qp 占   Y

Bill DME/MAC

Capped rental

DMEPOS Modifier(s): RR

* **K0855** Power wheelchair, group 3 extra heavy duty, captains chair, patient weight capacity 601 pounds or more Qp 占   Y

Bill DME/MAC

Capped rental

DMEPOS Modifier(s): RR

* **K0856** Power wheelchair, group 3 standard, single power option, sling/solid seat/back, patient weight capacity up to and including 300 pounds Qp 占   Y

Bill DME/MAC

Capped rental

DMEPOS Modifier(s): RR

* **K0857** Power wheelchair, group 3 standard, single power option, captains chair, patient weight capacity up to and including 300 pounds Qp 占   Y

Bill DME/MAC

Capped rental

DMEPOS Modifier(s): RR

* **K0858** Power wheelchair, group 3 heavy duty, single power option, sling/solid seat/back, patient weight 301 to 450 pounds Qp 占   Y

Bill DME/MAC

Capped rental

DMEPOS Modifier(s): RR

* **K0859** Power wheelchair, group 3 heavy duty, single power option, captains chair, patient weight capacity 301 to 450 pounds Qp 占   Y

Bill DME/MAC

Capped rental

DMEPOS Modifier(s): RR

* **K0860** Power wheelchair, group 3 very heavy duty, single power option, sling/solid seat/back, patient weight capacity 451 to 600 pounds Qp 占   Y

Bill DME/MAC

Capped rental

DMEPOS Modifier(s): RR

* **K0861** Power wheelchair, group 3 standard, multiple power option, sling/solid seat/back, patient weight capacity up to and including 300 pounds Qp 占   Y

Bill DME/MAC

Capped rental

DMEPOS Modifier(s): KF, RR

* **K0862** Power wheelchair, group 3 heavy duty, multiple power option, sling/solid seat/back, patient weight capacity 301 to 450 pounds Qp 占   Y

Bill DME/MAC

Capped rental

DMEPOS Modifier(s): RR

* **K0863** Power wheelchair, group 3 very heavy duty, multiple power option, sling/solid seat/back, patient weight capacity 451 to 600 pounds Qp 占   Y

Bill DME/MAC

Capped rental

DMEPOS Modifier(s): RR

* **K0864** Power wheelchair, group 3 extra heavy duty, multiple power option, sling/solid seat/back, patient weight capacity 601 pounds or more Qp 占   Y

Bill DME/MAC

Capped rental

DMEPOS Modifier(s): RR

* **K0868** Power wheelchair, group 4 standard, sling/solid seat/back, patient weight capacity up to and including 300 pounds Qp   Y

Bill DME/MAC

Capped rental

* **K0869** Power wheelchair, group 4 standard, captains chair, patient weight capacity up to and including 300 pounds Qp   Y

Bill DME/MAC

Capped rental

* **K0870** Power wheelchair, group 4 heavy duty, sling/solid seat/back, patient weight capacity 301 to 450 pounds   Y

Bill DME/MAC

Capped rental

* **K0871** Power wheelchair, group 4 very heavy duty, sling/solid seat/back, patient weight capacity 451 to 600 pounds   Y

Bill DME/MAC

Capped rental

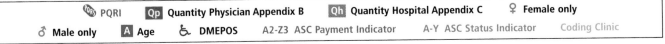

ⓟ PQRI	Qp Quantity Physician Appendix B	Qh Quantity Hospital Appendix C	♀ Female only
♂ Male only	A Age	占 DMEPOS	A2-Z3 ASC Payment Indicator A-Y ASC Status Indicator Coding Clinic

✳ **K0877** Power wheelchair, group 4 standard, single power option, sling/solid seat/back, patient weight capacity up to and including 300 pounds `Qp`   Y

Bill DME/MAC

Capped rental

✳ **K0878** Power wheelchair, group 4 standard, single power option, captains chair, patient weight capacity up to and including 300 pounds   Y

Bill DME/MAC

Capped rental

✳ **K0879** Power wheelchair, group 4 heavy duty, single power option, sling/solid seat/back, patient weight capacity 301 to 450 pounds   Y

Bill DME/MAC

Capped rental

✳ **K0880** Power wheelchair, group 4 very heavy duty, single power option, sling/solid seat/back, patient weight 451 to 600 pounds `Qp`   Y

Bill DME/MAC

Capped rental

✳ **K0884** Power wheelchair, group 4 standard, multiple power option, sling/solid seat/back, patient weight capacity up to and including 300 pounds `Qp`   Y

Bill DME/MAC

Capped rental

✳ **K0885** Power wheelchair, group 4 standard, multiple power option, captains chair, patient weight capacity up to and including 300 pounds   Y

Bill DME/MAC

Capped rental

✳ **K0886** Power wheelchair, group 4 heavy duty, multiple power option, sling/solid seat/back, patient weight capacity 301 to 450 pounds   Y

Bill DME/MAC

Capped rental

✳ **K0890** Power wheelchair, group 5 pediatric, single power option, sling/solid seat/back, patient weight capacity up to and including 125 pounds `A`   Y

Bill DME/MAC

Capped rental

✳ **K0891** Power wheelchair, group 5 pediatric, multiple power option, sling/solid seat/back, patient weight capacity up to and including 125 pounds `A`   Y

Bill DME/MAC

Capped rental

✳ **K0898** Power wheelchair, not otherwise classified   Y

Bill DME/MAC

→ ✳ **K0899** Power mobility device, not coded by **DME PDAC** or does not meet criteria   Y

Bill DME/MAC

▶ **New** → **Revised** ✔ **Reinstated** ~~deleted~~ **Deleted**

✪ **Special coverage instructions** ◆ **Not covered or valid by Medicare** ✳ **Carrier discretion**

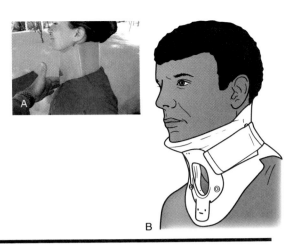

Figure 22 **A.** Flexible cervical collar. **B.** Adjustable cervical collar.

ORTHOTICS (L0100-L4999)

DMEPOS fee schedule:
www.cms.gov/DMEPOSFeeSched/LSDMEPOSFEE/list.asp#TopOfPage

Orthotic Devices: Spinal

Cervical

L0112-L0220:   Bill DME/MAC

* **L0112**   Cranial cervical orthosis, congenital torticollis type, with or without soft interface material, adjustable range of motion joint, custom fabricated Qp Qh &   A

* **L0113**   Cranial cervical orthosis, torticollis type, with or without joint, with or without soft interface material, prefabricated, includes fitting and adjustment Qp Qh &   A

* **L0120**   Cervical, flexible, non-adjustable (foam collar) Qp Qh &   A

   Cervical orthoses, including soft and rigid devices may be used as nonoperative management for cervical trauma

* **L0130**   Cervical, flexible, thermoplastic collar, molded to patient Qp Qh &   A

* **L0140**   Cervical, semi-rigid, adjustable (plastic collar) Qp Qh &   A

* **L0150**   Cervical, semi-rigid, adjustable molded chin cup (plastic collar with mandibular/occipital piece) Qp Qh &   A

* **L0160**   Cervical, semi-rigid, wire frame occipital/mandibular support Qp Qh &   A

* **L0170**   Cervical, collar, molded to patient model Qp Qh &   A

* **L0172**   Cervical, collar, semi-rigid thermoplastic foam, two piece Qp Qh &   A

* **L0174**   Cervical, collar, semi-rigid, thermoplastic foam, two piece with thoracic extension Qp Qh &   A

Multiple Post Collar

* **L0180**   Cervical, multiple post collar, occipital/mandibular supports, adjustable Qp Qh &   A

* **L0190**   Cervical, multiple post collar, occipital/mandibular supports, adjustable cervical bars (SOMI, Guilford, Taylor types) Qp Qh &   A

* **L0200**   Cervical, multiple post collar, occipital/mandibular supports, adjustable cervical bars, and thoracic extension Qp Qh &   A

Thoracic

* **L0220**   Thoracic, rib belt, custom fabricated Qp Qh &   A

Thoracic-Lumbar-Sacral

Anterior-Posterior-Lateral Rotary-Control

L0430-L0492:   Bill DME/MAC

* **L0430**   Spinal orthosis, anterior-posterior-lateral control, with interface material, custom fitted (Dewall posture protector only) Qp Qh &   A

* **L0450**   TLSO, flexible, provides trunk support, upper thoracic region, produces intracavitary pressure to reduce load on the intervertebral disks with rigid stays or panel(s), includes shoulder straps and closures, prefabricated, includes fitting and adjustment Qp Qh &   A

   Used to immobilize specified area of spine, and is generally worn under clothing

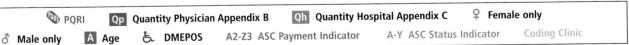

PQRI   Qp **Quantity Physician Appendix B**   Qh **Quantity Hospital Appendix C**   ♀ **Female only**
♂ **Male only**   A **Age**   & **DMEPOS**   A2-Z3 ASC Payment Indicator   A-Y ASC Status Indicator   Coding Clinic

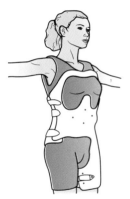

Figure 23 Thoracic-Lumbar-Sacral orthosis (TLSO).

* **L0452** TLSO, flexible, provides trunk support, upper thoracic region, produces intracavitary pressure to reduce load on the intervertebral disks with rigid stays or panel(s), includes shoulder straps and closures, custom fabricated Qp Qh 占 A

* **L0454** TLSO flexible, provides trunk support, extends from sacrococcygeal junction to above T-9 vertebra, restricts gross trunk motion in the sagittal plane, produces intracavitary pressure to reduce load on the intervertebral disks with rigid stays or panel(s), includes shoulder straps and closures, prefabricated, includes fitting and adjustment Qp Qh 占 A

Used to immobilize specified areas of spine; and is generally designed to be worn under clothing; not specifically designed for patients in wheelchairs

* **L0456** TLSO, flexible, provides trunk support, thoracic region, rigid posterior panel and soft anterior apron, extends from the sacrococcygeal junction and terminates just inferior to the scapular spine, restricts gross trunk motion in the sagittal plane, produces intracavitary pressure to reduce load on the intervertebral disks, includes straps and closures, prefabricated, includes fitting and adjustment Qp Qh 占 A

* **L0458** TLSO, triplanar control, modular segmented spinal system, two rigid plastic shells, posterior extends from the sacrococcygeal junction and terminates just inferior to the scapular spine, anterior extends from the symphysis pubis to the xiphoid, soft liner, restricts gross trunk motion in the sagittal, coronal, and transverse planes, lateral strength is provided by overlapping plastic and stabilizing closures, includes straps and closures, prefabricated, includes fitting and adjustment Qp Qh 占 A

To meet Medicare's definition of body jacket, orthosis has to have rigid plastic shell that circles trunk with overlapping edges and stabilizing closures, and entire circumference of shell must be made of same rigid material

* **L0460** TLSO, triplanar control, modular segmented spinal system, two rigid plastic shells, posterior extends from the sacrococcygeal junction and terminates just inferior to the scapular spine, anterior extends from the symphysis pubis to the sternal notch, soft liner, restricts gross trunk motion in the sagittal, coronal, and transverse planes, lateral strength is provided by overlapping plastic and stabilizing closures, includes straps and closures, prefabricated, includes fitting and adjustment Qp Qh 占 A

* **L0462** TLSO, triplanar control, modular segmented spinal system, three rigid plastic shells, posterior extends from the sacrococcygeal junction and terminates just inferior to the scapular spine, anterior extends from the symphysis pubis to the sternal notch, soft liner, restricts gross trunk motion in the sagittal, coronal, and transverse planes, lateral strength is provided by overlapping plastic and stabilizing closures, includes straps and closures, prefabricated, includes fitting and adjustment Qp Qh 占 A

▶ New　→ Revised　✔ Reinstated　deleted Deleted

☺ Special coverage instructions　◆ Not covered or valid by Medicare　* Carrier discretion

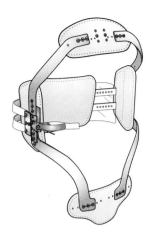

Figure 24 Thoracic-Lumbar-Sacral orthosis (TLSO) Jewett flexion control.

✳ **L0464** TLSO, triplanar control, modular segmented spinal system, four rigid plastic shells, posterior extends from sacrococcygeal junction and terminates just inferior to scapular spine, anterior extends from symphysis pubis to the sternal notch, soft liner, restricts gross trunk motion in sagittal, coronal, and transverse planes, lateral strength is provided by overlapping plastic and stabilizing closures, includes straps and closures, prefabricated, includes fitting and adjustment Qp Qh ♿   A

✳ **L0466** TLSO, sagittal control, rigid posterior frame and flexible soft anterior apron with straps, closures and padding, restricts gross trunk motion in sagittal plane, produces intracavitary pressure to reduce load on intervertebral disks, includes fitting and shaping the frame, prefabricated, includes fitting and adjustment Qp Qh ♿   A

✳ **L0468** TLSO, sagittal-coronal control, rigid posterior frame and flexible soft anterior apron with straps, closures and padding, extends from sacrococcygeal junction over scapulae, lateral strength provided by pelvic, thoracic, and lateral frame pieces, restricts gross trunk motion in sagittal, and coronal planes, produces intracavitary pressure to reduce load on intervertebral disks, includes fitting and shaping the frame, prefabricated, includes fitting and adjustment Qp Qh ♿   A

✳ **L0470** TLSO, triplanar control, rigid posterior frame and flexible soft anterior apron with straps, closures and padding, extends from sacrococcygeal junction to scapula, lateral strength provided by pelvic, thoracic, and lateral frame pieces, rotational strength provided by subclavicular extensions, restricts gross trunk motion in sagittal, coronal, and transverse planes, provides intracavitary pressure to reduce load on the intervertebral disks, includes fitting and shaping the frame, prefabricated, includes fitting and adjustment Qp Qh ♿   A

✳ **L0472** TLSO, triplanar control, hyperextension, rigid anterior and lateral frame extends from symphysis pubis to sternal notch with two anterior components (one pubic and one sternal), posterior and lateral pads with straps and closures, limits spinal flexion, restricts gross trunk motion in sagittal, coronal, and transverse planes, includes fitting and shaping the frame, prefabricated, includes fitting and adjustment Qp Qh ♿   A

✳ **L0480** TLSO, triplanar control, one piece rigid plastic shell without interface liner, with multiple straps and closures, posterior extends from sacrococcygeal junction and terminates just inferior to scapular spine, anterior extends from symphysis pubis to sternal notch, anterior or posterior opening, restricts gross trunk motion in sagittal, coronal, and transverse planes, includes a carved plaster or CAD-CAM model, custom fabricated Qp Qh ♿   A

✳ **L0482** TLSO, triplanar control, one piece rigid plastic shell with interface liner, multiple straps and closures, posterior extends from sacrococcygeal junction and terminates just inferior to scapular spine, anterior extends from symphysis pubis to sternal notch, anterior or posterior opening, restricts gross trunk motion in sagittal, coronal, and transverse planes, includes a carved plaster or CAD-CAM model, custom fabricated Qp Qh ♿   A

| 🅿 PQRI | Qp Quantity Physician Appendix B | Qh Quantity Hospital Appendix C | ♀ Female only |
| ♂ Male only | A Age | ♿ DMEPOS | A2-Z3 ASC Payment Indicator | A-Y ASC Status Indicator | Coding Clinic |

ORTHOTICS L0464 – L0482

263

✳ **L0484** TLSO, triplanar control, two piece rigid plastic shell without interface liner, with multiple straps and closures, posterior extends from sacrococcygeal junction and terminates just inferior to scapular spine, anterior extends from symphysis pubis to sternal notch, lateral strength is enhanced by overlapping plastic, restricts gross trunk motion in the sagittal, coronal, and transverse planes, includes a carved plaster or CAD-CAM model, custom fabricated `Qp` `Qh` & A

✳ **L0486** TLSO, triplanar control, two piece rigid plastic shell with interface liner, multiple straps and closures, posterior extends from sacrococcygeal junction and terminates just inferior to scapular spine, anterior extends from symphysis pubis to sternal notch, lateral strength is enhanced by overlapping plastic, restricts gross trunk motion in the sagittal, coronal, and transverse planes, includes a carved plaster or CAD-CAM model, custom fabricated `Qp` `Qh` & A

✳ **L0488** TLSO, triplanar control, one piece rigid plastic shell with interface liner, multiple straps and closures, posterior extends from sacrococcygeal junction and terminates just inferior to scapular spine, anterior extends from symphysis pubis to sternal notch, anterior or posterior opening, restricts gross trunk motion in sagittal, coronal, and transverse planes, prefabricated, includes fitting and adjustment `Qp` `Qh` & A

✳ **L0490** TLSO, sagittal-coronal control, one piece rigid plastic shell, with overlapping reinforced anterior, with multiple straps and closures, posterior extends from sacrococcygeal junction and terminates at or before the T-9 vertebra, anterior extends from symphysis pubis to xiphoid, anterior opening, restricts gross trunk motion in sagittal and coronal planes, prefabricated, includes fitting and adjustment `Qp` `Qh` & A

✳ **L0491** TLSO, sagittal-coronal control, modular segmented spinal system, two rigid plastic shells, posterior extends from the sacrococcygeal junction and terminates just inferior to the scapular spine, anterior extends from the symphysis pubis to the xiphoid, soft liner, restricts gross trunk motion in the sagittal and coronal planes, lateral strength is provided by overlapping plastic and stabilizing closures, includes straps and closures, prefabricated, includes fitting and adjustment `Qp` `Qh` & A

✳ **L0492** TLSO, sagittal-coronal control, modular segmented spinal system, three rigid plastic shells, posterior extends from the sacrococcygeal junction and terminates just inferior to the scapular spine, anterior extends from the symphysis pubis to the xiphoid, soft liner, restricts gross trunk motion in the sagittal and coronal planes, lateral strength is provided by overlapping plastic and stabilizing closures, includes straps and closures, prefabricated, includes fitting and adjustment `Qp` `Qh` & A

Sacroilliac, Lumbar, Sacral Orthosis

L0621-L0640: Bill DME/MAC

✳ **L0621** Sacroiliac orthosis, flexible, provides pelvic-sacral support, reduces motion about the sacroiliac joint, includes straps, closures, may include pendulous abdomen design, prefabricated, includes fitting and adjustment `Qp` `Qh` & A

✳ **L0622** Sacroiliac orthosis, flexible, provides pelvic-sacral support, reduces motion about the sacroiliac joint, includes straps, closures, may include pendulous abdomen design, custom fabricated `Qp` `Qh` & A

Type of custom-fabricated device for which impression of specific body part is made (e.g., by means of plaster cast, or CAD-CAM [computer-aided design] technology); impression then used to make specific patient model

▶ New   → Revised   ✔ Reinstated   ~~deleted~~ Deleted
♲ Special coverage instructions   ◆ Not covered or valid by Medicare   ✳ Carrier discretion

✳ **L0623** Sacroiliac orthosis, provides pelvic-sacral support, with rigid or semi-rigid panels over the sacrum and abdomen, reduces motion about the sacroiliac joint, includes straps, closures, may include pendulous abdomen design, prefabricated, includes fitting and adjustment `Qp` `Qh` ♿   A

✳ **L0624** Sacroiliac orthosis, provides pelvic-sacral support, with rigid or semi-rigid panels placed over the sacrum and abdomen, reduces motion about the sacroiliac joint, includes straps, closures, may include pendulous abdomen design, custom fabricated `Qp` `Qh` ♿   A

Custom fitted

✳ **L0625** Lumbar orthosis, flexible, provides lumbar support, posterior extends from L-1 to below L-5 vertebra, produces intracavitary pressure to reduce load on the intervertebral discs, includes straps, closures, may include pendulous abdomen design, shoulder straps, stays, prefabricated, includes fitting and adjustment `Qp` `Qh` ♿   A

✳ **L0626** Lumbar orthosis, sagittal control, with rigid posterior panel(s), posterior extends from L-1 to below L-5 vertebra, produces intracavitary pressure to reduce load on the intervertebral discs, includes straps, closures, may include padding, stays, shoulder straps, pendulous abdomen design, prefabricated, includes fitting and adjustment `Qp` `Qh` ♿   A

✳ **L0627** Lumbar orthosis, sagittal control, with rigid anterior and posterior panels, posterior extends from L-1 to below L-5 vertebra, produces intracavitary pressure to reduce load on the intervertebral discs, includes straps, closures, may include padding, shoulder straps, pendulous abdomen design, prefabricated, includes fitting and adjustment `Qp` `Qh` ♿   A

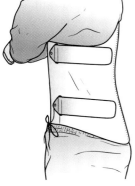

Figure 25 Lumbar-sacral orthosis.

✳ **L0628** Lumbar-sacral orthosis, flexible, provides lumbo-sacral support, posterior extends from sacrococcygeal junction to T-9 vertebra, produces intracavitary pressure to reduce load on the intervertebral discs, includes straps, closures, may include stays, shoulder straps, pendulous abdomen design, prefabricated, includes fitting and adjustment `Qp` `Qh` ♿   A

✳ **L0629** Lumbar-sacral orthosis, flexible, provides lumbo-sacral support, posterior extends from sacrococcygeal junction to T-9 vertebra, produces intracavitary pressure to reduce load on the intervertebral discs, includes straps, closures, may include stays, shoulder straps, pendulous abdomen design, custom fabricated `Qp` `Qh` ♿   A

Custom fitted

✳ **L0630** Lumbar-sacral orthosis, sagittal control, with rigid posterior panel(s), posterior extends from sacrococcygeal junction to T-9 vertebra, produces intracavitary pressure to reduce load on the intervertebral discs, includes straps, closures, may include padding, stays, shoulder straps, pendulous abdomen design, prefabricated, includes fitting and adjustment `Qp` `Qh` ♿   A

✳ **L0631** Lumbar-sacral orthosis, sagittal control, with rigid anterior and posterior panels, posterior extends from sacrococcygeal junction to T-9 vertebra, produces intracavitary pressure to reduce load on the intervertebral discs, includes straps, closures, may include padding, shoulder straps, pendulous abdomen design, prefabricated, includes fitting and adjustment `Qp` `Qh` ♿   A

✳ **L0632** Lumbar-sacral orthosis, sagittal control, with rigid anterior and posterior panels, posterior extends from sacrococcygeal junction to T-9 vertebra, produces intracavitary pressure to reduce load on the intervertebral discs, includes straps, closures, may include padding, shoulder straps, pendulous abdomen design, custom fabricated `Qp` `Qh` ♿   A

Custom fitted

✳ **L0633** Lumbar-sacral orthosis, sagittal-coronal control, with rigid posterior frame/panel(s), posterior extends from sacrococcygeal junction to T-9 vertebra, lateral strength provided by rigid lateral frame/panels, produces intracavitary pressure to reduce load on intervertebral discs, includes straps, closures, may include padding, stays, shoulder straps, pendulous abdomen design, prefabricated, includes fitting and adjustment `Qp` `Qh` ᕐ A

✳ **L0634** Lumbar-sacral orthosis, sagittal-coronal control, with rigid posterior frame/panel(s), posterior extends from sacrococcygeal junction to T-9 vertebra, lateral strength provided by rigid lateral frame/panel(s), produces intracavitary pressure to reduce load on intervertebral discs, includes straps, closures, may include padding, stays, shoulder straps, pendulous abdomen design, custom fabricated `Qp` `Qh` ᕐ A
Custom fitted

✳ **L0635** Lumbar-sacral orthosis, sagittal-coronal control, lumbar flexion, rigid posterior frame/panel(s), lateral articulating design to flex the lumbar spine, posterior extends from sacrococcygeal junction to T-9 vertebra, lateral strength provided by rigid lateral frame/panel(s), produces intracavitary pressure to reduce load on intervertebral discs, includes straps, closures, may include padding, anterior panel, pendulous abdomen design, prefabricated, includes fitting and adjustment `Qp` `Qh` ᕐ A

✳ **L0636** Lumbar sacral orthosis, sagittal-coronal control, lumbar flexion, rigid posterior frame/panels, lateral articulating design to flex the lumbar spine, posterior extends from sacrococcygeal junction to T-9 vertebra, lateral strength provided by rigid lateral frame/panels, produces intracavitary pressure to reduce load on intervertebral discs, includes straps, closures, may include padding, anterior panel, pendulous abdomen design, custom fabricated `Qp` `Qh` ᕐ A
Custom fitted

✳ **L0637** Lumbar-sacral orthosis, sagittal-coronal control, with rigid anterior and posterior frame/panels, posterior extends from sacrococcygeal junction to T-9 vertebra, lateral strength provided by rigid lateral frame/panels, produces intracavitary pressure to reduce load on intervertebral discs, includes straps, closures, may include padding, shoulder straps, pendulous abdomen design, prefabricated, includes fitting and adjustment `Qp` `Qh` ᕐ A

✳ **L0638** Lumbar-sacral orthosis, sagittal-coronal control, with rigid anterior and posterior frame/panels, posterior extends from sacrococcygeal junction to T-9 vertebra, lateral strength provided by rigid lateral frame/panels, produces intracavitary pressure to reduce load on intervertebral discs, includes straps, closures, may include padding, shoulder straps, pendulous abdomen design, custom fabricated `Qp` `Qh` ᕐ A

✳ **L0639** Lumbar-sacral orthosis, sagittal-coronal control, rigid shell(s)/panel(s), posterior extends from sacrococcygeal junction to T-9 vertebra, anterior extends from symphysis pubis to xyphoid, produces intracavitary pressure to reduce load on the intervertebral discs, overall strength is provided by overlapping rigid material and stabilizing closures, includes straps, closures may include soft interface, pendulous abdomen design, prefabricated, includes fitting and adjustment `Qp` `Qh` ᕐ A
Characterized by rigid plastic shell that encircles trunk with overlapping edges and stabilizing closures and provides high degree of immobility

✳ **L0640** Lumbar-sacral orthosis, sagittal-coronal control, rigid shell(s)/panel(s), posterior extends from sacrococcygeal junction to T-9 vertebra, anterior extends from symphysis pubis to xyphoid, produces intracavitary pressure to reduce load on the intervertebral discs, overall strength is provided by overlapping rigid material and stabilizing closures, includes straps, closures, may include soft interface, pendulous abdomen design, custom fabricated `Qp` `Qh` ᕐ A
Custom fitted

▶ New   → Revised   ✔ Reinstated   ~~deleted~~ Deleted
⊗ Special coverage instructions   ◆ Not covered or valid by Medicare   ✳ Carrier discretion

Cervical-Thoracic-Lumbar-Sacral

Anterior-Posterior-Lateral Control

L0700-L0710: Bill DME/MAC

- ✻ **L0700** Cervical-thoracic-lumbar-sacral-orthoses (CTLSO), anterior-posterior-lateral control, molded to patient model, (Minerva type) Qp Qh ♿ A
- ✻ **L0710** CTLSO, anterior-posterior-lateral-control, molded to patient model, with interface material, (Minerva type) Qp Qh ♿ A

HALO Procedure

L0810-L0861: Bill DME/MAC

- ✻ **L0810** HALO procedure, cervical halo incorporated into jacket vest Qp Qh ♿ A
- ✻ **L0820** HALO procedure, cervical halo incorporated into plaster body jacket Qp Qh ♿ A
- ✻ **L0830** HALO procedure, cervical halo incorporated into Milwaukee type orthosis Qp Qh ♿ A
- ✻ **L0859** Addition to HALO procedure, magnetic resonance image compatible systems, rings and pins, any material Qp Qh ♿ A
- ✻ **L0861** Addition to HALO procedure, replacement liner/interface material Qp Qh ♿ A

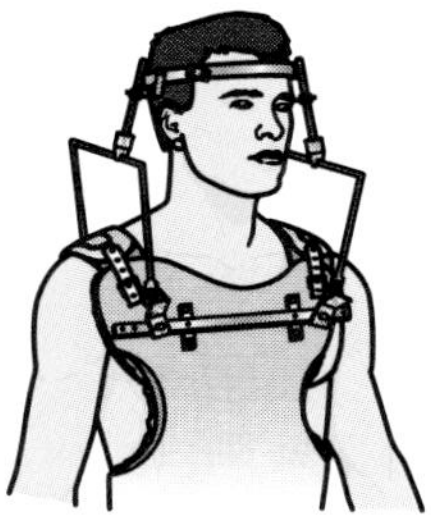

Figure 26 Halo device.

Additions to Spinal Orthoses

L0970-L0999: Bill DME/MAC

TLSO - Thoraci-lumbar-sacral orthoses

Spinal orthoses may be prefabricated, prefitted, or custom fabricated. Conservative treatment for back pain may include the use of spinal orthoses.

- ✻ **L0970** TLSO, corset front Qp Qh ♿ A
- ✻ **L0972** LSO, corset front Qp Qh ♿ A
- ✻ **L0974** TLSO, full corset Qp Qh ♿ A
- ✻ **L0976** LSO, full corset Qp Qh ♿ A
- ✻ **L0978** Axillary crutch extension Qp Qh ♿ A
- ✻ **L0980** Peroneal straps, pair Qp Qh ♿ A
- ✻ **L0982** Stocking supporter grips, set of four (4) ♿ A

  Convenience item
- ✻ **L0984** Protective body sock, each ♿ A

  Convenience item

  Garment made of cloth or similar material that is worn under spinal orthosis and is not primarily medical in nature
- ✻ **L0999** Addition to spinal orthosis, not otherwise specified A

Orthotic Devices: Scoliosis Procedures (L1000-L1520)

Note: Orthotic care of scoliosis differs from other orthotic care in that the treatment is more dynamic in nature and uses ongoing continual modification of the orthosis to the patient's changing condition. This coding structure uses the proper names, or eponyms, of the procedures because they have historic and universal acceptance in the profession. It should be recognized that variations to the basic procedures described by the founders/developers are accepted in various medical and orthotic practices throughout the country. All procedures include a model of patient when indicated.

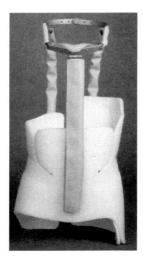

Figure 27 Milwaukee CTLSO.

Scoliosis: Cervical-Thoracic-Lumbar-Sacral (CTLSO) (Milwaukee)

L1000-L1520: Bill DME/MAC

* **L1000** Cervical-thoracic-lumbar-sacral orthosis (CTLSO) (Milwaukee), inclusive of furnishing initial orthosis, including model Qp Qh 👤   A

* **L1001** Cervical thoracic lumbar sacral orthosis, immobilizer, infant size, prefabricated, includes fitting and adjustment 👤   A

* **L1005** Tension based scoliosis orthosis and accessory pads, includes fitting and adjustment Qp Qh 👤   A

* **L1010** Addition to cervical-thoracic-lumbar-sacral orthosis (CTLSO) or scoliosis orthosis, axilla sling Qp Qh 👤   A

Correction Pads

* **L1020** Addition to CTLSO or scoliosis orthosis, kyphosis pad Qp Qh 👤   A

* **L1025** Addition to CTLSO or scoliosis orthosis, kyphosis pad, floating Qp Qh 👤   A

* **L1030** Addition to CTLSO or scoliosis orthosis, lumbar bolster pad Qp Qh 👤   A

* **L1040** Addition to CTLSO or scoliosis orthosis, lumbar or lumbar rib pad Qp Qh 👤   A

* **L1050** Addition to CTLSO or scoliosis orthosis, sternal pad Qp Qh 👤   A

* **L1060** Addition to CTLSO or scoliosis orthosis, thoracic pad Qp Qh 👤   A

* **L1070** Addition to CTLSO or scoliosis orthosis, trapezius sling Qp Qh 👤   A

* **L1080** Addition to CTLSO or scoliosis orthosis, outrigger Qp Qh 👤   A

* **L1085** Addition to CTLSO or scoliosis orthosis, outrigger, bilateral with vertical extensions Qp Qh 👤   A

* **L1090** Addition to CTLSO or scoliosis orthosis, lumbar sling Qp Qh 👤   A

* **L1100** Addition to CTLSO or scoliosis orthosis, ring flange, plastic or leather Qp Qh 👤   A

* **L1110** Addition to CTLSO or scoliosis orthosis, ring flange, plastic or leather, molded to patient model Qp Qh 👤   A

* **L1120** Addition to CTLSO, scoliosis orthosis, cover for upright, each Qp Qh 👤   A

Scoliosis: Thoracic-Lumbar-Sacral (Low Profile)

* **L1200** Thoracic-lumbar-sacral-orthosis (TLSO), inclusive of furnishing initial orthosis only Qp Qh 👤   A

* **L1210** Addition to TLSO, (low profile), lateral thoracic extension Qp Qh 👤   A

* **L1220** Addition to TLSO, (low profile), anterior thoracic extension Qp Qh 👤   A

* **L1230** Addition to TLSO, (low profile), Milwaukee type superstructure Qp Qh 👤   A

* **L1240** Addition to TLSO, (low profile), lumbar derotation pad Qp Qh 👤   A

* **L1250** Addition to TLSO, (low profile), anterior ASIS pad Qp Qh 👤   A

* **L1260** Addition to TLSO, (low profile), anterior thoracic derotation pad Qp Qh 👤   A

* **L1270** Addition to TLSO, (low profile), abdominal pad Qp Qh 👤   A

* **L1280** Addition to TLSO, (low profile), rib gusset (elastic), each Qp Qh 👤   A

* **L1290** Addition to TLSO, (low profile), lateral trochanteric pad Qp Qh 👤   A

Other Scoliosis Procedures

* **L1300** Other scoliosis procedure, body jacket molded to patient model Qp Qh 👤   A

* **L1310** Other scoliosis procedure, postoperative body jacket Qp Qh 👤   A

▶ New   → Revised   ✔ Reinstated   ~~deleted~~ Deleted

⊘ Special coverage instructions   ◆ Not covered or valid by Medicare   * Carrier discretion

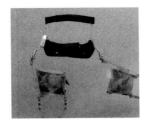

Figure 28 Thoracic-hip-knee-ankle orthosis (THKAO).

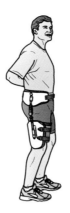

Figure 29 Hip orthosis.

* **L1499**   Spinal orthosis, not otherwise specified   A

~~L1500~~   ~~Thoracic-hip-knee ankle orthosis (THKAO), mobility frame (Newington, Parapodium types)~~   ✖

~~L1510~~   ~~THKAO, standing frame, with or without tray and accessories~~   ✖

~~L1520~~   ~~THKAO, swivel walker~~   ✖

Orthotic Devices: Lower Limb

NOTE: the procedures in L1600-L2999 are considered as *base* or *basic procedures* and may be modified by listing procedure from the Additions Sections and adding them to the base procedure.

Hip: Flexible

L1600-L2999:   Bill DME/MAC

* **L1600**   Hip orthosis (HO), abduction control of hip joints, flexible, Frejka type with cover, prefabricated, includes fitting and adjustment `Qp` `Qh` &   A

* **L1610**   Hip orthosis, abduction control of hip joints, flexible, (Frejka cover only) prefabricated, includes fitting and adjustment `Qp` `Qh` &   A

* **L1620**   Hip orthosis, abduction control of hip joints, flexible, (Pavlik harness), prefabricated, includes fitting and adjustment `Qp` `Qh` &   A

* **L1630**   Hip orthosis, abduction control of hip joints, semi-flexible (Von Rosen type), custom-fabricated `Qp` `Qh` &   A

* **L1640**   Hip orthosis, abduction control of hip joints, static, pelvic band or spreader bar, thigh cuffs, custom-fabricated `Qp` `Qh` &   A

* **L1650**   Hip orthosis, abduction control of hip joints, static, adjustable, (Ilfled type), prefabricated, includes fitting and adjustment `Qp` `Qh` &   A

* **L1652**   Hip orthosis, bilateral thigh cuffs with adjustable abductor spreader bar, adult size, prefabricated, includes fitting and adjustment, any type `Qp` `Qh` &   A

* **L1660**   Hip orthosis, abduction control of hip joints, static, plastic, prefabricated, includes fitting and adjustment `Qp` `Qh` &   A

* **L1680**   Hip orthosis, abduction control of hip joints, dynamic, pelvic control, adjustable hip motion control, thigh cuffs (Rancho hip action type), custom fabrication `Qp` `Qh` &   A

* **L1685**   Hip orthosis, abduction control of hip joint, postoperative hip abduction type, custom fabricated `Qp` `Qh` &   A

* **L1686**   Hip orthosis, abduction control of hip joint, postoperative hip abduction type, prefabricated, includes fitting and adjustment `Qp` `Qh` &   A

* **L1690**   Combination, bilateral, lumbo-sacral, hip, femur orthosis providing adduction and internal rotation control, prefabricated, includes fitting and adjustment `Qp` `Qh` &   A

Legg Perthes

* **L1700**   Legg-Perthes orthosis, (Toronto type), custom-fabricated `Qp` `Qh` &   A

* **L1710**   Legg-Perthes orthosis, (Newington type), custom-fabricated `Qp` `Qh` &   A

* **L1720**   Legg-Perthes orthosis, trilateral, (Tachdjian type), custom-fabricated `Qp` `Qh` &   A

* **L1730**   Legg-Perthes orthosis, (Scottish Rite type), custom-fabricated `Qp` `Qh` &   A

* **L1755**   Legg-Perthes orthosis, (Patten bottom type), custom-fabricated `Qp` `Qh` &   A

🅟 PQRI	`Qp` **Quantity Physician Appendix B**	`Qh` **Quantity Hospital Appendix C**	♀ **Female only**
♂ **Male only**	`A` **Age**	& **DMEPOS** A2-Z3 ASC Payment Indicator	A-Y ASC Status Indicator Coding Clinic

Knee (KO)

* **L1810** Knee orthosis, elastic with joints, prefabricated, includes fitting and adjustment `Qp` `Qh` ♿   A

* **L1820** Knee orthosis, elastic with condylar pads and joints, with or without patellar control, prefabricated, includes fitting and adjustment `Qp` `Qh` ♿   A

* **L1830** Knee orthosis, immobilizer, canvas longitudinal, prefabricated, includes fitting and adjustment `Qp` `Qh` ♿   A

* **L1831** Knee orthosis, locking knee joint(s), positional orthosis, prefabricated, includes fitting and adjustment `Qp` `Qh` ♿   A

* **L1832** Knee orthrosis, adjustable knee joints (unicentric or polycentric), positional orthosis, rigid support, prefabricated, includes fitting and adjustment `Qp` `Qh` ♿   A

* **L1834** Knee orthosis, without knee joint, rigid, custom-fabricated `Qp` `Qh` ♿   A

* **L1836** Knee orthosis, rigid, without joint(s), includes soft interface material, prefabricated, includes fitting and adjustment `Qp` `Qh` ♿   A

* **L1840** Knee orthosis, derotation, medial-lateral, anterior cruciate ligament, custom fabricated `Qp` `Qh` ♿   A

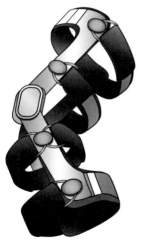

Figure 30 Knee Orthosis.

* **L1843** Knee orthosis, single upright, thigh and calf, with adjustable flexion and extension joint (unicentric or polycentric), medial-lateral and rotation control, with or without varus/valgus adjustment; prefabricated, includes fitting and adjustment `Qp` `Qh` ♿   A

* **L1844** Knee orthosis, single upright, thigh and calf, with adjustable flexion and extension joint (unicentric or polycentric), medial-lateral and rotation control, with or without varus/valgus adjustment, custom fabricated `Qp` `Qh` ♿   A

* **L1845** Knee orthrosis, double upright, thigh and calf, with adjustable flexion and extension joint (unicentric or polycentric), medial-lateral and rotation control, with or without varus/valgus adjustment, prefabricated, includes fitting and adjustment `Qp` `Qh` ♿   A

* **L1846** Knee orthrosis, double upright, thigh and calf, with adjustable flexion and extension joint (unicentric or polycentric), medial-lateral and rotation control, with or without varus/valgus adjustment, custom fabricated `Qp` `Qh` ♿   A

* **L1847** Knee orthosis, double upright with adjustable joint, with inflatable air support chambers, prefabricated, includes fitting and adjustment `Qp` `Qh` ♿   A

* **L1850** Knee orthosis, Swedish type, prefabricated, includes fitting and adjustment `Qp` `Qh` ♿   A

* **L1860** Knee orthosis, modification of supracondylar prosthetic socket, custom fabricated (SK) `Qp` `Qh` ♿   A

Ankle-Foot (AFO)

* **L1900** Ankle foot orthosis (AFO), spring wire, dorsiflexion assist calf band, custom-fabricated `Qp` `Qh` ♿   A

* **L1902** Ankle foot orthosis, ankle gauntlet, prefabricated, includes fitting and adjustment `Qp` `Qh` ♿   A

* **L1904** Ankle foot orthosis, molded ankle gauntlet, custom-fabricated `Qp` `Qh` ♿   A

* **L1906** Ankle-foot orthosis, multiligamentus ankle support, prefabricated, includes fitting and adjustment `Qp` `Qh` ♿   A

▶ New   → Revised   ✔ Reinstated   <del>deleted</del> Deleted

⚛ Special coverage instructions   ◆ Not covered or valid by Medicare   * Carrier discretion

✳ **L1907** AFO, supramalleolar with straps, with or without interface/pads, custom fabricated Qp Qh ♿   A

✳ **L1910** Ankle foot orthosis, posterior, single bar, clasp attachment to shoe counter, prefabricated, includes fitting and adjustment Qp Qh ♿   A

✳ **L1920** Ankle foot orthosis, single upright with static or adjustable stop (Phelps or Perlstein type), custom-fabricated Qp Qh ♿   A

✳ **L1930** Ankle-foot orthosis, plastic or other material, prefabricated, includes fitting and adjustment Qp Qh ♿   A

✳ **L1932** AFO, rigid anterior tibial section, total carbon fiber or equal material, prefabricated, includes fitting and adjustment Qp Qh ♿   A

✳ **L1940** Ankle foot orthosis, plastic or other material, custom-fabricated Qp Qh ♿   A

✳ **L1945** Ankle foot orthosis, plastic, rigid anterior tibial section (floor reaction), custom-fabricated Qp Qh ♿   A

✳ **L1950** Ankle foot orthosis, spiral, (Institute of Rehabilitation Medicine type), plastic, custom-fabricated Qp Qh ♿   A

✳ **L1951** Ankle foot orthosis, spiral, (Institute of Rehabilitative Medicine type), plastic or other material, prefabricated, includes fitting and adjustment Qp Qh ♿   A

✳ **L1960** Ankle foot orthosis, posterior solid ankle, plastic, custom-fabricated Qp Qh ♿   A

✳ **L1970** Ankle foot orthosis, plastic, with ankle joint, custom-fabricated Qp Qh ♿   A

✳ **L1971** Ankle foot orthosis, plastic or other material with ankle joint, prefabricated, includes fitting and adjustment Qp Qh ♿   A

✳ **L1980** Ankle foot orthosis, single upright free plantar dorsiflexion, solid stirrup, calf band/cuff (single bar 'BK' orthosis), custom-fabricated Qp Qh ♿   A

✳ **L1990** Ankle foot orthosis, double upright free plantar dorsiflexion, solid stirrup, calf band/cuff (double bar 'BK' orthosis), custom-fabricated Qp Qh ♿   A

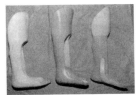

Figure 31 Ankle foot orthosis (AFO).

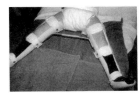

Figure 32 Knee ankle foot orthosis (KAFO).

Hip-Knee-Ankle-Foot (or Any Combination)

NOTE: L2000, L2020, and L2036 are base procedures to be used with any knee joint. L2010 and L2030 are to be used only with no knee joint.

✳ **L2000** Knee ankle foot orthosis, single upright, free knee, free ankle, solid stirrup, thigh and calf bands/cuffs (single bar 'AK' orthosis), custom-fabricated Qp Qh ♿   A

→ ✳ **L2005** Knee ankle foot orthosis, any material, single or double upright, stance control, automatic lock and swing phase release, any type activation; includes ankle joint, any type, custom fabricated Qp Qh ♿   A

✳ **L2010** Knee ankle foot orthosis, single upright, free ankle, solid stirrup, thigh and calf bands/cuffs (single bar 'AK' orthosis), without knee joint, custom-fabricated Qp Qh ♿   A

✳ **L2020** Knee ankle foot orthosis, double upright, free knee, free ankle, solid stirrup, thigh and calf bands/cuffs (double bar 'AK' orthosis), custom-fabricated Qp Qh ♿   A

✳ **L2030** Knee ankle foot orthosis, double upright, free ankle, solid stirrup, thigh and calf bands/cuffs (double bar 'AK' orthosis), without knee joint, custom fabricated Qp Qh ♿   A

✳ **L2034** Knee ankle foot orthosis, full plastic, single upright, with or without free motion knee, medial lateral rotation control, with or without free motion ankle, custom fabricated Qp Qh ♿   A

✳ **L2035** Knee ankle foot orthosis, full plastic, static (pediatric size), without free motion ankle, prefabricated, includes fitting and adjustment Qp Qh A ♿   A

✳ **L2036** Knee ankle foot orthosis, full plastic, double upright, with or without free motion knee, with or without free motion ankle, custom fabricated Qp Qh ♿   A

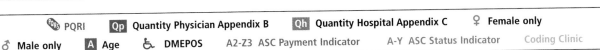

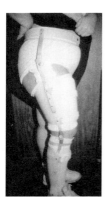

Figure 33 Hip-knee-ankle-foot orthosis (HKAFO).

* **L2037**   Knee ankle foot orthosis, full plastic, single upright, with or without free motion knee, with or without free motion ankle, custom fabricated `Qp` `Qh` ⬧   A

* **L2038**   Knee ankle foot orthosis, full plastic, with or without free motion knee, multi-axis ankle, custom fabricated `Qp` `Qh` ⬧   A

Torsion Control

* **L2040**   Hip knee ankle foot orthosis, torsion control, bilateral rotation straps, pelvic band/belt, custom fabricated `Qp` `Qh` ⬧   A

* **L2050**   Hip knee ankle foot orthosis, torsion control, bilateral torsion cables, hip joint, pelvic band/belt, custom-fabricated `Qp` `Qh` ⬧   A

* **L2060**   Hip knee ankle foot orthosis, torsion control, bilateral torsion cables, ball bearing hip joint, pelvic band/belt, custom-fabricated `Qp` `Qh` ⬧   A

* **L2070**   Hip knee ankle foot orthosis, torsion control, unilateral rotation straps, pelvic band/belt, custom-fabricated `Qp` `Qh` ⬧   A

* **L2080**   Hip knee ankle foot orthosis, torsion control, unilateral torsion cable, hip joint, pelvic band/belt, custom-fabricated `Qp` `Qh` ⬧   A

* **L2090**   Hip knee ankle foot orthosis, torsion control, unilateral torsion cable, ball bearing hip joint, pelvic band/belt, custom-fabricated `Qp` `Qh` ⬧   A

Fracture Orthoses

* **L2106**   Ankle foot orthosis, fracture orthosis, tibial fracture cast orthosis, thermoplastic type casting material, custom-fabricated `Qp` `Qh` ⬧   A

* **L2108**   Ankle foot orthosis, fracture orthosis, tibial fracture cast orthosis, custom-fabricated `Qp` `Qh` ⬧   A

* **L2112**   Ankle foot orthosis, fracture orthosis, tibial fracture orthosis, soft, prefabricated, includes fitting and adjustment `Qp` `Qh` ⬧   A

* **L2114**   Ankle foot orthosis, fracture orthosis, tibial fracture orthosis, semi-rigid, prefabricated, includes fitting and adjustment `Qp` `Qh` ⬧   A

* **L2116**   Ankle foot orthosis, fracture orthosis, tibial fracture orthosis, rigid, prefabricated, includes fitting and adjustment `Qp` `Qh` ⬧   A

* **L2126**   Knee ankle foot orthosis, fracture orthosis, femoral fracture cast orthosis, thermoplastic type casting material, custom-fabricated `Qp` `Qh` ⬧   A

* **L2128**   Knee ankle foot orthosis, fracture orthosis, femoral fracture cast orthosis, custom-fabricated `Qp` `Qh` ⬧   A

* **L2132**   KAFO, femoral fracture cast orthosis, soft, prefabricated, includes fitting and adjustment `Qp` `Qh` ⬧   A

* **L2134**   KAFO, femoral fracture cast orthosis, semi-rigid, prefabricated, includes fitting and adjustment `Qp` `Qh` ⬧   A

* **L2136**   KAFO, fracture orthosis, femoral fracture cast orthosis, rigid, prefabricated, includes fitting and adjustment `Qp` `Qh` ⬧   A

Additions to Fracture Orthosis

* **L2180**   Addition to lower extremity fracture orthosis, plastic shoe insert with ankle joints `Qp` `Qh` ⬧   A

* **L2182**   Addition to lower extremity fracture orthosis, drop lock knee joint ⬧   A

* **L2184**   Addition to lower extremity fracture orthosis, limited motion knee joint ⬧   A

* **L2186**   Addition to lower extremity fracture orthosis, adjustable motion knee joint, Lerman type ⬧   A

* **L2188**   Addition to lower extremity fracture orthosis, quadrilateral brim `Qp` `Qh` ⬧   A

▶ New   → Revised   ✔ Reinstated   ~~deleted~~ Deleted

⊙ Special coverage instructions   ◆ Not covered or valid by Medicare   * Carrier discretion

* **L2190** Addition to lower extremity fracture orthosis, waist belt `Qp` `Qh` ♿   A

* **L2192** Addition to lower extremity fracture orthosis, hip joint, pelvic band, thigh flange, and pelvic belt `Qp` `Qh` ♿   A

Additions to Lower Extremity Orthosis

Shoe-Ankle-Shin-Knee

* **L2200** Addition to lower extremity, limited ankle motion, each joint ♿   A

* **L2210** Addition to lower extremity, dorsiflexion assist (plantar flexion resist), each joint ♿   A

* **L2220** Addition to lower extremity, dorsiflexion and plantar flexion assist/ resist, each joint ♿   A

* **L2230** Addition to lower extremity, split flat caliper stirrups and plate attachment `Qp` `Qh` ♿   A

* **L2232** Addition to lower extremity orthosis, rocker bottom for total contact ankle foot orthosis, for custom fabricated orthosis only `Qp` `Qh` ♿   A

* **L2240** Addition to lower extremity, round caliper and plate attachment `Qp` `Qh` ♿   A

* **L2250** Addition to lower extremity, foot plate, molded to patient model, stirrup attachment `Qp` `Qh` ♿   A

* **L2260** Addition to lower extremity, reinforced solid stirrup (Scott-Craig type) `Qp` `Qh` ♿   A

* **L2265** Addition to lower extremity, long tongue stirrup `Qp` `Qh` ♿   A

* **L2270** Addition to lower extremity, varus/ valgus correction ('T') strap, padded/ lined or malleolus pad `Qp` `Qh` ♿   A

* **L2275** Addition to lower extremity, varus/ valgus correction, plastic modification, padded/lined `Qp` `Qh` ♿   A

* **L2280** Addition to lower extremity, molded inner boot `Qp` `Qh` ♿   A

* **L2300** Addition to lower extremity, abduction bar (bilateral hip involvement), jointed, adjustable `Qp` `Qh` ♿   A

* **L2310** Addition to lower extremity, abduction bar-straight `Qp` `Qh` ♿   A

* **L2320** Addition to lower extremity, non-molded lacer, for custom fabricated orthosis only `Qp` `Qh` ♿   A

* **L2330** Addition to lower extremity, lacer molded to patient model, for custom fabricated orthosis only `Qp` `Qh` ♿   A

    Used whether closure is lacer or Velcro

* **L2335** Addition to lower extremity, anterior swing band `Qp` `Qh` ♿   A

* **L2340** Addition to lower extremity, pre-tibial shell, molded to patient model `Qp` `Qh` ♿   A

* **L2350** Addition to lower extremity, prosthetic type, (BK) socket, molded to patient model, (used for 'PTB' and 'AFO' orthoses) `Qp` `Qh` ♿   A

* **L2360** Addition to lower extremity, extended steel shank `Qp` `Qh` ♿   A

* **L2370** Addition to lower extremity, Patten bottom `Qp` `Qh` ♿   A

* **L2375** Addition to lower extremity, torsion control, ankle joint and half solid stirrup `Qp` `Qh` ♿   A

* **L2380** Addition to lower extremity, torsion control, straight knee joint, each joint `Qp` `Qh` ♿   A

* **L2385** Addition to lower extremity, straight knee joint, heavy duty, each joint ♿   A

* **L2387** Addition to lower extremity, polycentric knee joint, for custom fabricated knee ankle foot orthosis, each joint ♿   A

* **L2390** Addition to lower extremity, offset knee joint, each joint ♿   A

* **L2395** Addition to lower extremity, offset knee joint, heavy duty, each joint ♿   A

* **L2397** Addition to lower extremity orthosis, suspension sleeve ♿   A

Additions to Straight Knee or Offset Knee Joints

* **L2405** Addition to knee joint, drop lock, each ♿   A

* **L2415** Addition to knee lock with integrated release mechanism (bail, cable, or equal), any material, each joint ♿   A

* **L2425** Addition to knee joint, disc or dial lock for adjustable knee flexion, each joint ♿   A

* **L2430** Addition to knee joint, ratchet lock for active and progressive knee extension, each joint ♿   A

* **L2492** Addition to knee joint, lift loop for drop lock ring ♿   A

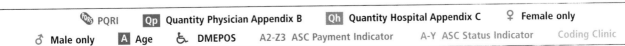

Additions to Thigh/Weight Bearing

Gluteal/Ischial Weight Bearing

✳ **L2500** Addition to lower extremity, thigh/weight bearing, gluteal/ischial weight bearing, ring `Qp` `Qh`   A

✳ **L2510** Addition to lower extremity, thigh/weight bearing, quadri-lateral brim, molded to patient model `Qp` `Qh`   A

✳ **L2520** Addition to lower extremity, thigh/weight bearing, quadri-lateral brim, custom fitted `Qp` `Qh`   A

✳ **L2525** Addition to lower extremity, thigh/weight bearing, ischial containment/narrow M-L brim molded to patient model `Qp` `Qh`   A

✳ **L2526** Addition to lower extremity, thigh/weight bearing, ischial containment/narrow M-L brim, custom fitted `Qp` `Qh`   A

✳ **L2530** Addition to lower extremity, thigh-weight bearing, lacer, non-molded `Qp` `Qh`   A

✳ **L2540** Addition to lower extremity, thigh/weight bearing, lacer, molded to patient model `Qp` `Qh`   A

✳ **L2550** Addition to lower extremity, thigh/weight bearing, high roll cuff `Qp` `Qh`   A

Additions to Pelvic and Thoracic Control

✳ **L2570** Addition to lower extremity, pelvic control, hip joint, Clevis type two position joint, each `Qp` `Qh`   A

✳ **L2580** Addition to lower extremity, pelvic control, pelvic sling `Qp` `Qh`   A

✳ **L2600** Addition to lower extremity, pelvic control, hip joint, Clevis type, or thrust bearing, free, each `Qp` `Qh`   A

✳ **L2610** Addition to lower extremity, pelvic control, hip joint, Clevis or thrust bearing, lock, each `Qp` `Qh`   A

✳ **L2620** Addition to lower extremity, pelvic control, hip joint, heavy duty, each `Qp` `Qh`   A

✳ **L2622** Addition to lower extremity, pelvic control, hip joint, adjustable flexion, each `Qp` `Qh`   A

✳ **L2624** Addition to lower extremity, pelvic control, hip joint, adjustable flexion, extension, abduction control, each `Qp` `Qh`   A

✳ **L2627** Addition to lower extremity, pelvic control, plastic, molded to patient model, reciprocating hip joint and cables `Qp` `Qh`   A

✳ **L2628** Addition to lower extremity, pelvic control, metal frame, reciprocating hip joint and cables `Qp` `Qh`   A

✳ **L2630** Addition to lower extremity, pelvic control, band and belt, unilateral `Qp` `Qh`   A

✳ **L2640** Addition to lower extremity, pelvic control, band and belt, bilateral `Qp` `Qh`   A

✳ **L2650** Addition to lower extremity, pelvic and thoracic control, gluteal pad, each `Qp` `Qh`   A

✳ **L2660** Addition to lower extremity, thoracic control, thoracic band `Qp` `Qh`   A

✳ **L2670** Addition to lower extremity, thoracic control, paraspinal uprights `Qp` `Qh`   A

✳ **L2680** Addition to lower extremity, thoracic control, lateral support uprights `Qp` `Qh`   A

General Additions

✳ **L2750** Addition to lower extremity orthosis, plating chrome or nickel, per bar   A

✳ **L2755** Addition to lower extremity orthosis, high strength, lightweight material, all hybrid lamination/prepreg composite, per segment, for custom fabricated orthosis only   A

✳ **L2760** Addition to lower extremity orthosis, extension, per extension, per bar (for lineal adjustment for growth)   A

✳ **L2768** Orthotic side bar disconnect device, per bar   A

✳ **L2780** Addition to lower extremity orthosis, non-corrosive finish, per bar   A

✳ **L2785** Addition to lower extremity orthosis, drop lock retainer, each   A

✳ **L2795** Addition to lower extremity orthosis, knee control, full kneecap `Qp` `Qh`   A

✳ **L2800** Addition to lower extremity orthosis, knee control, knee cap, medial or lateral pull, for use with custom fabricated orthosis only `Qp` `Qh`   A

✳ **L2810** Addition to lower extremity orthosis, knee control, condylar pad   A

▶ New   → Revised   ✔ Reinstated   ~~deleted~~ Deleted

⊘ Special coverage instructions   ◆ Not covered or valid by Medicare   ✳ Carrier discretion

✳ **L2820** Addition to lower extremity orthosis, soft interface for molded plastic, below knee section `Qp` `Qh` ᕕ A

Only report if soft interface provided, either leather or other material

✳ **L2830** Addition to lower extremity orthosis, soft interface for molded plastic, above knee section `Qp` `Qh` ᕕ A

✳ **L2840** Addition to lower extremity orthosis, tibial length sock, fracture or equal, each ᕕ A

✳ **L2850** Addition to lower extremity orthosis, femoral length sock, fracture or equal, each ᕕ A

◆ **L2861** Addition to lower extremity joint, knee or ankle, concentric adjustable torsion style mechanism for custom fabricated orthotics only, each E

✳ **L2999** Lower extremity orthoses, not otherwise specified A

Foot (Orthopedic Shoes)

Insert, Removable, Molded to Patient Model

L3000-L3649: Bill DME/MAC

⊛ **L3000** Foot, insert, removable, molded to patient model, 'UCB' type, Berkeley shell, each `Qp` `Qh` ᕕ A

If both feet casted and supplied with an orthosis, bill L3000-LT and L3000-RT

IOM: 100-02, 15, 290

⊛ **L3001** Foot, insert, removable, molded to patient model, Spenco, each `Qp` `Qh` ᕕ A

IOM: 100-02, 15, 290

⊛ **L3002** Foot, insert, removable, molded to patient model, Plastazote or equal, each `Qp` `Qh` ᕕ A

IOM: 100-02, 15, 290

⊛ **L3003** Foot, insert, removable, molded to patient model, silicone gel, each `Qp` `Qh` ᕕ A

IOM: 100-02, 15, 290

⊛ **L3010** Foot, insert, removable, molded to patient model, longitudinal arch support, each `Qp` `Qh` ᕕ A

IOM: 100-02, 15, 290

⊛ **L3020** Foot, insert, removable, molded to patient model, longitudinal/metatarsal support, each `Qp` `Qh` ᕕ A

IOM: 100-02, 15, 290

⊛ **L3030** Foot, insert, removable, formed to patient foot, each `Qp` `Qh` ᕕ A

IOM: 100-02, 15, 290

✳ **L3031** Foot, insert/plate, removable, addition to lower extremity orthosis, high strength, lightweight material, all hybrid lamination/prepreg composite, each `Qp` `Qh` ᕕ A

Arch Support, Removable, Premolded

⊛ **L3040** Foot, arch support, removable, premolded, longitudinal, each `Qp` `Qh` ᕕ A

IOM: 100-02, 15, 290

⊛ **L3050** Foot, arch support, removable, premolded, metatarsal, each `Qp` `Qh` ᕕ A

IOM: 100-02, 15, 290

⊛ **L3060** Foot, arch support, removable, premolded, longitudinal/metatarsal, each `Qp` `Qh` ᕕ A

IOM: 100-02, 15, 290

Arch Support, Non-removable, Attached to Shoe

⊛ **L3070** Foot, arch support, non-removable attached to shoe, longitudinal, each `Qp` `Qh` ᕕ A

IOM: 100-02, 15, 290

⊛ **L3080** Foot, arch support, non-removable attached to shoe, metatarsal, each `Qp` `Qh` ᕕ A

IOM: 100-02, 15, 290

⊛ **L3090** Foot, arch support, non-removable attached to shoe, longitudinal/metatarsal, each `Qp` `Qh` ᕕ A

IOM: 100-02, 15, 290

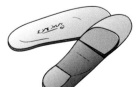

Figure 34 Foot inserts.

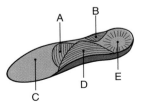

Figure 35 Arch support.

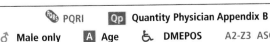

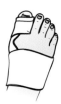

Figure 36 Hallux valgus splint.

⊛ **L3100** Hallus-valgus night dynamic splint Qp Qh ⴲ   A
    IOM: 100-02, 15, 290

Abduction and Rotation Bars

⊛ **L3140** Foot, abduction rotation bar, including shoes Qp Qh ♿   A
    IOM: 100-02, 15, 290

⊛ **L3150** Foot, abduction rotation bar, without shoes Qp Qh ♿   A
    IOM: 100-02, 15, 290

✳ **L3160** Foot, adjustable shoe-styled positioning device Qp Qh   A

⊛ **L3170** Foot, plastic, silicone or equal, heel stabilizer, each Qp Qh ♿   A
    IOM: 100-02, 15, 290

Orthopedic Footwear

⊛ **L3201** Orthopedic shoe, oxford with supinator or pronator, infant A   A
    IOM: 100-02, 15, 290

⊛ **L3202** Orthopedic shoe, oxford with supinator or pronator, child A   A
    IOM: 100-02, 15, 290

⊛ **L3203** Orthopedic shoe, oxford with supinator or pronator, junior A   A
    IOM: 100-02, 15, 290

⊛ **L3204** Orthopedic shoe, hightop with supinator or pronator, infant A   A
    IOM: 100-02, 15, 290

⊛ **L3206** Orthopedic shoe, hightop with supinator or pronator, child A   A
    IOM: 100-02, 15, 290

⊛ **L3207** Orthopedic shoe, hightop with supinator or pronator, junior A   A
    IOM: 100-02, 15, 290

⊛ **L3208** Surgical boot, infant, each A   A
    IOM: 100-02, 15, 100

⊛ **L3209** Surgical boot, each, child A   A
    IOM: 100-02, 15, 100

⊛ **L3211** Surgical boot, each, junior A   A
    IOM: 100-02, 15, 100

⊛ **L3212** Benesch boot, pair, infant A   A
    IOM: 100-02, 15, 100

⊛ **L3213** Benesch boot, pair, child A   A
    IOM: 100-02, 15, 100

⊛ **L3214** Benesch boot, pair, junior A   A
    IOM: 100-02, 15, 100

◆ **L3215** Orthopedic footwear, ladies shoe, oxford, each Qp Qh ♀   E
    Medicare Statute 1862a8

◆ **L3216** Orthopedic footwear, ladies shoe, depth inlay, each Qp Qh ♀   E
    Medicare Statute 1862a8

◆ **L3217** Orthopedic footwear, ladies shoe, hightop, depth inlay, each Qp Qh ♀   E
    Medicare Statute 1862a8

◆ **L3219** Orthopedic footwear, mens shoe, oxford, each Qp Qh ♂   E
    Medicare Statute 1862a8

◆ **L3221** Orthopedic footwear, mens shoe, depth inlay, each Qp Qh ♂   E
    Medicare Statute 1862a8

◆ **L3222** Orthopedic footwear, mens shoe, hightop, depth inlay, each Qp Qh ♂   E
    Medicare Statute 1862a8

⊛ **L3224** Orthopedic footwear, ladies shoe, oxford, used as an integral part of a brace (orthosis) Qp Qh ♀ ♿   A
    IOM: 100-02, 15, 290

⊛ **L3225** Orthopedic footwear, mens shoe, oxford, used as an integral part of a brace (orthosis) Qp Qh ♂ ♿   A
    IOM: 100-02, 15, 290

⊛ **L3230** Orthopedic footwear, custom shoe, depth inlay, each Qp Qh   A
    IOM: 100-02, 15, 290

⊛ **L3250** Orthopedic footwear, custom molded shoe, removable inner mold, prosthetic shoe, each Qp Qh   A
    IOM: 100-02, 15, 290

⊛ **L3251** Foot, shoe molded to patient model, silicone shoe, each Qp Qh   A
    IOM: 100-02, 15, 290

⊛ **L3252** Foot, shoe molded to patient model, Plastazote (or similar), custom fabricated, each Qp Qh   A
    IOM: 100-02, 15, 290

▶ **New**   → **Revised**   ✔ **Reinstated**   ~~deleted~~ **Deleted**

⊛ **Special coverage instructions**   ◆ **Not covered or valid by Medicare**   ✳ **Carrier discretion**

⊛ **L3253** Foot, molded shoe Plastazote (or similar), custom fitted, each `Qp` `Qh` A

IOM: 100-02, 15, 290

⊛ **L3254** Non-standard size or width A

IOM: 100-02, 15, 290

⊛ **L3255** Non-standard size or length A

IOM: 100-02, 15, 290

⊛ **L3257** Orthopedic footwear, additional charge for split size A

IOM: 100-02, 15, 290

⊛ **L3260** Surgical boot/shoe, each E

IOM: 100-02, 15, 100

✳ **L3265** Plastazote sandal, each A

Shoe Modifications
Lifts

⊛ **L3300** Lift, elevation, heel, tapered to metatarsals, per inch ♿ A

IOM: 100-02, 15, 290

⊛ **L3310** Lift, elevation, heel and sole, Neoprene, per inch ♿ A

IOM: 100-02, 15, 290

⊛ **L3320** Lift, elevation, heel and sole, cork, per inch A

IOM: 100-02, 15, 290

⊛ **L3330** Lift, elevation, metal extension (skate) `Qp` `Qh` ♿ A

IOM: 100-02, 15, 290

⊛ **L3332** Lift, elevation, inside shoe, tapered, up to one-half inch `Qp` `Qh` ♿ A

IOM: 100-02, 15, 290

⊛ **L3334** Lift, elevation, heel, per inch ♿ A

IOM: 100-02, 15, 290

Wedges

⊛ **L3340** Heel wedge, SACH `Qp` `Qh` ♿ A

IOM: 100-02, 15, 290

⊛ **L3350** Heel wedge `Qp` `Qh` ♿ A

IOM: 100-02, 15, 290

⊛ **L3360** Sole wedge, outside sole `Qp` `Qh` ♿ A

IOM: 100-02, 15, 290

⊛ **L3370** Sole wedge, between sole `Qp` `Qh` ♿ A

IOM: 100-02, 15, 290

⊛ **L3380** Clubfoot wedge `Qp` `Qh` ♿ A

IOM: 100-02, 15, 290

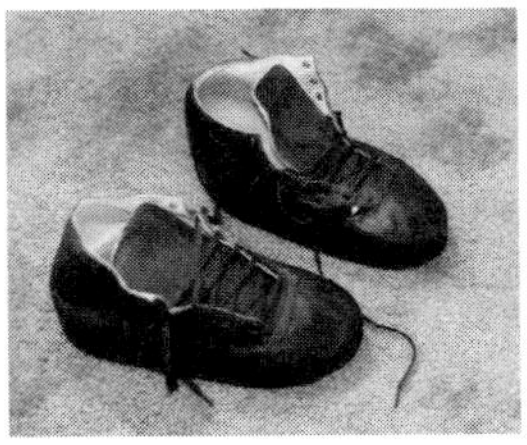

Figure 37 Molded custom shoe.

⊛ **L3390** Outflare wedge `Qp` `Qh` ♿ A

IOM: 100-02, 15, 290

⊛ **L3400** Metatarsal bar wedge, rocker `Qp` `Qh` ♿ A

IOM: 100-02, 15, 290

⊛ **L3410** Metatarsal bar wedge, between sole `Qp` `Qh` ♿ A

IOM: 100-02, 15, 290

⊛ **L3420** Full sole and heel wedge, between sole `Qp` `Qh` ♿ A

IOM: 100-02, 15, 290

Heels

⊛ **L3430** Heel, counter, plastic reinforced `Qp` `Qh` ♿ A

IOM: 100-02, 15, 290

⊛ **L3440** Heel, counter, leather reinforced `Qp` `Qh` ♿ A

IOM: 100-02, 15, 290

⊛ **L3450** Heel, SACH cushion type `Qp` `Qh` ♿ A

IOM: 100-02, 15, 290

⊛ **L3455** Heel, new leather, standard `Qp` `Qh` ♿ A

IOM: 100-02, 15, 290

⊛ **L3460** Heel, new rubber, standard `Qp` `Qh` ♿ A

IOM: 100-02, 15, 290

⊛ **L3465** Heel, Thomas with wedge `Qp` `Qh` ♿ A

IOM: 100-02, 15, 290

⊛ **L3470** Heel, Thomas extended to ball `Qp` `Qh` ♿ A

IOM: 100-02, 15, 290

⊛ **L3480** Heel, pad and depression for spur `Qp` `Qh` ♿ A

IOM: 100-02, 15, 290

⊛ **L3485** Heel, pad, removable for spur `Qp` `Qh` A

IOM: 100-02, 15, 290

Additions to Orthopedic Shoes

✪ **L3500** Orthopedic shoe addition, insole, leather `Qp` `Qh` ♿   A
IOM: 100-02, 15, 290

✪ **L3510** Orthopedic shoe addition, insole, rubber `Qp` `Qh` ♿   A
IOM: 100-02, 15, 290

✪ **L3520** Orthopedic shoe addition, insole, felt covered with leather `Qp` `Qh` ♿   A
IOM: 100-02, 15, 290

✪ **L3530** Orthopedic shoe addition, sole, half `Qp` `Qh` ♿   A
IOM: 100-02, 15, 290

✪ **L3540** Orthopedic shoe addition, sole, full `Qp` `Qh` ♿   A
IOM: 100-02, 15, 290

✪ **L3550** Orthopedic shoe addition, toe tap standard `Qp` `Qh` ♿   A
IOM: 100-02, 15, 290

✪ **L3560** Orthopedic shoe addition, toe tap, horseshoe `Qp` `Qh` ♿   A
IOM: 100-02, 15, 290

✪ **L3570** Orthopedic shoe addition, special extension to instep (leather with eyelets) `Qp` `Qh` ♿   A
IOM: 100-02, 15, 290

✪ **L3580** Orthopedic shoe addition, convert instep to Velcro closure `Qp` `Qh` ♿   A
IOM: 100-02, 15, 290

✪ **L3590** Orthopedic shoe addition, convert firm shoe counter to soft counter `Qp` `Qh` ♿   A
IOM: 100-02, 15, 290

✪ **L3595** Orthopedic shoe addition, March bar `Qp` `Qh` ♿   A
IOM: 100-02, 15, 290

Transfer or Replacement

✪ **L3600** Transfer of an orthosis from one shoe to another, caliper plate, existing `Qp` `Qh` ♿   A
IOM: 100-02, 15, 290

✪ **L3610** Transfer of an orthosis from one shoe to another, caliper plate, new `Qp` `Qh` ♿   A
IOM: 100-02, 15, 290

✪ **L3620** Transfer of an orthosis from one shoe to another, solid stirrup, existing `Qp` `Qh` ♿   A

IOM: 100-02, 15, 290

✪ **L3630** Transfer of an orthosis from one shoe to another, solid stirrup, new `Qp` `Qh` ♿   A
IOM: 100-02, 15, 290

✪ **L3640** Transfer of an orthosis from one shoe to another, Dennis Browne splint (Riveton), both shoes `Qp` `Qh` ♿   A
IOM: 100-02, 15, 290

✪ **L3649** Orthopedic shoe, modification, addition or transfer, not otherwise specified   A
IOM: 100-02, 15, 290

Orthotic Devices: Upper Limb

NOTE: The procedures in this section are considered as *base* or *basic procedures* and may be modified by listing procedures from the Additions section and adding them to the base procedure.

L3650-L3956: Bill DME/MAC

Shoulder

* **L3650** Shoulder orthosis, (SO), figure of eight design abduction restrainer, prefabricated, includes fitting and adjustment `Qp` `Qh` ♿   A

* **L3660** Shoulder orthosis, figure of eight design abduction restrainer, canvas and webbing, prefabricated, includes fitting and adjustment `Qh`

* **L3670** Shoulder orthosis, acromio/clavicular (canvas and webbing type), prefabricated, includes fitting and adjustment `Qh`

→ * **L3671** Shoulder orthosis, shoulder joint design, without joints, may include soft interface, straps, custom fabricated, includes fitting and adjustment `Qp` `Qh` ♿   A

▶ * **L3674** Shoulder orthosis, abduction positioning (airplane design), thoracic component and support bar, with or without nontorsion joint/turnbuckle, may include soft interface, straps, custom fabricated, includes fitting and adjustment `Qp` `Qh`   A

* **L3675** Shoulder orthosis, vest type abduction restrainer, canvas webbing type or equal, prefabricated, includes fitting and adjustment `Qp`

→ ✪ **L3677** Shoulder orthosis, shoulder joint design, without joints, may include soft interface, straps, pre-fabricated, includes fitting and adjustment `Qp` `Qh`   A

▶ New   → Revised   ✔ Reinstated   ~~deleted~~ Deleted
✪ Special coverage instructions   ◆ Not covered or valid by Medicare   * Carrier discretion

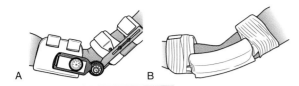

Figure 38 Elbow orthoses.

Elbow

⚹ **L3702** Elbow orthosis, without joints, may include soft interface, straps, custom fabricated, includes fitting and adjustment `Qp` `Qh` ⌖   A

⚹ **L3710** Elbow orthosis, elastic with metal joints, prefabricated, includes fitting and adjustment `Qp` `Qh` ⌖   A

⚹ **L3720** Elbow orthosis, double upright with forearm/arm cuffs, free motion, custom-fabricated `Qp` `Qh` ⌖   A

⚹ **L3730** Elbow orthosis, double upright with forearm/arm cuffs, extension/flexion assist, custom-fabricated `Qp` `Qh` ⌖   A

⚹ **L3740** Elbow orthosis, double upright with forearm/arm cuffs, adjustable position lock with active control, custom-fabricated `Qp` `Qh` ⌖   A

⚹ **L3760** Elbow orthosis, with adjustable position locking joint(s), prefabricated, includes fitting and adjustments, any type `Qp` `Qh` ⌖   A

⚹ **L3762** Elbow orthosis, rigid, without joints, includes soft interface material, prefabricated, includes fitting and adjustment `Qp` `Qh` ⌖   A

⚹ **L3763** Elbow wrist hand orthosis, rigid, without joints, may include soft interface, straps, custom fabricated, includes fitting and adjustment `Qp` `Qh` ⌖   A

⚹ **L3764** Elbow wrist hand orthosis, includes one or more nontorsion joints, elastic bands, turnbuckles, may include soft interface, straps, custom fabricated, includes fitting and adjustment `Qp` `Qh` ⌖   A

⚹ **L3765** Elbow wrist hand finger orthosis, rigid, without joints, may include soft interface, straps, custom fabricated, includes fitting and adjustment `Qp` `Qh` ⌖   A

⚹ **L3766** Elbow wrist hand finger orthosis, includes one or more nontorsion joints, elastic bands, turnbuckles, may include soft interface, straps, custom fabricated, includes fitting and adjustment `Qp` `Qh` ⌖   A

Wrist-Hand-Finger Orthosis (WHFO)

⚹ **L3806** Wrist hand finger orthosis, includes one or more nontorsion joint(s), turnbuckles, elastic bands/springs, may include soft interface material, straps, custom fabricated, includes fitting and adjustment `Qp` `Qh` ⌖   A

⚹ **L3807** Wrist hand finger orthosis, without joint(s), prefabricated, includes fitting and adjustments, any type `Qp` `Qh` ⌖   A

⚹ **L3808** Wrist hand finger orthosis, rigid without joints, may include soft interface material; straps, custom fabricated, includes fitting and adjustment `Qp` `Qh` ⌖   A

Additions and Extensions

◆ **L3891** Addition to upper extremity joint, wrist or elbow, concentric adjustable torsion style mechanism for custom fabricated orthotics only, each   E

⚹ **L3900** Wrist hand finger orthosis, dynamic flexor hinge, reciprocal wrist extension/flexion, finger flexion/extension, wrist or finger driven, custom-fabricated `Qp` `Qh` ⌖   A

⚹ **L3901** Wrist hand finger orthosis, dynamic flexor hinge, reciprocal wrist extension/flexion, finger flexion/extension, cable driven, custom-fabricated `Qp` `Qh` ⌖   A

External Power

⚹ **L3904** Wrist hand finger orthosis, external powered, electric, custom-fabricated `Qp` `Qh` ⌖   A

⚹ **L3905** Wrist hand orthosis, includes one or more nontorsion joints, elastic bands, turnbuckles, may include soft interface, straps, custom fabricated, includes fitting and adjustment `Qp` `Qh` ⌖   A

Other Wrist-Hand-Finger Orthoses: Custom Fitted

⚹ **L3906** Wrist hand orthosis, without joints, may include soft interface, straps, custom fabricated, includes fitting and adjustment `Qp` `Qh` ⌖   A

⚹ **L3908** Wrist hand orthosis, wrist extension control cock-up, non molded, prefabricated, includes fitting and adjustment `Qp` `Qh` ⌖   A

⊕ PQRI	`Qp` Quantity Physician Appendix B	`Qh` Quantity Hospital Appendix C ♀ Female only
♂ Male only `A` Age ⌖ DMEPOS	A2-Z3 ASC Payment Indicator	A-Y ASC Status Indicator Coding Clinic

* **L3912** Hand finger orthosis, flexion glove with elastic finger control, prefabricated, includes fitting and adjustment `Qp` `Qh` A

* **L3913** Hand finger orthosis, without joints, may include soft interface, straps, custom fabricated, includes fitting and adjustment `Qp` `Qh` A

* **L3915** Wrist hand orthosis, includes one or more nontorsion joint(s), elastic bands, turnbuckles, may include soft interface, straps, prefabricated, includes fitting and adjustment A

* **L3917** Hand orthosis, metacarpal fracture orthosis, prefabricated, includes fitting and adjustment `Qp` `Qh` A

* **L3919** Hand orthosis, without joints, may include soft interface, straps, custom fabricated, includes fitting and adjustment `Qp` `Qh` A

* **L3921** Hand finger orthosis, includes one or more nontorsion joints, elastic bands, turnbuckles, may include soft interface, straps, custom fabricated, includes fitting and adjustment `Qp` `Qh` A

* **L3923** Hand finger orthosis, without joints, may include soft interface, straps, prefabricated, includes fitting and adjustments `Qp` `Qh` A

* **L3925** Finger orthosis, proximal interphalangeal (PIP)/distal interphalangeal (DIP), non torsion joint/spring, extension/flexion, may include soft interface material, prefabricated, includes fitting and adjustment A

* **L3927** Finger orthosis, proximal interphalangeal (PIP)/distal interphalangeal (DIP), without joint/spring, extension/flexion (e.g. static or ring type), may include soft interface material, prefabricated, includes fitting and adjustment A

* **L3929** Hand finger orthosis, includes one or more nontorsion joint(s), turnbuckles, elastic bands/springs, may include soft interface material, straps, prefabricated, includes fitting and adjustment `Qp` `Qh` A

* **L3931** Wrist hand finger orthosis, includes one or more nontorsion joint(s), turnbuckles, elastic bands/springs, may include soft interface material, straps, prefabricated, includes fitting and adjustment `Qp` `Qh` A

* **L3933** Finger orthosis, without joints, may include soft interface, custom fabricated, includes fitting and adjustment `Qp` `Qh` A

* **L3935** Finger orthosis, nontorsion joint, may include soft interface, custom fabricated, includes fitting and adjustment `Qp` `Qh` A

* **L3956** Addition of joint to upper extremity orthosis, any material, per joint A

Shoulder-Elbow-Wrist-Hand Orthosis (SEWHO)

Abduction Positioning: Custom Fitted

L3960-L4631: Bill DME/MAC

* **L3960** Shoulder elbow wrist hand orthosis, abduction positioning, airplane design, prefabricated, includes fitting and adjustment `Qp` `Qh` A

* **L3961** Shoulder elbow wrist hand orthosis, shoulder cap design, without joints, may include soft interface, straps, custom fabricated, includes fitting and adjustment `Qp` `Qh` A

* **L3962** Shoulder elbow wrist hand orthosis, abduction positioning, Erbs palsy design, prefabricated, includes fitting and adjustment `Qp` `Qh` A

~~L3964~~ ~~Shoulder elbow orthosis, mobile arm support attached to wheelchair, balanced, adjustable, prefabricated, includes fitting and adjustment~~ ✖

~~L3965~~ ~~Shoulder elbow orthosis, mobile arm support attached to wheelchair, balanced, adjustable Rancho type, prefabricated, includes fitting and adjustment~~ ✖

~~L3966~~ ~~Shoulder elbow orthosis, mobile arm support attached to wheelchair, balanced, reclining, prefabricated, includes fitting and adjustment~~ ✖

* **L3967** Shoulder elbow wrist hand orthosis, abduction positioning (airplane design), thoracic component and support bar, without joints, may include soft interface, straps, custom fabricated, includes fitting and adjustment `Qp` `Qh` A

~~L3968~~ ~~Shoulder elbow orthosis, mobile arm support attached to wheelchair, balanced, friction arm support (friction dampening to proximal and distal joints), prefabricated, includes fitting and adjustment~~ ✖

▶ New   → Revised   ✔ Reinstated   ~~deleted~~ Deleted
⊘ Special coverage instructions   ◆ Not covered or valid by Medicare   * Carrier discretion

~~L3969 Shoulder elbow orthosis, mobile arm support, monosuspension arm and hand support, overhead elbow forearm hand sling support, yoke type suspension support, prefabricated, includes fitting and adjustment~~ ✖

Additions to Mobile Arm Supports and SEWHO

~~L3970 SEO, addition to mobile arm support, elevating proximal arm~~ ✖

✻ **L3971** Shoulder elbow wrist hand orthosis, shoulder cap design, includes one or more nontorsion joints, elastic bands, turnbuckles, may include soft interface, straps, custom fabricated, includes fitting and adjustment Qp Qh ♿ A

~~L3972 SEO, addition to mobile arm support, offset or lateral rocker arm with elastic balance control~~ ✖

✻ **L3973** Shoulder elbow wrist hand orthosis, abduction positioning (airplane design), thoracic component and support bar, includes one or more nontorsion joints, elastic bands, turnbuckles, may include soft interface, straps, custom fabricated, includes fitting and adjustment Qp Qh ♿ A

~~L3974 SEO, addition to mobile arm support, supinator~~ ✖

✻ **L3975** Shoulder elbow wrist hand finger orthosis, shoulder cap design, without joints, may include soft interface, straps, custom fabricated, includes fitting and adjustment Qp Qh ♿ A

✻ **L3976** Shoulder elbow wrist hand finger orthosis, abduction positioning (airplane design), thoracic component and support bar, without joints, may include soft interface, straps, custom fabricated, includes fitting and adjustment Qp Qh ♿ A

✻ **L3977** Shoulder elbow wrist hand finger orthosis, shoulder cap design, includes one or more nontorsion joints, elastic bands, turnbuckles, may include soft interface, straps, custom fabricated, includes fitting and adjustment Qp Qh ♿ A

✻ **L3978** Shoulder elbow wrist hand finger orthosis, abduction positioning (airplane design), thoracic component and support bar, includes one or more nontorsion joints, elastic bands, turnbuckles, may include soft interface, straps, custom fabricated, includes fitting and adjustment Qp Qh ♿ A

Fracture Orthoses

✻ **L3980** Upper extremity fracture orthosis, humeral, prefabricated, includes fitting and adjustment Qp Qh ♿ A

✻ **L3982** Upper extremity fracture orthosis, radius/ulnar, prefabricated, includes fitting and adjustment Qp Qh ♿ A

✻ **L3984** Upper extremity fracture orthosis, wrist, prefabricated, includes fitting and adjustment Qp Qh ♿ A

✻ **L3995** Addition to upper extremity orthosis, sock, fracture or equal, each ♿ A

✻ **L3999** Upper limb orthosis, not otherwise specified A

Specific Repair

✻ **L4000** Replace girdle for spinal orthosis (CTLSO or SO) Qp Qh ♿ A

✻ **L4002** Replacement strap, any orthosis, includes all components, any length, any type ♿ A

✻ **L4010** Replace trilateral socket brim Qp Qh ♿ A

✻ **L4020** Replace quadrilateral socket brim, molded to patient model Qp Qh ♿ A

✻ **L4030** Replace quadrilateral socket brim, custom fitted Qp Qh ♿ A

✻ **L4040** Replace molded thigh lacer, for custom fabricated orthosis only Qp Qh ♿ A

✻ **L4045** Replace non-molded thigh lacer, for custom fabricated orthosis only Qp Qh ♿ A

✻ **L4050** Replace molded calf lacer, for custom fabricated orthosis only Qp Qh ♿ A

✻ **L4055** Replace non-molded calf lacer, for custom fabricated orthosis only Qp Qh ♿ A

✻ **L4060** Replace high roll cuff Qp Qh ♿ A

✻ **L4070** Replace proximal and distal upright for KAFO Qp Qh ♿ A

✻ **L4080** Replace metal bands KAFO, proximal thigh Qp Qh ♿ A

✻ **L4090** Replace metal bands KAFO-AFO, calf or distal thigh ♿ A

✻ **L4100** Replace leather cuff KAFO, proximal thigh Qp Qh ♿ A

✻ **L4110** Replace leather cuff KAFO-AFO, calf or distal thigh ♿ A

✻ **L4130** Replace pretibial shell Qp Qh ♿ A

Repairs

⊕ **L4205** Repair of orthotic device, labor component, per 15 minutes   A
IOM: 100-02, 15, 110.2

⊕ **L4210** Repair of orthotic device, repair or replace minor parts   A
IOM: 100-02, 15, 110.2; 100-02, 15, 120

Ancillary Orthotic Services

✻ **L4350** Ankle control orthosis, stirrup style, rigid, includes any type interface (e.g., pneumatic, gel), prefabricated, includes fitting and adjustment `Qp` `Qh` 🦽   A

✻ **L4360** Walking boot, pneumatic, and/or vacuum, with or without joints, with or without interface material, prefabricated, includes fitting and adjustment `Qp` `Qh` 🦽   A

Noncovered when walking boots used primarily to relieve pressure, especially on sole of foot, or are used for patients with foot ulcers

✻ **L4370** Pneumatic full leg splint, prefabricated, includes fitting and adjustment `Qp` `Qh` 🦽   A

~~L4380~~ ~~Pneumatic knee splint, prefabricated, includes fitting and adjustment~~   ✖

✻ **L4386** Walking boot, non-pneumatic, with or without joints, with or without interface material, prefabricated, includes fitting and adjustment `Qp` `Qh` 🦽   A

✻ **L4392** Replacement, soft interface material, static AFO `Qp` `Qh` 🦽   A

✻ **L4394** Replace soft interface material, foot drop splint `Qp` `Qh` 🦽   A

✻ **L4396** Static or dynamic ankle foot orthosis, including soft interface material, adjustable for fit, for positioning, may be used for minimal ambulation, prefabricated, includes fitting and adjustment `Qp` `Qh` 🦽   A

✻ **L4398** Foot drop splint, recumbent positioning device, prefabricated, includes fitting and adjustment `Qp` `Qh` 🦽   A

▶ ✻ **L4631** Ankle foot orthosis, walking boot type, varus/valgus correction, rocker bottom, anterior tibial shell, soft interface, custom arch support, plastic or other material, includes straps and closures, custom fabricated `Qp` `Qh` 🦽   A

PROSTHETICS (L5000-L9999)

Lower Limb (L5000-L5999)

NOTE: The procedures in this section are considered as *base* or *basic procedures* and may be modified by listing items/procedures or special materials from the Additions section and adding them to the base procedure.

Partial Foot

L5000-L5999:   Bill DME/MAC

⊕ **L5000** Partial foot, shoe insert with longitudinal arch, toe filler `Qp` `Qh` 🦽   A
IOM: 100-02, 15, 290

⊕ **L5010** Partial foot, molded socket, ankle height, with toe filler `Qp` `Qh` 🦽   A
IOM: 100-02, 15, 290

⊕ **L5020** Partial foot, molded socket, tibial tubercle height, with toe filler `Qp` `Qh` 🦽   A
IOM: 100-02, 15, 290

Ankle

✻ **L5050** Ankle, Symes, molded socket, SACH foot `Qp` `Qh` 🦽   A

✻ **L5060** Ankle, Symes, metal frame, molded leather socket, articulated ankle/foot `Qp` `Qh` 🦽   A

Below Knee

✻ **L5100** Below knee, molded socket, shin, SACH foot `Qp` `Qh` 🦽   A

✻ **L5105** Below knee, plastic socket, joints and thigh lacer, SACH foot `Qp` `Qh` 🦽   A

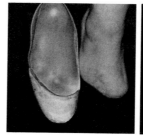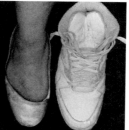

Figure 39 Partial foot.

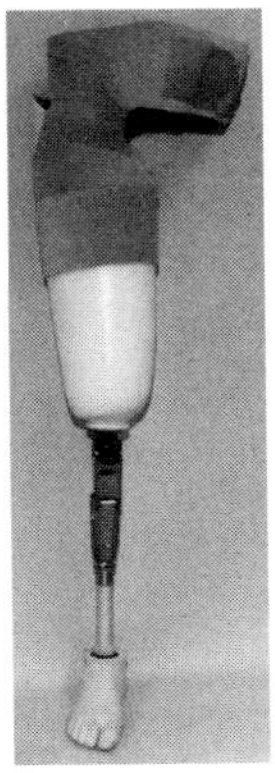

Figure 40 Above knee.

Knee Disarticulation

✻ **L5150** Knee disarticulation (or through knee), molded socket, external knee joints, shin, SACH foot Qp Qh ♿ A

✻ **L5160** Knee disarticulation (or through knee), molded socket, bent knee configuration, external knee joints, shin, SACH foot Qp Qh ♿ A

Above Knee

✻ **L5200** Above knee, molded socket, single axis constant friction knee, shin, SACH foot Qp Qh ♿ A

✻ **L5210** Above knee, short prosthesis, no knee joint ('stubbies'), with foot blocks, no ankle joints, each Qp Qh ♿ A

✻ **L5220** Above knee, short prosthesis, no knee joint ('stubbies'), with articulated ankle/foot, dynamically aligned, each Qp Qh ♿ A

✻ **L5230** Above knee, for proximal femoral focal deficiency, constant friction knee, shin, SACH foot Qp Qh ♿ A

Hip Disarticulation

✻ **L5250** Hip disarticulation, Canadian type; molded socket, hip joint, single axis constant friction knee, shin, SACH foot Qp Qh ♿ A

✻ **L5270** Hip disarticulation, tilt table type; molded socket, locking hip joint, single axis constant friction knee, shin, SACH foot Qp Qh ♿ A

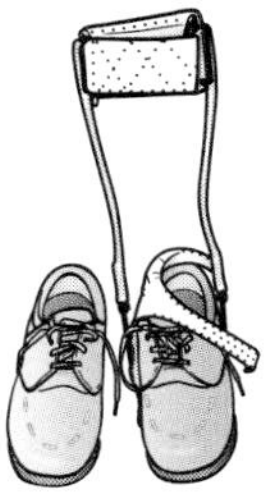

Figure 41 Ankle symes.

Hemipelvectomy

✻ **L5280** Hemipelvectomy, Canadian type; molded socket, hip joint, single axis constant friction knee, shin, SACH foot Qp Qh ♿ A

Endoskeleton: Below Knee

✻ **L5301** Below knee, molded socket, shin, SACH foot, endoskeletal system Qp Qh ♿ A

~~**L5311** Knee disarticulation (or through knee), molded socket, external knee joints, shin, SACH foot, endoskeletal system~~ ✖

▶ ✻ **L5312** Knee disarticulation (or through knee), molded socket, single axis knee, pylon, sach foot, endoskeletal system A

Endoskeletal: Above Knee

✻ **L5321** Above knee, molded socket, open end, SACH foot, endoskeletal system, single axis knee Qp Qh ♿ A

Endoskeletal: Hip Disarticulation

✻ **L5331** Hip disarticulation, Canadian type, molded socket, endoskeletal system, hip joint, single axis knee, SACH foot Qp Qh ♿ A

Endoskeletal: Hemipelvectomy

✻ **L5341** Hemipelvectomy, Canadian type, molded socket, endoskeletal system, hip joint, single axis knee, SACH foot Qp Qh ♿ A

Immediate Postsurgical or Early Fitting Procedures

* **L5400** Immediate post surgical or early fitting, application of initial rigid dressing, including fitting, alignment, suspension, and one cast change, below knee `Qp` `Qh` ⌖ A

* **L5410** Immediate post surgical or early fitting, application of initial rigid dressing, including fitting, alignment and suspension, below knee, each additional cast change and realignment `Qp` `Qh` ⌖ A

* **L5420** Immediate post surgical or early fitting, application of initial rigid dressing, including fitting, alignment and suspension and one cast change 'AK' or knee disarticulation `Qp` `Qh` ⌖ A

* **L5430** Immediate postsurgical or early fitting, application of initial rigid dressing, including fitting, alignment, and suspension, 'AK' or knee disarticulation, each additional cast change and realignment `Qp` `Qh` ⌖ A

* **L5450** Immediate post surgical or early fitting, application of non-weight bearing rigid dressing, below knee `Qp` `Qh` ⌖ A

* **L5460** Immediate post surgical or early fitting, application of non-weight bearing rigid dressing, above knee `Qp` `Qh` ⌖ A

Initial Prosthesis

* **L5500** Initial, below knee 'PTB' type socket, non-alignable system, pylon, no cover, SACH foot, plaster socket, direct formed `Qp` `Qh` ⌖ A

* **L5505** Initial, above knee–knee disarticulation, ischial level socket, non-alignable system, pylon, no cover, SACH foot, plaster socket, direct formed `Qp` `Qh` ⌖ A

Preparatory Prosthesis

* **L5510** Preparatory, below knee 'PTB' type socket, non-alignable system, pylon, no cover, SACH foot, plaster socket, molded to model `Qp` `Qh` ⌖ A

* **L5520** Preparatory, below knee 'PTB' type socket, non-alignable system, pylon, no cover, SACH foot, thermoplastic or equal, direct formed `Qp` `Qh` ⌖ A

* **L5530** Preparatory, below knee 'PTB' type socket, non-alignable system, pylon, no cover, SACH foot, thermoplastic or equal, molded to model `Qp` `Qh` ⌖ A

* **L5535** Preparatory, below knee 'PTB' type socket, non-alignable system, no cover, SACH foot, prefabricated, adjustable open end socket `Qp` `Qh` ⌖ A

* **L5540** Preparatory, below knee 'PTB' type socket, non-alignable system, pylon, no cover, SACH foot, laminated socket, molded to model `Qp` `Qh` ⌖ A

* **L5560** Preparatory, above knee - knee disarticulation, ischial level socket, non-alignable system, pylon, no cover, SACH foot, plaster socket, molded to model `Qp` `Qh` ⌖ A

* **L5570** Preparatory, above knee - knee disarticulation, ischial level socket, non-alignable system, pylon, no cover, SACH foot, thermoplastic or equal, direct formed `Qp` `Qh` ⌖ A

* **L5580** Preparatory, above knee - knee disarticulation, ischial level socket, non-alignable system, pylon, no cover, SACH foot, thermoplastic or equal, molded to model `Qp` `Qh` ⌖ A

* **L5585** Preparatory, above knee - knee disarticulation, ischial level socket, non-alignable system, pylon, no cover, SACH foot, prefabricated adjustable open end socket `Qp` `Qh` ⌖ A

* **L5590** Preparatory, above knee - knee disarticulation, ischial level socket, non-alignable system, pylon, no cover, SACH foot, laminated socket, molded to model `Qp` `Qh` ⌖ A

* **L5595** Preparatory, hip disarticulation-hemipelvectomy, pylon, no cover, SACH foot, thermoplastic or equal, molded to patient model `Qp` `Qh` ⌖ A

* **L5600** Preparatory, hip disarticulation-hemipelvectomy, pylon, no cover, SACH foot, laminated socket, molded to patient model `Qp` `Qh` ⌖ A

Additions to Lower Extremity

* **L5610** Addition to lower extremity, endoskeletal system, above knee, hydracadence system `Qp` `Qh` ⌖ A

* **L5611** Addition to lower extremity, endoskeletal system, above knee-knee disarticulation, 4 bar linkage, with friction swing phase control `Qp` `Qh` ⌖ A

* **L5613** Addition to lower extremity, endoskeletal system, above knee-knee disarticulation, 4 bar linkage, with hydraulic swing phase control `Qp` `Qh` ⌖ A

▶ New → Revised ✔ Reinstated ~~deleted~~ Deleted
☼ Special coverage instructions ◆ Not covered or valid by Medicare * Carrier discretion

✳ **L5614** Addition to lower extremity, exoskeletal system, above knee-knee disarticulation, 4 bar linkage, with pneumatic swing phase control `Qp` `Qh` ♿ A

✳ **L5616** Addition to lower extremity, endoskeletal system, above knee, universal multiplex system, friction swing phase control `Qp` `Qh` ♿ A

✳ **L5617** Addition to lower extremity, quick change self-aligning unit, above knee or below knee, each `Qp` `Qh` ♿ A

Additions to Test Sockets

✳ **L5618** Addition to lower extremity, test socket, Symes ♿ A

✳ **L5620** Addition to lower extremity, test socket, below knee ♿ A

✳ **L5622** Addition to lower extremity, test socket, knee disarticulation ♿ A

✳ **L5624** Addition to lower extremity, test socket, above knee ♿ A

✳ **L5626** Addition to lower extremity, test socket, hip disarticulation ♿ A

✳ **L5628** Addition to lower extremity, test socket, hemipelvectomy `Qp` `Qh` ♿ A

✳ **L5629** Addition to lower extremity, below knee, acrylic socket `Qp` `Qh` ♿ A

Additions to Socket Variations

✳ **L5630** Addition to lower extremity, Symes type, expandable wall socket `Qp` `Qh` ♿ A

✳ **L5631** Addition to lower extremity, above knee or knee disarticulation, acrylic socket `Qp` `Qh` ♿ A

✳ **L5632** Addition to lower extremity, Symes type, 'PTB' brim design socket `Qp` `Qh` ♿ A

✳ **L5634** Addition to lower extremity, Symes type, posterior opening (Canadian) socket `Qp` `Qh` ♿ A

✳ **L5636** Addition to lower extremity, Symes type, medial opening socket `Qp` `Qh` ♿ A

✳ **L5637** Addition to lower extremity, below knee, total contact `Qp` `Qh` ♿ A

✳ **L5638** Addition to lower extremity, below knee, leather socket `Qp` `Qh` ♿ A

✳ **L5639** Addition to lower extremity, below knee, wood socket `Qp` `Qh` ♿ A

✳ **L5640** Addition to lower extremity, knee disarticulation, leather socket `Qp` `Qh` ♿ A

✳ **L5642** Addition to lower extremity, above knee, leather socket `Qp` `Qh` ♿ A

✳ **L5643** Addition to lower extremity, hip disarticulation, flexible inner socket, external frame `Qp` `Qh` ♿ A

✳ **L5644** Addition to lower extremity, above knee, wood socket `Qp` `Qh` ♿ A

✳ **L5645** Addition to lower extremity, below knee, flexible inner socket, external frame `Qp` `Qh` ♿ A

✳ **L5646** Addition to lower extremity, below knee, air, fluid, gel or equal, cushion socket `Qp` `Qh` ♿ A

✳ **L5647** Addition to lower extremity, below knee, suction socket `Qp` `Qh` ♿ A

✳ **L5648** Addition to lower extremity, above knee, air, fluid, gel or equal, cushion socket `Qp` `Qh` ♿ A

✳ **L5649** Addition to lower extremity, ischial containment/narrow M-L socket `Qp` `Qh` ♿ A

✳ **L5650** Additions to lower extremity, total contact, above knee or knee disarticulation socket `Qp` `Qh` ♿ A

✳ **L5651** Addition to lower extremity, above knee, flexible inner socket, external frame `Qp` `Qh` ♿ A

✳ **L5652** Addition to lower extremity, suction suspension, above knee or knee disarticulation socket `Qp` `Qh` ♿ A

✳ **L5653** Addition to lower extremity, knee disarticulation, expandable wall socket `Qp` `Qh` ♿ A

Additions to Socket Insert and Suspension

✳ **L5654** Addition to lower extremity, socket insert, Symes, (Kemblo, Pelite, Aliplast, Plastazote or equal) `Qp` `Qh` ♿ A

✳ **L5655** Addition to lower extremity, socket insert, below knee (Kemblo, Pelite, Aliplast, Plastazote or equal) `Qp` `Qh` ♿ A

✳ **L5656** Addition to lower extremity, socket insert, knee disarticulation (Kemblo, Pelite, Aliplast, Plastazote or equal) `Qp` `Qh` ♿ A

✳ **L5658** Addition to lower extremity, socket insert, above knee (Kemblo, Pelite, Aliplast, Plastazote or equal) `Qp` `Qh` ♿ A

* **L5661** Addition to lower extremity, socket insert, multi-durometer Symes `Qp` `Qh` 🦽   A

* **L5665** Addition to lower extremity, socket insert, multi-durometer, below knee `Qp` `Qh` 🦽   A

* **L5666** Addition to lower extremity, below knee, cuff suspension `Qp` `Qh` 🦽   A

* **L5668** Addition to lower extremity, below knee, molded distal cushion `Qp` `Qh` 🦽   A

* **L5670** Addition to lower extremity, below knee, molded supracondylar suspension ('PTS' or similar) `Qp` `Qh` 🦽   A

* **L5671** Addition to lower extremity, below knee/above knee suspension locking mechanism (shuttle, lanyard or equal), excludes socket insert `Qp` `Qh` 🦽   A

* **L5672** Addition to lower extremity, below knee, removable medial brim suspension `Qp` `Qh` 🦽   A

* **L5673** Addition to lower extremity, below knee/above knee, custom fabricated from existing mold or prefabricated, socket insert, silicone gel, elastomeric or equal, for use with locking mechanism 🦽   A

* **L5676** Additions to lower extremity, below knee, knee joints, single axis, pair `Qp` `Qh` 🦽   A

* **L5677** Additions to lower extremity, below knee, knee joints, polycentric, pair `Qp` `Qh` 🦽   A

* **L5678** Additions to lower extremity, below knee, joint covers, pair `Qp` `Qh` 🦽   A

* **L5679** Addition to lower extremity, below knee/above knee, custom fabricated from existing mold or prefabricated, socket insert, silicone gel, elastomeric or equal, not for use with locking mechanism 🦽   A

* **L5680** Addition to lower extremity, below knee, thigh lacer, nonmolded `Qp` `Qh` 🦽   A

* **L5681** Addition to lower extremity, below knee/above knee, custom fabricated socket insert for congenital or atypical traumatic amputee, silicone gel, elastomeric or equal, for use with or without locking mechanism, initial only (for other than initial, use code L5673 or L5679) `Qp` `Qh` 🦽   A

* **L5682** Addition to lower extremity, below knee, thigh lacer, gluteal/ischial, molded `Qp` `Qh` 🦽   A

* **L5683** Addition to lower extremity, below knee/above knee, custom fabricated socket insert for other than congenital or atypical traumatic amputee, silicone gel, elastomeric, or equal, for use with or without locking mechanism, initial only (for other than initial, use code L5673 or L5679) `Qp` `Qh` 🦽   A

* **L5684** Addition to lower extremity, below knee, fork strap `Qp` `Qh` 🦽   A

* **L5685** Addition to lower extremity prosthesis, below knee, suspension/sealing sleeve, with or without valve, any material, each 🦽   A

* **L5686** Addition to lower extremity, below knee, back check (extension control) `Qp` `Qh` 🦽   A

* **L5688** Addition to lower extremity, below knee, waist belt, webbing `Qp` `Qh` 🦽   A

* **L5690** Addition to lower extremity, below knee, waist belt, padded and lined `Qp` `Qh` 🦽   A

* **L5692** Addition to lower extremity, above knee, pelvic control belt, light `Qp` `Qh` 🦽   A

* **L5694** Addition to lower extremity, above knee, pelvic control belt, padded and lined `Qp` `Qh` 🦽   A

* **L5695** Addition to lower extremity, above knee, pelvic control, sleeve suspension, neoprene or equal, each `Qp` `Qh` 🦽   A

* **L5696** Addition to lower extremity, above knee or knee disarticulation, pelvic joint `Qp` `Qh` 🦽   A

* **L5697** Addition to lower extremity, above knee or knee disarticulation, pelvic band `Qp` `Qh` 🦽   A

* **L5698** Addition to lower extremity, above knee or knee disarticulation, Silesian bandage `Qp` `Qh` 🦽   A

* **L5699** All lower extremity prostheses, shoulder harness `Qp` `Qh` 🦽   A

Additions/Replacements to Feet-Ankle Units

* **L5700** Replacement, socket, below knee, molded to patient model `Qp` `Qh` 🦽   A

* **L5701** Replacement, socket, above knee/knee disarticulation, including attachment plate, molded to patient model `Qp` `Qh` 🦽   A

* **L5702** Replacement, socket, hip disarticulation, including hip joint, molded to patient model `Qp` `Qh` 🦽   A

▶ New   → Revised   ✔ Reinstated   ~~deleted~~ Deleted

⊘ Special coverage instructions   ◆ Not covered or valid by Medicare   * Carrier discretion

✳ **L5703** Ankle, Symes, molded to patient model, socket without solid ankle cushion heel (SACH) foot, replacement only Qp Qh ㅊ A

✳ **L5704** Custom shaped protective cover, below knee Qp Qh ㅊ A

✳ **L5705** Custom shaped protective cover, above knee Qp Qh ㅊ A

✳ **L5706** Custom shaped protective cover, knee disarticulation Qp Qh ㅊ A

✳ **L5707** Custom shaped protective cover, hip disarticulation Qp Qh ㅊ A

Additions to Exoskeletal–Knee-Shin System

✳ **L5710** Addition, exoskeletal knee-shin system, single axis, manual lock Qp Qh ㅊ A

✳ **L5711** Additions exoskeletal knee-shin system, single axis, manual lock, ultra-light material Qp Qh ㅊ A

✳ **L5712** Addition, exoskeletal knee-shin system, single axis, friction swing and stance phase control (safety knee) Qp Qh ㅊ A

✳ **L5714** Addition, exoskeletal knee-shin system, single axis, variable friction swing phase control Qp Qh ㅊ A

✳ **L5716** Addition, exoskeletal knee-shin system, polycentric, mechanical stance phase lock Qp Qh ㅊ A

✳ **L5718** Addition, exoskeletal knee-shin system, polycentric, friction swing and stance phase control Qp Qh ㅊ A

✳ **L5722** Addition, exoskeletal knee-shin system, single axis, pneumatic swing, friction stance phase control Qp Qh ㅊ A

✳ **L5724** Addition, exoskeletal knee-shin system, single axis, fluid swing phase control Qp Qh ㅊ A

✳ **L5726** Addition, exoskeletal knee-shin system, single axis, external joints, fluid swing phase control Qp Qh ㅊ A

✳ **L5728** Addition, exoskeletal knee-shin system, single axis, fluid swing and stance phase control Qp Qh ㅊ A

✳ **L5780** Addition, exoskeletal knee-shin system, single axis, pneumatic/hydra pneumatic swing phase control Qp Qh ㅊ A

✳ **L5781** Addition to lower limb prosthesis, vacuum pump, residual limb volume management and moisture evacuation system Qp Qh ㅊ A

✳ **L5782** Addition to lower limb prosthesis, vacuum pump, residual limb volume management and moisture evacuation system, heavy duty Qp Qh ㅊ A

Component Modification

✳ **L5785** Addition, exoskeletal system, below knee, ultra-light material (titanium, carbon fiber, or equal) Qp Qh ㅊ A

✳ **L5790** Addition, exoskeletal system, above knee, ultra-light material (titanium, carbon fiber, or equal) Qp Qh ㅊ A

✳ **L5795** Addition, exoskeletal system, hip disarticulation, ultra-light material (titanium, carbon fiber, or equal) Qp Qh ㅊ A

Endoskeletal

✳ **L5810** Addition, endoskeletal knee-shin system, single axis, manual lock Qp Qh ㅊ A

✳ **L5811** Addition, endoskeletal knee-shin system, single axis, manual lock, ultralight material Qp Qh ㅊ A

✳ **L5812** Addition, endoskeletal knee-shin system, single axis, friction swing and stance phase control (safety knee) Qp Qh ㅊ A

✳ **L5814** Addition, endoskeletal knee-shin system, polycentric, hydraulic swing phase control, mechanical stance phase lock Qp Qh ㅊ A

✳ **L5816** Addition, endoskeletal knee-shin system, polycentric, mechanical stance phase lock Qp Qh ㅊ A

✳ **L5818** Addition, endoskeletal knee-shin system, polycentric, friction swing, and stance phase control Qp Qh ㅊ A

✳ **L5822** Addition, endoskeletal knee-shin system, single axis, pneumatic swing, friction stance phase control Qp Qh ㅊ A

✳ **L5824** Addition, endoskeletal knee-shin system, single axis, fluid swing phase control Qp Qh ㅊ A

✳ **L5826** Addition, endoskeletal knee-shin system, single axis, hydraulic swing phase control, with miniature high activity frame Qp Qh ㅊ A

✳ **L5828** Addition, endoskeletal knee-shin system, single axis, fluid swing and stance phase control Qp Qh ㅊ A

✳ **L5830** Addition, endoskeletal knee-shin system, single axis, pneumatic/swing phase control Qp Qh ㅊ A

✳ **L5840** Addition, endoskeletal knee/shin system, 4-bar linkage or multiaxial, pneumatic swing phase control Qp Qh ㅊ A

PQRS PQRI | Qp **Quantity Physician Appendix B** | Qh **Quantity Hospital Appendix C** | ♀ **Female only**
♂ **Male only** | A **Age** | ㅊ **DMEPOS** | A2-Z3 **ASC Payment Indicator** | A-Y **ASC Status Indicator** | Coding Clinic

✳ **L5845** Addition, endoskeletal, knee-shin system, stance flexion feature, adjustable `Qp` `Qh` ♿ A

✳ **L5848** Addition to endoskeletal, knee-shin system, fluid stance extension, dampening feature, with or without adjustability `Qp` `Qh` ♿ A

✳ **L5850** Addition, endoskeletal system, above knee or hip disarticulation, knee extension assist `Qp` `Qh` ♿ A

✳ **L5855** Addition, endoskeletal system, hip disarticulation, mechanical hip extension assist `Qp` `Qh` ♿ A

✳ **L5856** Addition to lower extremity prosthesis, endoskeletal knee-shin system, microprocessor control feature, swing and stance phase; includes electronic sensor(s), any type `Qp` `Qh` ♿ A

✳ **L5857** Addition to lower extremity prosthesis, endoskeletal knee-shin system, microprocessor control feature, swing phase only; includes electronic sensor(s), any type `Qp` `Qh` ♿ A

✳ **L5858** Addition to lower extremity prosthesis, endoskeletal knee shin system, microprocessor control feature, stance phase only, includes electronic sensor(s), any type `Qp` `Qh` ♿ A

✳ **L5910** Addition, endoskeletal system, below knee, alignable system `Qp` `Qh` ♿ A

✳ **L5920** Addition, endoskeletal system, above knee or hip disarticulation, alignable system `Qp` `Qh` ♿ A

✳ **L5925** Addition, endoskeletal system, above knee, knee disarticulation or hip disarticulation, manual lock `Qp` `Qh` ♿ A

✳ **L5930** Addition, endoskeletal system, high activity knee control frame `Qp` `Qh` ♿ A

✳ **L5940** Addition, endoskeletal system, below knee, ultra-light material (titanium, carbon fiber or equal) `Qp` `Qh` ♿ A

✳ **L5950** Addition, endoskeletal system, above knee, ultra-light material (titanium, carbon fiber or equal) `Qp` `Qh` ♿ A

✳ **L5960** Addition, endoskeletal system, hip disarticulation, ultra-light material (titanium, carbon fiber, or equal) `Qp` `Qh` ♿ A

▶ ✳ **L5961** Addition, endoskeletal system, polycentric hip joint, pneumatic or hydraulic control, rotation control, with or without flexion, and/or extension control `Qp` `Qh` ♿ A

✳ **L5962** Addition, endoskeletal system, below knee, flexible protective outer surface covering system `Qp` `Qh` ♿ A

✳ **L5964** Addition, endoskeletal system, above knee, flexible protective outer surface covering system `Qp` `Qh` ♿ A

✳ **L5966** Addition, endoskeletal system, hip disarticulation, flexible protective outer surface covering system `Qp` `Qh` ♿ A

✳ **L5968** Addition to lower limb prosthesis, multiaxial ankle with swing phase active dorsiflexion feature `Qp` `Qh` ♿ A

✳ **L5970** All lower extremity prostheses, foot, external keel, SACH foot `Qp` `Qh` ♿ A

✳ **L5971** All lower extremity prosthesis, solid ankle cushion keel (SACH) foot, replacement only `Qp` `Qh` ♿ A

✳ **L5972** All lower extremity prostheses, flexible heel foot (Safe, Sten, Bock Dynamic or equal) `Qp` `Qh` ♿ A

✳ **L5973** Endoskeletal ankle foot system, microprocessor controlled feature, dorsiflexion and/or plantar flexion control, includes power source `Qh` ♿ A

✳ **L5974** All lower extremity prostheses, foot, single axis ankle/foot `Qp` `Qh` ♿ A

✳ **L5975** All lower extremity prostheses, combination single axis ankle and flexible keel foot `Qp` `Qh` ♿ A

✳ **L5976** All lower extremity prostheses, energy storing foot (Seattle Carbon Copy II or equal) `Qp` `Qh` ♿ A

✳ **L5978** All lower extremity prostheses, foot, multiaxial ankle/foot `Qp` `Qh` ♿ A

✳ **L5979** All lower extremity prostheses, multiaxial ankle, dynamic response foot, one piece system `Qp` `Qh` ♿ A

✳ **L5980** All lower extremity prostheses, flex foot system `Qp` `Qh` ♿ A

✳ **L5981** All lower extremity prostheses, flexwalk system or equal `Qp` `Qh` ♿ A

✳ **L5982** All exoskeletal lower extremity prostheses, axial rotation unit `Qp` `Qh` ♿ A

✳ **L5984** All endoskeletal lower extremity prostheses, axial rotation unit, with or without adjustability `Qp` `Qh` ♿ A

✳ **L5985** All endoskeletal lower extremity prostheses, dynamic prosthetic pylon `Qp` `Qh` ♿ A

✳ **L5986** All lower extremity prostheses, multiaxial rotation unit ('MCP' or equal) `Qp` `Qh` ♿ A

▶ New → Revised ✔ Reinstated ~~deleted~~ Deleted

⊘ Special coverage instructions ◆ Not covered or valid by Medicare ✳ Carrier discretion

* **L5987** All lower extremity prostheses, shank foot system with vertical loading pylon `Qp` `Qh` 🔥   A

* **L5988** Addition to lower limb prosthesis, vertical shock reducing pylon feature `Qp` `Qh` 🔥   A

* **L5990** Addition to lower extremity prosthesis, user adjustable heel height `Qp` `Qh` 🔥   A

* **L5999** Lower extremity prosthesis, not otherwise specified   A

Upper Limb

NOTE: The procedures in L6000-L6599 are considered as base or basic procedures and may be modified by listing procedures from the additions sections. The base procedures include only standard friction wrist and control cable system unless otherwise specified.

Partial Hand

L6000-L6698: Bill DME/MAC

→ * **L6000** Partial hand, thumb remaining `Qp` `Qh` 🔥   A

→ * **L6010** Partial hand, little and/or ring finger remaining `Qp` `Qh` 🔥   A

→ * **L6020** Partial hand, no finger remaining `Qp` `Qh` 🔥   A

* **L6025** Transcarpal/metacarpal or partial hand disarticulation prosthesis, external power, self-suspended, inner socket with removable forearm section, electrodes and cables, two batteries, charger, myoelectric control of terminal device `Qp` `Qh` 🔥   A

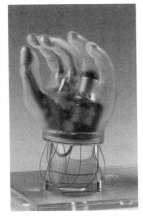

Figure 42 Partial hand.

Wrist Disarticulation

* **L6050** Wrist disarticulation, molded socket, flexible elbow hinges, triceps pad `Qp` `Qh` 🔥   A

* **L6055** Wrist disarticulation, molded socket with expandable interface, flexible elbow hinges, triceps pad `Qp` `Qh` 🔥   A

Below Elbow

* **L6100** Below elbow, molded socket, flexible elbow hinge, triceps pad `Qp` `Qh` 🔥   A

* **L6110** Below elbow, molded socket, (Muenster or Northwestern suspension types) `Qp` `Qh` 🔥   A

* **L6120** Below elbow, molded double wall split socket, step-up hinges, half cuff `Qp` `Qh` 🔥   A

* **L6130** Below elbow, molded double wall split socket, stump activated locking hinge, half cuff `Qp` `Qh` 🔥   A

Elbow Disarticulation

* **L6200** Elbow disarticulation, molded socket, outside locking hinge, forearm `Qp` `Qh` 🔥   A

* **L6205** Elbow disarticulation, molded socket with expandable interface, outside locking hinges, forearm `Qp` `Qh` 🔥   A

Above Elbow

* **L6250** Above elbow, molded double wall socket, internal locking elbow, forearm `Qp` `Qh` 🔥   A

Shoulder Disarticulation

* **L6300** Shoulder disarticulation, molded socket, shoulder bulkhead, humeral section, internal locking elbow, forearm `Qp` `Qh` 🔥   A

* **L6310** Shoulder disarticulation, passive restoration (complete prosthesis) `Qp` `Qh` 🔥   A

* **L6320** Shoulder disarticulation, passive restoration (shoulder cap only) `Qp` `Qh` 🔥   A

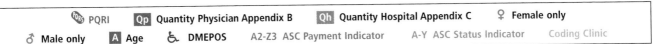

Interscapular Thoracic

∗ **L6350** Interscapular thoracic, molded socket, shoulder bulkhead, humeral section, internal locking elbow, forearm Qp Qh ✦   A

∗ **L6360** Interscapular thoracic, passive restoration (complete prosthesis) Qp Qh ✦   A

∗ **L6370** Interscapular thoracic, passive restoration (shoulder cap only) Qp Qh ✦   A

Immediate and Early Postsurgical Procedures

∗ **L6380** Immediate post surgical or early fitting, application of initial rigid dressing, including fitting alignment and suspension of components, and one cast change, wrist disarticulation or below elbow Qp Qh ✦   A

∗ **L6382** Immediate post surgical or early fitting, application of initial rigid dressing including fitting alignment and suspension of components, and one cast change, elbow disarticulation or above elbow Qp Qh ✦   A

∗ **L6384** Immediate post surgical or early fitting, application of initial rigid dressing including fitting alignment and suspension of components, and one cast change, shoulder disarticulation or interscapular thoracic Qp Qh ✦   A

∗ **L6386** Immediate post surgical or early fitting, each additional cast change and realignment Qp Qh ✦   A

∗ **L6388** Immediate post surgical or early fitting, application of rigid dressing only Qp Qh ✦   A

Endoskeletal: Below Elbow

∗ **L6400** Below elbow, molded socket, endoskeletal system, including soft prosthetic tissue shaping Qp Qh ✦   A

Endoskeletal: Elbow Disarticulation

∗ **L6450** Elbow disarticulation, molded socket, endoskeletal system, including soft prosthetic tissue shaping Qp Qh ✦   A

Endoskeletal: Above Elbow

∗ **L6500** Above elbow, molded socket, endoskeletal system, including soft prosthetic tissue shaping Qp Qh ✦   A

Endoskeletal: Shoulder Disarticulation

∗ **L6550** Shoulder disarticulation, molded socket, endoskeletal system, including soft prosthetic tissue shaping Qp Qh ✦   A

Endoskeletal: Interscapular Thoracic

∗ **L6570** Interscapular thoracic, molded socket, endoskeletal system, including soft prosthetic tissue shaping Qp Qh ✦   A

∗ **L6580** Preparatory, wrist disarticulation or below elbow, single wall plastic socket, friction wrist, flexible elbow hinges, figure of eight harness, humeral cuff, Bowden cable control, USMC or equal pylon, no cover, molded to patient model Qp Qh ✦   A

∗ **L6582** Preparatory, wrist disarticulation or below elbow, single wall socket, friction wrist, flexible elbow hinges, figure of eight harness, humeral cuff, Bowden cable control, USMC or equal pylon, no cover, direct formed Qp Qh ✦   A

∗ **L6584** Preparatory, elbow disarticulation or above elbow, single wall plastic socket, friction wrist, locking elbow, figure of eight harness, fair lead cable control, USMC or equal pylon, no cover, molded to patient model Qp Qh ✦   A

∗ **L6586** Preparatory, elbow disarticulation or above elbow, single wall socket, friction wrist, locking elbow, figure of eight harness, fair lead cable control, USMC or equal pylon, no cover, direct formed Qp Qh ✦   A

∗ **L6588** Preparatory, shoulder disarticulation or interscapular thoracic, single wall plastic socket, shoulder joint, locking elbow, friction wrist, chest strap, fair lead cable control, USMC or equal pylon, no cover, molded to patient model Qp Qh ✦   A

∗ **L6590** Preparatory, shoulder disarticulation or interscapular thoracic, single wall socket, shoulder joint, locking elbow, friction wrist, chest strap, fair lead cable control, USMC or equal pylon, no cover, direct formed Qp Qh ✦   A

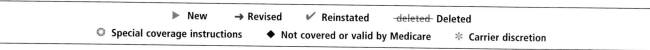

▶ New   → Revised   ✔ Reinstated   ~~deleted~~ Deleted

⊘ Special coverage instructions   ◆ Not covered or valid by Medicare   ∗ Carrier discretion

L6350 – L6590 PROSTHETICS

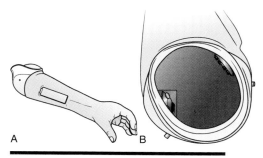

Figure 43 Upper extremity addition.

Additions to Upper Limb

NOTE: The following procedures/modifications/components may be added to other base procedures. The items in this section should reflect the additional complexity of each modification procedure, in addition to base procedure, at the time of the original order.

✳ **L6600**   Upper extremity additions, polycentric hinge, pair `Qp` `Qh` ♿   A

✳ **L6605**   Upper extremity additions, single pivot hinge, pair `Qp` `Qh` ♿   A

✳ **L6610**   Upper extremity additions, flexible metal hinge, pair `Qp` `Qh` ♿   A

✳ **L6611**   Addition to upper extremity prosthesis, external powered, additional switch, any type ♿   A

✳ **L6615**   Upper extremity addition, disconnect locking wrist unit `Qp` `Qh` ♿   A

✳ **L6616**   Upper extremity addition, additional disconnect insert for locking wrist unit, each `Qp` `Qh` ♿   A

✳ **L6620**   Upper extremity addition, flexion/extension wrist unit, with or without friction `Qp` `Qh` ♿   A

✳ **L6621**   Upper extremity prosthesis addition, flexion/extension wrist with or without friction, for use with external powered terminal device `Qp` `Qh` ♿   A

✳ **L6623**   Upper extremity addition, spring assisted rotational wrist unit with latch release `Qp` `Qh` ♿   A

✳ **L6624**   Upper extremity addition, flexion/extension and rotation wrist unit ♿   A

✳ **L6625**   Upper extremity addition, rotation wrist unit with cable lock `Qp` `Qh` ♿   A

✳ **L6628**   Upper extremity addition, quick disconnect hook adapter, Otto Bock or equal `Qp` `Qh` ♿   A

✳ **L6629**   Upper extremity addition, quick disconnect lamination collar with coupling piece, Otto Bock or equal `Qp` `Qh` ♿   A

✳ **L6630**   Upper extremity addition, stainless steel, any wrist `Qp` `Qh` ♿   A

✳ **L6632**   Upper extremity addition, latex suspension sleeve, each ♿   A

✳ **L6635**   Upper extremity addition, lift assist for elbow `Qp` `Qh` ♿   A

✳ **L6637**   Upper extremity addition, nudge control elbow lock `Qp` `Qh` ♿   A

✳ **L6638**   Upper extremity addition to prosthesis, electric locking feature, only for use with manually powered elbow `Qp` `Qh` ♿   A

✳ **L6640**   Upper extremity additions, shoulder abduction joint, pair `Qp` `Qh` ♿   A

✳ **L6641**   Upper extremity addition, excursion amplifier, pulley type `Qp` `Qh` ♿   A

✳ **L6642**   Upper extremity addition, excursion amplifier, lever type `Qp` `Qh` ♿   A

✳ **L6645**   Upper extremity addition, shoulder flexion-abduction joint, each `Qp` `Qh` ♿   A

✳ **L6646**   Upper extremity addition, shoulder joint, multipositional locking, flexion, adjustable abduction friction control, for use with body powered or external powered system `Qp` `Qh` ♿   A

✳ **L6647**   Upper extremity addition, shoulder lock mechanism, body powered actuator `Qp` `Qh` ♿   A

✳ **L6648**   Upper extremity addition, shoulder lock mechanism, external powered actuator `Qp` `Qh` ♿   A

✳ **L6650**   Upper extremity addition, shoulder universal joint, each `Qp` `Qh` ♿   A

✳ **L6655**   Upper extremity addition, standard control cable, extra ♿   A

✳ **L6660**   Upper extremity addition, heavy duty control cable ♿   A

✳ **L6665**   Upper extremity addition, Teflon, or equal, cable lining ♿   A

✳ **L6670**   Upper extremity addition, hook to hand, cable adapter `Qp` `Qh` ♿   A

✳ **L6672**   Upper extremity addition, harness, chest or shoulder, saddle type `Qp` `Qh` ♿   A

✳ **L6675**   Upper extremity addition, harness, (e.g. figure of eight type), single cable design `Qp` `Qh` ♿   A

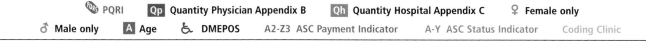

PQRI   `Qp` **Quantity Physician Appendix B**   `Qh` **Quantity Hospital Appendix C**   ♀ **Female only**

♂ **Male only**   `A` **Age**   ♿ **DMEPOS**   A2-Z3 **ASC Payment Indicator**   A-Y **ASC Status Indicator**   Coding Clinic

* **L6676** Upper extremity addition, harness, (e.g. figure of eight type), dual cable design `Qp` `Qh`   A

* **L6677** Upper extremity addition, harness, triple control, simultaneous operation of terminal device and elbow `Qp` `Qh`   A

* **L6680** Upper extremity addition, test socket, wrist disarticulation or below elbow   A

* **L6682** Upper extremity addition, test socket, elbow disarticulation or above elbow   A

* **L6684** Upper extremity addition, test socket, shoulder disarticulation or interscapular thoracic   A

* **L6686** Upper extremity addition, suction socket `Qp` `Qh`   A

* **L6687** Upper extremity addition, frame type socket, below elbow or wrist disarticulation `Qp` `Qh`   A

* **L6688** Upper extremity addition, frame type socket, above elbow or elbow disarticulation `Qp` `Qh`   A

* **L6689** Upper extremity addition, frame type socket, shoulder disarticulation `Qp` `Qh`   A

* **L6690** Upper extremity addition, frame type socket, interscapular-thoracic `Qp` `Qh`   A

* **L6691** Upper extremity addition, removable insert, each   A

* **L6692** Upper extremity addition, silicone gel insert or equal, each   A

* **L6693** Upper extremity addition, locking elbow, forearm counterbalance `Qp` `Qh`   A

* **L6694** Addition to upper extremity prosthesis, below elbow/above elbow, custom fabricated from existing mold or prefabricated, socket insert, silicone gel, elastomeric or equal, for use with locking mechanism `Qp` `Qh`   A

* **L6695** Addition to upper extremity prosthesis, below elbow/above elbow, custom fabricated from existing mold or prefabricated, socket insert, silicone gel, elastomeric or equal, not for use with locking mechanism `Qp` `Qh`   A

* **L6696** Addition to upper extremity prosthesis, below elbow/above elbow, custom fabricated socket insert for congenital or atypical traumatic amputee, silicone gel, elastomeric or equal, for use with or without locking mechanism, initial only (for other than initial, use code L6694 or L6695) `Qp` `Qh`   A

* **L6697** Addition to upper extremity prosthesis, below elbow/above elbow, custom fabricated socket insert for other than congenital or atypical traumatic amputee, silicone gel, elastomeric or equal, for use with or without locking mechanism, initial only (for other than initial, use code L6694 or L6695) `Qp` `Qh`   A

* **L6698** Addition to upper extremity prosthesis, below elbow/above elbow, lock mechanism, excludes socket insert `Qp` `Qh`   A

Terminal Devices

Hooks

L6703-L6915:   Bill DME/MAC

* **L6703** Terminal device, passive hand/mitt, any material, any size   A

* **L6704** Terminal device, sport/recreational/work attachment, any material, any size   A

* **L6706** Terminal device, hook, mechanical, voluntary opening, any material, any size, lined or unlined   A

* **L6707** Terminal device, hook, mechanical, voluntary closing, any material, any size, lined or unlined   A

* **L6708** Terminal device, hand, mechanical, voluntary opening, any material, any size   A

* **L6709** Terminal device, hand, mechanical, voluntary closing, any material, any size   A

* **L6711** Terminal device, hook, mechanical, voluntary opening, any material, any size, lined or unlined, pediatric `Qp` `Qh` `A`   A

* **L6712** Terminal device, hook, mechanical, voluntary closing, any material, any size, lined or unlined, pediatric `Qp` `Qh` `A`   A

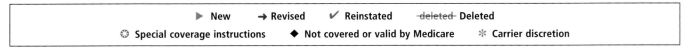

▶ **New** → **Revised** ✔ **Reinstated** ~~deleted~~ **Deleted**

⊗ **Special coverage instructions** ◆ **Not covered or valid by Medicare** ∗ **Carrier discretion**

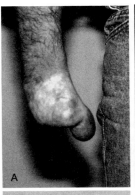
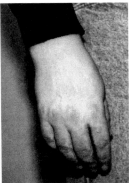
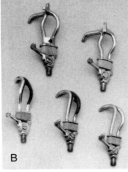

Figure 44 Terminal device.

* **L6713** Terminal device, hand, mechanical, voluntary opening, any material, any size, pediatric Qp Qh A   A

* **L6714** Terminal device, hand, mechanical, voluntary closing, any material, any size, pediatric Qp Qh A   A

▶ * **L6715** Terminal device, multiple articulating digit, includes motor(s), initial issue or replacement   A

* **L6721** Terminal device, hook or hand, heavy duty, mechanical, voluntary opening, any material, any size, lined or unlined Qp Qh   A

* **L6722** Terminal device, hook or hand, heavy duty, mechanical, voluntary closing, any material, any size, lined or unlined Qp Qh   A

○ **L6805** Addition to terminal device, modifier wrist unit Qp Qh   A
  IOM: 100-02, 15, 120; 100-04, 3, 10.4

○ **L6810** Addition to terminal device, precision pinch device Qp Qh   A
  IOM: 100-02, 15, 120; 100-04, 3, 10.4

Hands

▶ * **L6880** Electric hand, switch or myoelectric controlled, independently articulating digits, any grasp pattern or combination of grasp patterns, includes motor(s)   A

* **L6881** Automatic grasp feature, addition to upper limb electric prosthetic terminal device Qp Qh   A

○ **L6882** Microprocessor control feature, addition to upper limb prosthetic terminal device Qp Qh   A
  IOM: 100-02, 15, 120; 100-04, 3, 10.4

Replacement Sockets

* **L6883** Replacement socket, below elbow/wrist disarticulation, molded to patient model, for use with or without external power Qp Qh   A

* **L6884** Replacement socket, above elbow/elbow disarticulation, molded to patient model, for use with or without external power Qp Qh   A

* **L6885** Replacement socket, shoulder disarticulation/interscapular thoracic, molded to patient model, for use with or without external power Qp Qh   A

Gloves for Above Hands

* **L6890** Addition to upper extremity prosthesis, glove for terminal device, any material, prefabricated, includes fitting and adjustment Qp Qh   A

* **L6895** Addition to upper extremity prosthesis, glove for terminal device, any material, custom fabricated Qp Qh   A

Hand Restoration

* **L6900** Hand restoration (casts, shading and measurements included), partial hand, with glove, thumb or one finger remaining Qp Qh   A

* **L6905** Hand restoration (casts, shading and measurements included), partial hand, with glove, multiple fingers remaining Qp Qh   A

* **L6910** Hand restoration (casts, shading and measurements included), partial hand, with glove, no fingers remaining Qp Qh   A

* **L6915** Hand restoration (shading, and measurements included), replacement glove for above `Qp` `Qh` ♿   A

External Power

Base Devices

* **L6920** Wrist disarticulation, external power, self-suspended inner socket, removable forearm shell, Otto Bock or equal switch, cables, two batteries and one charger, switch control of terminal device `Qp` `Qh` ♿   A
Bill DME/MAC

* **L6925** Wrist disarticulation, external power, self-suspended inner socket, removable forearm shell, Otto Bock or equal electrodes, cables, two batteries and one charger, myoelectronic control of terminal device `Qp` `Qh` ♿   A
Bill DME/MAC

* **L6930** Below elbow, external power, self-suspended inner socket, removable forearm shell, Otto Bock or equal switch, cables, two batteries and one charger, switch control of terminal device `Qp` `Qh` ♿   A
Bill DME/MAC

* **L6935** Below elbow, external power, self-suspended inner socket, removable forearm shell, Otto Bock or equal electrodes, cables, two batteries and one charger, myoelectronic control of terminal device `Qp` `Qh` ♿   A
Bill DME/MAC

* **L6940** Elbow disarticulation, external power, molded inner socket, removable humeral shell, outside locking hinges, forearm, Otto Bock or equal switch, cables, two batteries and one charger, switch control of terminal device `Qp` `Qh` ♿   A
Bill DME/MAC

* **L6945** Elbow disarticulation, external power, molded inner socket, removable humeral shell, outside locking hinges, forearm, Otto Bock or equal electrodes, cables, two batteries and one charger, myoelectronic control of terminal device `Qp` `Qh` ♿   A
Bill DME/MAC

* **L6950** Above elbow, external power, molded inner socket, removable humeral shell, internal locking elbow, forearm, Otto Bock or equal switch, cables, two batteries and one charger, switch control of terminal device `Qp` `Qh` ♿   A
Bill DME/MAC

* **L6955** Above elbow, external power, molded inner socket, removable humeral shell, internal locking elbow, forearm, Otto Bock or equal electrodes, cables, two batteries and one charger, myoelectronic control of terminal device `Qp` `Qh` ♿   A
Bill DME/MAC

* **L6960** Shoulder disarticulation, external power, molded inner socket, removable shoulder shell, shoulder bulkhead, humeral section, mechanical elbow, forearm, Otto Bock or equal switch, cables, two batteries and one charger, switch control of terminal device `Qp` `Qh` ♿   A
Bill DME/MAC

* **L6965** Shoulder disarticulation, external power, molded inner socket, removable shoulder shell, shoulder bulkhead, humeral section, mechanical elbow, forearm, Otto Bock or equal electrodes, cables, two batteries and one charger, myoelectronic control of terminal device `Qp` `Qh` ♿   A
Bill DME/MAC

* **L6970** Interscapular-thoracic, external power, molded inner socket, removable shoulder shell, shoulder bulkhead, humeral section, mechanical elbow, forearm, Otto Bock or equal switch, cables, two batteries and one charger, switch control of terminal device `Qp` `Qh` ♿   A
Bill DME/MAC

* **L6975** Interscapular-thoracic, external power, molded inner socket, removable shoulder shell, shoulder bulkhead, humeral section, mechanical elbow, forearm, Otto Bock or equal electrodes, cables, two batteries and one charger, myoelectronic control of terminal device `Qp` `Qh` ♿   A
Bill DME/MAC

▶ **New**   → **Revised**   ✔ **Reinstated**   ~~deleted~~ **Deleted**

⊗ **Special coverage instructions**   ◆ **Not covered or valid by Medicare**   * **Carrier discretion**

Terminal Devices

❋ L7007 Electric hand, switch or myoelectric controlled, adult **A** ♿   A

    Bill DME/MAC

❋ L7008 Electric hand, switch or myoelectric controlled, pediatric **A** ♿   A

    Bill DME/MAC

❋ L7009 Electric hook, switch or myoelectric controlled, adult **A** ♿   A

    Bill DME/MAC

❋ L7040 Prehensile actuator, switch controlled **Qp** **Qh** ♿   A

    Bill DME/MAC

❋ L7045 Electric hook, switch or myoelectric controlled, pediatric **Qp** **Qh** **A** ♿ A

    Bill DME/MAC

Elbow

❋ L7170 Electronic elbow, Hosmer or equal, switch controlled **Qp** **Qh** ♿ A

    Bill DME/MAC

❋ L7180 Electronic elbow, microprocessor sequential control of elbow and terminal device **Qp** **Qh** ♿ A

    Bill DME/MAC

❋ L7181 Electronic elbow, microprocessor simultaneous control of elbow and terminal device **Qp** **Qh** ♿ A

    Bill DME/MAC

❋ L7185 Electronic elbow, adolescent, Variety Village or equal, switch controlled **Qp** **Qh** ♿ A

    Bill DME/MAC

❋ L7186 Electronic elbow, child, Variety Village or equal, switch controlled **Qp** **Qh** **A** ♿ A

    Bill DME/MAC

❋ L7190 Electronic elbow, adolescent, Variety Village or equal, myoelectronically controlled **Qp** **Qh** ♿ A

    Bill DME/MAC

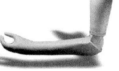

Figure 45 Electronic elbow.

❋ L7191 Electronic elbow, child, Variety Village or equal, myoelectronically controlled **Qp** **Qh** **A** ♿ A

    Bill DME/MAC

❋ L7260 Electronic wrist rotator, Otto Bock or equal **Qp** **Qh** ♿ A

    Bill DME/MAC

❋ L7261 Electronic wrist rotator, for Utah arm **Qp** **Qh** ♿ A

    Bill DME/MAC

~~L7266~~ ~~Servo control, Steeper or equal~~ **Qp** **Qh** ♿ ✖

~~L7272~~ ~~Analogue control, UNB or equal~~ **Qp** **Qh** ♿ ✖

~~L7274~~ ~~Proportional control, 6-12 volt, Liberty, Utah or equal~~ ✖

Battery Components

❋ L7360 Six volt battery, each ♿ A

    Bill DME/MAC

❋ L7362 Battery charger, six volt, each **Qp** **Qh** ♿ A

    Bill DME/MAC

❋ L7364 Twelve volt battery, each ♿ A

    Bill DME/MAC

❋ L7366 Battery charger, twelve volt, each **Qp** **Qh** ♿ A

    Bill DME/MAC

❋ L7367 Lithium ion battery, replacement ♿ A

    Bill DME/MAC

→ ❋ L7368 Lithium ion battery charger, replacement only **Qp** **Qh** ♿ A

    Bill DME/MAC

Other/Repair

❋ L7400 Addition to upper extremity prosthesis, below elbow/wrist disarticulation, ultralight material (titanium, carbon fiber or equal) **Qp** **Qh** ♿ A

    Bill DME/MAC

❋ L7401 Addition to upper extremity prosthesis, above elbow disarticulation, ultralight material (titanium, carbon fiber or equal) **Qp** **Qh** ♿ A

    Bill DME/MAC

ⓅⓆⓇⓈ PQRI	**Qp** Quantity Physician Appendix B	**Qh** Quantity Hospital Appendix C	♀ Female only
♂ Male only	**A** Age ♿ DMEPOS	A2-Z3 ASC Payment Indicator A-Y ASC Status Indicator	Coding Clinic

* **L7402** Addition to upper extremity prosthesis, shoulder disarticulation/interscapular thoracic, ultralight material (titanium, carbon fiber or equal) `Qp` `Qh` ♿ A

Bill DME/MAC

* **L7403** Addition to upper extremity prosthesis, below elbow/wrist disarticulation, acrylic material `Qp` `Qh` ♿ A

Bill DME/MAC

* **L7404** Addition to upper extremity prosthesis, above elbow disarticulation, acrylic material `Qp` `Qh` ♿ A

Bill DME/MAC

* **L7405** Addition to upper extremity prosthesis, shoulder disarticulation/interscapular thoracic, acrylic material `Qp` `Qh` ♿ A

Bill DME/MAC

* **L7499** Upper extremity prosthesis, not otherwise specified A

Bill DME/MAC

~~L7500~~ ~~Repair of prosthetic device, hourly rate (excludes V5335 repair of oral or laryngeal prosthesis or artificial larynx)~~ ✖

☺ **L7510** Repair of prosthetic device, repair or replace minor parts A

Bill local carrier if repair of implanted prosthetic device. If other, bill DME/MAC

IOM: 100-02, 15, 110.2; 100-02, 15, 120; 100-04, 32, 100

* **L7520** Repair prosthetic device, labor component, per 15 minutes A

Bill local carrier if repair of implanted prosthetic device. If other, bill DME/MAC

◆ **L7600** Prosthetic donning sleeve, any material, each E

Bill DME/MAC

Medicare Statute 1862(1)(a)

General

* **L7900** Male vacuum erection system `Qp` `Qh` ♂ ♿ A

Bill DME/MAC

Breast Prostheses

☺ **L8000** Breast prosthesis, mastectomy bra ♀ ♿ A

Bill DME/MAC

IOM: 100-02, 15, 120

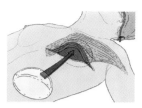

Figure 46 Implant breast prosthesis.

☺ **L8001** Breast prosthesis, mastectomy bra, with integrated breast prosthesis form, unilateral ♀ ♿ A

Bill DME/MAC

IOM: 100-02, 15, 120

☺ **L8002** Breast prosthesis, mastectomy bra, with integrated breast prosthesis form, bilateral ♀ ♿ A

Bill DME/MAC

IOM: 100-02, 15, 120

☺ **L8010** Breast prosthesis, mastectomy sleeve ♀ A

Bill DME/MAC

IOM: 100-02, 15, 120

☺ **L8015** External breast prosthesis garment, with mastectomy form, post mastectomy ♀ ♿ A

Bill DME/MAC

IOM: 100-02, 15, 120

☺ **L8020** Breast prosthesis, mastectomy form ♀ ♿ A

Bill DME/MAC

IOM: 100-02, 15, 120

* **L8030** Breast prosthesis, silicone or equal, without integral adhesive `Qp` `Qh` ♀ ♿ A

Bill DME/MAC

IOM: 100-02, 15, 120

☺ **L8031** Breast prosthesis, silicone or equal, with integral adhesive `Qp` `Qh` ♿ A

Bill DME/MAC

IOM: 100-02, 15, 120

* **L8032** Nipple prosthesis, reusable, any type, each `Qp` `Qh` ♿ A

Bill DME/MAC

☺ **L8035** Custom breast prosthesis, post mastectomy, molded to patient model `Qp` `Qh` ♀ ♿ A

Bill DME/MAC

IOM: 100-02, 15, 120

▶ New → Revised ✔ Reinstated ~~deleted~~ Deleted

☺ Special coverage instructions ◆ Not covered or valid by Medicare * Carrier discretion

L7402 – L8035 PROSTHETICS

✳ **L8039** Breast prosthesis, not otherwise specified [Qp] [Qh] ♀ A

Bill DME/MAC

Nasal, Orbital, Auricular Prosthesis

✳ **L8040** Nasal prosthesis, provided by a non-physician [Qp] [Qh] & A

Bill DME/MAC

DMEPOS Modifier(s): KM, KN

✳ **L8041** Midfacial prosthesis, provided by a non-physician [Qp] [Qh] & A

Bill DME/MAC

DMEPOS Modifier(s): KM, KN

✳ **L8042** Orbital prosthesis, provided by a non-physician [Qp] [Qh] & A

Bill DME/MAC

DMEPOS Modifier(s): KM, KN

✳ **L8043** Upper facial prosthesis, provided by a non-physician [Qp] [Qh] & A

Bill DME/MAC

DMEPOS Modifier(s): KM, KN

✳ **L8044** Hemi-facial prosthesis, provided by a non-physician [Qp] [Qh] & A

Bill DME/MAC

DMEPOS Modifier(s): KM, KN

✳ **L8045** Auricular prosthesis, provided by a non-physician [Qp] [Qh] & A

Bill DME/MAC

DMEPOS Modifier(s): KM, KN

✳ **L8046** Partial facial prosthesis, provided by a non-physician [Qp] [Qh] & A

Bill DME/MAC

DMEPOS Modifier(s): KM, KN

✳ **L8047** Nasal septal prosthesis, provided by a non-physician [Qp] [Qh] & A

Bill DME/MAC

DMEPOS Modifier(s): KM, KN

✳ **L8048** Unspecified maxillofacial prosthesis, by report, provided by a non-physician A

Bill DME/MAC

✳ **L8049** Repair or modification of maxillofacial prosthesis, labor component, 15 minute increments, provided by a non-physician A

Bill DME/MAC

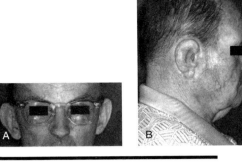

Figure 47 **A**. Nasal prosthesis. **B**. Auricular prosthesis.

Trusses

⊘ **L8300** Truss, single with standard pad [Qp] [Qh] & A

Bill DME/MAC

IOM: 100-02, 15, 120; 100-03, 4, 280.11; 100-03, 4, 280.12; 100-04, 4, 240

⊘ **L8310** Truss, double with standard pads [Qp] [Qh] & A

Bill DME/MAC

IOM: 100-02, 15, 120; 100-03, 4, 280.11; 100-03, 4, 280.12; 100-04, 4, 240

⊘ **L8320** Truss, addition to standard pad, water pad [Qp] [Qh] & A

Bill DME/MAC

IOM: 100-02, 15, 120; 100-03, 4, 280.11; 100-03, 4, 280.12; 100-04, 4, 240

⊘ **L8330** Truss, addition to standard pad, scrotal pad [Qp] [Qh] ♂ & A

Bill DME/MAC

IOM: 100-02, 15, 120; 100-03, 4, 280.11; 100-03, 4, 280.12; 100-04, 4, 240

Prosthetic Socks

⊘ **L8400** Prosthetic sheath, below knee, each & A

Bill DME/MAC

IOM: 100-02, 15, 200

⊘ **L8410** Prosthetic sheath, above knee, each & A

Bill DME/MAC

IOM: 100-02, 15, 200

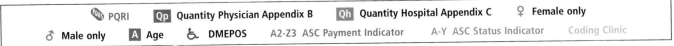

◎ **L8415** Prosthetic sheath, upper limb, each ✑   A

Bill DME/MAC

IOM: 100-02, 15, 200

✳ **L8417** Prosthetic sheath/sock, including a gel cushion layer, below knee or above knee, each ✑   A

Bill DME/MAC

◎ **L8420** Prosthetic sock, multiple ply, below knee, each ✑   A

Bill DME/MAC

IOM: 100-02, 15, 200

◎ **L8430** Prosthetic sock, multiple ply, above knee, each ✑   A

Bill DME/MAC

IOM: 100-02, 15, 200

◎ **L8435** Prosthetic sock, multiple ply, upper limb, each ✑   A

Bill DME/MAC

IOM: 100-02, 15, 200

◎ **L8440** Prosthetic shrinker, below knee, each ✑   A

Bill DME/MAC

IOM: 100-02, 15, 200

◎ **L8460** Prosthetic shrinker, above knee, each ✑   A

Bill DME/MAC

IOM: 100-02, 15, 200

◎ **L8465** Prosthetic shrinker, upper limb, each ✑   A

Bill DME/MAC

IOM: 100-02, 15, 200

◎ **L8470** Prosthetic sock, single ply, fitting, below knee, each ✑   A

Bill DME/MAC

IOM: 100-02, 15, 200

◎ **L8480** Prosthetic sock, single ply, fitting, above knee, each ✑   A

Bill DME/MAC

IOM: 100-02, 15, 200

◎ **L8485** Prosthetic sock, single ply, fitting, upper limb, each ✑   A

Bill DME/MAC

IOM: 100-02, 15, 200

✳ **L8499** Unlisted procedure for miscellaneous prosthetic services   A

Bill local carrier if repair of implanted prosthetic device. If other, bill DME/MAC

Prosthetic Implants

Larynx, Tracheoesophageal

◎ **L8500** Artificial larynx, any type `Qp` `Qh` ✑   A

Bill DME/MAC

IOM: 100-02, 15, 120; 100-03, 1, 50.2; 100-04, 4, 240

◎ **L8501** Tracheostomy speaking valve `Qp` `Qh` ✑   A

Bill DME/MAC

IOM: 100-03, 1, 50.4

✳ **L8505** Artificial larynx replacement battery/accessory, any type   A

Bill DME/MAC

✳ **L8507** Tracheo-esophageal voice prosthesis, patient inserted, any type, each `Qp` `Qh` ✑   A

Bill DME/MAC

✳ **L8509** Tracheo-esophageal voice prosthesis, inserted by a licensed health care provider, any type `Qp` `Qh` ✑   A

Bill DME/MAC

◎ **L8510** Voice amplifier `Qp` `Qh` ✑   A

Bill DME/MAC

IOM: 100-03, 1, 50.2

✳ **L8511** Insert for indwelling tracheoesophageal prosthesis, with or without valve, replacement only, each `Qp` `Qh` ✑   A

Bill DME/MAC

✳ **L8512** Gelatin capsules or equivalent, for use with tracheoesophageal voice prosthesis, replacement only, per 10 ✑   A

Bill DME/MAC

✳ **L8513** Cleaning device used with tracheoesophageal voice prosthesis, pipet, brush, or equal, replacement only, each ✑   A

Bill DME/MAC

✳ **L8514** Tracheoesophageal puncture dilator, replacement only, each `Qp` `Qh` ✑   A

Bill DME/MAC

▶ New   → Revised   ✔ Reinstated   ~~deleted~~ Deleted

◎ Special coverage instructions   ◆ Not covered or valid by Medicare   ✳ Carrier discretion

* **L8515** Gelatin capsule, application device for use with tracheoesophageal voice prosthesis, each `Qp` `Qh`   A

Bill DME/MAC

Breast

☼ **L8600** Implantable breast prosthesis, silicone or equal `Qp` `Qh` ♀   N1 N

Bill local carrier

IOM: 100-02, 15, 120; 100-3, 2, 140.2

Urinary System

☼ **L8603** Injectable bulking agent, collagen implant, urinary tract, 2.5 ml syringe, includes shipping and necessary supplies   N1 N

Bill local carrier

Bill on paper, acquisition cost invoice required

IOM: 100-03, 4, 280.1

* **L8604** Injectable bulking agent, dextranomer/hyaluronic acid copolymer implant, urinary tract, 1 ml, includes shipping and necessary supplies `Qp` `Qh`   N1 N

Bill local carrier

☼ **L8606** Injectable bulking agent, synthetic implant, urinary tract, 1 ml syringe, includes shipping and necessary supplies   N1 N

Bill local carrier

Bill on paper, acquisition cost invoice required

IOM: 100-03, 4, 280.1

Head (Skull, Facial Bones, and Temporomandibular Joint)

* **L8609** Artificial cornea   N1 N

Bill local carrier

☼ **L8610** Ocular implant `Qp` `Qh`   N1 N

Bill local carrier

IOM: 100-02, 15, 120

☼ **L8612** Aqueous shunt `Qp` `Qh`   N1 N

Bill local carrier

IOM: 100-02, 15, 120

Cross Reference Q0074

☼ **L8613** Ossicula implant `Qp` `Qh`   N1 N

Bill local carrier

IOM: 100-02, 15, 120

☼ **L8614** Cochlear device, includes all internal and external components `Qp` `Qh`   N1 N

Bill local carrier

IOM: 100-02, 15, 120; 100-03, 1, 50.3

☼ **L8615** Headset/headpiece for use with cochlear implant device, replacement `Qp` `Qh`   A

Bill local carrier

IOM: 100-03, 1, 50.3

☼ **L8616** Microphone for use with cochlear implant device, replacement `Qp` `Qh`   A

Bill local carrier

IOM: 100-03, 1, 50.3

☼ **L8617** Transmitting coil for use with cochlear implant device, replacement `Qp` `Qh`   A

Bill local carrier

IOM: 100-03, 1, 50.3

☼ **L8618** Transmitter cable for use with cochlear implant device, replacement `Qp` `Qh`   A

Bill local carrier

IOM: 100-03, 1, 50.3

* **L8619** Cochlear implant, external speech processor and controller, integrated system, replacement `Qp` `Qh`   A

Bill local carrier

IOM: 100-03, 1, 50.3

* **L8621** Zinc air battery for use with cochlear implant device, replacement, each   A

Bill local carrier

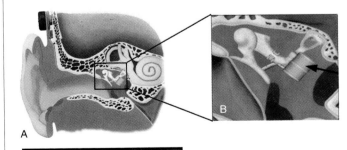

Figure 48 Cochlear device.

PQRI	`Qp` Quantity Physician Appendix B	`Qh` Quantity Hospital Appendix C	♀ Female only
♂ Male only	`A` Age	& DMEPOS	A2-Z3 ASC Payment Indicator	A-Y ASC Status Indicator	Coding Clinic

❋ **L8622** Alkaline battery for use with cochlear implant device, any size, replacement, each `Qp` `Qh` ♿ A

Bill local carrier

❋ **L8623** Lithium ion battery for use with cochlear implant device speech processor, other than ear level, replacement, each ♿ A

Bill local carrier

❋ **L8624** Lithium ion battery for use with cochlear implant device speech processor, ear level, replacement, each ♿ A

Bill local carrier

⊙ **L8627** Cochlear implant, external speech processor, component, replacement `Qp` `Qh` ♿ A

Bill local carrier

IOM: 103-03, Part 1, 50.3

⊙ **L8628** Cochlear implant, external controller component, replacement `Qp` `Qh` ♿ A

Bill local carrier

IOM: 103-03, Part 1, 50.3

⊙ **L8629** Transmitting coil and cable, integrated, for use with cochlear implant device, replacement `Qp` `Qh` ♿ A

Bill local carrier

IOM: 103-03, Part 1, 50.3

Upper Extremity

⊙ **L8630** Metacarpophalangeal joint implant ♿ N1 N

Bill local carrier

IOM: 100-02, 15, 120

⊙ **L8631** Metacarpal phalangeal joint replacement, two or more pieces, metal (e.g., stainless steel or cobalt chrome), ceramic-like material (e.g., pyrocarbon), for surgical implantation (all sizes, includes entire system) `Qp` `Qh` ♿ N1 N

Bill local carrier

IOM: 100-02, 15, 120

Lower Extremity (Joint: Knee, Ankle, Toe)

⊙ **L8641** Metatarsal joint implant `Qp` `Qh` ♿ N1 N

Bill local carrier

IOM: 100-02, 15, 120

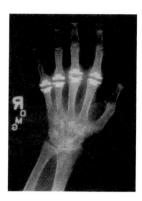

Figure 49 Metacarpophalangeal implant.

⊙ **L8642** Hallux implant `Qp` `Qh` ♿ N1 N

Bill local carrier

May be billed by ambulatory surgical center or surgeon

IOM: 100-02, 15, 120

Cross Reference CPT Q0073

Miscellaneous Muscular-Skeletal

⊙ **L8658** Interphalangeal joint spacer, silicone or equal, each `Qp` `Qh` ♿ N1 N

Bill local carrier

IOM: 100-02, 15, 120

⊙ **L8659** Interphalangeal finger joint replacement, 2 or more pieces, metal (e.g., stainless steel or cobalt chrome), ceramic-like material (e.g., pyrocarbon) for surgical implantation, any size `Qp` `Qh` ♿ N1 N

Bill local carrier

IOM: 100-02, 15, 120

Cardiovascular System

⊙ **L8670** Vascular graft material, synthetic, implant `Qp` `Qh` ♿ N1 N

Bill local carrier

IOM: 100-02, 15, 120

Neurostimulator

⊙ **L8680** Implantable neurostimulator electrode, each ♿ N

Bill local carrier

Related CPT codes: 43647, 63650, 63655, 64553, 64555, 64560, 64561, 64565, 64573, 64575, 64577, 64580, 64581.

IOM: 100-03, 4, 280.4

▶ **New**   → **Revised**   ✔ **Reinstated**   ~~deleted~~ **Deleted**

⊙ **Special coverage instructions**   ◆ **Not covered or valid by Medicare**   ❋ **Carrier discretion**

⊛ **L8681** Patient programmer (external) for use with implantable programmable neurostimulator pulse generator, replacement only `Qp` `Qh` ♿   A

Bill local carrier

IOM: 100-03, 4, 280.4

⊛ **L8682** Implantable neurostimulator radiofrequency receiver `Qp` ♿   N1   N

Bill local carrier

IOM: 100-03, 4, 280.4

⊛ **L8683** Radiofrequency transmitter (external) for use with implantable neurostimulator radiofrequency receiver `Qp` `Qh` ♿   A

Bill local carrier

IOM: 100-03, 4, 280.4

⊛ **L8684** Radiofrequency transmitter (external) for use with implantable sacral root neurostimulator receiver for bowel and bladder management, replacement `Qp` `Qh` ♿   A

Bill local carrier

IOM: 100-03, 4, 280.4

⊛ **L8685** Implantable neurostimulator pulse generator, single array, rechargeable, includes extension `Qp` ♿   N

Bill local carrier

Related CPT codes: 61885, 64590, 63685.

IOM: 100-03, 4, 280.4

⊛ **L8686** Implantable neurostimulator pulse generator, single array, non-rechargeable, includes extension `Qp` `Qh` ♿   N

Bill local carrier

Related CPT codes: 61885, 64590, 63685.

IOM: 100-03, 4, 280.4

⊛ **L8687** Implantable neurostimulator pulse generator, dual array, rechargeable, includes extension `Qp` `Qh` ♿   N

Bill local carrier

Related CPT codes: 64590, 63685, 61886.

IOM: 100-03, 4, 280.4

⊛ **L8688** Implantable neurostimulator pulse generator, dual array, non-rechargeable, includes extension `Qp` ♿   N

Bill local carrier

Related CPT codes: 61885, 64590, 63685.

IOM: 100-03, 4, 280.4

⊛ **L8689** External recharging system for battery (internal) for use with implantable neurostimulator, replacement only `Qp` `Qh` ♿   A

Bill local carrier

IOM: 100-03, 4, 280.4

✳ **L8690** Auditory osseointegrated device, includes all internal and external components `Qp` `Qh` ♿   N1   N

Bill local carrier

Related CPT codes: 69714, 69715, 69717, 69718.

✳ **L8691** Auditory osseointegrated device, external sound processor, replacement `Qp` `Qh` ♿   A

Bill local carrier

◆ **L8692** Auditory osseointegrated device, external sound processor, used without osseointegration, body worn, includes headband or other means of external attachment   E

Bill local carrier

Medicare Statute 1862(a)(7)

▶ ✳ **L8693** Auditory osseointegrated device abutment, any length, replacement only `Qp` `Qh` ♿   A

Bill local carrier

⊛ **L8695** External recharging system for battery (external) for use with implantable neurostimulator, replacement only `Qp` `Qh` ♿   A

Bill local carrier

IOM: 100-03, 4, 280.4

Genital

✳ **L8699** Prosthetic implant, not otherwise specified   N1   N

Bill local carrier

✳ **L9900** Orthotic and prosthetic supply, accessory, and/or service component of another HCPCS "L" code   N

Bill local carrier if repair of implanted prosthetic device. If other, bill DME/MAC

OTHER MEDICAL SERVICES (M0000-M0301)

M0064-M0301: Bill DME/MAC

⚙ **M0064** Brief office visit for the sole purpose of monitoring or changing drug prescriptions used in the treatment of mental psychoneurotic and personality disorders **Qp** **Qh**   Q3

Not to be reported separately from CPT codes 90801-90857

◆ **M0075** Cellular therapy   E

◆ **M0076** Prolotherapy   E

Prolotherapy stimulates production of new ligament tissue. Not covered by Medicare

◆ **M0100** Intragastric hypothermia using gastric freezing   E

◆ **M0300** IV chelation therapy (chemical endarterectomy)   E

Non-covered by Medicare

◆ **M0301** Fabric wrapping of abdominal aneurysm   E

Treatment for abdominal aneurysms that involves wrapping aneurysms with cellophane or fascia lata. Fabric wrapping of abdominal aneurysms is not a covered Medicare procedure.

▶ New   → Revised   ✔ Reinstated   ~~deleted~~ Deleted
⚙ Special coverage instructions   ◆ Not covered or valid by Medicare   ✳ Carrier discretion

LABORATORY SERVICES (P0000-P9999)

Chemistry and Toxicology Tests

P2028-P2038: Bill local carrier

⚙ **P2028** Cephalin floculation, blood Qp Qh   A

IOM: 100-03, 4, 300.1

⚙ **P2029** Congo red, blood Qp Qh   A

IOM: 100-03, 4, 300.1

◆ **P2031** Hair analysis (excluding arsenic)   E

IOM: 100-03, 4, 300.1

⚙ **P2033** Thymol turbidity, blood Qp Qh   A

IOM: 100-03, 4, 300.1

⚙ **P2038** Mucoprotein, blood (seromucoid) (medical necessity procedure) Qp Qh   A

IOM: 100-03, 4, 300.1

Pathology Screening Tests

P3000-P7001: Bill local carrier

⚙ **P3000** Screening Papanicolaou smear, cervical or vaginal, up to three smears, by technician under physician supervision Qp Qh ♀   A

Co-insurance and deductible waived

Assign for Pap smear ordered for screening purposes only, conventional method, performed by technician

IOM: 100-03, 3, 190.2,

Laboratory Certification: Cytology

⚙ **P3001** Screening Papanicolaou smear, cervical or vaginal, up to three smears, requiring interpretation by physician Qp Qh ♀   B

Co-insurance and deductible waived

Report professional component for Pap smears requiring physician interpretation. There are CPT codes assigned for diagnostic Paps, such as, 88141; HCPCS are for screening Paps

IOM: 100-03, 3, 190.2

Laboratory Certification: Cytology

Microbiology Tests

◆ **P7001** Culture, bacterial, urine; quantitative, sensitivity study   E

Cross Reference CPT

Laboratory Certification: Bacteriology

Miscellaneous Pathology

P9010-P9615: Bill local carrier

⚙ **P9010** Blood (whole), for transfusion, per unit   R

Blood furnished on an outpatient basis, subject to Medicare Part B blood deductible; applicable to first 3 pints of whole blood or equivalent units of packed red cells in calendar year

IOM: 100-01, 3, 20.5; 100-02, 1, 10

OPPS recognized blood/blood products

⚙ **P9011** Blood, split unit   R

Reports all splitting activities of any blood component

IOM: 100-01, 3, 20.5; 100-02, 1, 10

OPPS recognized blood/blood products

⚙ **P9012** Cryoprecipitate, each unit   R

IOM: 100-01, 3, 20.5; 100-02, 1, 10

OPPS recognized blood/blood products

⚙ **P9016** Red blood cells, leukocytes reduced, each unit   R

IOM: 100-01, 3, 20.5; 100-02, 1, 10

OPPS recognized blood/blood products

⚙ **P9017** Fresh frozen plasma (single donor), frozen within 8 hours of collection, each unit   R

IOM: 100-01, 3, 20.5; 100-02, 1, 10

OPPS recognized blood/blood products

⚙ **P9019** Platelets, each unit   R

IOM: 100-01, 3, 20.5; 100-02, 1, 10

OPPS recognized blood/blood products

⚙ **P9020** Platelet rich plasma, each unit   R

IOM: 100-01, 3, 20.5; 100-02, 1, 10

OPPS recognized blood/blood products

⚙ **P9021** Red blood cells, each unit   R

IOM: 100-01, 3, 20.5; 100-02, 1, 10

OPPS recognized blood/blood products

⚙ **P9022** Red blood cells, washed, each unit   R

IOM: 100-01, 3, 20.5; 100-02, 1, 10

OPPS recognized blood/blood products

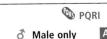 PQRI   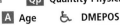 Qp **Quantity Physician Appendix B**   Qh **Quantity Hospital Appendix C**   ♀ **Female only**

♂ **Male only**   A **Age**   ♿ **DMEPOS**   A2-Z3 **ASC Payment Indicator**   A-Y **ASC Status Indicator**   Coding Clinic

⊗ **P9023** Plasma, pooled multiple donor, solvent/detergent treated, frozen, each unit R

IOM: 100-01, 3, 20.5; 100-02, 1, 10

OPPS recognized blood/blood products

⊗ **P9031** Platelets, leukocytes reduced, each unit R

IOM: 100-01, 3, 20.5; 100-02, 1, 10

OPPS recognized blood/blood products

⊗ **P9032** Platelets, irradiated, each unit R

IOM: 100-01, 3, 20.5; 100-02, 1, 10

OPPS recognized blood/blood products

⊗ **P9033** Platelets, leukocytes reduced, irradiated, each unit R

IOM: 100-01, 3, 20.5; 100-02, 1, 10

OPPS recognized blood/blood products

⊗ **P9034** Platelets, pheresis, each unit R

IOM: 100-01, 3, 20.5; 100-02, 1, 10

OPPS recognized blood/blood products

⊗ **P9035** Platelets, pheresis, leukocytes reduced, each unit R

IOM: 100-01, 3, 20.5; 100-02, 1, 10

OPPS recognized blood/blood products

⊗ **P9036** Platelets, pheresis, irradiated, each unit R

IOM: 100-01, 3, 20.5; 100-02, 1, 10

OPPS recognized blood/blood products

⊗ **P9037** Platelets, pheresis, leukocytes reduced, irradiated, each unit R

IOM: 100-01, 3, 20.5; 100-02, 1, 10

OPPS recognized blood/blood products

⊗ **P9038** Red blood cells, irradiated, each unit R

IOM: 100-01, 3, 20.5; 100-02, 1, 10

OPPS recognized blood/blood products

⊗ **P9039** Red blood cells, deglycerolized, each unit R

IOM: 100-01, 3, 20.5; 100-02, 1, 10

OPPS recognized blood/blood products

⊗ **P9040** Red blood cells, leukocytes reduced, irradiated, each unit R

IOM: 100-01, 3, 20.5; 100-02, 1, 10

OPPS recognized blood/blood products

✳ **P9041** Infusion, albumin (human), 5%, 50 ml K2 K

⊗ **P9043** Infusion, plasma protein fraction (human), 5%, 50 ml R

IOM: 100-01, 3, 20.5; 100-02, 1, 10

OPPS recognized blood/blood products

⊗ **P9044** Plasma, cryoprecipitate reduced, each unit R

IOM: 100-01, 3, 20.5; 100-02, 1, 10

OPPS recognized blood/blood products

✳ **P9045** Infusion, albumin (human), 5%, 250 ml K2 K

✳ **P9046** Infusion, albumin (human), 25%, 20 ml K2 K

✳ **P9047** Infusion, albumin (human), 25%, 50 ml K2 K

✳ **P9048** Infusion, plasma protein fraction (human), 5%, 250 ml R

OPPS recognized blood/blood products

✳ **P9050** Granulocytes, pheresis, each unit R

OPPS recognized blood/blood products

⊗ **P9051** Whole blood or red blood cells, leukocytes reduced, CMV-negative, each unit R

Medicare Statute 1833(t)

OPPS recognized blood/blood products

⊗ **P9052** Platelets, HLA-matched leukocytes reduced, apheresis/pheresis, each unit R

Medicare Statute 1833(t)

OPPS recognized blood/blood products

⊗ **P9053** Platelets, pheresis, leukocytes reduced, CMV-negative, irradiated, each unit R

Freezing and thawing are reported separately, see Transmittal 1487 (Hospital outpatient)

Medicare Statute 1833(t)

OPPS recognized blood/blood products

▶ New   → Revised   ✔ Reinstated   ~~deleted~~ Deleted

⊗ Special coverage instructions   ◆ Not covered or valid by Medicare   ✳ Carrier discretion

✿ **P9054** Whole blood or red blood cells, leukocytes reduced, frozen, deglycerol, washed, each unit   R

Medicare Statute 1833(t)

OPPS recognized blood/blood products

✿ **P9055** Platelets, leukocytes reduced, CMV-negative, apheresis/pheresis, each unit   R

Medicare Statute 1833(t)

OPPS recognized blood/blood products

✿ **P9056** Whole blood, leukocytes reduced, irradiated, each unit   R

Medicare Statute 1833(t)

OPPS recognized blood/blood products

✿ **P9057** Red blood cells, frozen/deglycerolized/washed, leukocytes reduced, irradiated, each unit   R

Medicare Statute 1833(t)

OPPS recognized blood/blood products

✿ **P9058** Red blood cells, leukocytes reduced, CMV-negative, irradiated, each unit   R

Medicare Statute 1833(t)

OPPS recognized blood/blood products

✿ **P9059** Fresh frozen plasma between 8-24 hours of collection, each unit   R

Medicare Statute 1833(t)

OPPS recognized blood/blood products

✿ **P9060** Fresh frozen plasma, donor retested, each unit   R

Medicare Statute 1833(t)

OPPS recognized blood/blood products

✿ **P9603** Travel allowance one way in connection with medically necessary laboratory specimen collection drawn from home bound or nursing home bound patient; prorated miles actually traveled   A

Fee for clinical laboratory travel (P9603) is $0.96 per mile for CY2011

IOM: 100-04, 16, 60

✿ **P9604** Travel allowance one way in connection with medically necessary laboratory specimen collection drawn from home bound or nursing home bound patient; prorated trip charge   A

For CY2010, the fee for clinical laboratory travel is $9.60 per flat rate trip for CY2011

IOM: 100-04, 16, 60

✿ **P9612** Catheterization for collection of specimen, single patient, all places of service `Qp` `Qh`   A

NCCI edits indicate that when 51701 is comprehensive or is a Column 1 code, P9612 cannot be reported. When the catheter insertion is a component of another procedure, do not report straight catheterization separately.

IOM: 100-04, 16, 60

Coding Clinic: 2007, Q3, P7

✿ **P9615** Catheterization for collection of specimen(s) (multiple patients) `Qp` `Qh`   N

IOM: 100-04, 16, 60

 PQRI   `Qp` **Quantity Physician Appendix B**   `Qh` **Quantity Hospital Appendix C**   ♀ **Female only**

♂ **Male only**   `A` **Age**   ♿ **DMEPOS**   A2-Z3 **ASC Payment Indicator**   A-Y **ASC Status Indicator**   Coding Clinic

TEMPORARY CODES ASSIGNED BY CMS (Q0000-Q9999)

Cardiokymography

⊛ **Q0035** Cardiokymography `Qp` `Qh` X

Bill local carrier

Report modifier 26 if professional component only

IOM: 100-03, 1, 20.24

Chemotherapy

Q0081-Q0085: Bill local carrier

⊛ **Q0081** Infusion therapy, using other than chemotherapeutic drugs, per visit B

IV piggyback only assigned one time per patient encounter per day. Report for hydration or the intravenous administration of antibiotics, anti-emetics, or analgesics. Bill on paper. Requires a report.

IOM: 100-03, 4, 280.14

Coding Clinic: 2004, Q2, P11; Q1, P5, 8; 2002, Q2, P10; Q1, P7

✳ **Q0083** Chemotherapy administration by other than infusion technique only (e.g., subcutaneous, intramuscular, push), per visit B

Coding Clinic: 2002, Q1, P7

⊛ **Q0084** Chemotherapy administration by infusion technique only, per visit B

IOM: 100-03, 4, 280.14

Coding Clinic: 2004, Q2, P11; 2002, Q1, P7

✳ **Q0085** Chemotherapy administration by both infusion technique and other technique(s) (e.g., subcutaneous, intramuscular, push), per visit `Qh` B

Coding Clinic: 2002, Q1, P7

Smear, Papanicolaou

⊛ **Q0091** Screening Papanicolaou smear; obtaining, preparing and conveyance of cervical or vaginal smear to laboratory `Qp` `Qh` ♀ T

Bill local carrier

Medicare does not cover comprehensive preventive medicine services; however, services described by G0101 and Q0091 (only for Medicare patients) are covered. Includes the services necessary to procure and transport the specimen to the laboratory.

IOM: 100-03, 3, 190.2

Coding Clinic: 2002, Q4, P8

Equipment, X-Ray, Portable

⊛ **Q0092** Set-up portable x-ray equipment N

Bill local carrier

IOM: 100-04, 13, 90

Laboratory

Q0111-Q0115: Bill local carrier

✳ **Q0111** Wet mounts, including preparations of vaginal, cervical or skin specimens `Qp` `Qh` A

Laboratory Certification: Bacteriology, Mycology, Parasitology

✳ **Q0112** All potassium hydroxide (KOH) preparations `Qp` `Qh` A

Laboratory Certification: Mycology A

✳ **Q0113** Pinworm examinations `Qp` `Qh` A

Laboratory Certification: Parasitology

✳ **Q0114** Fern test `Qp` `Qh` ♀ A

Laboratory certification: Routine chemistry A

✳ **Q0115** Post-coital direct, qualitative examinations of vaginal or cervical mucous `Qp` `Qh` ♀ A

Laboratory Certification: Hematology

Drugs

✳ **Q0138** Injection, ferumoxytol, for treatment of iron deficiency anemia, 1 mg (non-ESRD use) K2 K

Feraheme is FDA approved for chronic kidney disease

NDC: Feraheme

▶ **New** → **Revised** ✔ **Reinstated** ~~deleted~~ **Deleted**

⊛ **Special coverage instructions** ◆ **Not covered or valid by Medicare** ✳ **Carrier discretion**

✳ **Q0139** Injection, ferumoxytol, for treatment of iron deficiency anemia, 1 mg (for ESRD on dialysis)   A

   NDC: Feraheme

◆ **Q0144** Azithromycin dihydrate, oral, capsules/powder, 1 gm   E

   If incident to a physician's service, do not bill; otherwise, bill DME/MAC.

   Other: Zithromax

▶ ⚙ **Q0162** Ondansetron 1 mg, oral, FDA-approved prescription anti-emetic, for use as a complete therapeutic substitute for an iv anti-emetic at the time of chemotherapy treatment, not to exceed a 48 hour dosage regimen   N1 N

   Medicare Statute 4557

⚙ **Q0163** Diphenhydramine hydrochloride, 50 mg, oral, FDA approved prescription anti-emetic, for use as a complete therapeutic substitute for an IV anti-emetic at time of chemotherapy treatment not to exceed a 48 hour dosage regimen   N1 N

   Bill DME/MAC

   NDC: Compoz, Dytuss

   Other: Alercap, Aler-Dryl, Allergy Children's, Allergy Relief Intense Strength, Allergy Relief Medicine, Allermax, Alertab, Anti-Hist, Antihistamine, Banophen, Complete Allergy Medication, Complete Allergy medicine, Diphedryl, Diphen, Diphenhist, Diphenyl, Dormin Sleep Aid, Geridryl, Good Sense Antihistamine Allergy Relief, Good Sense Nighttime Sleep Aid, Genahist, Hydramine, Medicine Shoppe Medi-Phedryl, Medicine Shoppe Nite Time Sleep, Mediphedryl, Night Time Sleep Aid, Nytol Quickcaps, Nytol Quickgels maximum strength, Q-Dryl, Quality Choice dye-free allergy medicine, Quality Choice Sleep Aid, Quality Choice Rest Simply, Quenalin, Rite Aid Allergy, Serabrina La France, Siladryl Allergy, Silphen, Simply Sleep, Sleep Formula, Sleep Tabs, Sleep-ettes D, Sleepinal, Sominex, Twilite, Valu-Dryl Allergy

   Medicare Statute 4557

⚙ **Q0164** Prochlorperazine maleate, 5 mg, oral, FDA approved prescription anti-emetic, for use as a complete therapeutic substitute for an IV anti-emetic at the time of chemotherapy treatment, not to exceed a 48 hour dosage regimen   N1 N

   Bill DME/MAC

   NDC: Compazine

   Medicare Statute 4557

⚙ **Q0165** Prochlorperazine maleate, 10 mg, oral, FDA approved prescription anti-emetic, for use as a complete therapeutic substitute for an IV anti-emetic at the time of chemotherapy treatment, not to exceed a 48 hour dosage regimen   N

   Bill DME/MAC

   NDC: Compazine

   Medicare Statute 4557

⚙ **Q0166** Granisetron hydrochloride, 1 mg, oral, FDA approved prescription anti-emetic, for use as a complete therapeutic substitute for an IV anti-emetic at the time of chemotherapy treatment, not to exceed a 24 hour dosage regimen   N1 N

   Bill DME/MAC

   NDC: Kytril

   Medicare Statute 4557

⚙ **Q0167** Dronabinol, 2.5 mg, oral, FDA approved prescription anti-emetic, for use as a complete therapeutic substitute for an IV anti-emetic at the time of chemotherapy treatment, not to exceed a 48 hour dosage regimen   N1 N

   Bill DME/MAC

   NDC: Marinol

   Medicare Statute 4557

⚙ **Q0168** Dronabinol, 5 mg, oral, FDA approved prescription anti-emetic, for use as a complete therapeutic substitute for an IV anti-emetic at the time of chemotherapy treatment, not to exceed a 48 hour dosage regimen   N

   Bill DME/MAC

   NDC: Marinol

   Medicare Statute 4557

⚙ **Q0169** Promethazine hydrochloride, 12.5 mg, oral, FDA approved prescription anti-emetic, for use as a complete therapeutic substitute for an IV anti-emetic at the time of chemotherapy treatment, not to exceed a 48 hour dosage regimen   N1 N

   Bill DME/MAC

   NDC: Phenergan

   Medicare Statute 4557

Ⓟ PQRI	Qp Quantity Physician Appendix B	Qh Quantity Hospital Appendix C	♀ Female only
♂ Male only A Age ♿ DMEPOS	A2-Z3 ASC Payment Indicator	A-Y ASC Status Indicator	Coding Clinic

◎ **Q0170** Promethazine hydrochloride, 25 mg, oral, FDA approved prescription anti-emetic, for use as a complete therapeutic substitute for an IV anti-emetic at the time of chemotherapy treatment, not to exceed a 48 hour dosage regimen   N

Bill DME/MAC

Other: Phenergan, Promacot

Medicare Statute 4557

◎ **Q0171** Chlorpromazine hydrochloride, 10 mg, oral, FDA approved prescription anti-emetic, for use as a complete therapeutic substitute for an IV anti-emetic at the time of chemotherapy treatment, not to exceed a 48 hour dosage regimen   N1   N

Bill DME/MAC

Medicare Statute 4557

◎ **Q0172** Chlorpromazine hydrochloride, 25 mg, oral, FDA approved prescription anti-emetic, for use as a complete therapeutic substitute for an IV anti-emetic at the time of chemotherapy treatment, not to exceed a 48 hour dosage regimen   N

Bill DME/MAC

Medicare Statute 4557

◎ **Q0173** Trimethobenzamide hydrochloride, 250 mg, oral, FDA approved prescription anti-emetic, for use as a complete therapeutic substitute for an IV anti-emetic at the time of chemotherapy treatment, not to exceed a 48 hour dosage regimen   N1   N

Bill DME/MAC

Other: Tigan

Medicare Statute 4557

◎ **Q0174** Thiethylperazine maleate, 10 mg, oral, FDA approved prescription anti-emetic, for use as a complete therapeutic substitute for an IV anti-emetic at the time of chemotherapy treatment, not to exceed a 48 hour dosage regimen   E

Bill DME/MAC

Other: Torecan

Medicare Statute 4557

◎ **Q0175** Perphenazine, 4 mg, oral, FDA approved prescription anti-emetic, for use as a complete therapeutic substitute for an IV anti-emetic at the time of chemotherapy treatment, not to exceed a 48 hour dosage regimen   N1   N

Bill DME/MAC

Medicare Statute 4557

◎ **Q0176** Perphenazine, 8mg, oral, FDA approved prescription anti-emetic, for use as a complete therapeutic substitute for an IV anti-emetic at the time of chemotherapy treatment, not to exceed a 48 hour dosage regimen   N

Bill DME/MAC

Medicare Statute 4557

◎ **Q0177** Hydroxyzine pamoate, 25 mg, oral, FDA approved prescription anti-emetic, for use as a complete therapeutic substitute for an IV anti-emetic at the time of chemotherapy treatment, not to exceed a 48 hour dosage regimen   N1   N

Bill DME/MAC

Other: Vistaril

Medicare Statute 4557

◎ **Q0178** Hydroxyzine pamoate, 50 mg, oral, FDA approved prescription anti-emetic, for use as a complete therapeutic substitute for an IV anti-emetic at the time of chemotherapy treatment, not to exceed a 48 hour dosage regimen   N

Bill DME/MAC

Other: Vistaril

Medicare Statute 4557

~~Q0179~~   ~~Ondansetron hydrochloride, 8 mg, oral, FDA approved prescription anti-emetic, for use as a complete therapeutic substitute for an IV anti-emetic at the time of chemotherapy treatment, not to exceed a 48 hour dosage regimen~~   ✖

◎ **Q0180** Dolasetron mesylate, 100 mg, oral, FDA approved prescription anti-emetic, for use as a complete therapeutic substitute for an IV anti-emetic at the time of chemotherapy treatment, not to exceed a 24 hour dosage regimen   N1   N

Bill DME/MAC

NDC: Anzemet

Medicare Statute 4557

◎ **Q0181** Unspecified oral dosage form, FDA approved prescription anti-emetic, for use as a complete therapeutic substitute for a IV anti-emetic at the time of chemotherapy treatment, not to exceed a 48 hour dosage regimen   E

Bill DME/MAC

Medicare Statute 4557

▶ New   → Revised   ✔ Reinstated   ~~deleted~~ Deleted

◎ Special coverage instructions   ◆ Not covered or valid by Medicare   ✳ Carrier discretion

Miscellaneous Devices

▶ ⊙ **Q0478** Power adapter for use with electric or electric/pneumatic ventricular assist device, vehicle type `Qp` `Qh` 🦽   A

CMS has determined the reasonable useful lifetime is one year. Add modifier -RA to claims to report when battery is replaced because it was lost, stolen, or irreparably damaged. (http://www.wpsmedicare.com/part_b/publications/communique/archived/_files/winter-2011-comm.pdf)

▶ ⊙ **Q0479** Power module for use with electric or electric/pneumatic ventricular assist device, replacemment only `Qp` `Qh` 🦽   A

CMS has determined the reasonable useful lifetime is one year. Add modifier -RA in cases where the battery is being replaced because it was lost, stolen, or irreparably damaged. (http://www.wpsmedicare.com/part_b/publications/communique/archived/_files/winter-2011-comm.pdf)

⊙ **Q0480** Driver for use with pneumatic ventricular assist device, replacement only `Qp` `Qh` 🦽   A

Bill local carrier

⊙ **Q0481** Microprocessor control unit for use with electric ventricular assist device, replacement only `Qp` `Qh` 🦽   A

Bill local carrier

⊙ **Q0482** Microprocessor control unit for use with electric/pneumatic combination ventricular assist device, replacement only `Qp` `Qh` 🦽   A

Bill local carrier

⊙ **Q0483** Monitor/display module for use with electric ventricular assist device, replacement only `Qp` `Qh` 🦽   A

Bill local carrier

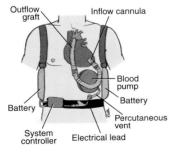

Outflow graft   Inflow cannula
Blood pump
Battery   Battery
Percutaneous vent
System controller   Electrical lead

Figure 50 Ventricular assist device.

⊙ **Q0484** Monitor/display module for use with electric or electric/pneumatic ventricular assist device, replacement only `Qp` `Qh` 🦽   A

Bill local carrier

⊙ **Q0485** Monitor control cable for use with electric ventricular assist device, replacement only `Qp` `Qh` 🦽   A

Bill local carrier

⊙ **Q0486** Monitor control cable for use with electric/pneumatic ventricular assist device, replacement only `Qp` `Qh` 🦽   A

Bill local carrier

⊙ **Q0487** Leads (pneumatic/electrical) for use with any type electric/pneumatic ventricular assist device, replacement only `Qp` `Qh` 🦽   A

Bill local carrier

⊙ **Q0488** Power pack base for use with electric ventricular assist device, replacement only `Qp` `Qh`   A

Bill local carrier

⊙ **Q0489** Power pack base for use with electric/pneumatic ventricular assist device, replacement only `Qp` `Qh` 🦽   A

Bill local carrier

⊙ **Q0490** Emergency power source for use with electric ventricular assist device, replacement only `Qp` `Qh` 🦽   A

Bill local carrier

⊙ **Q0491** Emergency power source for use with electric/pneumatic ventricular assist device, replacement only `Qp` `Qh` 🦽   A

Bill local carrier

⊙ **Q0492** Emergency power supply cable for use with electric ventricular assist device, replacement only `Qp` `Qh` 🦽   A

Bill local carrier

⊙ **Q0493** Emergency power supply cable for use with electric/pneumatic ventricular assist device, replacement only `Qp` `Qh` 🦽   A

Bill local carrier

⊙ **Q0494** Emergency hand pump for use with electric or electric/pneumatic ventricular assist device, replacement only `Qp` `Qh` 🦽   A

Bill local carrier

⊙ **Q0495** Battery/power pack charger for use with electric or electric/pneumatic ventricular assist device, replacement only `Qp` `Qh` 🦽   A

Bill local carrier

🔵 PQRI	`Qp` **Quantity Physician Appendix B**	`Qh` **Quantity Hospital Appendix C**	♀ **Female only**
♂ **Male only**	A **Age**	🦽 **DMEPOS** A2-Z3 **ASC Payment Indicator**	A-Y **ASC Status Indicator** Coding Clinic

* **Q0496** Battery, other than lithium-ion, for use with electric or electric/pneumatic ventricular assist device, replacement only ♿   A

Bill local carrier

Reasonable useful lifetime is 6 months (CR3931).

⊛ **Q0497** Battery clips for use with electric or electric/pneumatic ventricular assist device, replacement only `Qp` `Qh` ♿   A

Bill local carrier

⊛ **Q0498** Holster for use with electric or electric/ pneumatic ventricular assist device, replacement only `Qp` `Qh` ♿   A

Bill local carrier

→ * **Q0499** Belt/vest/bag for use to carry external peripheral components of any type ventricular assist device, replacement only `Qp` `Qh` ♿   A

Bill local carrier

⊛ **Q0500** Filters for use with electric or electric/ pneumatic ventricular assist device, replacement only ♿   A

Bill local carrier

⊛ **Q0501** Shower cover for use with electric or electric/pneumatic ventricular assist device, replacement only `Qp` `Qh` ♿   A

Bill local carrier

⊛ **Q0502** Mobility cart for pneumatic ventricular assist device, replacement only `Qp` `Qh` ♿   A

Bill local carrier

⊛ **Q0503** Battery for pneumatic ventricular assist device, replacement only, each `Qp` `Qh` ♿   A

Bill local carrier

Reasonable useful lifetime is 6 months (CR3931).

⊛ **Q0504** Power adapter for pneumatic ventricular assist device, replacement only, vehicle type `Qp` `Qh` ♿   A

Bill local carrier

⊛ **Q0505** Miscellaneous supply or accessory for use with ventricular assist device   A

Bill local carrier

⊛ **Q0506** Battery, lithium-ion, for use with electric or electric/pneumatic, ventricular assist device, replacement only ♿   A

Reasonable useful lifetime is 12 months. Add -RA for replacement if lost, stolen, or irreparable damage.

Fee, Pharmacy

Q0510-Q0515: Bill DME/MAC

⊛ **Q0510** Pharmacy supply fee for initial immunosuppressive drug(s), first month following transplant   B

⊛ **Q0511** Pharmacy supply fee for oral anti-cancer, oral anti-emetic or immunosuppressive drug(s); for the first prescription in a 30-day period   B

⊛ **Q0512** Pharmacy supply fee for oral anti-cancer, oral anti-emetic or immunosuppressive drug(s); for a subsequent prescription in a 30-day period   B

⊛ **Q0513** Pharmacy dispensing fee for inhalation drug(s); per 30 days   B

⊛ **Q0514** Pharmacy dispensing fee for inhalation drug(s); per 90 days   B

⊛ **Q0515** Injection, sermorelin acetate, 1 microgram   K2   K

NDC: Geref Diagnostic

IOM: 100-02, 15, 50

Lens, Intraocular

Q1004-Q1005: Bill local carrier

~~Q1003~~ ~~New technology intraocular lens category 3 (reduced spherical aberration)~~   ✖

⊛ **Q1004** New technology intraocular lens category 4 as defined in Federal Register notice `Qp`   E

⊛ **Q1005** New technology intraocular lens category 5 as defined in Federal Register notice `Qp`   E

Solutions and Drugs

⊛ **Q2004** Irrigation solution for treatment of bladder calculi, for example renacidin, per 500 ml   N

Bill local carrier

IOM: 100-02, 15, 50

Medicare Statute 1861S2B

* **Q2009** Injection, fosphenytoin, 50 mg phenytoin equivalent   N1   N

Bill local carrier

NDC: Cerebyx

IOM: 100-02, 15, 50

Medicare Statute 1861S2B

▶ New   → Revised   ✔ Reinstated   ~~deleted~~ Deleted

⊛ Special coverage instructions   ◆ Not covered or valid by Medicare   * Carrier discretion

⊙ **Q2017** Injection, teniposide, 50 mg   K2   K

Bill local carrier

NDC: Vumon

IOM: 100-02, 15, 50

Medicare Statute 1861S2B

▶ ⊙ **Q2026** Injection, radiesse, 0.1 ml   B

Coding Clinic: 2010, Q3, P8

▶ ⊙ **Q2027** Injection, sculptra, 0.1 ml   B

Coding Clinic: 2010, Q3, P8

▶ ⊙ **Q2035** Influenza virus vaccine, split virus, when administered to individuals 3 years of age and older, for intramuscular use (Afluria) Qp Qh A   L1   L

IOM: 100-02, 15, 50

Coding Clinic: 2011, Q1, P7; 2010, Q4, P8-9

▶ ⊙ **Q2036** Influenza virus vaccine, split virus, when administered to individuals 3 years of age and older, for intramuscular use (Flulaval) Qp Qh A   L1   L

IOM: 100-02, 15, 50

Coding Clinic: 2011, Q1, P7; 2010, Q4, P8-9

▶ ⊙ **Q2037** Influenza virus vaccine, split virus, when administered to individuals 3 years of age and older, for intramuscular use (Fluvirin) Qp Qh A   L1   L

IOM: 100-02, 15, 50

Coding Clinic: 2011, Q1, P7; 2010, Q4, P8-9

▶ ⊙ **Q2038** Influenza virus vaccine, split virus, when administered to individuals 3 years of age or older, for intramuscular use (Fluzone) Qp Qh A   L1   L

IOM: 100-02, 15, 50

Coding Clinic: 2011, Q1, P7; 2010, Q4, P8-9

▶ ⊙ **Q2039** Influenza virus vaccine, split virus, when administered to individuals 3 years of age and older, for intramuscular use (not otherwise specified) Qp Qh A   L1   L

IOM: 100-02, 15, 50

Coding Clinic: 2011, Q1, P7; 2010, Q4, P8-9

~~Q2040~~ ~~Injection, incobotulinumtoxin-A, 1 unit~~   ✖

~~Q2041~~ ~~Injection, von Willebrand factor complex (human), Wilate, 1 I.U., VWF:RCO~~   ✖

~~Q2042~~ ~~Injection, hydroxyprojesterone caproate, 1 mg~~   ✖

▶ ⊙ **Q2043** Sipuleucel-T, minimum of 50 million autologous CD54+ cells activated with PAP-GM-CSF, including leukapheresis and all other preparatory procedures, per infusion Qp Qh   G

~~Q2044~~ ~~Injection, belimumab, 10 mg~~   ✖

Brachytherapy Radioelements

⊙ **Q3001** Radioelements for brachytherapy, any type, each   B

IOM: 100-04, 12, 70; 100-04, 13, 20

Telehealth

✳ **Q3014** Telehealth originating site facility fee   A

Bill local carrier

Effective January of each year, the fee for telehealth services is increased by the Medicare Economic Index (MEI). The telehealth originating facility site fee (HCPCS code Q3014) for 2011 was 80 percent of the lesser of the actual charge or $24.10.

Drugs

Q3025-Q3026: Bill local carrier

⊙ **Q3025** Injection, interferon beta-1a, 11 mcg for intramuscular use   K2   K

NDC: Avonex

IOM: 100-02, 15, 50

Coding Clinic: 2011, Q2, P9

◆ **Q3026** Injection, interferon beta-1a, 11 mcg for subcutaneous use   E

Other: Rebif

Coding Clinic: 2011, Q2, P9

Test, Skin

⊙ **Q3031** Collagen skin test   N

Bill local carrier

IOM: 100-03, 4, 280.1

PQRI   Qp **Quantity Physician Appendix B**   Qh **Quantity Hospital Appendix C**   ♀ **Female only**

♂ **Male only**   A **Age**   ♿ **DMEPOS**   A2-Z3 ASC Payment Indicator   A-Y ASC Status Indicator   Coding Clinic

Supplies, Cast

Q4001-Q4051: Bill local carrier

Payment on a reasonable charge basis is required for splints, casts by regulations contained in 42 CFR 405.501.

✳ **Q4001** Casting supplies, body cast adult, with or without head, plaster `Qp` `Qh` `A`　　B

✳ **Q4002** Cast supplies, body cast adult, with or without head, fiberglass `Qp` `Qh` `A`　　B

✳ **Q4003** Cast supplies, shoulder cast, adult (11 years +), plaster `Qp` `Qh` `A`　　B

✳ **Q4004** Cast supplies, shoulder cast, adult (11 years +), fiberglass `Qp` `Qh` `A`　　B

✳ **Q4005** Cast supplies, long arm cast, adult (11 years +), plaster `A`　　B

✳ **Q4006** Cast supplies, long arm cast, adult (11 years +), fiberglass `A`　　B

✳ **Q4007** Cast supplies, long arm cast, pediatric (0-10 years), plaster `A`　　B

✳ **Q4008** Cast supplies, long arm cast, pediatric (0-10 years), fiberglass `A`　　B

✳ **Q4009** Cast supplies, short arm cast, adult (11 years +), plaster `A`　　B

✳ **Q4010** Cast supplies, short arm cast, adult (11 years +), fiberglass `A`　　B

✳ **Q4011** Cast supplies, short arm cast, pediatric (0-10 years), plaster `A`　　B

✳ **Q4012** Cast supplies, short arm cast, pediatric (0-10 years), fiberglass `A`　　B

✳ **Q4013** Cast supplies, gauntlet cast (includes lower forearm and hand), adult (11 years +), plaster `A`　　B

✳ **Q4014** Cast supplies, gauntlet cast (includes lower forearm and hand), adult (11 years +), fiberglass `A`　　B

✳ **Q4015** Cast supplies, gauntlet cast (includes lower forearm and hand), pediatric (0-10 years), plaster `A`　　B

✳ **Q4016** Cast supplies, gauntlet cast (includes lower forearm and hand), pediatric (0-10 years), fiberglass `A`　　B

✳ **Q4017** Cast supplies, long arm splint, adult (11 years +), plaster `A`　　B

✳ **Q4018** Cast supplies, long arm splint, adult (11 years +), fiberglass `A`　　B

✳ **Q4019** Cast supplies, long arm splint, pediatric (0-10 years), plaster `A`　　B

✳ **Q4020** Cast supplies, long arm splint, pediatric (0-10 years), fiberglass `A`

✳ **Q4021** Cast supplies, short arm splint, adult (11 years +), plaster `A`　　B

✳ **Q4022** Cast supplies, short arm splint, adult (11 years +), fiberglass `A`　　B

✳ **Q4023** Cast supplies, short arm splint, pediatric (0-10 years), plaster `A`　　B

✳ **Q4024** Cast supplies, short arm splint, pediatric (0-10 years), fiberglass `A`　　B

✳ **Q4025** Cast supplies, hip spica (one or both legs), adult (11 years +), plaster `Qp` `Qh` `A`　　B

✳ **Q4026** Cast supplies, hip spica (one or both legs), adult (11 years +), fiberglass `Qp` `Qh` `A`　　B

✳ **Q4027** Cast supplies, hip spica (one or both legs), pediatric (0-10 years), plaster `Qp` `Qh` `A`　　B

✳ **Q4028** Cast supplies, hip spica (one or both legs), pediatric (0-10 years), fiberglass `Qp` `Qh` `A`　　B

✳ **Q4029** Cast supplies, long leg cast, adult (11 years +), plaster `A`　　B

✳ **Q4030** Cast supplies, long leg cast, adult (11 years +), fiberglass `A`　　B

✳ **Q4031** Cast supplies, long leg cast, pediatric (0-10 years), plaster `A`　　B

✳ **Q4032** Cast supplies, long leg cast, pediatric (0-10 years), fiberglass `A`　　B

✳ **Q4033** Cast supplies, long leg cylinder cast, adult (11 years +), plaster `A`　　B

✳ **Q4034** Cast supplies, long leg cylinder cast, adult (11 years +), fiberglass `A`　　B

✳ **Q4035** Cast supplies, long leg cylinder cast, pediatric (0-10 years), plaster `A`　　B

✳ **Q4036** Cast supplies, long leg cylinder cast, pediatric (0-10 years), fiberglass `A`　　B

✳ **Q4037** Cast supplies, short leg cast, adult (11 years +), plaster `A`　　B

✳ **Q4038** Cast supplies, short leg cast, adult (11 years +), fiberglass `A`　　B

✳ **Q4039** Cast supplies, short leg cast, pediatric (0-10 years), plaster `A`　　B

✳ **Q4040** Cast supplies, short leg cast, pediatric (0-10 years), fiberglass `A`　　B

✳ **Q4041** Cast supplies, long leg splint, adult (11 years +), plaster `A`　　B

✳ **Q4042** Cast supplies, long leg splint, adult (11 years +), fiberglass `A`　　B

✳ **Q4043** Cast supplies, long leg splint, pediatric (0-10 years), plaster `A`　　B

✳ **Q4044** Cast supplies, long leg splint, pediatric (0-10 years), fiberglass `A`　　B

▶ New　→ Revised　✔ Reinstated　~~deleted~~ Deleted
○ Special coverage instructions　◆ Not covered or valid by Medicare　✳ Carrier discretion

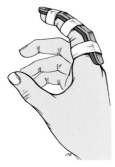

Figure 51 Finger splint.

* **Q4045** Cast supplies, short leg splint, adult (11 years +), plaster [A] B

* **Q4046** Cast supplies, short leg splint, adult (11 years +), fiberglass [A] B

* **Q4047** Cast supplies, short leg splint, pediatric (0-10 years), plaster [A] B

* **Q4048** Cast supplies, short leg splint, pediatric (0-10 years), fiberglass [A] B

* **Q4049** Finger splint, static B

* **Q4050** Cast supplies, for unlisted types and materials of casts B

* **Q4051** Splint supplies, miscellaneous (includes thermoplastics, strapping, fasteners, padding and other supplies) B

Drugs

* **Q4074** Iloprost, inhalation solution, FDA-approved final product, non-compounded, administered through DME, unit dose form, up to 20 micrograms Y

NDC: Ventavis

☯ **Q4081** Injection, epoetin alfa, 100 units (for ESRD on dialysis) A

Bill DME/MAC for method II home dialysis. If other, bill DME/MAC.

NDC: Epogen, Procrit

* **Q4082** Drug or biological, not otherwise classified, Part B drug competitive acquisition program (CAP) B

Bill local carrier

Skin Substitutes

* **Q4100** Skin substitute, not otherwise specified N1 N

Bill local carrier

Other: Orcel, Surgimend collagen matrix

→ * **Q4101** Apligraf, per square centimeter K2 K

Bill local carrier

Coding Clinic: 2011, Q1, P9

→ * **Q4102** Oasis Wound Matrix, per square centimeter K2 K

Bill local carrier

Coding Clinic: 2011, Q1, P9

→ * **Q4103** Oasis Burn Matrix, per square centimeter K2 K

Bill local carrier

Coding Clinic: 2011, Q1, P9

→ * **Q4104** Integra Bilayer Matrix Wound Dressing (BMWD), per square centimeter K2 K

Bill local carrier

Coding Clinic: 2011, Q1, P9; 2010, Q2, P8

→ * **Q4105** Integra Dermal Regeneration Template (DRT), per square centimeter K2 K

Bill local carrier

Coding Clinic: 2011, Q1, P9; 2010, Q2, P8

→ * **Q4106** Dermagraft, per square centimeter K2 K

Bill local carrier

Coding Clinic: 2011, Q1, P9

→ * **Q4107** Graftjacket, per square centimeter K2 K

Bill local carrier

NDC: Graftjacket Maxstrip, Graftjacket Small Ligament Repair Matrix, Graftjacket STD, Handjacket Scaffold Thin, Maxforce Thick, Ulcerjacket Scaffold, Ultra Maxforce

Coding Clinic: 2011, Q1, P9

→ * **Q4108** Integra Matrix, per square centimeter K2 K

Bill local carrier

Coding Clinic: 2011, Q1, P9; 2010, Q2, P8

→ * **Q4110** Primatrix, per square centimeter K2 K

Bill local carrier

Coding Clinic: 2011, Q1, P9

→ * **Q4111** GammaGraft, per square centimeter K2 K

Bill local carrier

Coding Clinic: 2011, Q1, P9

→ * **Q4112** Cymetra, injectable, 1cc K2 K

Coding Clinic: 2011, Q1, P9

→ * **Q4113** GraftJacket Xpress, injectable, 1cc K2 K

Bill local carrier

Coding Clinic: 2011, Q1, P9

🄟 PQRI	**Qp** Quantity Physician Appendix B	**Qh** Quantity Hospital Appendix C ♀ Female only
♂ Male only [A] Age 🦽 DMEPOS	A2-Z3 ASC Payment Indicator	A-Y ASC Status Indicator Coding Clinic

✳ **Q4114** Integra Flowable Wound Matrix, injectable, 1cc   K2   K

Bill local carrier

Coding Clinic: 2010, Q2, P8

→ ✳ **Q4115** Alloskin, per square centimeter   K2   K

Bill local carrier

Coding Clinic: 2011, Q1, P9

→ ✳ **Q4116** Alloderm, per square centimeter   K2   K

Bill local carrier

Coding Clinic: 2011, Q1, P9

▶ ✳ **Q4117** Hyalomatrix, per square centimeter   E

IOM: 100-02, 15, 50

▶ ✳ **Q4118** Matristem micromatrix, 1 mg   K2   K

Coding Clinic: 2011, Q1, P6

▶ ✳ **Q4119** Matristem wound matrix, per square centimeter   K2   K

Coding Clinic: 2011, Q1, P6

▶ ✳ **Q4120** Matristem burn matrix, per square centimeter   E

▶ ✳ **Q4121** Theraskin, per square centimeter   K2   K

Coding Clinic: 2011, Q1, P6

▶ ✳ **Q4122** Dermacell, per square centimeter   K2   K

▶ ✳ **Q4123** AlloSkin RT, per square centimeter   E

▶ ✳ **Q4124** Oasis Ultra Tri-layer Wound Matrix, per square centimeter   K2   G

▶ ✳ **Q4125** Arthroflex, per square centimeter   E

▶ ✳ **Q4126** Memoderm, per square centimeter   E

▶ ✳ **Q4127** Talymed, per square centimeter   E

▶ ✳ **Q4128** FlexHD or Allopatch HD, per square centimeter   E

▶ ✳ **Q4129** Unite Biomatrix, per square centimeter   E

▶ ✳ **Q4130** Strattice TM, per square centimeter   N1   N

Hospice Care

☺ **Q5001** Hospice care provided in patient's home/residence   B

Bill local carrier

☺ **Q5002** Hospice care provided in assisted living facility   B

Bill local carrier

☺ **Q5003** Hospice care provided in nursing long term care facility (LTC) or non-skilled nursing facility (NF)   B

Bill local carrier

☺ **Q5004** Hospice care provided in skilled nursing facility (SNF)   B

Bill local carrier

☺ **Q5005** Hospice care provided in inpatient hospital   B

Bill local carrier

☺ **Q5006** Hospice care provided in inpatient hospice facility   B

Bill local carrier

Hospice care provided in an inpatient hospice facility. These are residential facilities, which are places for patients to live while receiving routine home care or continuous home care. These hospice residential facilities are not certified by Medicare or Medicaid for provision of General Inpatient (GIP) or respite care, and regulations at 42 CFR 418.202(e) do not allow provision of GIP or respite care at hospice residential facilities. (http://www.palmettogba.com/Palmetto/Providers.Nsf/files/Hospice_Coalition_QAs_03-2011.pdf/$File/Hospice_Coalition_QAs_03-2011.pdf)

☺ **Q5007** Hospice care provided in long term care facility   B

Bill local carrier

☺ **Q5008** Hospice care provided in inpatient psychiatric facility   B

Bill local carrier

☺ **Q5009** Hospice care provided in place not otherwise specified (NOS)   B

Bill local carrier

▶ ☺ **Q5010** Hospice home care provided in a hospice facility   B

Contrast

☺ **Q9951** Low osmolar contrast material, 400 or greater mg/ml iodine concentration, per ml   N1   N

Bill local carrier

IOM: 100-04, 12, 70; 100-04, 13, 20; 100-04, 13, 90

☺ **Q9953** Injection, iron-based magnetic resonance contrast agent, per ml   N1   N

Bill local carrier

IOM: 100-04, 12, 70; 100-04, 13, 20; 100-04, 13, 90

▶ New   → Revised   ✔ Reinstated   ~~deleted~~ Deleted

☺ Special coverage instructions   ◆ Not covered or valid by Medicare   ✳ Carrier discretion

✪ **Q9954** Oral magnetic resonance contrast agent, per 100 ml   N1   N

Bill local carrier

NDC: Gastromark

IOM: 100-04, 12, 70; 100-04, 13, 20; 100-04, 13, 90

✳ **Q9955** Injection, perflexane lipid microspheres, per ml   N1   N

Bill local carrier

✳ **Q9956** Injection, octafluoropropane microspheres, per ml   N1   N

Bill local carrier

NDC: Optison

✳ **Q9957** Injection, perflutren lipid microspheres, per ml   N1   N

Bill local carrier

NDC: Definity

✪ **Q9958** High osmolar contrast material, up to 149 mg/ml iodine concentration, per ml   N1   N

Bill local carrier

NDC: Conray 30, Cysto-Conray II, Cystografin, Cystografin-Dilute, Hypaque Sodium Oral, Reno-30, Reno-Dip

IOM: 100-04, 12, 70; 100-04, 13, 20; 100-04, 13, 90

Coding Clinic: 2007, Q1, P6

✪ **Q9959** High osmolar contrast material, 150-199 mg/ml iodine concentration, per ml   N1   N

Bill local carrier

IOM: 100-04, 12, 70; 100-04, 13, 20; 100-04, 13, 90

Coding Clinic: 2007, Q1, P6

✪ **Q9960** High osmolar contrast material, 200-249 mg/ml iodine concentration, per ml   N1   N

Bill local carrier

NDC: Conray 43

IOM: 100-04, 12, 70; 100-04, 13, 20; 100-04, 13, 90

Coding Clinic: 2007, Q1, P6

✪ **Q9961** High osmolar contrast material, 250-299 mg/ml iodine concentration, per ml   N1   N

Bill local carrier

NDC: Conray, Cholografin Meglumine, Renografin-60, Reno-M60

IOM: 100-04, 12, 70; 100-04, 13, 20; 100-04, 13, 90

Coding Clinic: 2007, Q1, P6

✪ **Q9962** High osmolar contrast material, 300-349 mg/ml iodine concentration, per ml   N1   N

Bill local carrier

IOM: 100-04, 12, 70; 100-04, 13, 20; 100-04, 13, 90

Coding Clinic: 2007, Q1, P6

✪ **Q9963** High osmolar contrast material, 350-399 mg/ml iodine concentration, per ml   N1   N

Bill local carrier

NDC: Gastrografin, Hypaque, Md-76R, Md Gastroview, Renocal-76, Sinografin

IOM: 100-04, 12, 70; 100-04, 13, 20; 100-04, 13, 90

Coding Clinic: 2007, Q1, P6

✪ **Q9964** High osmolar contrast material, 400 or greater mg/ml iodine concentration, per ml   N1   N

Bill local carrier

IOM: 100-04, 12, 70; 100-04, 13, 20; 100-04, 13, 90

Coding Clinic: 2007, Q1, P6

✪ **Q9965** Low osmolar contrast material, 100-199 mg/ml iodine concentration, per ml   N1   N

Bill local carrier

NDC: Omnipaque, Ultravist

IOM: 100-04, 12, 70; 100-04, 13, 20; 100-04, 13, 90

✪ **Q9966** Low osmolar contrast material, 200-299 mg/ml iodine concentration, per ml   N1   N

Bill local carrier

NDC: Isovue, Omnipaque, Optiray, Ultravist, Visipaque

IOM: 100-04, 12, 70; 100-04, 13, 20; 100-04, 13, 90

✪ **Q9967** Low osmolar contrast material, 300-399 mg/ml iodine concentration, per ml   N1   N

Bill local carrier

NDC: Hexabrix 320, Isovue-300, Isovue-370, Omnipaque 300, Omnipaque 350, Optiray, Oxilan, Ultravist, Vispaque

IOM: 100-04, 12, 70; 100-04, 13, 20; 100-04, 13, 90

✳ **Q9968** Injection, non-radioactive, non-contrast, visualization adjunct (e.g., Methylene Blue, Isosulfan Blue), 1 mg   N1   N

🅟 PQRI	**Qp Quantity Physician Appendix B**	**Qh Quantity Hospital Appendix C** ♀ **Female only**
♂ **Male only** **A Age** ♿ **DMEPOS**	A2-Z3 **ASC Payment Indicator**	A-Y **ASC Status Indicator** Coding Clinic

DIAGNOSTIC RADIOLOGY SERVICES (R0000-R9999)

Transportation/Setup of Portable Equipment

R0070-R0076: Bill local carrier

⊗ **R0070** Transportation of portable x-ray equipment and personnel to home or nursing home, per trip to facility or location, one patient seen `Qp` `Qh`   B

CMS Transmittal B03-049; specific instructions to contractors on pricing

IOM: 100-04, 13, 90; 100-04, 13, 90.3

⊗ **R0075** Transportation of portable x-ray equipment and personnel to home or nursing home, per trip to facility or location, more than one patient seen `Qp` `Qh`   B

This code would not apply to the x-ray equipment if stored at the location where the x-ray was performed (e.g., a nursing home).

IOM: 100-04, 13, 90; 100-04, 13, 90.3

⊗ **R0076** Transportation of portable ECG to facility or location, per patient `Qh`   B

EKG procedure code 93000 or 93005 must be submitted on same claim as transportation code. Bundled status on physician fee schedule

IOM: 100-01, 5, 90.2; 100-02, 15, 80; 100-03, 1, 20.15; 100-04, 13, 90; 100-04, 16, 10; 100-04, 16, 110.4

▶ New   → Revised   ✔ Reinstated   ~~deleted~~ Deleted
⊗ Special coverage instructions   ◆ Not covered or valid by Medicare   ✳ Carrier discretion

TEMPORARY NATIONAL CODES ESTABLISHED BY PRIVATE PAYERS (S0000-S9999)

Medicare and other federal payers do not recognize "S" codes; however, S codes may be useful for claims to some private insurers.

◆ **S0012** Butorphanol tartrate, nasal spray, **25 mg**

◆ **S0014** Tacrine hydrochloride, **10 mg**

◆ **S0017** Injection, aminocaproic acid, **5 grams**

◆ **S0020** Injection, bupivacaine hydrochloride, **30 ml**

◆ **S0021** Injection, cefoperazone sodium, **1 gram**

◆ **S0023** Injection, cimetidine hydrochloride, **300 mg**

◆ **S0028** Injection, famotidine, **20 mg**

◆ **S0030** Injection, metronidazole, **500 mg**

◆ **S0032** Injection, nafcillin sodium, **2 grams**

◆ **S0034** Injection, ofloxacin, **400 mg**

◆ **S0039** Injection, sulfamethoxazole and trimethoprim, **10 ml**

◆ **S0040** Injection, ticarcillin disodium and clavulanate potassium, **3.1 grams**

◆ **S0073** Injection, aztreonam, **500 mg**

◆ **S0074** Injection, cefotetan disodium, **500 mg**

◆ **S0077** Injection, clindamycin phosphate, **300 mg**

◆ **S0078** Injection, fosphenytoin sodium, **750 mg**

◆ **S0080** Injection, pentamidine isethionate, **300 mg**

◆ **S0081** Injection, piperacillin sodium, **500 mg**

◆ **S0088** Imatinib, **100 mg**

◆ **S0090** Sildenafil citrate, **25 mg**

◆ **S0091** Granisetron hydrochloride, **1 mg** (for circumstances falling under the Medicare Statute, use Q0166)

◆ **S0092** Injection, hydromorphone hydrochloride, **250 mg** (loading dose for infusion pump)

◆ **S0093** Injection, morphine sulfate, **500 mg** (loading dose for infusion pump)

◆ **S0104** Zidovudine, oral, **100 mg**

◆ **S0106** Bupropion HCl sustained release tablet, **150 mg,** per bottle of 60 tablets

◆ **S0108** Mercaptopurine, oral, **50 mg**

◆ **S0109** Methadone, oral, **5 mg**

◆ **S0117** Tretinoin, topical, **5 grams**

▶ ◆ **S0119** Ondansetron, oral, 4 mg (for circumstances falling under the medicare statute, use HCPCS Q code)

◆ **S0122** Injection, menotropins, **75 IU**

◆ **S0126** Injection, follitropin alfa, **75 IU** ♀

◆ **S0128** Injection, follitropin beta, **75 IU**

◆ **S0132** Injection, ganirelix acetate, **250 mcg** ♀

◆ **S0136** Clozapine, **25 mg**

◆ **S0137** Didanosine (DDI), **25 mg**

◆ **S0138** Finasteride, **5 mg** ♂

◆ **S0139** Minoxidil, **10 mg**

◆ **S0140** Saquinavir, **200 mg**

◆ **S0142** Colistimethate sodium, inhalation solution administered through DME, concentrated form, **per mg**

◆ **S0145** Injection, pegylated interferon alfa-2a, **180 mcg per ml**

▶ ◆ **S0148** Injection, pegylated interferon ALFA-2b, **10 mcg**

◆ **S0155** Sterile dilutant for epoprostenol, **50 ml**

◆ **S0156** Exemestane, **25 mg**

◆ **S0157** Becaplermin gel 0.01%, **0.5 gm**

◆ **S0160** Dextroamphetamine sulfate, **5 mg**

◆ **S0164** Injection, pantoprazole sodium, **40 mg**

◆ **S0166** Injection, olanzapine, **2.5 mg**

▶ ◆ **S0169** Calcitrol, **0.25 microgram**

◆ **S0170** Anastrozole, oral, **1mg**

◆ **S0171** Injection, bumetanide, **0.5 mg**

◆ **S0172** Chlorambucil, oral, **2 mg**

◆ **S0174** Dolasetron mesylate, oral **50 mg** (for circumstances falling under the Medicare Statute, use Q0180)

◆ **S0175** Flutamide, oral, **125 mg**

◆ **S0176** Hydroxyurea, oral, **500 mg**

◆ **S0177** Levamisole hydrochloride, oral, **50 mg**

◆ **S0178** Lomustine, oral, **10 mg**

◆ **S0179** Megestrol acetate, oral, **20 mg**

~~S0181~~ ~~Ondansetron hydrochloride, oral, 4 mg (for circumstances falling under the Medicare Statute, use Q0179)~~ ✖

◆ **S0182** Procarbazine hydrochloride, oral, **50 mg**

◆ **S0183** Prochlorperazine maleate, oral, **5 mg** (for circumstances falling under the Medicare Statute, use Q0164-Q0165)

◆ **S0187** Tamoxifen citrate, oral, **10 mg**

◆ **S0189** Testosterone pellet, **75 mg**

◆ **S0190** Mifepristone, oral, **200 mg** ♀

◆ **S0191** Misoprostol, oral **200 mcg**

◆ **S0194** Dialysis/stress vitamin supplement, oral, **100 capsules**

◆ **S0195** Pneumococcal conjugate vaccine, polyvalent, intramuscular, for children from five years to nine years of age who have not previously received the vaccine Ⓐ

◆ **S0197** Prenatal vitamins, 30-day supply ♀

◆ **S0199** Medically induced abortion by oral ingestion of medication including all associated services and supplies (e.g., patient counseling, office visits, confirmation of pregnancy by HCG, ultrasound to confirm duration of pregnancy, ultrasound to confirm completion of abortion) except drugs ♀

◆ **S0201** Partial hospitalization services, less than 24 hours, per diem

◆ **S0207** Paramedic intercept, non-hospital-based ALS service (non-voluntary), non-transport

◆ **S0208** Paramedic intercept, hospital-based ALS service (non-voluntary), non-transport

◆ **S0209** Wheelchair van, mileage, per mile

◆ **S0215** Non-emergency transportation; mileage per mile

◆ **S0220** Medical conference by a physician with interdisciplinary team of health professionals or representatives of community agencies to coordinate activities of patient care (patient is present); approximately 30 minutes

◆ **S0221** Medical conference by a physician with interdisciplinary team of health professionals or representatives of community agencies to coordinate activities of patient care (patient is present); approximately 60 minutes

◆ **S0250** Comprehensive geriatric assessment and treatment planning performed by assessment team Ⓐ

◆ **S0255** Hospice referral visit (advising patient and family of care options) performed by nurse, social worker, or other designated staff

◆ **S0257** Counseling and discussion regarding advance directives or end of life care planning and decisions, with patient and/or surrogate (list separately in addition to code for appropriate evaluation and management service)

◆ **S0260** History and physical (outpatient or office) related to surgical procedure (list separately in addition to code for appropriate evaluation and management service)

◆ **S0265** Genetic counseling, under physician supervision, each 15 minutes

◆ **S0270** Physician management of patient home care, standard monthly case rate (per 30 days)

◆ **S0271** Physician management of patient home care, hospice monthly case rate (per 30 days)

◆ **S0272** Physician management of patient home care, episodic care monthly case rate (per 30 days)

◆ **S0273** Physician visit at member's home, outside of a capitation arrangement

◆ **S0274** Nurse practitioner visit at member's home, outside of a capitation arrangement

◆ **S0280** Medical home program, comprehensive care coordination and planning, initial plan

◆ **S0281** Medical home program, comprehensive care coordination and planning, maintenance of plan

◆ **S0302** Completed Early Periodic Screening Diagnosis and Treatment (EPSDT) service (list in addition to code for appropriate evaluation and management service) Ⓐ

◆ **S0310** Hospitalist services (list separately in addition to code for appropriate evaluation and management service)

◆ **S0315** Disease management program; initial assessment and initiation of the program

◆ **S0316** Disease management program; follow-up/reassessment

◆ **S0317** Disease management program; per diem

▶ New   → Revised   ✔ Reinstated   ~~deleted~~ Deleted

☺ Special coverage instructions   ◆ Not covered or valid by Medicare   ✳ Carrier discretion

◆ **S0320** Telephone calls by a registered nurse to a disease management program member for monitoring purposes; per month

◆ **S0340** Lifestyle modification program for management of coronary artery disease, including all supportive services; first quarter/stage

◆ **S0341** Lifestyle modification program for management of coronary artery disease, including all supportive services; second or third quarter/stage

◆ **S0342** Lifestyle modification program for management of coronary artery disease, including all supportive services; fourth quarter/stage

◆ **S0390** Routine foot care; removal and/or trimming of corns, calluses and/or nails and preventive maintenance in specific medical conditions (e.g. diabetes), per visit

◆ **S0395** Impression casting of a foot performed by a practitioner other than the manufacturer of the orthotic

◆ **S0400** Global fee for extracorporeal shock wave lithotripsy treatment of kidney stone(s)

◆ **S0500** Disposable contact lens, per lens

◆ **S0504** Single vision prescription lens (safety, athletic, or sunglass), per lens

◆ **S0506** Bifocal vision prescription lens (safety, athletic, or sunglass), per lens

◆ **S0508** Trifocal vision prescription lens (safety, athletic, or sunglass), per lens

◆ **S0510** Non-prescription lens (safety, athletic, or sunglass), per lens

◆ **S0512** Daily wear specialty contact lens, per lens

◆ **S0514** Color contact lens, per lens

◆ **S0515** Scleral lens, liquid bandage device, per lens

◆ **S0516** Safety eyeglass frames

◆ **S0518** Sunglasses frames

◆ **S0580** Polycarbonate lens (list this code in addition to the basic code for the lens)

◆ **S0581** Nonstandard lens (list this code in addition to the basic code for the lens)

◆ **S0590** Integral lens service, miscellaneous services reported separately

◆ **S0592** Comprehensive contact lens evaluation

◆ **S0595** Dispensing new spectacle lenses for patient supplied frame

◆ **S0601** Screening proctoscopy

◆ **S0610** Annual gynecological examination, new patient ♀

◆ **S0612** Annual gynecological examination, established patient ♀

◆ **S0613** Annual gynecological examination; clinical breast examination without pelvic evaluation ♀

◆ **S0618** Audiometry for hearing aid evaluation to determine the level and degree of hearing loss

◆ **S0620** Routine ophthalmological examination including refraction; new patient

Many non-Medicare vision plans may require code for routine encounter, no complaints

◆ **S0621** Routine ophthalmological examination including refraction; established patient

Many non-Medicare vision plans may require code for routine encounter, no complaints

◆ **S0622** Physical exam for college, new or established patient (list separately) in addition to appropriate evaluation and management code **A**

~~S0625~~ ~~Retinal telescreening by digital imaging of multiple different fundus areas to screen for vision-threatening conditions, including imaging, interpretation and report~~ ✖

◆ **S0630** Removal of sutures; by a physician other than the physician who originally closed the wound

◆ **S0800** Laser in situ keratomileusis (LASIK)

◆ **S0810** Photorefractive keratectomy (PRK)

◆ **S0812** Phototherapeutic keratectomy (PTK)

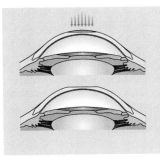

Figure 52
Phototherapeutic keratectomy (PRK).

◆ **S1001** Deluxe item, patient aware (list in addition to code for basic item)

◆ **S1002** Customized item (list in addition to code for basic item)

◆ **S1015** IV tubing extension set

◆ **S1016** Non-PVC (polyvinyl chloride) intravenous administration set, for use with drugs that are not stable in PVC e.g. paclitaxel

◆ **S1030** Continuous noninvasive glucose monitoring device, purchase (for physician interpretation of data, use CPT code)

◆ **S1031** Continuous noninvasive glucose monitoring device, rental, including sensor, sensor replacement, and download to monitor (for physician interpretation of data, use CPT code)

◆ **S1040** Cranial remolding orthosis, pediatric, rigid, with soft interface material, custom fabricated, includes fitting and adjustment(s) Ⓐ

◆ **S2053** Transplantation of small intestine and liver allografts

◆ **S2054** Transplantation of multivisceral organs

◆ **S2055** Harvesting of donor multivisceral organs, with preparation and maintenance of allografts; from cadaver donor

◆ **S2060** Lobar lung transplantation

◆ **S2061** Donor lobectomy (lung) for transplantation, living donor

◆ **S2065** Simultaneous pancreas kidney transplantation

◆ **S2066** Breast reconstruction with gluteal artery perforator (GAP) flap, including harvesting of the flap, microvascular transfer, closure of donor site and shaping the flap into a breast, unilateral ♀

◆ **S2067** Breast reconstruction of a single breast with "stacked" deep inferior epigastric perforator (DIEP) flap(s) and/or gluteal artery perforator (GAP) flap(s), including harvesting of the flap(s), microvascular transfer, closure of donor site(s) and shaping the flap into a breast, unilateral ♀

◆ **S2068** Breast reconstruction with deep inferior epigastric perforator (DIEP) flap, or superficial inferior epigastric artery (SIEA) flap, including harvesting of the flap, microvascular transfer, closure of donor site and shaping the flap into a breast, unilateral ♀

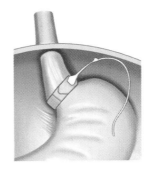

Figure 53 Gastric band.

◆ **S2070** Cystourethroscopy, with ureteroscopy and/or pyeloscopy; with endoscopic laser treatment of ureteral calculi (includes ureteral catheterization)

◆ **S2079** Laparoscopic esophagomyotomy (Heller type)

◆ **S2080** Laser-assisted uvulopalatoplasty (LAUP)

◆ **S2083** Adjustment of gastric band diameter via subcutaneous port by injection or aspiration of saline

◆ **S2095** Transcatheter occlusion or embolization for tumor destruction, percutaneous, any method, using yttrium-90 microspheres

◆ **S2102** Islet cell tissue transplant from pancreas; allogeneic

◆ **S2103** Adrenal tissue transplant to brain

◆ **S2107** Adoptive immunotherapy i.e. development of specific anti-tumor reactivity (e.g. tumor-infiltrating lymphocyte therapy) per course of treatment

◆ **S2112** Arthroscopy, knee, surgical for harvesting of cartilage (chondrocyte cells)

◆ **S2115** Osteotomy, periacetabular, with internal fixation

◆ **S2117** Arthroereisis, subtalar

◆ **S2118** Metal-on-metal total hip resurfacing, including acetabular and femoral components

◆ **S2120** Low density lipoprotein (LDL) apheresis using heparin-induced extracorporeal LDL precipitation

◆ **S2140** Cord blood harvesting for transplantation, allogeneic

◆ **S2142** Cord blood-derived stem cell transplantation, allogeneic

---

▶ New　→ Revised　✔ Reinstated　~~deleted~~ Deleted
⊙ Special coverage instructions　◆ Not covered or valid by Medicare　✳ Carrier discretion

◆ **S2150** Bone marrow or blood-derived stem cells (peripheral or umbilical), allogeneic or autologous, harvesting, transplantation, and related complications; including: pheresis and cell preparation/storage; marrow ablative therapy; drugs, supplies, hospitalization with outpatient follow-up; medical/surgical, diagnostic, emergency, and rehabilitative services; and the number of days of pre- and post-transplant care in the global definition

◆ **S2152** Solid organ(s), complete or segmental, single organ or combination of organs; deceased or living donor(s), procurement, transplantation, and related complications; including: drugs; supplies; hospitalization with outpatient follow-up; medical/surgical, diagnostic, emergency, and rehabilitative services, and the number of days of pre- and post-transplant care in the global definition

◆ **S2202** Echosclerotherapy

◆ **S2205** Minimally invasive direct coronary artery bypass surgery involving mini-thoracotomy or mini-sternotomy surgery, performed under direct vision; using arterial graft(s), single coronary arterial graft

◆ **S2206** Minimally invasive direct coronary artery bypass surgery involving mini-thoracotomy or mini-sternotomy surgery, performed under direct vision; using arterial graft(s), two coronary arterial grafts

◆ **S2207** Minimally invasive direct coronary artery bypass surgery involving mini-thoracotomy or mini-sternotomy surgery, performed under direct vision; using venous graft only, single coronary venous graft

◆ **S2208** Minimally invasive direct coronary artery bypass surgery involving mini-thoracotomy or mini-sternotomy surgery, performed under direct vision; using single arterial and venous graft(s), single venous graft

◆ **S2209** Minimally invasive direct coronary artery bypass surgery involving mini-thoracotomy or mini-sternotomy surgery, performed under direct vision; using two arterial grafts and single venous graft

◆ **S2225** Myringotomy, laser-assisted

◆ **S2230** Implantation of magnetic component of semi-implantable hearing device on ossicles in middle ear

◆ **S2235** Implantation of auditory brain stem implant

◆ **S2260** Induced abortion, 17 to 24 weeks ♀

◆ **S2265** Induced abortion, 25 to 28 weeks ♀

◆ **S2266** Induced abortion, 29 to 31 weeks ♀

◆ **S2267** Induced abortion, 32 weeks or greater ♀

~~S2270~~ ~~Insertion of vaginal cylinder for application of radiation source or clinical brachytherapy (report separately in addition to radiation source delivery)~~ ✖

◆ **S2300** Arthroscopy, shoulder, surgical; with thermally-induced capsulorrhaphy

◆ **S2325** Hip core decompression

◆ **S2340** Chemodenervation of abductor muscle(s) of vocal cord

◆ **S2341** Chemodenervation of adductor muscle(s) of vocal cord

◆ **S2342** Nasal endoscopy for post-operative debridement following functional endoscopic sinus surgery, nasal and/or sinus cavity(s), unilateral or bilateral

~~S2344~~ ~~Nasal/sinus endoscopy, surgical; with enlargement of sinus ostium opening using inflatable device (i.e., balloon sinuplasty)~~ ✖

◆ **S2348** Decompression procedure, percutaneous, of nucleus pulpous of intervertebral disc, using radiofrequency energy, single or multiple levels, lumbar

◆ **S2350** Diskectomy, anterior, with decompression of spinal cord and/or nerve root(s), including osteophytectomy; lumbar, single interspace

◆ **S2351** Diskectomy, anterior, with decompression of spinal cord and/or nerve root(s) including osteophytectomy; lumbar, each additional interspace (list separately in addition to code for primary procedure)

◆ **S2360** Percutaneous vertebroplasty, one vertebral body, unilateral or bilateral injection; cervical

◆ **S2361** Each additional cervical vertebral body (list separately in addition to code for primary procedure)

◆ **S2400** Repair, congenital diaphragmatic hernia in the fetus using temporary tracheal occlusion, procedure performed in utero ♀ A

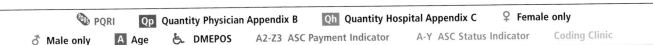

PQRI · Qp Quantity Physician Appendix B · Qh Quantity Hospital Appendix C · ♀ Female only · ♂ Male only · A Age · DMEPOS · A2-Z3 ASC Payment Indicator · A-Y ASC Status Indicator · Coding Clinic

321

◆ **S2401**   Repair, urinary tract obstruction in the fetus, procedure performed in utero ♀ A

◆ **S2402**   Repair, congenital cystic adenomatoid malformation in the fetus, procedure performed in utero ♀ A

◆ **S2403**   Repair, extralobar pulmonary sequestration in the fetus, procedure performed in utero ♀ A

◆ **S2404**   Repair, myelomeningocele in the fetus, procedure performed in utero ♀ A

◆ **S2405**   Repair of sacrococcygeal teratoma in the fetus, procedure performed in utero ♀ A

◆ **S2409**   Repair, congenital malformation of fetus, procedure performed in utero, not otherwise classified ♀ A

◆ **S2411**   Fetoscopic laser therapy for treatment of twin-to-twin transfusion syndrome A

◆ **S2900**   Surgical techniques requiring use of robotic surgical system (list separately in addition to code for primary procedure)

Coding Clinic: 2010, Q2, P6

◆ **S3000**   Diabetic indicator; retinal eye exam, dilated, bilateral

◆ **S3005**   Performance measurement, evaluation of patient self assessment, depression

◆ **S3600**   STAT laboratory request (situations other than S3601)

◆ **S3601**   Emergency STAT laboratory charge for patient who is homebound or residing in a nursing facility

◆ **S3620**   Newborn metabolic screening panel, includes test kit, postage and the laboratory tests specified by the state for inclusion in this panel (e.g. galactose; hemoglobin, electrophoresis; hydroxyprogesterone, 17-D; phenylalanine (PKU); and thyroxine, total) A

◆ **S3625**   Maternal serum triple marker screen including alpha-fetoprotein (AFP), estriol, and human chorionic gonadotropin (HCG) ♀

◆ **S3626**   Maternal serum quadruple marker screen including alpha-fetoprotein (AFP), estriol, human chorionic gonadotropin (HCG) and inhibin a ♀

~~S3628   Placental alpha microglobulin-1 rapidimmunoassay for detection of rupture of fetal membranes~~   ✖

◆ **S3630**   Eosinophil count, blood, direct

◆ **S3645**   HIV-1 antibody testing of oral mucosal transudate

◆ **S3650**   Saliva test, hormone level; during menopause ♀

◆ **S3652**   Saliva test, hormone level; to assess preterm labor risk ♀

◆ **S3655**   Antisperm antibodies test (immunobead) ♀

◆ **S3708**   Gastrointestinal fat absorption study

◆ **S3711**   Circulating tumor cell test

◆ **S3713**   KRAS mutation analysis testing

▶ ◆ **S3722**   Dose optimization by area under the curve (AUC) analysis, for infusional 5-fluorouracil

◆ **S3800**   Genetic testing for amyotrophic lateral sclerosis (ALS)

◆ **S3818**   Complete gene sequence analysis; BRCA1 gene

◆ **S3819**   Complete gene sequence analysis; BRCA2 gene

◆ **S3820**   Complete BRCA1 and BRCA2 gene sequence analysis for susceptibility to breast and ovarian cancer ♀

◆ **S3822**   Single mutation analysis (in individual with a known BRCA1 or BRCA2 mutation in the family) for susceptibility to breast and ovarian cancer

◆ **S3823**   Three-mutation BRCA1 and BRCA2 analysis for susceptibility to breast and ovarian cancer in Ashkenazi individuals ♀

◆ **S3828**   Complete gene sequence analysis; MLH1 gene

◆ **S3829**   Complete gene sequence analysis; MSH2 gene

◆ **S3830**   Complete MLH and MSH2 gene sequence analysis for hereditary nonpolyposis colorectal cancer (HNPCC) genetic testing

◆ **S3831**   Single-mutation analysis (in individual with a known MLH and MSH2 mutation in the family) for hereditary nonpolyposis colorectal cancer (HNPCC) genetic testing

◆ **S3833**   Complete APC gene sequence analysis for susceptibility to familial adenomatous polyposis (FAP) and attenuated FAP

◆ **S3834**   Single-mutation analysis (in individual with a known APC mutation in the family) for susceptibility to familial adenomatous polyposis (FAP) and attenuated FAP

▶ New   → Revised   ✔ Reinstated   ~~deleted~~ Deleted
⊗ Special coverage instructions   ◆ Not covered or valid by Medicare   ✳ Carrier discretion

◆ **S3835**   Complete gene sequence analysis for cystic fibrosis genetic testing

◆ **S3837**   Complete gene sequence analysis for hemochromatosis genetic testing

◆ **S3840**   DNA analysis for germline mutations of the RET proto-oncogene for susceptibility to multiple endocrine neoplasia type 2

◆ **S3841**   Genetic testing for retinoblastoma

◆ **S3842**   Genetic testing for von Hippel-Lindau disease

◆ **S3843**   DNA analysis of the F5 gene for susceptibility to Factor V Leiden thrombophilia

◆ **S3844**   DNA analysis of the connexin 26 gene (GJB2) for susceptibility to congenital, profound deafness

◆ **S3845**   Genetic testing for alpha-thalassemia

◆ **S3846**   Genetic testing for hemoglobin E beta-thalassemia

◆ **S3847**   Genetic testing for Tay-Sachs disease

◆ **S3848**   Genetic testing for Gaucher disease

◆ **S3849**   Genetic testing for Niemann-Pick disease

◆ **S3850**   Genetic testing for sickle cell anemia

◆ **S3851**   Genetic testing for Canavan disease

◆ **S3852**   DNA analysis for APOE epilson 4 allele for susceptibility to Alzheimer's disease

◆ **S3853**   Genetic testing for myotonic muscular dystrophy

◆ **S3854**   Gene expression profiling panel for use in the management of breast cancer treatment ♀

◆ **S3855**   Genetic testing for detection of mutations in the presenilin - 1 gene

◆ **S3860**   Genetic testing, comprehensive cardiac ion channel analysis, for variants in 5 major cardiac ion channel genes for individuals with high index of suspicion for familial long QT syndrome (LQTS) or related syndromes

◆ **S3861**   Genetic testing, sodium channel, voltage-gated, type V, alpha subunit (SCN5A) and variants for suspected Brugada syndrome

◆ **S3862**   Genetic testing, family-specific ion channel analysis, for blood-relatives of individuals (index case) who have previously tested positive for a genetic variant of a cardiac ion channel syndrome using either one of the above test configurations or confirmed results from another laboratory

◆ **S3865**   Comprehensive gene sequence analysis for hypertrophic cardiomyopathy

◆ **S3866**   Genetic analysis for a specific gene mutation for hypertrophic cardiomyopathy (HCM) in an individual with a known HCM mutation in the family

◆ **S3870**   Comparative genomic hybrization (CGH) microarray testing for developmental delay, autism spectrum disorder and/or mental retardation

◆ **S3890**   DNA analysis, fecal, for colorectal cancer screening

◆ **S3900**   Surface electromyography (EMG)

◆ **S3902**   Ballistrocardiogram

◆ **S3904**   Masters two step

Bill on paper. Requires a report.

~~S3905   Non-invasive electrodiagnostic testing with automatic computerized hand-held device to stimulate and measure neuromuscular signals in diagnosing and evaluating systemic and entrapment neuropathies~~ ✖

◆ **S4005**   Interim labor facility global (labor occurring but not resulting in delivery) ♀

◆ **S4011**   In vitro fertilization; including but not limited to identification and incubation of mature oocytes, fertilization with sperm, incubation of embryo(s), and subsequent visualization for determination of development ♀

◆ **S4013**   Complete cycle, gamete intrafallopian transfer (GIFT), case rate ♀

◆ **S4014**   Complete cycle, zygote intrafallopian transfer (ZIFT), case rate ♀

◆ **S4015**   Complete in vitro fertilization cycle, not otherwise specified, case rate ♀

◆ **S4016**   Frozen in vitro fertilization cycle, case rate ♀

◆ **S4017**   Incomplete cycle, treatment cancelled prior to stimulation, case rate ♀

◆ **S4018**   Frozen embryo transfer procedure cancelled before transfer, case rate ♀

(PQRI) PQRI	Qp Quantity Physician Appendix B	Qh Quantity Hospital Appendix C	♀ Female only
♂ Male only A Age ⴲ DMEPOS	A2-Z3 ASC Payment Indicator	A-Y ASC Status Indicator	Coding Clinic

◆ **S4020** In vitro fertilization procedure cancelled before aspiration, case rate ♀

◆ **S4021** In vitro fertilization procedure cancelled after aspiration, case rate ♀

◆ **S4022** Assisted oocyte fertilization, case rate ♀

◆ **S4023** Donor egg cycle, incomplete, case rate ♀

◆ **S4025** Donor services for in vitro fertilization (sperm or embryo), case rate

◆ **S4026** Procurement of donor sperm from sperm bank ♂

◆ **S4027** Storage of previously frozen embryos ♀

◆ **S4028** Microsurgical epididymal sperm aspiration (MESA) ♂

◆ **S4030** Sperm procurement and cryopreservation services; initial visit ♂

◆ **S4031** Sperm procurement and cryopreservation services; subsequent visit ♂

◆ **S4035** Stimulated intrauterine insemination (IUI), case rate ♀

◆ **S4037** Cryopreserved embryo transfer, case rate ♀

◆ **S4040** Monitoring and storage of cryopreserved embryos, per 30 days ♀

◆ **S4042** Management of ovulation induction (interpretation of diagnostic tests and studies, non-face-to-face medical management of the patient), per cycle ♀

◆ **S4981** Insertion of levonorgestrel-releasing intrauterine system ♀

◆ **S4989** Contraceptive intrauterine device (e.g. Progestasert IUD), including implants and supplies ♀

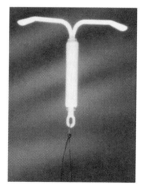

Figure 54 IUD.

◆ **S4990** Nicotine patches, legend

◆ **S4991** Nicotine patches, non-legend

◆ **S4993** Contraceptive pills for birth control ♀
  Only billed by Family Planning Clinics

◆ **S4995** Smoking cessation gum

◆ **S5000** Prescription drug, generic

◆ **S5001** Prescription drug, brand name

◆ **S5010** 5% dextrose and 0.45% normal saline, **1000 ml**

◆ **S5011** 5% dextrose in lactated Ringer's, **1000 ml**

◆ **S5012** 5% dextrose with potassium chloride, **1000 ml**

◆ **S5013** 5% dextrose/0.45% normal saline with potassium chloride and magnesium sulfate, **1000 ml**

◆ **S5014** 5% dextrose/0.45% normal saline with potassium chloride and magnesium sulfate, **1500 ml**

◆ **S5035** Home infusion therapy, routine service of infusion device (e.g. pump maintenance)

◆ **S5036** Home infusion therapy, repair of infusion device (e.g. pump repair)

◆ **S5100** Day care services, adult; per 15 minutes **A**

◆ **S5101** Day care services, adult; per half day **A**

◆ **S5102** Day care services, adult; per diem **A**

◆ **S5105** Day care services, center-based; services not included in program fee, per diem

◆ **S5108** Home care training to home care client, per 15 minutes

◆ **S5109** Home care training to home care client, per session

◆ **S5110** Home care training, family; per 15 minutes

◆ **S5111** Home care training, family; per session

◆ **S5115** Home care training, non-family; per 15 minutes

◆ **S5116** Home care training, non-family; per session

◆ **S5120** Chore services; per 15 minutes

◆ **S5121** Chore services; per diem

◆ **S5125** Attendant care services; per 15 minutes

◆ **S5126** Attendant care services; per diem

▶ New   → Revised   ✔ Reinstated   ~~deleted~~ Deleted
⊙ Special coverage instructions   ◆ Not covered or valid by Medicare   ✳ Carrier discretion

◆ **S5130** Homemaker service, NOS; per 15 minutes

◆ **S5131** Homemaker service, NOS; per diem

◆ **S5135** Companion care, adult (e.g. IADL/ADL); per 15 minutes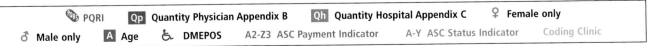

◆ **S5136** Companion care, adult (e.g. IADL/ADL); per diem A

◆ **S5140** Foster care, adult; per diem A

◆ **S5141** Foster care, adult; per month A

◆ **S5145** Foster care, therapeutic, child; per diem A

◆ **S5146** Foster care, therapeutic, child; per month A

◆ **S5150** Unskilled respite care, not hospice; per 15 minutes

◆ **S5151** Unskilled respite care, not hospice; per diem

◆ **S5160** Emergency response system; installation and testing

◆ **S5161** Emergency response system; service fee, per month (excludes installation and testing)

◆ **S5162** Emergency response system; purchase only

◆ **S5165** Home modifications; per service

◆ **S5170** Home delivered meals, including preparation; per meal

◆ **S5175** Laundry service, external, professional; per order

◆ **S5180** Home health respiratory therapy, initial evaluation

◆ **S5181** Home health respiratory therapy, NOS, per diem

◆ **S5185** Medication reminder service, non-face-to-face; per month

◆ **S5190** Wellness assessment, performed by non-physician

◆ **S5199** Personal care item, NOS, each

◆ **S5497** Home infusion therapy, catheter care/maintenance, not otherwise classified; includes administrative services, professional pharmacy services, care coordination, and all necessary supplies and equipment (drugs and nursing visits coded separately), per diem

◆ **S5498** Home infusion therapy, catheter care/maintenance, simple (single lumen), includes administrative services, professional pharmacy services, care coordination and all necessary supplies and equipment, (drugs and nursing visits coded separately), per diem

◆ **S5501** Home infusion therapy, catheter care/maintenance, complex (more than one lumen), includes administrative services, professional pharmacy services, care coordination, and all necessary supplies and equipment (drugs and nursing visits coded separately), per diem

◆ **S5502** Home infusion therapy, catheter care/maintenance, implanted access device, includes administrative services, professional pharmacy services, care coordination, and all necessary supplies and equipment, (drugs and nursing visits coded separately), per diem (use this code for interim maintenance of vascular access not currently in use)

◆ **S5517** Home infusion therapy, all supplies necessary for restoration of catheter patency or declotting

◆ **S5518** Home infusion therapy, all supplies necessary for catheter repair

◆ **S5520** Home infusion therapy, all supplies (including catheter) necessary for a peripherally inserted central venous catheter (PICC) line insertion

Bill on paper. Requires a report.

◆ **S5521** Home infusion therapy, all supplies (including catheter) necessary for a midline catheter insertion

◆ **S5522** Home infusion therapy, insertion of peripherally inserted central venous catheter (PICC), nursing services only (no supplies or catheter included)

◆ **S5523** Home infusion therapy, insertion of midline central venous catheter, nursing services only (no supplies or catheter included)

◆ **S5550** Insulin, rapid onset, **5 units**

◆ **S5551** Insulin, most rapid onset (Lispro or Aspart); **5 units**

◆ **S5552** Insulin, intermediate acting (NPH or Lente); **5 units**

◆ **S5553** Insulin, long acting; **5 units**

◆ **S5560** Insulin delivery device, reusable pen; **1.5 ml** size

◆ **S5561** Insulin delivery device, reusable pen; **3 ml** size

◆ **S5565** Insulin cartridge for use in insulin delivery device other than pump; **150 units**

◆ **S5566** Insulin cartridge for use in insulin delivery device other than pump; **300 units**

◆ **S5570** Insulin delivery device, disposable pen (including insulin); **1.5 ml** size

◆ **S5571** Insulin delivery device, disposable pen (including insulin); **3 ml** size

◆ **S8030** Scleral application of tantalum ring(s) for localization of lesions for proton beam therapy

◆ **S8035** Magnetic source imaging

◆ **S8037** Magnetic resonance cholangiopancreatography (MRCP)

◆ **S8040** Topographic brain mapping

◆ **S8042** Magnetic resonance imaging (MRI), low-field

◆ **S8049** Intraoperative radiation therapy (single administration)

◆ **S8055** Ultrasound guidance for multifetal pregnancy reduction(s), technical component (only to be used when the physician doing the reduction procedure does not perform the ultrasound, guidance is included in the CPT code for multifetal pregnancy reduction - 59866) ♀

◆ **S8080** Scintimammography (radioimmunoscintigraphy of the breast), unilateral, including supply of radiopharmaceutical ♀

◆ **S8085** Fluorine-18 fluorodeoxyglucose (F-18 FDG) imaging using dual-head coincidence detection system (non-dedicated PET scan)

◆ **S8092** Electron beam computed tomography (also known as ultrafast CT, cine CT)

◆ **S8096** Portable peak flow meter

◆ **S8097** Asthma kit (including but not limited to portable peak expiratory flow meter, instructional video, brochure, and/or spacer)

◆ **S8100** Holding chamber or spacer for use with an inhaler or nebulizer; without mask

◆ **S8101** Holding chamber or spacer for use with an inhaler or nebulizer; with mask

◆ **S8110** Peak expiratory flow rate (physician services)

◆ **S8120** Oxygen contents, gaseous, 1 unit equals 1 cubic foot

◆ **S8121** Oxygen contents, liquid, 1 unit equals 1 pound

▶◆ **S8130** Interferential current stimulator, 2 channel

▶◆ **S8131** Interferential current stimulator, 4 channel

◆ **S8185** Flutter device

◆ **S8186** Swivel adaptor

◆ **S8189** Tracheostomy supply, not otherwise classified

◆ **S8210** Mucus trap

◆ **S8262** Mandibular orthopedic repositioning device, each

◆ **S8265** Haberman feeder for cleft lip/palate

◆ **S8270** Enuresis alarm, using auditory buzzer and/or vibration device

◆ **S8301** Infection control supplies, not otherwise specified

◆ **S8415** Supplies for home delivery of infant **A**

◆ **S8420** Gradient pressure aid (sleeve and glove combination), custom made

◆ **S8421** Gradient pressure aid (sleeve and glove combination), ready made

◆ **S8422** Gradient pressure aid (sleeve), custom made, medium weight

◆ **S8423** Gradient pressure aid (sleeve), custom made, heavy weight

◆ **S8424** Gradient pressure aid (sleeve), ready made

◆ **S8425** Gradient pressure aid (glove), custom made, medium weight

◆ **S8426** Gradient pressure aid (glove), custom made, heavy weight

◆ **S8427** Gradient pressure aid (glove), ready made

◆ **S8428** Gradient pressure aid (gauntlet), ready made

◆ **S8429** Gradient pressure exterior wrap

◆ **S8430** Padding for compression bandage, roll

◆ **S8431** Compression bandage, roll

◆ **S8450** Splint, prefabricated, digit (specify digit by use of modifier)

◆ **S8451** Splint, prefabricated, wrist or ankle

◆ **S8452** Splint, prefabricated, elbow

◆ **S8460** Camisole, post-mastectomy

◆ **S8490** Insulin syringes (100 syringes, any size)

◆ **S8940** Equestrian/Hippotherapy, per session

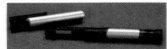

Figure 55 Nova Pen.

▶ New   → Revised   ✔ Reinstated   ~~deleted~~ Deleted

○ Special coverage instructions   ◆ Not covered or valid by Medicare   ✳ Carrier discretion

◆ **S8948**   Application of a modality (requiring constant provider attendance) to one or more areas; low-level laser; each 15 minutes

◆ **S8950**   Complex lymphedema therapy, each 15 minutes

◆ **S8990**   Physical or manipulative therapy performed for maintenance rather than restoration

◆ **S8999**   Resuscitation bag (for use by patient on artificial respiration during power failure or other catastrophic event)

◆ **S9001**   Home uterine monitor with or without associated nursing services ♀

◆ **S9007**   Ultrafiltration monitor

◆ **S9015**   Automated EEG monitoring

◆ **S9024**   Paranasal sinus ultrasound

◆ **S9025**   Omnicardiogram/cardiointegram

◆ **S9034**   Extracorporeal shockwave lithotripsy for gall stones (if performed with ERCP, use 43265)

◆ **S9055**   Procuren or other growth factor preparation to promote wound healing

◆ **S9056**   Coma stimulation per diem

◆ **S9061**   Home administration of aerosolized drug therapy (e.g., pentamidine); administrative services, professional pharmacy services, care coordination, all necessary supplies and equipment (drugs and nursing visits coded separately), per diem

~~S9075   Smoking cessation treatment~~ ✖

◆ **S9083**   Global fee urgent care centers

◆ **S9088**   Services provided in an urgent care center (list in addition to code for service)

◆ **S9090**   Vertebral axial decompression, per session

◆ **S9097**   Home visit for wound care

◆ **S9098**   Home visit, phototherapy services (e.g. Bili-Lite), including equipment rental, nursing services, blood draw, supplies, and other services, per diem

◆ **S9109**   Congestive heart failure telemonitoring, equipment rental, including telescale, computer system and software, telephone connections, and maintenance, per month

◆ **S9117**   Back school, per visit

◆ **S9122**   Home health aide or certified nurse assistant, providing care in the home; per hour

◆ **S9123**   Nursing care, in the home; by registered nurse, per hour (use for general nursing care only, not to be used when CPT codes 99500-99602 can be used)

◆ **S9124**   Nursing care, in the home; by licensed practical nurse, per hour

◆ **S9125**   Respite care, in the home, per diem

◆ **S9126**   Hospice care, in the home, per diem

◆ **S9127**   Social work visit, in the home, per diem

◆ **S9128**   Speech therapy, in the home, per diem

◆ **S9129**   Occupational therapy, in the home, per diem

◆ **S9131**   Physical therapy; in the home, per diem

◆ **S9140**   Diabetic management program, follow-up visit to non-MD provider

◆ **S9141**   Diabetic management program, follow-up visit to MD provider

◆ **S9145**   Insulin pump initiation, instruction in initial use of pump (pump not included)

◆ **S9150**   Evaluation by ocularist

◆ **S9152**   Speech therapy, re-evaluation

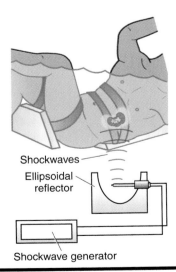

Shockwaves
Ellipsoidal reflector
Shockwave generator

Figure 56   Extracorporeal shockwave lithotripsy (ESWL).

ⓅQRS PQRI	Qp **Quantity Physician Appendix B**	Qh **Quantity Hospital Appendix C**	♀ **Female only**
♂ **Male only** A **Age** ♿ **DMEPOS**	A2-Z3 **ASC Payment Indicator**	A-Y **ASC Status Indicator**	Coding Clinic

◆ **S9208** Home management of preterm labor, including administrative services, professional pharmacy services, care coordination, and all necessary supplies or equipment (drugs and nursing visits coded separately), per diem (do not use this code with any home infusion per diem code) ♀

◆ **S9209** Home management of preterm premature rupture of membranes (PPROM), including administrative services, professional pharmacy services, care coordination, and all necessary supplies or equipment (drugs and nursing visits coded separately), per diem (do not use this code with any home infusion per diem code) ♀

◆ **S9211** Home management of gestational hypertension, includes administrative services, professional pharmacy services, care coordination, and all necessary supplies and equipment (drugs and nursing visits coded separately); per diem (do not use this code with any home infusion per diem code) ♀

◆ **S9212** Home management of postpartum hypertension, includes administrative services, professional pharmacy services, care coordination, and all necessary supplies and equipment (drugs and nursing visits coded separately), per diem (do not use this code with any home infusion per diem code) ♀

◆ **S9213** Home management of preeclampsia, includes administrative services, professional pharmacy services, care coordination, and all necessary supplies and equipment (drugs and nursing services coded separately); per diem (do not use this code with any home infusion per diem code) ♀

◆ **S9214** Home management of gestational diabetes, includes administrative services, professional pharmacy services, care coordination, and all necessary supplies and equipment (drugs and nursing visits coded separately); per diem (do not use this code with any home infusion per diem code) ♀

◆ **S9325** Home infusion therapy, pain management infusion; administrative services, professional pharmacy services, care coordination, and all necessary supplies and equipment, (drugs and nursing visits coded separately), per diem (do not use this code with S9326, S9327 or S9328)

◆ **S9326** Home infusion therapy, continuous (twenty-four hours or more) pain management infusion; administrative services, professional pharmacy services, care coordination, and all necessary supplies and equipment (drugs and nursing visits coded separately), per diem

◆ **S9327** Home infusion therapy, intermittent (less than twenty-four hours) pain management infusion; administrative services, professional pharmacy services, care coordination, and all necessary supplies and equipment (drugs and nursing visits coded separately), per diem

◆ **S9328** Home infusion therapy, implanted pump pain management infusion; administrative services, professional pharmacy services, care coordination, and all necessary supplies and equipment (drugs and nursing visits coded separately), per diem

◆ **S9329** Home infusion therapy, chemotherapy infusion; administrative services, professional pharmacy services, care coordination, and all necessary supplies and equipment (drugs and nursing visits coded separately), per diem (do not use this code with S9330 or S9331)

◆ **S9330** Home infusion therapy, continuous (twenty-four hours or more) chemotherapy infusion; administrative services, professional pharmacy services, care coordination, and all necessary supplies and equipment (drugs and nursing visits coded separately), per diem

◆ **S9331** Home infusion therapy, intermittent (less than twenty-four hours) chemotherapy infusion; administrative services, professional pharmacy services, care coordination, and all necessary supplies and equipment (drugs and nursing visits coded separately), per diem

◆ **S9335** Home therapy, hemodialysis; administrative services, professional pharmacy services, care coordination, and all necessary supplies and equipment (drugs and nursing services coded separately), per diem

▶ New   → Revised   ✔ Reinstated   ~~deleted~~ Deleted
✪ Special coverage instructions   ◆ Not covered or valid by Medicare   ✳ Carrier discretion

◆ **S9336** Home infusion therapy, continuous anticoagulant infusion therapy (e.g. heparin), administrative services, professional pharmacy services, care coordination, and all necessary supplies and equipment (drugs and nursing visits coded separately), per diem

◆ **S9338** Home infusion therapy, immunotherapy, administrative services, professional pharmacy services, care coordination, and all necessary supplies and equipment (drug and nursing visits coded separately), per diem

◆ **S9339** Home therapy; peritoneal dialysis, administrative services, professional pharmacy services, care coordination and all necessary supplies and equipment (drugs and nursing visits coded separately), per diem

◆ **S9340** Home therapy; enteral nutrition; administrative services, professional pharmacy services, care coordination, and all necessary supplies and equipment (enteral formula and nursing visits coded separately), per diem

◆ **S9341** Home therapy; enteral nutrition via gravity; administrative services, professional pharmacy services, care coordination, and all necessary supplies and equipment (enteral formula and nursing visits coded separately), per diem

◆ **S9342** Home therapy; enteral nutrition via pump; administrative services, professional pharmacy services, care coordination, and all necessary supplies and equipment (enteral formula and nursing visits coded separately), per diem

◆ **S9343** Home therapy; enteral nutrition via bolus; administrative services, professional pharmacy services, care coordination, and all necessary supplies and equipment (enteral formula and nursing visits coded separately), per diem

◆ **S9345** Home infusion therapy, anti-hemophilic agent infusion therapy (e.g. Factor VIII); administrative services, professional pharmacy services, care coordination, and all necessary supplies and equipment (drugs and nursing visits coded separately), per diem

◆ **S9346** Home infusion therapy, alpha-1-proteinase inhibitor (e.g., Prolastin); administrative services, professional pharmacy services, care coordination, and all necessary supplies and equipment (drugs and nursing visits coded separately), per diem

◆ **S9347** Home infusion therapy, uninterrupted, long-term, controlled rate intravenous or subcutaneous infusion therapy (e.g. Epoprostenol); administrative services, professional pharmacy services, care coordination, and all necessary supplies and equipment (drugs and nursing visits coded separately), per diem

◆ **S9348** Home infusion therapy, sympathomimetic/inotropic agent infusion therapy (e.g., Dobutamine); administrative services, professional pharmacy services, care coordination, all necessary supplies and equipment (drugs and nursing visits coded separately), per diem

◆ **S9349** Home infusion therapy, tocolytic infusion therapy; administrative services, professional pharmacy services, care coordination, and all necessary supplies and equipment (drugs and nursing visits coded separately), per diem

◆ **S9351** Home infusion therapy, continuous or intermittent anti-emetic infusion therapy; administrative services, professional pharmacy services, care coordination, and all necessary supplies and equipment (drugs and visits coded separately), per diem

◆ **S9353** Home infusion therapy, continuous insulin infusion therapy; administrative services, professional pharmacy services, care coordination, and all necessary supplies and equipment (drugs and nursing visits coded separately), per diem

◆ **S9355** Home infusion therapy, chelation therapy; administrative services, professional pharmacy services, care coordination, and all necessary supplies and equipment (drugs and nursing visits coded separately), per diem

◆ **S9357** Home infusion therapy, enzyme replacement intravenous therapy; (e.g. Imiglucerase); administrative services, professional pharmacy services, care coordination, and all necessary supplies and equipment (drugs and nursing visits coded separately), per diem

PQRI	**Qp** Quantity Physician Appendix B	**Qh** Quantity Hospital Appendix C	♀ Female only
♂ Male only	**A** Age ♿ DMEPOS	A2-Z3 ASC Payment Indicator A-Y ASC Status Indicator	Coding Clinic

◆ **S9359** Home infusion therapy, anti-tumor necrosis factor intravenous therapy; (e.g. Infliximab); administrative services, professional pharmacy services, care coordination, and all necessary supplies and equipment (drugs and nursing visits coded separately), per diem

◆ **S9361** Home infusion therapy, diuretic intravenous therapy; administrative services, professional pharmacy services, care coordination, and all necessary supplies and equipment (drugs and nursing visits coded separately), per diem

◆ **S9363** Home infusion therapy, anti-spasmotic therapy; administrative services, professional pharmacy services, care coordination, and all necessary supplies and equipment (drugs and nursing visits coded separately), per diem

◆ **S9364** Home infusion therapy, total parenteral nutrition (TPN); administrative services, professional pharmacy services, care coordination, and all necessary supplies and equipment including standard TPN formula (lipids, specialty amino acid formulas, drugs other than in standard formula, and nursing visits coded separately) per diem (do not use with home infusion codes S9365-S9368 using daily volume scales)

◆ **S9365** Home infusion therapy, total parenteral nutrition (TPN); one liter per day, administrative services, professional pharmacy services, care coordination, and all necessary supplies and equipment including standard TPN formula (lipids, specialty amino acid formulas, drugs other than in standard formula and nursing visits coded separately), per diem

◆ **S9366** Home infusion therapy, total parenteral nutrition (TPN); more than one liter but no more than two liters per day, administrative services, professional pharmacy services, care coordination, and all necessary supplies and equipment including standard TPN formula; (lipids, specialty amino acid formulas, drugs other than in standard formula and nursing visits coded separately), per diem

◆ **S9367** Home infusion therapy, total parenteral nutrition (TPN); more than two liters but no more than three liters per day, administrative services, professional pharmacy services, care coordination, and all necessary supplies and equipment including standard TPN formula; (lipids, specialty amino acid formulas, drugs other than in standard formula and nursing visits coded separately), per diem

◆ **S9368** Home infusion therapy, total parenteral nutrition (TPN); more than three liters per day, administrative services, professional pharmacy services, care coordination, and all necessary supplies and equipment (including standard TPN formula; lipids, specialty amino acid formulas, drugs other than in standard formula and nursing visits coded separately), per diem

◆ **S9370** Home therapy, intermittent anti-emetic injection therapy; administrative services, professional pharmacy services, care coordination, and all necessary supplies and equipment (drugs and nursing visits coded separately), per diem

◆ **S9372** Home therapy; intermittent anticoagulant injection therapy (e.g., heparin); administrative services, professional pharmacy services, care coordination, and all necessary supplies and equipment (drugs and nursing visits coded separately), per diem (do not use this code for flushing of infusion devices with heparin to maintain patency)

◆ **S9373** Home infusion therapy, hydration therapy; administrative services, professional pharmacy services, care coordination, and all necessary supplies and equipment (drugs and nursing visits coded separately), per diem (do not use with hydration therapy codes S9374-S9377 using daily volume scales)

◆ **S9374** Home infusion therapy, hydration therapy; one liter per day, administrative services, professional pharmacy services, care coordination, and all necessary supplies and equipment (drugs and nursing visits coded separately), per diem

◆ **S9375** Home infusion therapy, hydration therapy; more than one liter but no more than two liters per day, administrative services, professional pharmacy services, care coordination, and all necessary supplies and equipment (drugs and nursing visits coded separately), per diem

◆ **S9376** Home infusion therapy, hydration therapy; more than two liters but no more than three liters per day, administrative services, professional pharmacy services, care coordination, and all necessary supplies and equipment (drugs and nursing visits coded separately), per diem

◆ **S9377** Home infusion therapy, hydration therapy; more than three liters per day, administrative services, professional pharmacy services, care coordination, and all necessary supplies (drugs and nursing visits coded separately), per diem

◆ **S9379** Home infusion therapy, infusion therapy, not otherwise classified; administrative services, professional pharmacy services, care coordination, and all necessary supplies and equipment (drugs and nursing visits coded separately), per diem

◆ **S9381** Delivery or service to high risk areas requiring escort or extra protection, per visit

◆ **S9401** Anticoagulation clinic, inclusive of all services except laboratory tests, per session

◆ **S9430** Pharmacy compounding and dispensing services

◆ **S9433** Medical food nutritionally complete, administered orally, providing 100% of nutritional intake

◆ **S9434** Modified solid food supplements for inborn errors of metabolism

◆ **S9435** Medical foods for inborn errors of metabolism

◆ **S9436** Childbirth preparation/Lamaze classes, non-physician provider, per session ♀

◆ **S9437** Childbirth refresher classes, non-physician provider, per session ♀

◆ **S9438** Cesarean birth classes, non-physician provider, per session ♀

◆ **S9439** VBAC (vaginal birth after cesarean) classes, non-physician provider, per session ♀

◆ **S9441** Asthma education, non-physician provider, per session

◆ **S9442** Birthing classes, non-physician provider, per session ♀

◆ **S9443** Lactation classes, non-physician provider, per session ♀

◆ **S9444** Parenting classes, non-physician provider, per session

◆ **S9445** Patient education, not otherwise classified, non-physician provider, individual, per session

◆ **S9446** Patient education, not otherwise classified, non-physician provider, group, per session

◆ **S9447** Infant safety (including CPR) classes, non-physician provider, per session

◆ **S9449** Weight management classes, non-physician provider, per session

◆ **S9451** Exercise classes, non-physician provider, per session

◆ **S9452** Nutrition classes, non-physician provider, per session

◆ **S9453** Smoking cessation classes, non-physician provider, per session

◆ **S9454** Stress management classes, non-physician provider, per session

◆ **S9455** Diabetic management program, group session

◆ **S9460** Diabetic management program, nurse visit

◆ **S9465** Diabetic management program, dietitian visit

◆ **S9470** Nutritional counseling, dietitian visit

◆ **S9472** Cardiac rehabilitation program, non-physician provider, per diem

◆ **S9473** Pulmonary rehabilitation program, non-physician provider, per diem

◆ **S9474** Enterostomal therapy by a registered nurse certified in enterostomal therapy, per diem

◆ **S9475** Ambulatory setting substance abuse treatment or detoxification services, per diem

◆ **S9476** Vestibular rehabilitation program, non-physician provider, per diem

◆ **S9480** Intensive outpatient psychiatric services, per diem

◆ **S9482** Family stabilization services, per 15 minutes

◆ **S9484** Crisis intervention mental health services, per hour

◆ **S9485** Crisis intervention mental health services, per diem

---

◆ **S9490** Home infusion therapy, corticosteroid infusion; administrative services, professional pharmacy services, care coordination, and all necessary supplies and equipment (drugs and nursing visits coded separately), per diem

◆ **S9494** Home infusion therapy, antibiotic, antiviral, or antifungal therapy; administrative services, professional pharmacy services, care coordination, and all necessary supplies and equipment (drugs and nursing visits coded separately) per diem, (do not use this code with home infusion codes for hourly dosing schedules S9497-S9504)

◆ **S9497** Home infusion therapy, antibiotic, antiviral, or antifungal therapy; once every 3 hours; administrative services, professional pharmacy services, care coordination, and all necessary supplies and equipment (drugs and nursing visits coded separately), per diem

◆ **S9500** Home infusion therapy, antibiotic, antiviral, or antifungal therapy; once every 24 hours; administrative services, professional pharmacy services, care coordination, and all necessary supplies and equipment (drugs and nursing visits coded separately), per diem

◆ **S9501** Home infusion therapy, antibiotic, antiviral, or antifungal therapy; once every 12 hours; administrative services, professional pharmacy services, care coordination, and all necessary supplies and equipment (drugs and nursing visits coded separately), per diem

◆ **S9502** Home infusion therapy, antibiotic, antiviral, or antifungal therapy; once every 8 hours, administrative services, professional pharmacy services, care coordination, and all necessary supplies and equipment (drugs and nursing visits coded separately), per diem

◆ **S9503** Home infusion therapy, antibiotic, antiviral, or antifungal; once every 6 hours; administrative services, professional pharmacy services, care coordination, and all necessary supplies and equipment (drugs and nursing visits coded separately), per diem

◆ **S9504** Home infusion therapy, antibiotic, antiviral, or antifungal; once every 4 hours; administrative services, professional pharmacy services, care coordination, and all necessary supplies and equipment (drugs and nursing visits coded separately), per diem

◆ **S9529** Routine venipuncture for collection of specimen(s), single home bound, nursing home, or skilled nursing facility patient

◆ **S9537** Home therapy; hematopoietic hormone injection therapy (e.g. erythropoietin, G-CSF, GM-CSF); administrative services, professional pharmacy services, care coordination, and all necessary supplies and equipment (drugs and nursing visits coded separately), per diem

◆ **S9538** Home transfusion of blood product(s); administrative services, professional pharmacy services, care coordination, and all necessary supplies and equipment (blood products, drugs, and nursing visits coded separately), per diem

◆ **S9542** Home injectable therapy; not otherwise classified, including administrative services, professional pharmacy services, care coordination, and all necessary supplies and equipment (drugs and nursing visits coded separately), per diem

◆ **S9558** Home injectable therapy; growth hormone, including administrative services, professional pharmacy services, care coordination, and all necessary supplies and equipment (drugs and nursing visits coded separately), per diem

◆ **S9559** Home injectable therapy; interferon, including administrative services, professional pharmacy services, care coordination, and all necessary supplies and equipment (drugs and nursing visits coded separately), per diem

◆ **S9560** Home injectable therapy; hormonal therapy (e.g., Leuprolide, Goserelin), including administrative services, professional pharmacy services, care coordination, and all necessary supplies and equipment (drugs and nursing visits coded separately), per diem

◆ **S9562** Home injectable therapy, palivizumab, including administrative services, professional pharmacy services, care coordination, and all necessary supplies and equipment (drugs and nursing visits coded separately), per diem

---

▶ New → Revised ✔ Reinstated ~~deleted~~ Deleted
⊙ Special coverage instructions ◆ Not covered or valid by Medicare ✳ Carrier discretion

◆ **S9590** Home therapy, irrigation therapy (e.g. sterile irrigation of an organ or anatomical cavity); including administrative services, professional pharmacy services, care coordination, and all necessary supplies and equipment (drugs and nursing visits coded separately), per diem

◆ **S9810** Home therapy; professional pharmacy services for provision of infusion, specialty drug administration, and/or disease state management, not otherwise classified, per hour (do not use this code with any per diem code)

→ ◆ **S9900** Services by journal-listed Christian Science Practitioner for the purpose of healing, per diem

◆ **S9970** Health club membership, annual

◆ **S9975** Transplant related lodging, meals and transportation, per diem

◆ **S9976** Lodging, per diem, not otherwise classified

◆ **S9977** Meals, per diem, not otherwise specified

◆ **S9981** Medical records copying fee, administrative

◆ **S9982** Medical records copying fee, per page

◆ **S9986** Not medically necessary service (patient is aware that service not medically necessary)

◆ **S9988** Services provided as part of a Phase I clinical trial

◆ **S9989** Services provided outside of the United States of America (list in addition to code(s) for services(s))

◆ **S9990** Services provided as part of a Phase II clinical trial

◆ **S9991** Services provided as part of a Phase III clinical trial

◆ **S9992** Transportation costs to and from trial location and local transportation costs (e.g., fares for taxicab or bus) for clinical trial participant and one caregiver/companion

◆ **S9994** Lodging costs (e.g., hotel charges) for clinical trial participant and one caregiver/companion

◆ **S9996** Meals for clinical trial participant and one caregiver/companion

◆ **S9999** Sales tax

🄟 PQRI	Qp **Quantity Physician Appendix B**	Qh **Quantity Hospital Appendix C**	♀ **Female only**
♂ **Male only**	A **Age**	♿ **DMEPOS**	A2-Z3 **ASC Payment Indicator** A-Y **ASC Status Indicator** Coding Clinic

TEMPORARY NATIONAL CODES ESTABLISHED BY PRIVATE PAYERS   S9590 – S9999

333

TEMPORARY NATIONAL CODES ESTABLISHED BY MEDICAID (T1000-T9999)

Not Valid For Medicare

◆ **T1000**   Private duty/independent nursing service(s) - licensed, up to 15 minutes

◆ **T1001**   Nursing assessment/evaluation

◆ **T1002**   RN services, up to 15 minutes

◆ **T1003**   LPN/LVN services, up to 15 minutes

◆ **T1004**   Services of a qualified nursing aide, up to 15 minutes

◆ **T1005**   Respite care services, up to 15 minutes

◆ **T1006**   Alcohol and/or substance abuse services, family/couple counseling

◆ **T1007**   Alcohol and/or substance abuse services, treatment plan development and/or modification

◆ **T1009**   Child sitting services for children of the individual receiving alcohol and/or substance abuse services

◆ **T1010**   Meals for individuals receiving alcohol and/or substance abuse services (when meals not included in the program)

◆ **T1012**   Alcohol and/or substance abuse services, skills development

◆ **T1013**   Sign language or oral interpretive services, per 15 minutes

◆ **T1014**   Telehealth transmission, per minute, professional services bill separately

◆ **T1015**   Clinic visit/encounter, all-inclusive

◆ **T1016**   Case Management, each 15 minutes

◆ **T1017**   Targeted Case Management, each 15 minutes

◆ **T1018**   School-based individualized education program (IEP) services, bundled

◆ **T1019**   Personal care services, per 15 minutes, not for an inpatient or resident of a hospital, nursing facility, ICF/MR or IMD, part of the individualized plan of treatment (code may not be used to identify services provided by home health aide or certified nurse assistant)

◆ **T1020**   Personal care services, per diem, not for an inpatient or resident of a hospital, nursing facility, ICF/MR or IMD, part of the individualized plan of treatment (code may not be used to identify services provided by home health aide or certified nurse assistant)

◆ **T1021**   Home health aide or certified nurse assistant, per visit

◆ **T1022**   Contracted home health agency services, all services provided under contract, per day

◆ **T1023**   Screening to determine the appropriateness of consideration of an individual for participation in a specified program, project or treatment protocol, per encounter

◆ **T1024**   Evaluation and treatment by an integrated, specialty team contracted to provide coordinated care to multiple or severely handicapped children, per encounter **A**

◆ **T1025**   Intensive, extended multidisciplinary services provided in a clinic setting to children with complex medical, physical, mental and psychosocial impairments, per diem **A**

◆ **T1026**   Intensive, extended multidisciplinary services provided in a clinic setting to children with complex medical, physical, medical and psychosocial impairments, per hour **A**

◆ **T1027**   Family training and counseling for child development, per 15 minutes

◆ **T1028**   Assessment of home, physical and family environment, to determine suitability to meet patient's medical needs

◆ **T1029**   Comprehensive environmental lead investigation, not including laboratory analysis, per dwelling

◆ **T1030**   Nursing care, in the home, by registered nurse, per diem

◆ **T1031**   Nursing care, in the home, by licensed practical nurse, per diem

◆ **T1502**   Administration of oral, intramuscular and/or subcutaneous medication by health care agency/professional, per visit

◆ **T1503**   Administration of medication, other than oral and/or injectable, by a health care agency/professional, per visit

◆ **T1505**   Electronic medication compliance management device, includes all components and accessories, not otherwise classified

---

▶ **New**   ➡ **Revised**   ✔ **Reinstated**   ~~deleted~~ **Deleted**

⊙ **Special coverage instructions**   ◆ **Not covered or valid by Medicare**   ✳ **Carrier discretion**

◆ **T1999** Miscellaneous therapeutic items and supplies, retail purchases, not otherwise classified; identify product in "remarks"

◆ **T2001** Non-emergency transportation; patient attendant/escort

◆ **T2002** Non-emergency transportation; per diem

◆ **T2003** Non-emergency transportation; encounter/trip

◆ **T2004** Non-emergency transport; commercial carrier, multi-pass

◆ **T2005** Non-emergency transportation: stretcher van

◆ **T2007** Transportation waiting time, air ambulance and non-emergency vehicle, one-half (1/2) hour increments

◆ **T2010** Preadmission screening and resident review (PASRR) level I identification screening, per screen

◆ **T2011** Preadmission screening and resident review (PASRR) level II evaluation, per evaluation

◆ **T2012** Habilitation, educational, waiver; per diem

◆ **T2013** Habilitation, educational, waiver; per hour

◆ **T2014** Habilitation, prevocational, waiver; per diem

◆ **T2015** Habilitation, prevocational, waiver; per hour

◆ **T2016** Habilitation, residential, waiver; per diem

◆ **T2017** Habilitation, residential, waiver; 15 minutes

◆ **T2018** Habilitation, supported employment, waiver; per diem

◆ **T2019** Habilitation, supported employment, waiver; per 15 minutes

◆ **T2020** Day habilitation, waiver; per diem

◆ **T2021** Day habilitation, waiver; per 15 minutes

◆ **T2022** Case management, per month

◆ **T2023** Targeted case management; per month

◆ **T2024** Service assessment/plan of care development, waiver

◆ **T2025** Waiver services; not otherwise specified (NOS)

◆ **T2026** Specialized childcare, waiver; per diem

◆ **T2027** Specialized childcare, waiver; per 15 minutes

◆ **T2028** Specialized supply, not otherwise specified, waiver

◆ **T2029** Specialized medical equipment, not otherwise specified, waiver

◆ **T2030** Assisted living, waiver; per month

◆ **T2031** Assisted living; waiver, per diem

◆ **T2032** Residential care, not otherwise specified (NOS), waiver; per month

◆ **T2033** Residential care, not otherwise specified (NOS), waiver; per diem

◆ **T2034** Crisis intervention, waiver; per diem

◆ **T2035** Utility services to support medical equipment and assistive technology/devices, waiver

◆ **T2036** Therapeutic camping, overnight, waiver; each session

◆ **T2037** Therapeutic camping, day, waiver; each session

◆ **T2038** Community transition, waiver; per service

◆ **T2039** Vehicle modifications, waiver; per service

◆ **T2040** Financial management, self-directed, waiver; per 15 minutes

◆ **T2041** Supports brokerage, self-directed, waiver; per 15 minutes

◆ **T2042** Hospice routine home care; per diem

◆ **T2043** Hospice continuous home care; per hour

◆ **T2044** Hospice inpatient respite care; per diem

◆ **T2045** Hospice general inpatient care; per diem

◆ **T2046** Hospice long term care, room and board only; per diem

◆ **T2048** Behavioral health; long-term care residential (non-acute care in a residential treatment program where stay is typically longer than 30 days), with room and board, per diem

◆ **T2049** Non-emergency transportation; stretcher van, mileage; per mile

◆ **T2101** Human breast milk processing, storage and distribution only ♀

◆ **T4521** Adult sized disposable incontinence product, brief/diaper, small, each

IOM: 100-03, 4, 280.1

◆ **T4522** Adult sized disposable incontinence product, brief/diaper, medium, each

IOM: 100-03, 4, 280.1

◆ **T4523** Adult sized disposable incontinence product, brief/diaper, large, each

IOM: 100-03, 4, 280.1

◆ **T4524** Adult sized disposable incontinence product, brief/diaper, extra large, each

IOM: 100-03, 4, 280.1

◆ **T4525** Adult sized disposable incontinence product, protective underwear/pull-on, small size, each

IOM: 100-03, 4, 280.1

◆ **T4526** Adult sized disposable incontinence product, protective underwear/pull-on, medium size, each

IOM: 100-03, 4, 280.1

◆ **T4527** Adult sized disposable incontinence product, protective underwear/pull-on, large size, each

IOM: 100-03, 4, 280.1

◆ **T4528** Adult sized disposable incontinence product, protective underwear/pull-on, extra large size, each

IOM: 100-03, 4, 280.1

◆ **T4529** Pediatric sized disposable incontinence product, brief/diaper, small/medium size, each A

IOM: 100-03, 4, 280.1

◆ **T4530** Pediatric sized disposable incontinence product, brief/diaper, large size, each A

IOM: 100-03, 4, 280.1

◆ **T4531** Pediatric sized disposable incontinence product, protective underwear/pull-on, small/medium size, each A

IOM: 100-03, 4, 280.1

◆ **T4532** Pediatric sized disposable incontinence product, protective underwear/pull-on, large size, each A

IOM: 100-03, 4, 280.1

◆ **T4533** Youth sized disposable incontinence product, brief/diaper, each

IOM: 100-03, 4, 280.1

◆ **T4534** Youth sized disposable incontinence product, protective underwear/pull-on, each

IOM: 100-03, 4, 280.1

◆ **T4535** Disposable liner/shield/guard/pad/undergarment, for incontinence, each

IOM: 100-03, 4, 280.1

◆ **T4536** Incontinence product, protective underwear/pull-on, reusable, any size, each

IOM: 100-03, 4, 280.1

◆ **T4537** Incontinence product, protective underpad, reusable, bed size, each

IOM: 100-03, 4, 280.1

◆ **T4538** Diaper service, reusable diaper, each diaper

IOM: 100-03, 4, 280.1

◆ **T4539** Incontinence product, diaper/brief, reusable, any size, each

IOM: 100-03, 4, 280.1

◆ **T4540** Incontinence product, protective underpad, reusable, chair size, each

IOM: 100-03, 4, 280.1

◆ **T4541** Incontinence product, disposable underpad, large, each

◆ **T4542** Incontinence product, disposable underpad, small size, each

◆ **T4543** Disposable incontinence product, brief/diaper, bariatric, each

IOM: 100-03, 4, 280.1

◆ **T5001** Positioning seat for persons with special orthopedic needs, supply, not otherwise specified

◆ **T5999** Supply, not otherwise specified

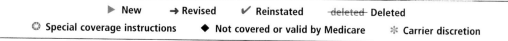

▶ New   → Revised   ✔ Reinstated   ~~deleted~~ Deleted
☺ Special coverage instructions   ◆ Not covered or valid by Medicare   ✳ Carrier discretion

VISION SERVICES (V0000-V2999)

Frames

V2020-V2025: Bill DME/MAC

⊙ **V2020** Frames, purchases `Qp` `Qh` ♿   A

Includes cost of frame/replacement and dispensing fee. One unit of service represents one frame.

IOM: 100-02, 15, 120

◆ **V2025** Deluxe frame   E

Not a benefit. Billing deluxe frames—submit V2020 on one line; V2025 on second line

IOM: 100-04, 1, 30.3.5

Spectacle Lenses

NOTE: If a CPT procedure code for supply of spectacles or a permanent prosthesis is reported, recode with the specific lens type listed below. For aphakic temporary spectacle correction, see CPT.

Single Vision, Glass or Plastic

✳ **V2100** Sphere, single vision, plano to plus or minus 4.00, per lens ♿   A

Bill DME/MAC

✳ **V2101** Sphere, single vision, plus or minus 4.12 to plus or minus 7.00d, per lens `Qp` `Qh` ♿   A

Bill DME/MAC

✳ **V2102** Sphere, single vision, plus or minus 7.12 to plus or minus 20.00d, per lens `Qp` `Qh` ♿   A

Bill DME/MAC

✳ **V2103** Spherocylinder, single vision, plano to plus or minus 4.00d sphere, .12 to 2.00d cylinder, per lens ♿   A

Bill DME/MAC

✳ **V2104** Spherocylinder, single vision, plano to plus or minus 4.00d sphere, 2.12 to 4.00d cylinder, per lens `Qp` `Qh` ♿   A

Bill DME/MAC

✳ **V2105** Spherocylinder, single vision, plano to plus or minus 4.00d sphere, 4.25 to 6.00d cylinder, per lens `Qp` `Qh` ♿   A

Bill DME/MAC

✳ **V2106** Spherocylinder, single vision, plano to plus or minus 4.00d sphere, over 6.00d cylinder, per lens `Qp` `Qh` ♿   A

Bill DME/MAC

✳ **V2107** Spherocylinder, single vision, plus or minus 4.25 to plus or minus 7.00 sphere, .12 to 2.00d cylinder, per lens `Qp` `Qh` ♿   A

Bill DME/MAC

✳ **V2108** Spherocylinder, single vision, plus or minus 4.25d to plus or minus 7.00d sphere, 2.12 to 4.00d cylinder, per lens `Qp` `Qh` ♿   A

Bill DME/MAC

✳ **V2109** Spherocylinder, single vision, plus or minus 4.25 to plus or minus 7.00 sphere, 4.25 to 6.00d cylinder, per lens `Qp` `Qh` ♿   A

Bill DME/MAC

✳ **V2110** Sperocylinder, single vision, plus or minus 4.25 to 7.00d sphere, over 6.00d cylinder, per lens `Qp` `Qh` ♿   A

Bill DME/MAC

✳ **V2111** Spherocylinder, single vision, plus or minus 7.25 to plus or minus 12.00d sphere, .25 to 2.25d cylinder, per lens `Qp` `Qh` ♿   A

Bill DME/MAC

✳ **V2112** Spherocylinder, single vision, plus or minus 7.25 to plus or minus 12.00d sphere, 2.25d to 4.00d cylinder, per lens `Qp` `Qh` ♿   A

Bill DME/MAC

✳ **V2113** Spherocylinder, single vision, plus or minus 7.25 to plus or minus 12.00d sphere, 4.25 to 6.00d cylinder, per lens `Qp` `Qh` ♿   A

Bill DME/MAC

✳ **V2114** Spherocylinder, single vision, sphere over plus or minus 12.00d, per lens `Qp` `Qh` ♿   A

Bill DME/MAC

✳ **V2115** Lenticular, (myodisc), per lens, single vision `Qp` `Qh` ♿   A

Bill DME/MAC

✳ **V2118** Aniseikonic lens, single vision `Qp` `Qh` ♿   A

Bill DME/MAC

⊙ **V2121** Lenticular lens, per lens, single `Qp` `Qh` ♿   A

Bill DME/MAC

IOM: 100-02, 15, 120; 100-04, 3, 10.4

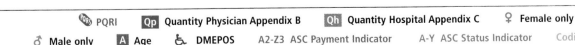

Ⓟ PQRI	`Qp` Quantity Physician Appendix B	`Qh` Quantity Hospital Appendix C	♀ Female only
♂ Male only `A` Age ♿ DMEPOS	A2-Z3 ASC Payment Indicator	A-Y ASC Status Indicator	Coding Clinic

✳ **V2199** Not otherwise classified, single vision lens
A

Bill DME/MAC

Bill on paper. Requires report of type of single vision lens and optical lab invoice.

Bifocal, Glass or Plastic

✳ **V2200** Sphere, bifocal, plano to plus or minus 4.00d, per lens `Qp` `Qh` ♿
A

Bill DME/MAC

✳ **V2201** Sphere, bifocal, plus or minus 4.12 to plus or minus 7.00d, per lens `Qp` `Qh` ♿
A

Bill DME/MAC

✳ **V2202** Sphere, bifocal, plus or minus 7.12 to plus or minus 20.00d, per lens `Qp` `Qh` ♿
A

Bill DME/MAC

✳ **V2203** Spherocylinder, bifocal, plano to plus or minus 4.00d sphere, .12 to 2.00d cylinder, per lens `Qp` `Qh` ♿
A

Bill DME/MAC

✳ **V2204** Spherocylinder, bifocal, plano to plus or minus 4.00d sphere, 2.12 to 4.00d cylinder, per lens `Qp` `Qh` ♿
A

Bill DME/MAC

✳ **V2205** Spherocylinder, bifocal, plano to plus or minus 4.00d sphere, 4.25 to 6.00d cylinder, per lens `Qp` `Qh` ♿
A

Bill DME/MAC

✳ **V2206** Spherocylinder, bifocal, plano to plus or minus 4.00d sphere, over 6.00d cylinder, per lens `Qp` `Qh` ♿
A

Bill DME/MAC

✳ **V2207** Spherocylinder, bifocal, plus or minus 4.25 to plus or minus 7.00d sphere, .12 to 2.00d cylinder, per lens `Qp` `Qh` ♿
A

Bill DME/MAC

✳ **V2208** Spherocylinder, bifocal, plus or minus 4.25 to plus or minus 7.00d sphere, 2.12 to 4.00d cylinder, per lens `Qp` `Qh` ♿
A

Bill DME/MAC

✳ **V2209** Spherocylinder, bifocal, plus or minus 4.25 to plus or minus 7.00d sphere, 4.25 to 6.00d cylinder, per lens `Qp` `Qh` ♿
A

Bill DME/MAC

✳ **V2210** Spherocylinder, bifocal, plus or minus 4.25 to plus or minus 7.00d sphere, over 6.00d cylinder, per lens `Qp` `Qh` ♿
A

Bill DME/MAC

✳ **V2211** Spherocylinder, bifocal, plus or minus 7.25 to plus or minus 12.00d sphere, .25 to 2.25d cylinder, per lens `Qp` `Qh` ♿
A

Bill DME/MAC

✳ **V2212** Spherocylinder, bifocal, plus or minus 7.25 to plus or minus 12.00d sphere, 2.25 to 4.00d cylinder, per lens `Qp` `Qh` ♿
A

Bill DME/MAC

✳ **V2213** Spherocylinder, bifocal, plus or minus 7.25 to plus or minus 12.00d sphere, 4.25 to 6.00d cylinder, per lens `Qp` `Qh` ♿
A

Bill DME/MAC

✳ **V2214** Spherocylinder, bifocal, sphere over plus or minus 12.00d, per lens `Qp` `Qh` ♿
A

Bill DME/MAC

✳ **V2215** Lenticular (myodisc), per lens, bifocal `Qp` `Qh` ♿
A

Bill DME/MAC

✳ **V2218** Aniseikonic, per lens, bifocal `Qp` `Qh` ♿
A

Bill DME/MAC

✳ **V2219** Bifocal seg width over 28mm `Qp` `Qh` ♿
A

Bill DME/MAC

✳ **V2220** Bifocal add over 3.25d `Qp` `Qh` ♿
A

Bill DME/MAC

⊙ **V2221** Lenticular lens, per lens, bifocal `Qp` `Qh` ♿
A

Bill DME/MAC

IOM: 100-02, 15, 120; 100-04, 3, 10.4

✳ **V2299** Specialty bifocal (by report) `Qp` `Qh`
A

Bill DME/MAC

Bill on paper. Requires report of type of specialty bifocal lens and optical lab invoice.

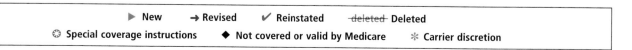

▶ New   → Revised   ✔ Reinstated   ~~deleted~~ Deleted
⊙ Special coverage instructions   ◆ Not covered or valid by Medicare   ✳ Carrier discretion

V2199 – V2299 VISION SERVICES

Trifocal, Glass or Plastic

✳ **V2300** Sphere, trifocal, plano to plus or minus 4.00d, per lens `Qp` `Qh` ♿   A

    Bill DME/MAC

✳ **V2301** Sphere, trifocal, plus or minus 4.12 to plus or minus 7.00d per lens `Qp` `Qh` ♿   A

    Bill DME/MAC

✳ **V2302** Sphere, trifocal, plus or minus 7.12 to plus or minus 20.00, per lens `Qp` `Qh` ♿   A

    Bill DME/MAC

✳ **V2303** Spherocylinder, trifocal, plano to plus or minus 4.00d sphere, .12 to 2.00d cylinder, per lens `Qp` `Qh` ♿   A

    Bill DME/MAC

✳ **V2304** Spherocylinder, trifocal, plano to plus or minus 4.00d sphere, 2.25-4.00d cylinder, per lens `Qp` `Qh` ♿   A

    Bill DME/MAC

✳ **V2305** Spherocylinder, trifocal, plano to plus or minus 4.00d sphere, 4.25 to 6.00 cylinder, per lens `Qp` `Qh` ♿   A

    Bill DME/MAC

✳ **V2306** Spherocylinder, trifocal, plano to plus or minus 4.00d sphere, over 6.00d cylinder, per lens `Qp` `Qh` ♿   A

    Bill DME/MAC

✳ **V2307** Spherocylinder, trifocal, plus or minus 4.25 to plus or minus 7.00d sphere, .12 to 2.00d cylinder, per lens `Qp` `Qh` ♿   A

    Bill DME/MAC

✳ **V2308** Spherocylinder, trifocal, plus or minus 4.25 to plus or minus 7.00d sphere, 2.12 to 4.00d cylinder, per lens `Qp` `Qh` ♿   A

    Bill DME/MAC

✳ **V2309** Spherocylinder, trifocal, plus or minus 4.25 to plus or minus 7.00d sphere, 4.25 to 6.00d cylinder, per lens `Qp` `Qh` ♿   A

    Bill DME/MAC

✳ **V2310** Spherocylinder, trifocal, plus or minus 4.25 to plus or minus 7.00d sphere, over 6.00d cylinder, per lens `Qp` `Qh` ♿   A

    Bill DME/MAC

✳ **V2311** Spherocylinder, trifocal, plus or minus 7.25 to plus or minus 12.00d sphere, .25 to 2.25d cylinder, per lens `Qp` `Qh` ♿   A

    Bill DME/MAC

✳ **V2312** Spherocylinder, trifocal, plus or minus 7.25 to plus or minus 12.00d sphere, 2.25 to 4.00d cylinder, per lens `Qp` `Qh` ♿   A

    Bill DME/MAC

✳ **V2313** Spherocylinder, trifocal, plus or minus 7.25 to plus or minus 12.00d sphere, 4.25 to 6.00d cylinder, per lens `Qp` `Qh` ♿   A

    Bill DME/MAC

✳ **V2314** Spherocylinder, trifocal, sphere over plus or minus 12.00d, per lens `Qp` `Qh` ♿   A

    Bill DME/MAC

✳ **V2315** Lenticular, (myodisc), per lens, trifocal `Qp` `Qh`   A

    Bill DME/MAC

✳ **V2318** Aniseikonic lens, trifocal `Qp` `Qh` ♿   A

    Bill DME/MAC

✳ **V2319** Trifocal seg width over 28 mm `Qp` `Qh` ♿   A

    Bill DME/MAC

✳ **V2320** Trifocal add over 3.25d `Qp` `Qh` ♿   A

    Bill DME/MAC

◑ **V2321** Lenticular lens, per lens, trifocal `Qp` `Qh` ♿   A

    Bill DME/MAC

    IOM: 100-02, 15, 120; 100-04, 3, 10.4

✳ **V2399** Specialty trifocal (by report) `Qp` `Qh`   A

    Bill DME/MAC

    Bill on paper. Requires report of type of trifocal lens and optical lab invoice.

Variable Asphericity

✳ **V2410** Variable asphericity lens, single vision, full field, glass or plastic, per lens `Qp` `Qh` ♿   A

    Bill DME/MAC

✳ **V2430** Variable asphericity lens, bifocal, full field, glass or plastic, per lens `Qp` `Qh` ♿   A

    Bill DME/MAC

✳ **V2499** Variable sphericity lens, other type   A

    Bill DME/MAC

    Bill on paper. Requires report of other type of lens and optical lab invoice.

🅟 PQRI	`Qp` Quantity Physician Appendix B	`Qh` Quantity Hospital Appendix C	♀ Female only
♂ Male only	`A` Age	♿ DMEPOS	A2-Z3 ASC Payment Indicator A-Y ASC Status Indicator Coding Clinic

Contact Lenses

If a CPT procedure code for supply of contact lens is reported, recode with specific lens type listed below (per lens).

✳ **V2500** Contact lens, PMMA, spherical, per lens `Qp` `Qh` ♿   A

Bill DME/MAC

Requires prior authorization for patients under age 21.

✳ **V2501** Contact lens, PMMA, toric or prism ballast, per lens `Qp` `Qh` ♿   A

Bill DME/MAC

Requires prior authorization for clients under age 21.

✳ **V2502** Contact lens PMMA, bifocal, per lens `Qp` `Qh` ♿   A

Bill DME/MAC

Requires prior authorization for clients under age 21. Bill on paper. Requires optical lab invoice.

✳ **V2503** Contact lens PMMA, color vision deficiency, per lens `Qp` `Qh` ♿   A

Bill DME/MAC

Requires prior authorization for clients under age 21. Bill on paper. Requires optical lab invoice.

✳ **V2510** Contact lens, gas permeable, spherical, per lens `Qp` `Qh` ♿   A

Bill DME/MAC

Requires prior authorization for clients under age 21.

✳ **V2511** Contact lens, gas permeable, toric, prism ballast, per lens `Qp` `Qh` ♿   A

Bill DME/MAC

Requires prior authorization for clients under age 21.

✳ **V2512** Contact lens, gas permeable, bifocal, per lens `Qp` `Qh` ♿   A

Bill DME/MAC

Requires prior authorization for clients under age 21.

✳ **V2513** Contact lens, gas permeable, extended wear, per lens `Qp` `Qh` ♿   A

Bill DME/MAC

Requires prior authorization for clients under age 21.

☮ **V2520** Contact lens, hydrophilic, spherical, per lens `Qp` `Qh` ♿   A

If "incident to" a physician service, do not bill; otherwise, bill DME/MAC

Requires prior authorization for clients under age 21.

IOM: 100-03, 1, 80.1; 100-03, 1, 80.4

☮ **V2521** Contact lens, hydrophilic, toric, or prism ballast, per lens `Qp` `Qh` ♿   A

If "incident to" a physician's service, do not bill; otherwise, bill DME/MAC.

Requires prior authorization for clients under age 21.

IOM: 100-03, 1, 80.1; 100-03, 1, 80.4

☮ **V2522** Contact lens, hydrophilic, bifocal, per lens `Qp` `Qh` ♿   A

If "incident to" a physician's service, do not bill; otherwise, bill DME/MAC.

Requires prior authorization for clients under age 21.

IOM: 100-03, 1, 80.1; 100-03, 1, 80.4

☮ **V2523** Contact lens, hydrophilic, extended wear, per lens `Qp` `Qh` ♿   A

If "incident to" a physician's service, do not bill; otherwise, bill DME/MAC.

Requires prior authorization for clients under age 21.

IOM: 100-03, 1, 80.1; 100-03, 1, 80.4

✳ **V2530** Contact lens, scleral, gas impermeable, per lens (for contact lens modification, see 92325) `Qp` `Qh` ♿   A

Bill DME/MAC

Requires prior authorization for clients under age 21.

☮ **V2531** Contact lens, scleral, gas permeable, per lens (for contact lens modification, see 92325) `Qp` `Qh` ♿   A

Bill DME/MAC

Requires prior authorization for clients under age 21. Bill on paper. Requires optical lab invoice.

IOM: 100-03, 1, 80.5

✳ **V2599** Contact lens, other type   A

If "incident to" a physician's service, do not bill; otherwise, bill DME/MAC.

Requires prior authorization for clients under age 21. Bill on paper. Requires report of other type of contact lens and optical invoice.

▶ New   → Revised   ✔ Reinstated   deleted Deleted

☮ Special coverage instructions   ◆ Not covered or valid by Medicare   ✳ Carrier discretion

Low Vision Aids

If a CPT procedure code for supply of low vision aid is reported, recode with specific systems listed below.

✳ **V2600**   Hand held low vision aids and other nonspectacle mounted aids `Qp` `Qh`   A

Bill DME/MAC

Requires prior authorization.

✳ **V2610**   Single lens spectacle mounted low vision aids `Qp` `Qh`   A

Bill DME/MAC

Requires prior authorization.

✳ **V2615**   Telescopic and other compound lens system, including distance vision telescopic, near vision telescopes and compound microscopic lens system `Qp` `Qh`   A

Bill DME/MAC

Requires prior authorization. Bill on paper. Requires optical lab invoice.

Prosthetic Eye

⊕ **V2623**   Prosthetic eye, plastic, custom `Qp` `Qh` ♿   A

Bill DME/MAC

DME regional carrier. Requires prior authorization. Bill on paper. Requires optical lab invoice.

✳ **V2624**   Polishing/resurfacing of ocular prosthesis `Qp` `Qh` ♿   A

Bill DME/MAC

Requires prior authorization. Bill on paper. Requires optical lab invoice.

✳ **V2625**   Enlargement of ocular prosthesis `Qp` `Qh` ♿   A

Bill DME/MAC

Requires prior authorization. Bill on paper. Requires optical lab invoice.

✳ **V2626**   Reduction of ocular prosthesis `Qp` `Qh` ♿   A

Bill DME/MAC

Requires prior authorization. Bill on paper. Requires optical lab invoice.

⊕ **V2627**   Scleral cover shell `Qp` `Qh` ♿   A

Bill DME/MAC

DME regional carrier

Requires prior authorization. Bill on paper. Requires optical lab invoice.

IOM: 100-03, 4, 280.2

✳ **V2628**   Fabrication and fitting of ocular conformer `Qp` `Qh` ♿   A

Bill DME/MAC

Requires prior authorization. Bill on paper. Requires optical lab invoice.

✳ **V2629**   Prosthetic eye, other type `Qp` `Qh`   A

Bill DME/MAC

Requires prior authorization. Bill on paper. Requires optical lab invoice.

Intraocular Lenses

⊕ **V2630**   Anterior chamber intraocular lens `Qp` `Qh`   N1   N

Bill local carrier

IOM: 100-02, 15, 120

⊕ **V2631**   Iris supported intraocular lens `Qp` `Qh`   N1   N

Bill local carrier

IOM: 100-02, 15, 120

Figure 57   Posterior intraocular lens.

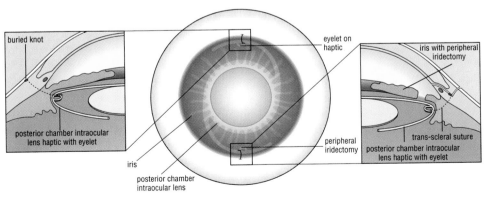

⊕ **V2632** Posterior chamber intraocular lens `Qp` `Qh` — N1 N
Bill local carrier
IOM: 100-02, 15, 120

Miscellaneous

✳ **V2700** Balance lens, per lens `Qp` `Qh` & — A
Bill DME/MAC

◆ **V2702** Deluxe lens feature — E
Bill DME/MAC
IOM: 100-02, 15, 120; 100-04, 3, 10.4

✳ **V2710** Slab off prism, glass or plastic, per lens `Qp` `Qh` & — A
Bill DME/MAC

✳ **V2715** Prism, per lens & — A
Bill DME/MAC

✳ **V2718** Press-on lens, Fresnel prism, per lens `Qp` `Qh` & — A
Bill DME/MAC

✳ **V2730** Special base curve, glass or plastic, per lens `Qp` `Qh` & — A
Bill DME/MAC

⊕ **V2744** Tint, photochromatic, per lens & — A
Bill DME/MAC
Requires prior authorization.
IOM: 100-02, 15, 120; 100-04, 3, 10.4

⊕ **V2745** Addition to lens, tint, any color, solid, gradient or equal, excludes photochroatic, any lens material, per lens & — A
Bill DME/MAC
Includes photochromatic lenses (V2744) used as sunglasses, which are prescribed in addition to regular prosthetic lenses for aphakic patient will be denied as not medically necessary.
IOM: 100-02, 15, 120; 100-04, 3, 10.4

⊕ **V2750** Anti-reflective coating, per lens & — A
Bill DME/MAC
Requires prior authorization.
IOM: 100-02, 15, 120; 100-04, 3, 10.4

⊕ **V2755** U-V lens, per lens & — A
Bill DME/MAC
IOM: 100-02, 15, 120; 100-04, 3, 10.4

✳ **V2756** Eye glass case — E
Bill DME/MAC

✳ **V2760** Scratch resistant coating, per lens & — A
Bill DME/MAC

⊕ **V2761** Mirror coating, any type, solid, gradient or equal, any lens material, per lens `Qp` — B
Bill DME/MAC
IOM: 100-02, 15, 120; 100-04, 3, 10.4

⊕ **V2762** Polarization, any lens material, per lens & — A
Bill DME/MAC
IOM: 100-02, 15, 120; 100-04, 3, 10.4

✳ **V2770** Occluder lens, per lens `Qp` `Qh` & — A
Bill DME/MAC
Requires prior authorization.

✳ **V2780** Oversize lens, per lens `Qp` `Qh` & — A
Bill DME/MAC
Requires prior authorization.

✳ **V2781** Progressive lens, per lens `Qp` — B
Bill DME/MAC
Requires prior authorization.

⊕ **V2782** Lens, index 1.54 to 1.65 plastic or 1.60 to 1.79 glass, excludes polycarbonate, per lens `Qp` `Qh` & — A
Bill DME/MAC
Do not bill in addition to V2784
IOM: 100-02, 15, 120; 100-04, 3, 10.4

⊕ **V2783** Lens, index greater than or equal to 1.66 plastic or greater than or equal to 1.80 glass, excludes polycarbonate, per lens `Qp` `Qh` & — A
Bill DME/MAC
Do not bill in addition to V2784
IOM: 100-02, 15, 120; 100-04, 3, 10.4

⊕ **V2784** Lens, polycarbonate or equal, any index, per lens & — A
Bill DME/MAC
Covered only for patients with functional vision in one eye—in this situation, an impact-resistant material is covered for both lenses if eyeglasses are covered. Claims with V2784 that do not meet this coverage criterion will be denied as not medically necessary.
IOM: 100-02, 15, 120; 100-04, 3, 10.4

✳ **V2785** Processing, preserving and transporting corneal tissue `Qp` `Qh` — F4 F
Bill local carrier
Bill on paper. Must attach eye bank invoice to claim.

▶ New → Revised ✔ Reinstated deleted Deleted
⊕ Special coverage instructions ◆ Not covered or valid by Medicare ✳ Carrier discretion

⚙ **V2786**   Specialty occupational multifocal lens, per lens ♿   A

Bill DME/MAC

IOM: 100-02, 15, 120; 100-04, 3, 10.4

◆ **V2787**   Astigmatism correcting function of intraocular lens   E

Bill local carrier

Medicare Statute 1862(a)(7)

◆ **V2788**   Presbyopia correcting function of intraocular lens   E

Bill local carrier

Medicare Statute 1862a7

✳ **V2790**   Amniotic membrane for surgical reconstruction, per procedure `Qp` `Qh`   N1 N

Bill local carrier

✳ **V2797**   Vision supply, accessory and/or service component of another HCPCS vision code `Qp` `Qh`   A

Bill DME/MAC

✳ **V2799**   Vision service, miscellaneous   A

Bill DME/MAC

Bill on paper. Requires report of miscellaneous service and optical lab invoice.

HEARING SERVICES (V5000-V5999)

NOTE: These codes are for non-physician services.

V5008-V5299:   Bill local carrier

◆ **V5008**   Hearing screening `Qp`   E

IOM: 100-02, 16, 90

◆ **V5010**   Assessment for hearing aid `Qp`   E

Medicare Statute 1862a7

◆ **V5011**   Fitting/orientation/checking of hearing aid `Qp`   E

Medicare Statute 1862a7

◆ **V5014**   Repair/modification of a hearing aid   E

Medicare Statute 1862a7

◆ **V5020**   Conformity evaluation   E

Medicare Statute 1862a7

◆ **V5030**   Hearing aid, monaural, body worn, air conduction   E

Medicare Statute 1862a7

◆ **V5040**   Hearing aid, monaural, body worn, bone conduction   E

Medicare Statute 1862a7

◆ **V5050**   Hearing aid, monaural, in the ear   E

Medicare Statute 1862a7

◆ **V5060**   Hearing aid, monaural, behind the ear   E

Medicare Statute 1862a7

◆ **V5070**   Glasses, air conduction   E

Medicare Statute 1862a7

◆ **V5080**   Glasses, bone conduction   E

Medicare Statute 1862a7

◆ **V5090**   Dispensing fee, unspecified hearing aid   E

Medicare Statute 1862a7

◆ **V5095**   Semi-implantable middle ear hearing prosthesis   E

Medicare Statute 1862a7

◆ **V5100**   Hearing aid, bilateral, body worn   E

Medicare Statute 1862a7

◆ **V5110**   Dispensing fee, bilateral   E

Medicare Statute 1862a7

◆ **V5120**   Binaural, body   E

Medicare Statute 1862a7

◆ **V5130**   Binaural, in the ear   E

Medicare Statute 1862a7

◆ **V5140**   Binaural, behind the ear   E

Medicare Statute 1862a7

◆ **V5150**   Binaural, glasses   E

Medicare Statute 1862a7

◆ **V5160**   Dispensing fee, binaural   E

Medicare Statute 1862a7

◆ **V5170**   Hearing aid, CROS, in the ear   E

Medicare Statute 1862a7

◆ **V5180**   Hearing aid, CROS, behind the ear   E

Medicare Statute 1862a7

◆ **V5190**   Hearing aid, CROS, glasses   E

Medicare Statute 1862a7

◆ **V5200**   Dispensing fee, CROS   E

Medicare Statute 1862a7

◆ **V5210**   Hearing aid, BICROS, in the ear   E

Medicare Statute 1862a7

◆ **V5220**   Hearing aid, BICROS, behind the ear   E

Medicare Statute 1862a7

◆ **V5230**   Hearing aid, BICROS, glasses   E

Medicare Statute 1862a7

PQRI	`Qp` Quantity Physician Appendix B	`Qh` Quantity Hospital Appendix C	♀ Female only
♂ Male only	`A` Age ♿ DMEPOS A2-Z3 ASC Payment Indicator	A-Y ASC Status Indicator	Coding Clinic

◆ **V5240** Dispensing fee, BICROS E
Medicare Statute 1862a7

◆ **V5241** Dispensing fee, monaural hearing aid, any type E
Medicare Statute 1862a7

◆ **V5242** Hearing aid, analog, monaural, CIC (completely in the ear canal) E
Medicare Statute 1862a7

◆ **V5243** Hearing aid, analog, monaural, ITC (in the canal) E
Medicare Statute 1862a9

◆ **V5244** Hearing aid, digitally programmable analog, monaural, CIC E
Medicare Statute 1862a7

◆ **V5245** Hearing aid, digitally programmable, analog, monaural, ITC E
Medicare Statute 1862a7

◆ **V5246** Hearing aid, digitally programmable analog, monaural, ITE (in the ear) E
Medicare Statute 1862a7

◆ **V5247** Hearing aid, digitally programmable analog, monaural, BTE (behind the ear) E
Medicare Statute 1862a7

◆ **V5248** Hearing aid, analog, binaural, CIC E
Medicare Statute 1862a7

◆ **V5249** Hearing aid, analog, binaural, ITC E
Medicare Statute 1862a7

◆ **V5250** Hearing aid, digitally programmable analog, binaural, CIC E
Medicare Statute 1862a7

◆ **V5251** Hearing aid, digitally programmable analog, binaural, ITC E
Medicare Statute 1862a7

◆ **V5252** Hearing aid, digitally programmable, binaural, ITE E
Medicare Statute 1862a7

◆ **V5253** Hearing aid, digitally programmable, binaural, BTE E
Medicare Statute 1862a7

◆ **V5254** Hearing aid, digital, monaural, CIC E
Medicare Statute 1862a7

◆ **V5255** Hearing aid, digital, monaural, ITC E
Medicare Statute 1862a7

◆ **V5256** Hearing aid, digital, monaural, ITE E
Medicare Statute 1862a7

◆ **V5257** Hearing aid, digital, monaural, BTE E
Medicare Statute 1862a7

◆ **V5258** Hearing aid, digital, binaural, CIC E
Medicare Statute 1862a7

◆ **V5259** Hearing aid, digital, binaural, ITC E
Medicare Statute 1862a7

◆ **V5260** Hearing aid, digital, binaural, ITE E
Medicare Statute 1862a7

◆ **V5261** Hearing aid, digital, binaural, BTE E
Medicare Statute 1862a7

◆ **V5262** Hearing aid, disposable, any type, monaural E
Medicare Statute 1862a7

◆ **V5263** Hearing aid, disposable, any type, binaural E
Medicare Statute 1862a7

◆ **V5264** Ear mold/insert, not disposable, any type E
Medicare Statute 1862a7

◆ **V5265** Ear mold/insert, disposable, any type E
Medicare Statute 1862a7

◆ **V5266** Battery for use in hearing device E
Medicare Statute 1862a7

◆ **V5267** Hearing aid supplies/accessories E
Medicare Statute 1862a7

◆ **V5268** Assistive listening device, telephone amplifier, any type E
Medicare Statute 1862a7

◆ **V5269** Assistive listening device, alerting, any type E
Medicare Statute 1862a7

◆ **V5270** Assistive listening device, television amplifier, any type E
Medicare Statute 1862a7

◆ **V5271** Assistive listening device, television caption decoder E
Medicare Statute 1862a7

◆ **V5272** Assistive listening device, TDD E
Medicare Statute 1862a7

◆ **V5273** Assistive listening device, for use with cochlear implant E
Medicare Statute 1862a7

◆ **V5274** Assistive listening device, not otherwise specified E
Medicare Statute 1862a7

▶ **New** → **Revised** ✔ **Reinstated** deleted **Deleted**

✪ **Special coverage instructions** ◆ **Not covered or valid by Medicare** ✳ **Carrier discretion**

V5240 – V5274 HEARING SERVICES

◆ **V5275**   Ear impression, each   E

Medicare Statute 1862a7

◆ **V5298**   Hearing aid, not otherwise classified   E

Medicare Statute 1862a7

✪ **V5299**   Hearing service, miscellaneous   B

IOM: 100-02, 16, 90

Speech-Language Pathology Services

NOTE: These codes are for non-physician services.

◆ **V5336**   Repair/modification of augmentative communicative system or device (excludes adaptive hearing aid)   E

Bill DME/MAC

Medicare Statute 1862a7

◆ **V5362**   Speech screening   E

Bill local carrier

Medicare Statute 1862a7

◆ **V5363**   Language screening   E

Bill local carrier

Medicare Statute 1862a7

◆ **V5364**   Dysphagia screening   E

Bill local carrier

Medicare Statute 1862a7

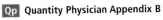 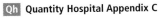

APPENDIX A

Physician/Provider Payment Edits

(Effective Date: 10/01/11-12/31/11, Version: 17.3)

Appendix B contains three sets of edits that provide guidance when reporting physician/provider services/procedures/supplies/equipment with HCPCS codes.

1. Practitioner/DME Supplier **Medically Unlikely Edits** (MUEs) units indicate the maximum allowable number of units of service per day, per patient. The purpose of the MUEs project is to detect and deny unlikely Medicare claims on a pre-payment basis in order to stop inappropriate payment. The MUE project is not meant to establish Medicare payment policy, but rather to improve the accuracy of the Medicare payments.

2. **Mutually Exclusive Code Edits** (MEEs) are National Correct Coding Initiative (NCCI) edits for physicians and list codes that are not reported together.

3. **Columns 1 and 2 Correct Coding Edits** are National Correct Coding Initiative (NCCI) edits for physicians and list codes that are not reported together.

2011 Practitioners/DME Suppliers Medically Unlikely Edits (MUEs)

CODE	MUE UNIT	CODE	MUE UNIT	CODE	MUE UNIT	CODE	MUE UNIT
A4221	1	A6511	1	A9545	1	E0140	1
A4253	1	A6513	1	A9546	1	E0141	1
A4255	1	A6545	2	A9550	1	E0143	1
A4258	1	A7017	1	A9551	1	E0144	1
A4259	1	A7020	1	A9552	1	E0147	1
A4470	1	A7025	1	A9553	1	E0148	1
A4480	1	A7026	1	A9554	1	E0149	1
A4557	2	A7027	1	A9555	3	E0153	2
A4561	1	A7035	1	A9557	2	E0154	2
A4562	1	A7036	1	A9559	1	E0155	1
A4614	1	A7039	1	A9560	2	E0156	1
A4640	1	A7040	2	A9561	1	E0157	2
A4642	1	A7041	2	A9562	2	E0158	1
A4650	3	A7042	2	A9566	1	E0163	1
A4660	1	A7043	2	A9567	2	E0165	1
A4663	1	A9284	1	A9569	1	E0167	1
A5500	2	A9500	3	A9570	1	E0168	1
A5501	2	A9501	3	A9571	1	E0170	1
A5503	2	A9502	3	A9580	1	E0171	1
A5505	2	A9503	1	A9582	1	E0175	2
A5506	2	A9504	1	A9604	1	E0181	1
A5507	2	A9507	1	A9700	2	E0182	1
A5508	2	A9510	1	E0100	1	E0184	1
A5510	2	A9521	2	E0105	1	E0185	1
A6501	1	A9526	2	E0110	1	E0186	1
A6502	1	A9536	1	E0111	2	E0187	1
A6503	1	A9537	1	E0112	1	E0188	1
A6504	2	A9538	1	E0113	2	E0189	1
A6505	2	A9539	2	E0114	1	E0193	1
A6506	2	A9540	2	E0116	2	E0194	1
A6507	2	A9541	1	E0117	2	E0196	1
A6508	2	A9542	1	E0118	2	E0197	1
A6509	1	A9543	1	E0130	1	E0198	1
A6510	1	A9544	1	E0135	1	E0199	1

CODE	MUE UNIT	CODE	MUE UNIT	CODE	MUE UNIT	CODE	MUE UNIT
E0200	1	E0350	1	E0585	1	E0693	1
E0202	1	E0371	1	E0600	1	E0694	1
E0205	1	E0372	1	E0601	1	E0705	1
E0210	1	E0373	1	E0605	1	E0720	1
E0215	1	E0424	1	E0606	1	E0730	1
E0217	1	E0431	1	E0607	1	E0731	1
E0218	1	E0434	1	E0610	1	E0740	1
E0225	1	E0439	1	E0615	1	E0744	1
E0235	1	E0441	1	E0616	1	E0745	1
E0236	1	E0442	1	E0617	1	E0746	1
E0239	1	E0443	1	E0618	1	E0747	1
E0249	1	E0444	1	E0619	1	E0748	1
E0250	1	E0450	2	E0620	1	E0749	1
E0251	1	E0455	1	E0621	1	E0755	1
E0255	1	E0457	1	E0627	1	E0760	1
E0256	1	E0459	1	E0628	1	E0762	1
E0260	1	E0460	1	E0629	1	E0764	1
E0261	1	E0461	1	E0630	1	E0765	1
E0265	1	E0462	1	E0635	1	E0776	1
E0266	1	E0463	1	E0636	1	E0779	1
E0270	1	E0464	1	E0637	1	E0780	1
E0271	1	E0470	1	E0638	1	E0781	1
E0272	1	E0471	1	E0639	1	E0782	1
E0275	1	E0472	1	E0640	1	E0783	1
E0276	1	E0480	1	E0641	1	E0784	1
E0277	1	E0481	1	E0642	1	E0785	1
E0280	1	E0482	1	E0650	1	E0786	1
E0290	1	E0483	1	E0651	1	E0791	1
E0291	1	E0484	1	E0652	1	E0840	1
E0292	1	E0485	1	E0655	2	E0849	1
E0293	1	E0486	1	E0656	1	E0850	1
E0294	1	E0500	1	E0657	1	E0855	1
E0295	1	E0550	1	E0660	2	E0856	1
E0296	1	E0555	1	E0665	2	E0860	1
E0297	1	E0560	1	E0666	2	E0870	1
E0300	1	E0561	1	E0667	2	E0880	1
E0301	1	E0562	1	E0668	2	E0890	1
E0302	1	E0565	1	E0669	2	E0900	1
E0303	1	E0570	1	E0671	2	E0910	1
E0304	1	E0571	1	E0672	2	E0911	1
E0310	2	E0572	1	E0673	2	E0912	1
E0316	1	E0574	1	E0675	1	E0920	1
E0325	1	E0575	1	E0691	1	E0930	1
E0326	1	E0580	1	E0692	1	E0940	1

CODE	MUE UNIT		CODE	MUE UNIT		CODE	MUE UNIT		CODE	MUE UNIT
E0941	1		E1014	1		E1223	1		E1610	1
E0942	1		E1015	2		E1224	1		E1615	1
E0944	1		E1016	2		E1225	1		E1620	1
E0945	2		E1017	2		E1226	1		E1625	1
E0946	1		E1018	2		E1228	1		E1630	1
E0947	1		E1020	2		E1230	1		E1635	1
E0948	1		E1028	4		E1231	1		E1639	1
E0950	1		E1029	1		E1232	1		E1700	1
E0951	2		E1030	1		E1233	1		E1800	2
E0952	2		E1031	1		E1234	1		E1801	2
E0955	1		E1035	1		E1235	1		E1802	2
E0957	2		E1037	1		E1236	1		E1805	2
E0958	2		E1038	1		E1237	1		E1806	2
E0959	2		E1039	1		E1238	1		E1810	2
E0960	2		E1050	1		E1240	1		E1811	2
E0961	2		E1060	1		E1250	1		E1812	2
E0966	1		E1070	1		E1260	1		E1815	2
E0967	2		E1083	1		E1270	1		E1816	2
E0968	1		E1084	1		E1280	1		E1818	2
E0970	2		E1085	1		E1285	1		E1820	2
E0971	2		E1086	1		E1290	1		E1821	1
E0973	2		E1087	1		E1295	1		E1825	2
E0974	2		E1088	1		E1310	1		E1830	2
E0978	1		E1089	1		E1353	1		E1831	2
E0981	1		E1090	1		E1355	1		E1840	2
E0982	1		E1092	1		E1372	1		E1841	2
E0983	1		E1093	1		E1390	1		E1902	1
E0984	1		E1100	1		E1391	1		E2000	1
E0985	1		E1110	1		E1392	1		E2100	1
E0986	1		E1130	1		E1405	1		E2101	1
E0990	2		E1140	1		E1406	1		E2120	1
E0992	1		E1150	1		E1500	1		E2201	1
E0994	2		E1160	1		E1510	1		E2202	1
E0995	2		E1161	1		E1520	1		E2203	1
E1002	1		E1170	1		E1530	1		E2204	1
E1003	1		E1171	1		E1540	1		E2205	2
E1004	1		E1172	1		E1550	1		E2206	2
E1005	1		E1180	1		E1560	1		E2207	2
E1006	1		E1190	1		E1570	1		E2208	1
E1007	1		E1195	1		E1580	1		E2209	2
E1008	1		E1200	1		E1590	1		E2211	2
E1009	2		E1220	1		E1592	1		E2212	2
E1010	1		E1221	1		E1594	1		E2213	2
E1011	1		E1222	1		E1600	1		E2214	2

CODE	MUE UNIT
E2215	2
E2216	2
E2217	2
E2218	2
E2219	2
E2220	2
E2221	2
E2222	2
E2224	2
E2225	2
E2226	2
E2227	2
E2228	2
E2231	1
E2295	1
E2300	1
E2301	1
E2310	1
E2311	1
E2312	1
E2313	1
E2321	1
E2322	1
E2323	1
E2324	1
E2325	1
E2326	1
E2327	1
E2328	1
E2329	1
E2330	1
E2331	1
E2340	1
E2341	1
E2342	1
E2343	1
E2351	1
E2361	2
E2363	2
E2365	2
E2366	1
E2367	1
E2368	2
E2369	2

CODE	MUE UNIT
E2370	2
E2371	2
E2375	1
E2381	2
E2382	2
E2383	2
E2384	4
E2385	4
E2387	4
E2389	4
E2391	4
E2392	4
E2395	4
E2396	4
E2397	1
E2402	1
E2500	1
E2502	1
E2504	1
E2506	1
E2508	1
E2510	1
E2511	1
E2512	1
E2601	1
E2602	1
E2603	1
E2604	1
E2605	1
E2606	1
E2607	1
E2608	1
E2609	1
E2611	1
E2612	1
E2613	1
E2614	1
E2615	1
E2616	1
E2617	1
E2619	2
E2620	1
E2621	1
E2622	1

CODE	MUE UNIT
E2623	1
E2624	1
E2625	1
G0008	1
G0009	1
G0010	2
G0027	1
G0101	1
G0102	1
G0103	1
G0104	1
G0105	1
G0106	1
G0117	1
G0118	1
G0120	1
G0121	1
G0123	1
G0124	1
G0127	1
G0128	1
G0130	1
G0141	1
G0143	1
G0144	1
G0145	1
G0147	1
G0148	1
G0166	2
G0168	2
G0173	1
G0175	1
G0179	1
G0180	1
G0181	1
G0182	1
G0186	1
G0202	1
G0204	1
G0206	1
G0239	1
G0245	1
G0246	1
G0247	1

CODE	MUE UNIT
G0248	1
G0249	1
G0250	1
G0251	1
G0259	2
G0260	2
G0268	1
G0275	1
G0278	1
G0281	1
G0283	1
G0288	1
G0289	2
G0290	1
G0291	2
G0293	1
G0294	1
G0302	1
G0303	1
G0304	1
G0305	1
G0306	2
G0307	2
G0328	1
G0329	1
G0333	1
G0337	1
G0339	1
G0340	1
G0341	1
G0342	1
G0343	1
G0364	2
G0365	2
G0372	1
G0389	1
G0396	1
G0397	1
G0398	1
G0399	1
G0400	1
G0406	1
G0407	1
G0408	1

CODE	MUE UNIT		CODE	MUE UNIT		CODE	MUE UNIT		CODE	MUE UNIT
G0416	1		K0052	2		K0836	1		L0450	1
G0417	1		K0053	2		K0837	1		L0452	1
G0418	1		K0056	1		K0838	1		L0454	1
G0419	1		K0065	2		K0839	1		L0456	1
G0425	1		K0069	2		K0840	1		L0458	1
G0426	1		K0070	2		K0841	1		L0460	1
G0427	1		K0071	2		K0842	1		L0462	1
G0429	1		K0072	2		K0843	1		L0464	1
G0431	1		K0073	2		K0848	1		L0466	1
G0432	1		K0077	2		K0849	1		L0468	1
G0433	1		K0105	1		K0850	1		L0470	1
G0434	1		K0195	2		K0851	1		L0472	1
G0435	1		K0455	1		K0852	1		L0480	1
G0436	1		K0462	1		K0854	1		L0482	1
G0437	1		K0606	1		K0855	1		L0484	1
G0438	1		K0607	1		K0856	1		L0486	1
G0439	1		K0608	1		K0857	1		L0488	1
G0440	1		K0609	1		K0858	1		L0490	1
K0001	1		K0730	1		K0859	1		L0491	1
K0002	1		K0733	2		K0860	1		L0492	1
K0003	1		K0738	1		K0861	1		L0621	1
K0004	1		K0800	1		K0862	1		L0622	1
K0005	1		K0801	1		K0863	1		L0623	1
K0006	1		K0802	1		K0864	1		L0624	1
K0007	1		K0806	1		K0868	1		L0625	1
K0009	1		K0807	1		K0869	1		L0626	1
K0015	2		K0808	1		K0877	1		L0627	1
K0017	2		K0813	1		K0880	1		L0628	1
K0018	2		K0814	1		K0884	1		L0629	1
K0019	2		K0815	1		L0112	1		L0630	1
K0020	1		K0816	1		L0113	1		L0631	1
K0037	2		K0820	1		L0120	1		L0632	1
K0038	2		K0821	1		L0130	1		L0633	1
K0039	2		K0822	1		L0140	1		L0634	1
K0040	2		K0823	1		L0150	1		L0635	1
K0041	2		K0824	1		L0160	1		L0636	1
K0042	2		K0825	1		L0170	1		L0637	1
K0043	2		K0826	1		L0172	1		L0638	1
K0044	2		K0827	1		L0174	1		L0639	1
K0045	2		K0828	1		L0180	1		L0640	1
K0046	2		K0829	1		L0190	1		L0700	1
K0047	2		K0830	1		L0200	1		L0710	1
K0050	2		K0831	1		L0220	1		L0810	1
K0051	2		K0835	1		L0430	1		L0820	1

CODE	MUE UNIT
L0830	1
L0859	1
L0861	1
L0970	1
L0972	1
L0974	1
L0976	1
L0978	2
L0980	1
L1000	1
L1005	1
L1010	2
L1020	2
L1025	1
L1030	1
L1040	1
L1050	1
L1060	1
L1070	2
L1080	2
L1085	1
L1090	1
L1100	2
L1110	2
L1120	3
L1200	1
L1210	2
L1220	1
L1230	1
L1240	1
L1250	2
L1260	1
L1270	3
L1280	2
L1290	2
L1300	1
L1310	1
L1500	1
L1510	1
L1520	1
L1600	1
L1610	1
L1620	1
L1630	1

CODE	MUE UNIT
L1640	1
L1650	1
L1652	1
L1660	1
L1680	1
L1685	1
L1686	1
L1690	1
L1700	1
L1710	1
L1720	2
L1730	1
L1755	2
L1810	2
L1820	2
L1830	2
L1831	2
L1832	2
L1834	2
L1836	2
L1840	2
L1843	2
L1844	2
L1845	2
L1846	2
L1847	2
L1850	2
L1860	2
L1900	2
L1902	2
L1904	2
L1906	2
L1907	2
L1910	2
L1920	2
L1930	2
L1932	2
L1940	2
L1945	2
L1950	2
L1951	2
L1960	2
L1970	2
L1971	2

CODE	MUE UNIT
L1980	2
L1990	2
L2000	2
L2005	2
L2010	2
L2020	2
L2030	2
L2034	2
L2035	2
L2036	2
L2037	2
L2038	2
L2040	1
L2050	1
L2060	1
L2070	1
L2080	1
L2090	1
L2106	2
L2108	2
L2112	2
L2114	2
L2116	2
L2126	2
L2128	2
L2132	2
L2134	2
L2136	2
L2180	2
L2188	2
L2190	2
L2192	2
L2230	2
L2232	2
L2240	2
L2250	2
L2260	2
L2265	2
L2270	2
L2275	2
L2280	2
L2300	1
L2310	1
L2320	2

CODE	MUE UNIT
L2330	2
L2335	2
L2340	2
L2350	2
L2360	2
L2370	2
L2375	2
L2380	2
L2500	2
L2510	2
L2520	2
L2525	2
L2526	2
L2530	2
L2540	2
L2550	2
L2570	2
L2580	2
L2600	2
L2610	2
L2620	2
L2622	2
L2624	2
L2627	1
L2628	1
L2630	1
L2640	1
L2650	2
L2660	1
L2670	2
L2680	2
L2795	2
L2800	2
L2820	2
L2830	2
L3000	2
L3001	2
L3002	2
L3003	2
L3010	2
L3020	2
L3030	2
L3031	2
L3040	2

CODE	MUE UNIT
L3050	2
L3060	2
L3070	2
L3080	2
L3090	2
L3100	2
L3140	1
L3150	1
L3160	2
L3170	2
L3215	2
L3216	2
L3217	2
L3219	2
L3221	2
L3222	2
L3224	2
L3225	2
L3230	2
L3250	2
L3251	2
L3252	2
L3253	2
L3330	2
L3332	2
L3340	2
L3350	2
L3360	2
L3370	2
L3380	2
L3390	2
L3400	2
L3410	2
L3420	2
L3430	2
L3440	2
L3450	2
L3455	2
L3460	2
L3465	2
L3470	2
L3480	2
L3485	2
L3500	2

CODE	MUE UNIT
L3510	2
L3520	2
L3530	2
L3540	2
L3550	2
L3560	2
L3570	2
L3580	2
L3590	2
L3595	2
L3600	2
L3610	2
L3620	2
L3630	2
L3640	1
L3650	1
L3660	1
L3670	1
L3671	1
L3674	2
L3675	1
L3677	1
L3702	2
L3710	2
L3720	2
L3730	2
L3740	2
L3760	2
L3762	2
L3763	2
L3764	2
L3765	2
L3766	2
L3806	2
L3807	2
L3808	2
L3900	2
L3901	2
L3904	2
L3905	2
L3906	2
L3908	2
L3912	2
L3913	2

CODE	MUE UNIT
L3917	2
L3919	2
L3921	2
L3923	2
L3929	2
L3931	2
L3933	3
L3935	3
L3960	1
L3961	1
L3962	1
L3964	2
L3965	2
L3966	2
L3967	1
L3968	2
L3969	2
L3970	2
L3971	1
L3972	2
L3973	1
L3974	2
L3975	1
L3976	1
L3977	1
L3978	1
L3980	2
L3982	2
L3984	2
L4000	1
L4010	2
L4020	2
L4030	2
L4040	2
L4045	2
L4050	2
L4055	2
L4060	2
L4070	2
L4080	2
L4100	2
L4130	2
L4350	2
L4360	2

CODE	MUE UNIT
L4370	2
L4380	2
L4386	2
L4392	2
L4394	2
L4396	2
L4398	2
L4631	2
L5000	2
L5010	2
L5020	2
L5050	2
L5060	2
L5100	2
L5105	2
L5150	2
L5160	2
L5200	2
L5210	2
L5220	2
L5230	2
L5250	2
L5270	2
L5280	2
L5301	2
L5311	2
L5321	2
L5331	2
L5341	2
L5400	2
L5410	2
L5420	2
L5430	2
L5450	2
L5460	2
L5500	2
L5505	2
L5510	2
L5520	2
L5530	2
L5535	2
L5540	2
L5560	2
L5570	2

CODE	MUE UNIT	CODE	MUE UNIT	CODE	MUE UNIT	CODE	MUE UNIT
L5580	2	L5672	2	L5811	2	L5987	2
L5585	2	L5676	2	L5812	2	L5988	2
L5590	2	L5677	2	L5814	2	L5990	2
L5595	2	L5678	2	L5816	2	L6000	2
L5600	2	L5680	2	L5818	2	L6010	2
L5610	2	L5681	2	L5822	2	L6020	2
L5611	2	L5682	2	L5824	2	L6025	2
L5613	2	L5683	2	L5826	2	L6050	2
L5614	2	L5684	2	L5828	2	L6055	2
L5616	2	L5686	2	L5830	2	L6100	2
L5617	2	L5688	2	L5840	2	L6110	2
L5628	2	L5690	2	L5845	2	L6120	2
L5629	2	L5692	2	L5848	2	L6130	2
L5630	2	L5694	2	L5850	2	L6200	2
L5631	2	L5695	2	L5855	2	L6205	2
L5632	2	L5696	2	L5856	2	L6250	2
L5634	2	L5697	2	L5857	2	L6300	2
L5636	2	L5698	2	L5858	2	L6310	2
L5637	2	L5699	2	L5910	2	L6320	2
L5638	2	L5700	2	L5920	2	L6350	2
L5639	2	L5701	2	L5925	2	L6360	2
L5640	2	L5702	2	L5930	2	L6370	2
L5642	2	L5703	2	L5940	2	L6380	2
L5643	2	L5704	2	L5950	2	L6382	2
L5644	2	L5705	2	L5960	2	L6384	2
L5645	2	L5706	2	L5961	2	L6386	2
L5646	2	L5707	2	L5962	2	L6388	2
L5647	2	L5710	2	L5964	2	L6400	2
L5648	2	L5711	2	L5966	2	L6450	2
L5649	2	L5712	2	L5968	2	L6500	2
L5650	2	L5714	2	L5970	2	L6550	2
L5651	2	L5716	2	L5971	2	L6570	2
L5652	2	L5718	2	L5972	2	L6580	2
L5653	2	L5722	2	L5974	2	L6582	2
L5654	2	L5724	2	L5975	2	L6584	2
L5655	2	L5726	2	L5976	2	L6586	2
L5656	2	L5728	2	L5978	2	L6588	2
L5658	2	L5780	2	L5979	2	L6590	2
L5661	2	L5781	2	L5980	2	L6600	2
L5665	2	L5782	2	L5981	2	L6605	2
L5666	2	L5785	2	L5982	2	L6610	2
L5668	2	L5790	2	L5984	2	L6615	2
L5670	2	L5795	2	L5985	2	L6616	2
L5671	2	L5810	2	L5986	2	L6620	2

CODE	MUE UNIT		CODE	MUE UNIT		CODE	MUE UNIT		CODE	MUE UNIT
L6621	2		L6884	2		L8030	2		L8659	4
L6623	2		L6885	2		L8031	2		L8670	4
L6625	2		L6890	2		L8032	2		L8681	1
L6628	2		L6895	2		L8035	2		L8682	2
L6629	2		L6900	2		L8039	2		L8683	1
L6630	2		L6905	2		L8040	1		L8684	1
L6635	2		L6910	2		L8041	1		L8685	1
L6637	2		L6915	2		L8042	2		L8686	2
L6638	2		L6920	2		L8043	1		L8687	2
L6640	2		L6925	2		L8044	1		L8688	2
L6641	2		L6930	2		L8045	2		L8689	1
L6642	2		L6935	2		L8046	1		L8690	1
L6645	2		L6940	2		L8047	1		L8691	1
L6646	2		L6945	2		L8300	1		L8693	1
L6647	2		L6950	2		L8310	1		L8695	1
L6648	2		L6955	2		L8320	2		M0064	1
L6650	2		L6960	2		L8330	2		P2028	1
L6670	2		L6965	2		L8500	1		P2029	1
L6672	2		L6970	2		L8501	2		P2033	1
L6675	2		L6975	2		L8507	3		P2038	1
L6676	2		L7040	2		L8509	1		P3000	1
L6677	2		L7045	2		L8510	1		P3001	1
L6686	2		L7170	2		L8511	1		P9612	1
L6687	2		L7180	2		L8514	1		P9615	1
L6688	2		L7181	2		L8515	1		Q0035	1
L6689	2		L7185	2		L8600	2		Q0091	1
L6690	2		L7186	2		L8604	3		Q0111	2
L6693	2		L7190	2		L8610	2		Q0112	3
L6694	2		L7191	2		L8612	2		Q0113	2
L6695	2		L7260	2		L8613	2		Q0114	1
L6696	2		L7261	2		L8614	2		Q0115	1
L6697	2		L7266	2		L8615	2		Q0478	1
L6698	2		L7272	2		L8616	2		Q0479	1
L6711	2		L7274	2		L8617	2		Q0480	1
L6712	2		L7362	1		L8618	2		Q0481	1
L6713	2		L7366	1		L8619	2		Q0482	1
L6714	2		L7368	1		L8622	2		Q0483	1
L6721	2		L7400	2		L8627	2		Q0484	1
L6722	2		L7401	2		L8628	2		Q0485	1
L6805	2		L7402	2		L8629	2		Q0486	1
L6810	2		L7403	2		L8631	4		Q0487	1
L6881	2		L7404	2		L8641	4		Q0488	1
L6882	2		L7405	2		L8642	2		Q0489	1
L6883	2		L7900	1		L8658	4		Q0490	1

CODE	MUE UNIT		CODE	MUE UNIT		CODE	MUE UNIT		CODE	MUE UNIT
Q0491	1		V2104	2		V2299	2		V2522	2
Q0492	1		V2105	2		V2300	2		V2523	2
Q0493	1		V2106	2		V2301	2		V2530	2
Q0494	1		V2107	2		V2302	2		V2531	2
Q0495	1		V2108	2		V2303	2		V2600	1
Q0497	2		V2109	2		V2304	2		V2610	1
Q0498	1		V2110	2		V2305	2		V2615	2
Q0499	1		V2111	2		V2306	2		V2623	2
Q0501	1		V2112	2		V2307	2		V2624	2
Q0502	1		V2113	2		V2308	2		V2625	2
Q0503	3		V2114	2		V2309	2		V2626	2
Q0504	1		V2115	2		V2310	2		V2627	2
Q1003	2		V2118	2		V2311	2		V2628	2
Q1004	2		V2121	2		V2312	2		V2629	2
Q1005	2		V2200	2		V2313	2		V2630	2
Q2035	1		V2201	2		V2314	2		V2631	2
Q2036	1		V2202	2		V2315	2		V2632	2
Q2037	1		V2203	2		V2318	2		V2700	2
Q2038	1		V2204	2		V2319	2		V2710	2
Q2039	1		V2205	2		V2320	2		V2718	2
Q2043	1		V2206	2		V2321	2		V2730	2
Q4001	1		V2207	2		V2399	2		V2761	2
Q4002	1		V2208	2		V2410	2		V2770	2
Q4003	2		V2209	2		V2430	2		V2780	2
Q4004	2		V2210	2		V2500	2		V2781	2
Q4025	1		V2211	2		V2501	2		V2782	2
Q4026	1		V2212	2		V2502	2		V2783	2
Q4027	1		V2213	2		V2503	2		V2785	2
Q4028	1		V2214	2		V2510	2		V2790	1
R0070	2		V2215	2		V2511	2		V2797	1
R0075	2		V2218	2		V2512	2		V5008	1
V2020	1		V2219	2		V2513	2		V5010	1
V2101	2		V2220	2		V2520	2		V5011	1
V2102	2		V2221	2		V2521	2			

NCCI Mutually Exclusive Edits (MEEs)—Physician
(Effective Date: 10/01/11-12/31/11, Version: 17.3)
Codes in Column 1 are not reported with codes in Column 2 if "0" or "9"

Column 1	Column 2	Modifier 0=not allowed 1=allowed 9=not applicable
C8928	C8923	1
C8928	C8924	1
C8928	C8925	1
C8928	C8927	0
C8928	C8929	1
C8928	93306	1
C8928	93307	1
C8928	93308	1
C8928	93312	1
C8928	93313	1
C8928	93314	1
C8928	93318	0
C8930	93303	1
C8930	93304	1
C8930	93313	1
C8931	72159	0
C8932	72159	0
C8933	72159	0
C8934	73225	0
C8935	73225	0
C8936	73225	0
C8930	93314	1
C8930	93797	1
C8930	93798	1
C8957	96415	0
C9716	46750	0
C9800	G0429	0
C9800	11950	1
C9800	11951	1
C9800	11952	1
C9800	11954	1
C9716	46751	0
C9716	46760	0
C9716	46761	0
C9716	46762	0
E0781	E0782	1
G0101	57410	1
G0103	84153	0

Column 1	Column 2	Modifier 0=not allowed 1=allowed 9=not applicable
G0103	84154	1
G0104	G0105	0
G0104	G0106	1
G0104	G0120	1
G0104	G0121	0
G0104	45300	0
G0104	45303	0
G0104	45305	0
G0104	45307	0
G0104	45308	0
G0104	45309	0
G0104	45315	0
G0104	45317	0
G0104	45320	0
G0104	45321	0
G0104	45327	0
G0104	45330	0
G0104	45331	0
G0104	45332	0
G0104	45333	0
G0104	45334	0
G0104	45335	0
G0104	45337	0
G0104	45338	0
G0104	45339	0
G0104	45340	0
G0104	45341	0
G0104	45342	0
G0104	45345	0
G0104	45355	0
G0104	45378	0
G0104	45379	0
G0104	45380	0
G0104	45381	0
G0104	45382	0
G0104	45383	0
G0104	45384	0
G0104	45385	0

Column 1	Column 2	Modifier 0=not allowed 1=allowed 9=not applicable
G0104	45386	0
G0104	45387	0
G0104	46604	0
G0104	46608	0
G0104	46614	0
G0105	45300	0
G0105	45303	0
G0105	45305	0
G0105	45307	0
G0105	45308	0
G0105	45309	0
G0105	45315	0
G0105	45317	0
G0105	45320	0
G0105	45321	0
G0105	45327	0
G0105	45330	0
G0105	45331	0
G0105	45332	0
G0105	45333	0
G0105	45334	0
G0105	45335	0
G0105	45337	0
G0105	45338	0
G0105	45339	0
G0105	45340	0
G0105	45341	0
G0105	45342	0
G0105	45345	0
G0105	45355	0
G0106	G0105	0
G0106	G0121	0
G0106	74270	1
G0106	74280	1
G0120	G0105	0
G0120	G0106	0
G0120	G0121	0
G0120	74270	1

Column 1	Column 2	Modifier 0=not allowed 1=allowed 9=not applicable	Column 1	Column 2	Modifier 0=not allowed 1=allowed 9=not applicable	Column 1	Column 2	Modifier 0=not allowed 1=allowed 9=not applicable
G0120	74280	1	G0127	99212	1	G0127	99334	1
G0121	G0105	0	G0127	99213	1	G0127	99335	1
G0121	45300	0	G0127	99214	1	G0127	99336	1
G0121	45303	0	G0127	99215	1	G0127	99337	1
G0121	45305	0	G0127	99217	1	G0127	99341	1
G0121	45307	0	G0127	99218	1	G0127	99342	1
G0121	45308	0	G0127	99219	1	G0127	99343	1
G0121	45309	0	G0127	99220	1	G0127	99344	1
G0121	45315	0	G0127	99221	1	G0127	99345	1
G0121	45317	0	G0127	99222	1	G0127	99347	1
G0121	45320	0	G0127	99223	1	G0127	99348	1
G0121	45321	0	G0127	99224	1	G0127	99349	1
G0121	45327	0	G0127	99225	1	G0127	99350	1
G0121	45330	0	G0127	99226	1	G0127	99354	1
G0121	45331	0	G0127	99231	1	G0127	99355	1
G0121	45332	0	G0127	99232	1	G0127	99356	1
G0121	45333	0	G0127	99233	1	G0127	99357	1
G0121	45334	0	G0127	99234	1	G0130	76977	0
G0121	45335	0	G0127	99235	1	G0130	77080	1
G0121	45337	0	G0127	99236	1	G0154	G0128	1
G0121	45338	0	G0127	99238	1	G0162	G0128	1
G0121	45339	0	G0127	99239	1	G0163	G0128	1
G0121	45340	0	G0127	99281	1	G0164	G0128	1
G0121	45341	0	G0127	99282	1	G0173	G0251	1
G0121	45342	0	G0127	99283	1	G0173	G0339	0
G0121	45345	0	G0127	99284	1	G0173	G0340	0
G0121	45355	0	G0127	99285	1	G0173	61304	1
G0127	G0380	1	G0127	99304	1	G0173	61305	1
G0127	G0381	1	G0127	99305	1	G0173	61312	1
G0127	G0382	1	G0127	99306	1	G0173	61313	1
G0127	G0383	1	G0127	99307	1	G0173	61314	1
G0127	G0384	1	G0127	99308	1	G0173	61315	1
G0127	G0406	1	G0127	99309	1	G0173	61320	1
G0127	G0407	1	G0127	99310	1	G0173	61321	1
G0127	G0408	1	G0127	99315	1	G0173	61330	1
G0127	G0425	1	G0127	99316	1	G0173	61332	1
G0127	G0426	1	G0127	99318	1	G0173	61333	1
G0127	G0427	1	G0127	99324	1	G0173	61440	1
G0127	99203	1	G0127	99325	1	G0173	61450	1
G0127	99204	1	G0127	99326	1	G0173	61458	1
G0127	99205	1	G0127	99327	1	G0173	61460	1
G0127	99211	1	G0127	99328	1	G0173	61470	1

Column 1	Column 2	Modifier 0=not allowed 1=allowed 9=not applicable
G0173	61480	1
G0173	61490	1
G0173	61500	1
G0173	61501	1
G0173	61510	1
G0173	61512	1
G0173	61514	1
G0173	61516	1
G0173	61518	1
G0173	61519	1
G0173	61520	1
G0173	61521	1
G0173	61522	1
G0173	61524	1
G0173	61526	1
G0173	61530	1
G0173	61563	1
G0173	61564	1
G0173	61720	1
G0173	61735	1
G0173	61790	1
G0173	61791	1
G0173	77371	1
G0173	77372	1
G0173	77373	1
G0173	77427	1
G0173	77431	1
G0173	77470	1
G0175	90804	1
G0175	90805	1
G0175	90806	1
G0175	90807	1
G0175	90808	1
G0175	90809	1
G0175	90810	1
G0175	90811	1
G0175	90812	1
G0175	90813	1
G0175	90814	1
G0175	90815	1
G0175	90816	1
G0175	90817	1

Column 1	Column 2	Modifier 0=not allowed 1=allowed 9=not applicable
G0175	90818	1
G0175	90819	1
G0175	90821	1
G0175	90822	1
G0175	90823	1
G0175	90824	1
G0175	90826	1
G0175	90827	1
G0175	90828	1
G0175	90829	1
G0175	90846	1
G0175	90847	1
G0179	G0180	0
G0181	G0182	1
G0186	67210	1
G0186	67228	1
G0251	G0339	0
G0251	G0340	0
G0251	20661	1
G0251	20693	1
G0251	20694	1
G0251	61304	1
G0251	61305	1
G0251	61312	1
G0251	61313	1
G0251	61314	1
G0251	61315	1
G0251	61320	1
G0251	61321	1
G0251	61330	1
G0251	61332	1
G0251	61333	1
G0251	61440	1
G0251	61450	1
G0251	61458	1
G0251	61460	1
G0251	61470	1
G0251	61480	1
G0251	61490	1
G0251	61500	1
G0251	61510	1
G0251	61512	1

Column 1	Column 2	Modifier 0=not allowed 1=allowed 9=not applicable
G0251	61514	1
G0251	61516	1
G0251	61518	1
G0251	61519	1
G0251	61520	1
G0251	61521	1
G0251	61522	1
G0251	61524	1
G0251	61530	1
G0251	61563	1
G0251	61564	1
G0251	61735	1
G0268	69210	0
G0270	G0271	0
G0281	G0283	1
G0281	G0329	0
G0328	82274	0
G0329	G0283	1
G0337	99201	0
G0337	99202	0
G0337	99203	0
G0337	99204	0
G0337	99205	0
G0337	99211	0
G0337	99212	0
G0337	99213	0
G0337	99214	0
G0337	99215	0
G0339	G0340	1
G0339	20661	1
G0339	20693	1
G0339	20694	1
G0339	61304	1
G0339	61305	1
G0339	61312	1
G0339	61313	1
G0339	61314	1
G0339	61315	1
G0339	61320	1
G0339	61321	1
G0339	61330	1
G0339	61332	1

Column 1	Column 2	Modifier 0=not allowed 1=allowed 9=not applicable
G0339	61333	1
G0339	61440	1
G0339	61450	1
G0339	61458	1
G0339	61460	1
G0339	61470	1
G0339	61480	1
G0339	61490	1
G0339	61500	1
G0339	61510	1
G0339	61512	1
G0339	61514	1
G0339	61516	1
G0339	61518	1
G0339	61519	1
G0339	61520	1
G0339	61521	1
G0339	61522	1
G0339	61524	1
G0339	61526	1
G0339	61530	1
G0339	61563	1
G0339	61564	1
G0339	61735	1
G0340	20661	1
G0340	20693	1
G0340	20694	1
G0340	61304	1
G0340	61305	1
G0340	61312	1
G0340	61313	1
G0340	61314	1
G0340	61315	1
G0340	61320	1
G0340	61321	1
G0340	61330	1
G0340	61332	1
G0340	61333	1
G0340	61440	1
G0340	61450	1
G0340	61458	1

Column 1	Column 2	Modifier 0=not allowed 1=allowed 9=not applicable
G0340	61460	1
G0340	61470	1
G0340	61480	1
G0340	61490	1
G0340	61500	1
G0340	61510	1
G0340	61512	1
G0340	61514	1
G0340	61516	1
G0340	61518	1
G0340	61519	1
G0340	61520	1
G0340	61521	1
G0340	61522	1
G0340	61524	1
G0340	61526	1
G0340	61530	1
G0340	61563	1
G0340	61564	1
G0340	61735	1
G0341	48554	0
G0342	48554	0
G0343	48554	0
G0365	76998	1
G0365	93971	1
G0380	99239	1
G0381	G0380	1
G0381	99239	1
G0382	G0380	1
G0382	G0381	1
G0382	99239	1
G0383	G0380	1
G0383	G0381	1
G0383	G0382	1
G0383	99463	1
G0384	G0380	1
G0384	G0381	1
G0384	G0382	1
G0384	G0383	1
G0384	99463	1
G0398	G0399	0

Column 1	Column 2	Modifier 0=not allowed 1=allowed 9=not applicable
G0398	G0400	0
G0399	G0400	0
G0402	G0380	1
G0402	G0381	1
G0402	G0382	1
G0402	G0383	1
G0402	G0384	1
G0402	G0438	0
G0402	G0439	0
G0402	99201	1
G0402	99202	1
G0402	99203	1
G0402	99204	1
G0402	99205	1
G0402	99211	1
G0402	99212	1
G0402	99213	1
G0402	99214	1
G0402	99215	1
G0402	99281	1
G0402	99282	1
G0402	99283	1
G0402	99284	1
G0402	99285	1
G0402	99304	1
G0402	99305	1
G0402	99306	1
G0402	99307	1
G0402	99308	1
G0402	99309	1
G0402	99310	1
G0402	99315	1
G0402	99316	1
G0402	99318	1
G0402	99324	1
G0402	99325	1
G0402	99326	1
G0402	99327	1
G0402	99328	1
G0402	99334	1
G0402	99335	1

Column 1	Column 2	Modifier 0=not allowed 1=allowed 9=not applicable
G0402	99336	1
G0402	99337	1
G0402	99341	1
G0402	99342	1
G0402	99343	1
G0402	99344	1
G0402	99345	1
G0402	99347	1
G0402	99348	1
G0402	99349	1
G0402	99350	1
G0403	93000	1
G0403	93005	1
G0403	93010	1
G0403	93040	1
G0403	93041	1
G0403	93042	1
G0404	93000	1
G0404	93005	1
G0404	93010	1
G0404	93040	1
G0404	93041	1
G0404	93042	1
G0405	93000	1
G0405	93005	1
G0405	93010	1
G0405	93040	1
G0405	93041	1
G0405	93042	1
G0409	G0155	1
G0409	G0176	1
G0409	G0177	1
G0409	90801	1
G0409	90802	1
G0409	90804	1
G0409	90805	1
G0409	90806	1
G0409	90807	1
G0409	90808	1
G0409	90809	1
G0409	90810	1

Column 1	Column 2	Modifier 0=not allowed 1=allowed 9=not applicable
G0409	90811	1
G0409	90812	1
G0409	90813	1
G0409	90814	1
G0409	90815	1
G0409	90816	1
G0409	90817	1
G0409	90818	1
G0409	90819	1
G0409	90821	1
G0409	90822	1
G0409	90823	1
G0409	90824	1
G0409	90826	1
G0409	90827	1
G0409	90828	1
G0409	90829	1
G0409	90845	1
G0409	90846	1
G0409	90847	1
G0409	90849	1
G0409	90853	1
G0409	90857	1
G0409	90862	1
G0409	90865	1
G0409	90870	1
G0409	90880	1
G0410	90801	1
G0410	90804	1
G0410	90805	1
G0410	90806	1
G0410	90807	1
G0410	90808	1
G0410	90809	1
G0410	90810	1
G0410	90811	1
G0410	90812	1
G0410	90813	1
G0410	90814	1
G0410	90815	1
G0410	90816	1

Column 1	Column 2	Modifier 0=not allowed 1=allowed 9=not applicable
G0410	90817	1
G0410	90818	1
G0410	90819	1
G0410	90821	1
G0410	90822	1
G0410	90823	1
G0410	90824	1
G0410	90826	1
G0410	90827	1
G0410	90828	1
G0410	90829	1
G0410	90845	1
G0410	90846	1
G0410	90847	1
G0410	90849	1
G0410	90853	1
G0410	90865	1
G0410	90870	1
G0411	G0410	1
G0411	90801	1
G0411	90804	1
G0411	90805	1
G0411	90806	1
G0411	90807	1
G0411	90808	1
G0411	90809	1
G0411	90810	1
G0411	90811	1
G0411	90812	1
G0411	90813	1
G0411	90814	1
G0411	90815	1
G0411	90816	1
G0411	90817	1
G0411	90818	1
G0411	90819	1
G0411	90821	1
G0411	90822	1
G0411	90823	1
G0411	90824	1
G0411	90826	1

Column 1	Column 2	Modifier 0=not allowed 1=allowed 9=not applicable
G0411	90827	1
G0411	90828	1
G0411	90829	1
G0411	90845	1
G0411	90846	1
G0411	90847	1
G0411	90849	1
G0411	90857	1
G0411	90865	1
G0411	90870	1
G0422	93015	1
G0422	93016	0
G0422	93017	1
G0422	93018	1
G0422	93025	1
G0423	93015	1
G0423	93016	0
G0423	93017	1
G0423	93018	1
G0423	93025	1
G0424	G0237	0
G0424	G0238	0
G0424	G0239	0
G0424	G0422	1
G0424	G0423	1
G0424	93015	1
G0424	93016	0
G0424	93017	1
G0424	93018	1
G0424	93025	1
G0424	93797	1
G0424	93798	1
G0428	29882	1
G0428	29883	1
G0429	11950	1
G0429	11951	1
G0429	11952	1
G0429	11954	1
G0436	99406	0
G0436	99407	0
G0437	99406	0
G0437	99407	0

Column 1	Column 2	Modifier 0=not allowed 1=allowed 9=not applicable
G0438	G0380	1
G0438	G0381	1
G0438	G0382	1
G0438	G0383	1
G0438	G0384	1
G0438	99201	1
G0438	99202	1
G0438	99203	1
G0438	99204	1
G0438	99205	1
G0438	99211	1
G0438	99212	1
G0438	99213	1
G0438	99214	1
G0438	99215	1
G0438	99281	1
G0438	99282	1
G0438	99283	1
G0438	99284	1
G0438	99285	1
G0438	99304	1
G0438	99305	1
G0438	99306	1
G0438	99307	1
G0438	99308	1
G0438	99309	1
G0438	99310	1
G0438	99315	1
G0438	99316	1
G0438	99318	1
G0438	99324	1
G0438	99325	1
G0438	99326	1
G0438	99327	1
G0438	99328	1
G0438	99334	1
G0438	99335	1
G0438	99336	1
G0438	99337	1
G0438	99341	1
G0438	99342	1
G0438	99343	1

Column 1	Column 2	Modifier 0=not allowed 1=allowed 9=not applicable
G0438	99344	1
G0438	99345	1
G0438	99347	1
G0438	99348	1
G0438	99349	1
G0438	99350	1
G0439	G0380	1
G0439	G0381	1
G0439	G0382	1
G0439	G0383	1
G0439	G0384	1
G0439	99201	1
G0439	99202	1
G0439	99203	1
G0439	99204	1
G0439	99205	1
G0439	99211	1
G0439	99212	1
G0439	99213	1
G0439	99214	1
G0439	99215	1
G0439	99281	1
G0439	99282	1
G0439	99283	1
G0439	99284	1
G0439	99285	1
G0439	99304	1
G0439	99305	1
G0439	99306	1
G0439	99307	1
G0439	99308	1
G0439	99309	1
G0439	99310	1
G0439	99315	1
G0439	99316	1
G0439	99318	1
G0439	99324	1
G0439	99325	1
G0439	99326	1
G0439	99327	1
G0439	99328	1
G0439	99334	1

Column 1	Column 2	Modifier 0=not allowed 1=allowed 9=not applicable
G0439	99335	1
G0439	99336	1
G0439	99337	1
G0439	99341	1
G0439	99342	1
G0439	99343	1
G0439	99344	1
G0439	99345	1
G0439	99347	1
G0439	99348	1
G0439	99349	1
G0439	99350	1
G0440	15170	1
G0440	15171	1
G0440	15175	1
G0440	15176	1
G0440	15300	1
G0440	15301	1
G0440	15320	1
G0440	15321	1
G0440	15330	1
G0440	15331	1

Column 1	Column 2	Modifier 0=not allowed 1=allowed 9=not applicable
G0440	15335	1
G0440	15336	1
G0440	15340	1
G0440	15341	1
G0440	15360	1
G0440	15361	1
G0440	15365	1
G0440	15366	1
G0441	15170	1
G0441	15171	1
G0441	15175	1
G0441	15176	1
G0441	15300	1
G0441	15301	1
G0441	15320	1
G0441	15321	1
G0441	15330	1
G0441	15331	1
G0441	15335	1
G0441	15336	1
G0441	15340	1
G0441	15341	1

Column 1	Column 2	Modifier 0=not allowed 1=allowed 9=not applicable
G0441	15360	1
G0441	15361	1
G0441	15365	1
G0441	15366	1
J2790	J2792	1
M0064	90862	0
P9011	P9010	1
P9011	P9021	0
P9011	P9022	0
P9011	P9039	0
P9022	P9010	1
P9022	P9016	1
P9022	P9021	1
P9022	P9039	1
P9039	P9010	1
P9039	P9016	1
P9039	P9021	1
P9603	P9604	1
P9612	P9615	0
Q1003	Q1004	1
Q1003	Q1005	1
Q1004	Q1005	1

NCCI Column 1/2 Edits—Physician
(Effective Date: 10/01/11-12/31/11, Version: 17.3)
Codes in Column 1 are not to be reported with codes in Column 2 if "0" or "9"

Column 1	Column 2	Modifier 0=not allowed 1=allowed 9=not applicable
A9500	A9512	1
A9501	A9512	0
A9502	A9512	0
A9503	A9512	0
A9504	A9512	0
A9510	A9512	0
A9521	A9512	0
A9536	A9512	0
A9537	A9512	0
A9538	A9512	0
A9539	A9512	0
A9540	A9512	1
A9541	A9512	1
A9550	A9512	0
A9551	A9512	0
A9557	A9512	0
A9560	A9512	0
A9561	A9512	0
A9562	A9512	0
A9566	A9512	0
A9567	A9512	0
A9568	A9512	0
A9569	A9512	0
C8900	01916	0
C8900	01922	0
C8900	01924	0
C8900	01925	0
C8900	01926	0
C8900	36000	1
C8900	36410	1
C8900	76000	1
C8900	76001	1
C8900	76350	0
C8900	76376	0
C8900	76377	0
C8900	76942	1
C8900	76998	1
C8900	77002	1

Column 1	Column 2	Modifier 0=not allowed 1=allowed 9=not applicable
C8900	96360	1
C8900	96365	1
C8900	96372	1
C8900	96374	1
C8900	96375	1
C8900	96376	1
C8901	01916	0
C8901	01922	0
C8901	01924	0
C8901	01925	0
C8901	01926	0
C8901	36000	1
C8901	36410	1
C8901	76000	1
C8901	76001	1
C8901	76350	0
C8901	76376	0
C8901	76377	0
C8901	76942	1
C8901	76998	1
C8901	77002	1
C8901	96360	1
C8901	96365	1
C8901	96372	1
C8901	96374	1
C8901	96375	1
C8901	96376	1
C8902	01916	0
C8902	01922	0
C8902	01924	0
C8902	01925	0
C8902	01926	0
C8902	36000	1
C8902	36410	1
C8902	76000	1
C8902	76001	1
C8902	76350	0
C8902	76376	0

Column 1	Column 2	Modifier 0=not allowed 1=allowed 9=not applicable
C8902	76377	0
C8902	76942	1
C8902	76998	1
C8902	77002	1
C8902	96360	1
C8902	96365	1
C8902	96372	1
C8902	96374	1
C8902	96375	1
C8902	96376	1
C8903	36000	1
C8903	36410	1
C8903	76000	1
C8903	76001	1
C8903	76350	0
C8903	76942	1
C8903	76998	1
C8903	77002	1
C8903	96360	1
C8903	96365	1
C8903	96372	1
C8903	96374	1
C8903	96375	1
C8903	96376	1
C8904	36000	1
C8904	36410	1
C8904	76000	1
C8904	76001	1
C8904	76350	0
C8904	76942	1
C8904	76998	1
C8904	77002	1
C8904	96360	1
C8904	96365	1
C8904	96372	1
C8904	96374	1
C8904	96375	1
C8904	96376	1

364

Column 1	Column 2	Modifier 0=not allowed 1=allowed 9=not applicable
C8905	36000	1
C8905	36410	1
C8905	76000	1
C8905	76001	1
C8905	76350	0
C8905	76942	1
C8905	76998	1
C8905	77002	1
C8905	96360	1
C8905	96365	1
C8905	96372	1
C8905	96374	1
C8905	96375	1
C8905	96376	1
C8906	C8903	1
C8906	C8904	1
C8906	C8905	1
C8906	36000	1
C8906	36410	1
C8906	76000	1
C8906	76001	1
C8906	76350	0
C8906	76942	1
C8906	76998	1
C8906	77002	1
C8906	96360	1
C8906	96365	1
C8906	96372	1
C8906	96374	1
C8906	96375	1
C8906	96376	1
C8907	C8903	1
C8907	C8904	1
C8907	C8905	1
C8907	36000	1
C8907	36410	1
C8907	76000	1
C8907	76001	1
C8907	76350	0
C8907	76942	1
C8907	76998	1
C8907	77002	1

Column 1	Column 2	Modifier 0=not allowed 1=allowed 9=not applicable
C8907	96360	1
C8907	96365	1
C8907	96372	1
C8907	96374	1
C8907	96375	1
C8907	96376	1
C8908	C8903	1
C8908	C8904	1
C8908	C8905	1
C8908	36000	1
C8908	36410	1
C8908	76000	1
C8908	76001	1
C8908	76350	0
C8908	76942	1
C8908	76998	1
C8908	77002	1
C8908	96360	1
C8908	96365	1
C8908	96372	1
C8908	96374	1
C8908	96375	1
C8908	96376	1
C8909	01916	0
C8909	01922	0
C8909	01924	0
C8909	01925	0
C8909	01926	0
C8909	36000	1
C8909	36410	1
C8909	76000	1
C8909	76001	1
C8909	76350	0
C8909	76376	0
C8909	76377	0
C8909	76942	1
C8909	76998	1
C8909	77002	1
C8909	96360	1
C8909	96365	1
C8909	96372	1
C8909	96374	1

Column 1	Column 2	Modifier 0=not allowed 1=allowed 9=not applicable
C8909	96375	1
C8909	96376	1
C8910	01916	0
C8910	01922	0
C8910	01924	0
C8910	01925	0
C8910	01926	0
C8910	36000	1
C8910	36410	1
C8910	76000	1
C8910	76001	1
C8910	76350	0
C8910	76376	0
C8910	76377	0
C8910	76942	1
C8910	76998	1
C8910	77002	1
C8910	96360	1
C8910	96365	1
C8910	96372	1
C8910	96374	1
C8910	96375	1
C8910	96376	1
C8911	01916	0
C8911	01922	0
C8911	01924	0
C8911	01925	0
C8911	01926	0
C8911	36000	1
C8911	36410	1
C8911	76000	1
C8911	76001	1
C8911	76350	0
C8911	76376	0
C8911	76377	0
C8911	76942	1
C8911	76998	1
C8911	77002	1
C8911	96360	1
C8911	96365	1
C8911	96372	1
C8911	96374	1

Column 1	Column 2	Modifier 0=not allowed 1=allowed 9=not applicable
C8911	96375	1
C8911	96376	1
C8912	01916	0
C8912	01922	0
C8912	01924	0
C8912	01925	0
C8912	01926	0
C8912	36000	1
C8912	36410	1
C8912	76000	1
C8912	76001	1
C8912	76350	0
C8912	76376	0
C8912	76377	0
C8912	76942	1
C8912	76998	1
C8912	77002	1
C8912	96360	1
C8912	96365	1
C8912	96372	1
C8912	96374	1
C8912	96375	1
C8912	96376	1
C8913	01916	0
C8913	01922	0
C8913	01924	0
C8913	01925	0
C8913	01926	0
C8913	36000	1
C8913	36410	1
C8913	76000	1
C8913	76001	1
C8913	76350	0
C8913	76376	0
C8913	76377	0
C8913	76942	1
C8913	76998	1
C8913	77002	1
C8913	96360	1
C8913	96365	1
C8913	96372	1
C8913	96374	1

Column 1	Column 2	Modifier 0=not allowed 1=allowed 9=not applicable
C8913	96375	1
C8913	96376	1
C8914	01916	0
C8914	01922	0
C8914	01924	0
C8914	01925	0
C8914	01926	0
C8914	36000	1
C8914	36410	1
C8914	76000	1
C8914	76001	1
C8914	76350	0
C8914	76376	0
C8914	76377	0
C8914	76942	1
C8914	76998	1
C8914	77002	1
C8914	96360	1
C8914	96365	1
C8914	96372	1
C8914	96374	1
C8914	96375	1
C8914	96376	1
C8918	01916	0
C8918	01922	0
C8918	01924	0
C8918	36000	1
C8918	36410	1
C8918	76000	1
C8918	76001	1
C8918	76350	0
C8918	76376	0
C8918	76377	0
C8918	76942	1
C8918	76998	1
C8918	77002	1
C8918	96372	1
C8918	96374	1
C8918	96375	1
C8918	96376	1
C8919	01916	0
C8919	01922	0

Column 1	Column 2	Modifier 0=not allowed 1=allowed 9=not applicable
C8919	01924	0
C8919	36000	1
C8919	36410	1
C8919	76000	1
C8919	76001	1
C8919	76350	0
C8919	76376	0
C8919	76377	0
C8919	76942	1
C8919	76998	1
C8919	77002	1
C8919	96372	1
C8919	96374	1
C8919	96375	1
C8919	96376	1
C8920	01916	0
C8920	01922	0
C8920	01924	0
C8920	36000	1
C8920	36410	1
C8920	76000	1
C8920	76001	1
C8920	76350	0
C8920	76376	0
C8920	76377	0
C8920	76942	1
C8920	76998	1
C8920	77002	1
C8920	96372	1
C8920	96374	1
C8920	96375	1
C8920	96376	1
C8921	C8922	1
C8921	36000	1
C8921	36005	1
C8921	36410	1
C8921	76998	1
C8921	93040	1
C8921	93041	1
C8921	93042	1
C8921	93303	0
C8921	93304	1

Column 1	Column 2	Modifier 0=not allowed 1=allowed 9=not applicable
C8921	96360	1
C8921	96365	1
C8921	96372	1
C8921	96374	1
C8921	96375	1
C8921	96376	1
C8922	36000	1
C8922	36005	1
C8922	36410	1
C8922	76998	1
C8922	93040	1
C8922	93041	1
C8922	93042	1
C8922	93304	1
C8922	96360	1
C8922	96365	1
C8922	96372	1
C8922	96374	1
C8922	96375	1
C8922	96376	1
C8923	C8924	1
C8923	C8929	0
C8923	36000	1
C8923	36005	1
C8923	36410	1
C8923	76998	1
C8923	93040	1
C8923	93041	1
C8923	93042	1
C8923	93306	0
C8923	93307	0
C8923	93308	1
C8923	96360	1
C8923	96365	1
C8923	96372	1
C8923	96374	1
C8923	96375	1
C8923	96376	1
C8924	36000	1
C8924	36005	1
C8924	36410	1
C8924	76998	1

Column 1	Column 2	Modifier 0=not allowed 1=allowed 9=not applicable
C8924	93040	1
C8924	93041	1
C8924	93042	1
C8924	93308	1
C8924	96360	1
C8924	96365	1
C8924	96372	1
C8924	96374	1
C8924	96375	1
C8924	96376	1
C8925	36000	1
C8925	36005	1
C8925	36410	1
C8925	76998	1
C8925	93040	1
C8925	93041	1
C8925	93042	1
C8925	93312	0
C8925	93313	0
C8925	93314	0
C8925	96360	1
C8925	96365	1
C8925	96372	1
C8925	96374	1
C8925	96375	1
C8925	96376	1
C8926	36000	1
C8926	36005	1
C8926	36410	1
C8926	76998	1
C8926	93040	1
C8926	93041	1
C8926	93042	1
C8926	93315	0
C8926	93316	0
C8926	93317	0
C8926	96360	1
C8926	96365	1
C8926	96372	1
C8926	96374	1
C8926	96375	1
C8926	96376	1

Column 1	Column 2	Modifier 0=not allowed 1=allowed 9=not applicable
C8927	36000	1
C8927	36005	1
C8927	36410	1
C8927	76998	1
C8927	93040	1
C8927	93041	1
C8927	93042	1
C8927	93318	0
C8927	96360	1
C8927	96365	1
C8927	96372	1
C8927	96374	1
C8927	96375	1
C8927	96376	1
C8928	C8930	0
C8928	36000	1
C8928	36005	1
C8928	36410	1
C8928	76998	1
C8928	93040	1
C8928	93041	1
C8928	93042	1
C8928	93350	0
C8928	93351	0
C8928	94761	0
C8928	96360	1
C8928	96365	1
C8928	96372	1
C8928	96374	1
C8928	96375	1
C8928	96376	1
C8929	C8924	1
C8929	36000	1
C8929	36005	1
C8929	36410	1
C8929	76604	1
C8929	76998	1
C8929	93040	1
C8929	93041	1
C8929	93042	1
C8929	93304	1
C8929	93307	0

Column 1	Column 2	Modifier 0=not allowed 1=allowed 9=not applicable
C8929	93308	1
C8929	93320	0
C8929	93321	0
C8929	93325	0
C8929	96360	1
C8929	96365	1
C8929	96372	1
C8929	96374	1
C8929	96375	1
C8929	96376	1
C8930	C8929	1
C8930	36000	1
C8930	36005	1
C8930	36410	1
C8930	76998	1
C8930	93000	1
C8930	93005	1
C8930	93010	1
C8930	93015	0
C8930	93016	0
C8930	93017	0
C8930	93018	0
C8930	93040	1
C8930	93041	1
C8930	93042	1
C8930	93306	1
C8930	93308	1
C8930	93350	0
C8930	93351	0
C8930	94620	1
C8930	94621	0
C8930	94760	0
C8930	94761	0
C8930	96360	1
C8930	96365	1
C8930	96372	1
C8930	96374	1
C8930	96375	1
C8930	96376	1
C8931	C8932	0
C8931	J1642	1
C8931	01916	0

Column 1	Column 2	Modifier 0=not allowed 1=allowed 9=not applicable
C8931	36000	1
C8931	36005	1
C8931	36410	1
C8931	72141	1
C8931	72142	1
C8931	72146	1
C8931	72147	1
C8931	72148	1
C8931	72149	1
C8931	72156	1
C8931	72157	1
C8931	72158	1
C8931	76000	1
C8931	76001	1
C8931	76376	0
C8931	76377	0
C8931	76942	1
C8931	76998	1
C8931	77002	1
C8931	96360	1
C8931	96365	1
C8931	96372	1
C8931	96374	1
C8931	96375	1
C8931	96376	1
C8932	J1642	1
C8932	01916	0
C8932	36000	1
C8932	36005	1
C8932	36410	1
C8932	72141	1
C8932	72142	1
C8932	72146	1
C8932	72147	1
C8932	72148	1
C8932	72149	1
C8932	72156	1
C8932	72157	1
C8932	72158	1
C8932	76000	1
C8932	76001	1
C8932	76376	0

Column 1	Column 2	Modifier 0=not allowed 1=allowed 9=not applicable
C8932	76377	0
C8932	76942	1
C8932	76998	1
C8932	77002	1
C8932	96360	1
C8932	96365	1
C8932	96372	1
C8932	96374	1
C8932	96375	1
C8932	96376	1
C8933	C8931	0
C8933	C8932	0
C8933	J1642	1
C8933	01916	0
C8933	36000	1
C8933	36005	1
C8933	36410	1
C8933	72141	1
C8933	72142	1
C8933	72146	1
C8933	72147	1
C8933	72148	1
C8933	72149	1
C8933	72156	1
C8933	72157	1
C8933	72158	1
C8933	76000	1
C8933	76001	1
C8933	76376	0
C8933	76377	0
C8933	76942	1
C8933	76998	1
C8933	77002	1
C8933	96360	1
C8933	96365	1
C8933	96372	1
C8933	96374	1
C8933	96375	1
C8933	96376	1
C8934	C8935	0
C8934	J1642	1
C8934	01916	0

Column 1	Column 2	Modifier 0=not allowed 1=allowed 9=not applicable
C8934	36000	1
C8934	36005	1
C8934	36410	1
C8934	73218	1
C8934	73219	1
C8934	73220	1
C8934	73221	1
C8934	73222	1
C8934	73223	1
C8934	76000	1
C8934	76001	1
C8934	76376	0
C8934	76377	0
C8934	76942	1
C8934	76998	1
C8934	77002	1
C8934	96360	1
C8934	96365	1
C8934	96372	1
C8934	96374	1
C8934	96375	1
C8934	96376	1
C8935	J1642	1
C8935	01916	0
C8935	36000	1
C8935	36005	1
C8935	36410	1
C8935	73218	1
C8935	73219	1
C8935	73220	1
C8935	73221	1
C8935	73222	1
C8935	73223	1
C8935	76000	1
C8935	76001	1
C8935	76376	0
C8935	76377	0
C8935	76942	1
C8935	76998	1
C8935	77002	1
C8935	96360	1
C8935	96365	1

Column 1	Column 2	Modifier 0=not allowed 1=allowed 9=not applicable
C8935	96372	1
C8935	96374	1
C8935	96375	1
C8935	96376	1
C8936	C8934	0
C8936	C8935	0
C8936	J1642	1
C8936	01916	0
C8936	36000	1
C8936	36005	1
C8936	36410	1
C8936	73218	1
C8936	73219	1
C8936	73220	1
C8936	73221	1
C8936	73222	1
C8936	73223	1
C8936	76000	1
C8936	76001	1
C8936	76376	0
C8936	76377	0
C8936	76942	1
C8936	76998	1
C8936	77002	1
C8936	96360	1
C8936	96365	1
C8936	96372	1
C8936	96374	1
C8936	96375	1
C8936	96376	1
C8957	36000	1
C8957	36410	1
C8957	64450	1
C8957	96360	1
C8957	96365	1
C8957	96372	1
C8957	96374	1
C8957	96521	0
C8957	96522	0
C8957	96523	0
C8957	99201	1
C8957	99202	1

Column 1	Column 2	Modifier 0=not allowed 1=allowed 9=not applicable
C8957	99203	1
C8957	99204	1
C8957	99205	1
C8957	99211	0
C8957	99212	1
C8957	99213	1
C8957	99214	1
C8957	99215	1
C9716	0213T	1
C9716	0216T	1
C9716	36000	1
C9716	36410	1
C9716	37202	1
C9716	43752	1
C9716	45900	0
C9716	45905	0
C9716	45910	0
C9716	45915	0
C9716	45990	0
C9716	46040	0
C9716	46080	0
C9716	46220	0
C9716	46600	0
C9716	46940	0
C9716	46942	0
C9716	62318	1
C9716	62319	1
C9716	64415	1
C9716	64416	1
C9716	64417	1
C9716	64450	1
C9716	64490	1
C9716	64493	1
C9716	96360	1
C9716	96365	1
C9716	96372	1
C9716	96374	1
C9716	96375	1
C9716	96376	1
C9724	0213T	1
C9724	0216T	1
C9724	31505	0

Column 1	Column 2	Modifier 0=not allowed 1=allowed 9=not applicable
C9724	31525	0
C9724	31575	0
C9724	36000	1
C9724	36410	1
C9724	37202	1
C9724	43200	0
C9724	43201	0
C9724	43202	0
C9724	43204	0
C9724	43205	0
C9724	43215	0
C9724	43216	0
C9724	43217	0
C9724	43219	0
C9724	43220	0
C9724	43226	0
C9724	43227	0
C9724	43228	0
C9724	43231	0
C9724	43232	0
C9724	43234	0
C9724	43235	0
C9724	43255	1
C9724	43752	1
C9724	62318	1
C9724	62319	1
C9724	64415	1
C9724	64416	1
C9724	64417	1
C9724	64450	1
C9724	64490	1
C9724	64493	1
C9724	89130	0
C9724	91000	0
C9724	91055	0
C9724	91105	1
C9724	92511	0
C9724	94760	0
C9724	94761	0
C9724	96360	1
C9724	96365	1
C9724	96372	1

Column 1	Column 2	Modifier 0=not allowed 1=allowed 9=not applicable
C9724	96374	1
C9724	96375	1
C9724	96376	1
C9725	0213T	1
C9725	0216T	1
C9725	36000	1
C9725	36410	1
C9725	37202	1
C9725	43752	1
C9725	45900	0
C9725	45905	0
C9725	45910	0
C9725	45915	0
C9725	45990	0
C9725	46040	0
C9725	46080	0
C9725	46220	0
C9725	46600	0
C9725	46940	0
C9725	46942	0
C9725	62318	1
C9725	62319	1
C9725	64415	1
C9725	64416	1
C9725	64417	1
C9725	64450	1
C9725	64490	1
C9725	64493	1
C9725	96360	1
C9725	96365	1
C9725	96372	1
C9725	96374	1
C9725	96375	1
C9725	96376	1
C9800	J2001	1
C9800	Q2026	0
C9800	Q2027	0
C9800	0213T	0
C9800	0216T	0
C9800	0228T	0
C9800	0230T	0
C9800	36000	1

Column 1	Column 2	Modifier 0=not allowed 1=allowed 9=not applicable
C9800	36400	1
C9800	36405	1
C9800	36406	1
C9800	36410	1
C9800	36420	1
C9800	36425	1
C9800	36430	1
C9800	36440	1
C9800	36600	1
C9800	36640	1
C9800	37202	1
C9800	43752	1
C9800	51701	1
C9800	51702	1
C9800	51703	1
C9800	62310	0
C9800	62311	0
C9800	62318	0
C9800	62319	0
C9800	64400	0
C9800	64402	0
C9800	64405	0
C9800	64408	0
C9800	64410	0
C9800	64412	0
C9800	64413	0
C9800	64415	0
C9800	64416	0
C9800	64417	0
C9800	64418	0
C9800	64420	0
C9800	64421	0
C9800	64425	0
C9800	64430	0
C9800	64435	0
C9800	64445	0
C9800	64446	0
C9800	64447	0
C9800	64448	0
C9800	64449	0
C9800	64450	1
C9800	64479	0

Column 1	Column 2	Modifier 0=not allowed 1=allowed 9=not applicable
C9800	64483	0
C9800	64490	0
C9800	64493	0
C9800	64505	0
C9800	64508	0
C9800	64510	0
C9800	64517	0
C9800	64520	0
C9800	64530	0
C9800	69990	0
C9800	93000	1
C9800	93005	1
C9800	93010	1
C9800	93040	1
C9800	93041	1
C9800	93042	1
C9800	93318	1
C9800	94002	1
C9800	94200	1
C9800	94250	1
C9800	94680	1
C9800	94681	1
C9800	94690	1
C9800	94770	1
C9800	95812	1
C9800	95813	1
C9800	95816	1
C9800	95819	1
C9800	95822	1
C9800	95829	1
C9800	95955	1
C9800	96360	1
C9800	96365	1
C9800	96372	1
C9800	96374	1
C9800	96375	1
C9800	96376	1
C9800	99148	0
C9800	99149	0
C9800	99150	0
G0008	99211	0
G0009	99211	0

Column 1	Column 2	Modifier 0=not allowed 1=allowed 9=not applicable
G0010	99211	0
G0027	80500	1
G0027	80502	1
G0027	89321	0
G0101	G0181	1
G0101	G0182	1
G0101	G0380	1
G0101	G0381	1
G0101	G0382	1
G0101	G0383	1
G0101	G0384	1
G0101	G0406	1
G0101	G0407	1
G0101	G0408	1
G0101	G0425	1
G0101	G0426	1
G0101	G0427	1
G0101	99201	1
G0101	99202	1
G0101	99203	1
G0101	99204	1
G0101	99205	1
G0101	99211	1
G0101	99212	1
G0101	99213	1
G0101	99214	1
G0101	99215	1
G0101	99217	1
G0101	99218	1
G0101	99219	1
G0101	99220	1
G0101	99221	1
G0101	99222	1
G0101	99223	1
G0101	99231	1
G0101	99232	1
G0101	99233	1
G0101	99234	1
G0101	99235	1
G0101	99236	1
G0101	99238	1
G0101	99239	1

Column 1	Column 2	Modifier 0=not allowed 1=allowed 9=not applicable
G0101	99281	1
G0101	99282	1
G0101	99283	1
G0101	99284	1
G0101	99285	1
G0101	99291	1
G0101	99292	1
G0101	99304	1
G0101	99305	1
G0101	99306	1
G0101	99307	1
G0101	99308	1
G0101	99309	1
G0101	99310	1
G0101	99315	1
G0101	99316	1
G0101	99318	1
G0101	99324	1
G0101	99325	1
G0101	99326	1
G0101	99327	1
G0101	99328	1
G0101	99334	1
G0101	99335	1
G0101	99336	1
G0101	99337	1
G0101	99341	1
G0101	99342	1
G0101	99343	1
G0101	99344	1
G0101	99345	1
G0101	99347	1
G0101	99348	1
G0101	99349	1
G0101	99350	1
G0101	99354	1
G0101	99355	1
G0101	99356	1
G0101	99357	1
G0101	99360	1
G0101	99455	1
G0101	99456	1

Column 1	Column 2	Modifier 0=not allowed 1=allowed 9=not applicable
G0101	99460	1
G0101	99461	1
G0101	99462	1
G0101	99463	1
G0101	99464	1
G0101	99465	1
G0101	99466	1
G0101	99468	1
G0101	99469	1
G0101	99471	1
G0101	99472	1
G0101	99475	1
G0101	99476	1
G0101	99477	1
G0101	99478	1
G0101	99479	1
G0101	99480	1
G0102	99463	0
G0104	G0181	1
G0104	G0182	1
G0104	G0380	1
G0104	G0381	1
G0104	G0382	1
G0104	G0383	1
G0104	G0384	1
G0104	G0406	1
G0104	G0407	1
G0104	G0408	1
G0104	G0425	1
G0104	G0426	1
G0104	G0427	1
G0104	0213T	0
G0104	0216T	0
G0104	0228T	0
G0104	0230T	0
G0104	36000	1
G0104	36400	1
G0104	36405	1
G0104	36406	1
G0104	36410	1
G0104	36420	1
G0104	36425	1

Column 1	Column 2	Modifier 0=not allowed 1=allowed 9=not applicable
G0104	36430	1
G0104	36440	1
G0104	36600	1
G0104	36640	1
G0104	43752	1
G0104	51701	1
G0104	51702	1
G0104	51703	1
G0104	62310	0
G0104	62311	0
G0104	62318	0
G0104	62319	0
G0104	64400	0
G0104	64402	0
G0104	64405	0
G0104	64408	0
G0104	64410	0
G0104	64412	0
G0104	64413	0
G0104	64415	0
G0104	64416	0
G0104	64417	0
G0104	64418	0
G0104	64420	0
G0104	64421	0
G0104	64425	0
G0104	64430	0
G0104	64435	0
G0104	64445	0
G0104	64446	0
G0104	64447	0
G0104	64448	0
G0104	64449	0
G0104	64450	0
G0104	64479	0
G0104	64483	0
G0104	64490	0
G0104	64493	0
G0104	64505	0
G0104	64508	0
G0104	64510	0
G0104	64517	0

Column 1	Column 2	Modifier 0=not allowed 1=allowed 9=not applicable
G0104	64520	0
G0104	64530	0
G0104	93000	1
G0104	93005	1
G0104	93010	1
G0104	93040	1
G0104	93041	1
G0104	93042	1
G0104	93318	1
G0104	94002	1
G0104	94200	1
G0104	94250	1
G0104	94680	1
G0104	94681	1
G0104	94690	1
G0104	94770	1
G0104	95812	1
G0104	95813	1
G0104	95816	1
G0104	95819	1
G0104	95822	1
G0104	95829	1
G0104	95955	1
G0104	96360	1
G0104	96365	1
G0104	96372	1
G0104	96374	1
G0104	96375	1
G0104	96376	1
G0104	99148	0
G0104	99149	0
G0104	99150	0
G0104	99201	1
G0104	99202	1
G0104	99203	1
G0104	99204	1
G0104	99205	1
G0104	99211	1
G0104	99212	1
G0104	99213	1
G0104	99214	1
G0104	99215	1

Column 1	Column 2	Modifier 0=not allowed 1=allowed 9=not applicable
G0104	99217	1
G0104	99218	1
G0104	99219	1
G0104	99220	1
G0104	99221	1
G0104	99222	1
G0104	99223	1
G0104	99231	1
G0104	99232	1
G0104	99233	1
G0104	99234	1
G0104	99235	1
G0104	99236	1
G0104	99238	1
G0104	99239	1
G0104	99281	1
G0104	99282	1
G0104	99283	1
G0104	99284	1
G0104	99285	1
G0104	99291	1
G0104	99292	1
G0104	99304	1
G0104	99305	1
G0104	99306	1
G0104	99307	1
G0104	99308	1
G0104	99309	1
G0104	99310	1
G0104	99315	1
G0104	99316	1
G0104	99318	1
G0104	99324	1
G0104	99325	1
G0104	99326	1
G0104	99327	1
G0104	99328	1
G0104	99334	1
G0104	99335	1
G0104	99336	1
G0104	99337	1
G0104	99341	1

Column 1	Column 2	Modifier 0=not allowed 1=allowed 9=not applicable
G0104	99342	1
G0104	99343	1
G0104	99344	1
G0104	99345	1
G0104	99347	1
G0104	99348	1
G0104	99349	1
G0104	99350	1
G0104	99354	1
G0104	99355	1
G0104	99356	1
G0104	99357	1
G0104	99360	1
G0104	99455	1
G0104	99456	1
G0104	99460	1
G0104	99461	1
G0104	99462	1
G0104	99463	1
G0104	99464	1
G0104	99465	1
G0104	99466	1
G0104	99468	1
G0104	99469	1
G0104	99471	1
G0104	99472	1
G0104	99475	1
G0104	99476	1
G0104	99477	1
G0104	99478	1
G0104	99479	1
G0104	99480	1
G0105	G0181	1
G0105	G0182	1
G0105	G0380	1
G0105	G0381	1
G0105	G0382	1
G0105	G0383	1
G0105	G0384	1
G0105	G0406	1
G0105	G0407	1
G0105	G0408	1

Column 1	Column 2	Modifier 0=not allowed 1=allowed 9=not applicable
G0105	G0425	1
G0105	G0426	1
G0105	G0427	1
G0105	0213T	0
G0105	0216T	0
G0105	0228T	0
G0105	0230T	0
G0105	36000	1
G0105	36400	1
G0105	36405	1
G0105	36406	1
G0105	36410	1
G0105	36420	1
G0105	36425	1
G0105	36430	1
G0105	36440	1
G0105	36600	1
G0105	36640	1
G0105	43752	1
G0105	51701	1
G0105	51702	1
G0105	51703	1
G0105	62310	0
G0105	62311	0
G0105	62318	0
G0105	62319	0
G0105	64400	0
G0105	64402	0
G0105	64405	0
G0105	64408	0
G0105	64410	0
G0105	64412	0
G0105	64413	0
G0105	64415	0
G0105	64416	0
G0105	64417	0
G0105	64418	0
G0105	64420	0
G0105	64421	0
G0105	64425	0
G0105	64430	0
G0105	64435	0

Column 1	Column 2	Modifier 0=not allowed 1=allowed 9=not applicable	Column 1	Column 2	Modifier 0=not allowed 1=allowed 9=not applicable	Column 1	Column 2	Modifier 0=not allowed 1=allowed 9=not applicable
G0105	64445	0	G0105	96376	1	G0105	99310	1
G0105	64446	0	G0105	99148	0	G0105	99315	1
G0105	64447	0	G0105	99149	0	G0105	99316	1
G0105	64448	0	G0105	99150	0	G0105	99318	1
G0105	64449	0	G0105	99201	1	G0105	99324	1
G0105	64450	0	G0105	99202	1	G0105	99325	1
G0105	64479	0	G0105	99203	1	G0105	99326	1
G0105	64483	0	G0105	99204	1	G0105	99327	1
G0105	64490	0	G0105	99205	1	G0105	99328	1
G0105	64493	0	G0105	99211	1	G0105	99334	1
G0105	64505	0	G0105	99212	1	G0105	99335	1
G0105	64508	0	G0105	99213	1	G0105	99336	1
G0105	64510	0	G0105	99214	1	G0105	99337	1
G0105	64517	0	G0105	99215	1	G0105	99341	1
G0105	64520	0	G0105	99217	1	G0105	99342	1
G0105	64530	0	G0105	99218	1	G0105	99343	1
G0105	93000	1	G0105	99219	1	G0105	99344	1
G0105	93005	1	G0105	99220	1	G0105	99345	1
G0105	93010	1	G0105	99221	1	G0105	99347	1
G0105	93040	1	G0105	99222	1	G0105	99348	1
G0105	93041	1	G0105	99223	1	G0105	99349	1
G0105	93042	1	G0105	99231	1	G0105	99350	1
G0105	93318	1	G0105	99232	1	G0105	99354	1
G0105	94002	1	G0105	99233	1	G0105	99355	1
G0105	94200	1	G0105	99234	1	G0105	99356	1
G0105	94250	1	G0105	99235	1	G0105	99357	1
G0105	94680	1	G0105	99236	1	G0105	99360	1
G0105	94681	1	G0105	99238	1	G0105	99455	1
G0105	94690	1	G0105	99239	1	G0105	99456	1
G0105	94770	1	G0105	99281	1	G0105	99460	1
G0105	95812	1	G0105	99282	1	G0105	99461	1
G0105	95813	1	G0105	99283	1	G0105	99462	1
G0105	95816	1	G0105	99284	1	G0105	99463	1
G0105	95819	1	G0105	99285	1	G0105	99464	1
G0105	95822	1	G0105	99291	1	G0105	99465	1
G0105	95829	1	G0105	99292	1	G0105	99466	1
G0105	95955	1	G0105	99304	1	G0105	99468	1
G0105	96360	1	G0105	99305	1	G0105	99469	1
G0105	96365	1	G0105	99306	1	G0105	99471	1
G0105	96372	1	G0105	99307	1	G0105	99472	1
G0105	96374	1	G0105	99308	1	G0105	99475	1
G0105	96375	1	G0105	99309	1	G0105	99476	1

Column 1	Column 2	Modifier 0=not allowed 1=allowed 9=not applicable
G0105	99477	1
G0105	99478	1
G0105	99479	1
G0105	99480	1
G0106	G0181	1
G0106	G0182	1
G0106	G0380	1
G0106	G0381	1
G0106	G0382	1
G0106	G0383	1
G0106	G0384	1
G0106	G0406	1
G0106	G0407	1
G0106	G0408	1
G0106	G0425	1
G0106	G0426	1
G0106	G0427	1
G0106	74010	1
G0106	76000	1
G0106	76001	1
G0106	99201	1
G0106	99202	1
G0106	99203	1
G0106	99204	1
G0106	99205	1
G0106	99211	1
G0106	99212	1
G0106	99213	1
G0106	99214	1
G0106	99215	1
G0106	99217	1
G0106	99218	1
G0106	99219	1
G0106	99220	1
G0106	99221	1
G0106	99222	1
G0106	99223	1
G0106	99231	1
G0106	99232	1
G0106	99233	1
G0106	99234	1
G0106	99235	1

Column 1	Column 2	Modifier 0=not allowed 1=allowed 9=not applicable
G0106	99236	1
G0106	99238	1
G0106	99239	1
G0106	99281	1
G0106	99282	1
G0106	99283	1
G0106	99284	1
G0106	99285	1
G0106	99291	1
G0106	99292	1
G0106	99304	1
G0106	99305	1
G0106	99306	1
G0106	99307	1
G0106	99308	1
G0106	99309	1
G0106	99310	1
G0106	99315	1
G0106	99316	1
G0106	99318	1
G0106	99324	1
G0106	99325	1
G0106	99326	1
G0106	99327	1
G0106	99328	1
G0106	99334	1
G0106	99335	1
G0106	99336	1
G0106	99337	1
G0106	99341	1
G0106	99342	1
G0106	99343	1
G0106	99344	1
G0106	99345	1
G0106	99347	1
G0106	99348	1
G0106	99350	1
G0106	99354	1
G0106	99355	1
G0106	99356	1
G0106	99357	1
G0106	99360	1

Column 1	Column 2	Modifier 0=not allowed 1=allowed 9=not applicable
G0106	99455	1
G0106	99456	1
G0106	99460	1
G0106	99461	1
G0106	99462	1
G0106	99463	1
G0106	99464	1
G0106	99465	1
G0106	99466	1
G0106	99468	1
G0106	99469	1
G0106	99471	1
G0106	99472	1
G0106	99475	1
G0106	99476	1
G0106	99477	1
G0106	99478	1
G0106	99479	1
G0106	99480	1
G0108	G0270	0
G0108	G0271	0
G0108	97802	0
G0108	97803	0
G0108	97804	0
G0109	G0270	0
G0109	G0271	0
G0109	97802	0
G0109	97803	0
G0109	97804	0
G0117	G0118	0
G0120	G0181	1
G0120	G0182	1
G0120	G0380	1
G0120	G0381	1
G0120	G0382	1
G0120	G0383	1
G0120	G0384	1
G0120	G0406	1
G0120	G0407	1
G0120	G0408	1
G0120	G0425	1
G0120	G0426	1

Column 1	Column 2	Modifier 0=not allowed 1=allowed 9=not applicable	Column 1	Column 2	Modifier 0=not allowed 1=allowed 9=not applicable	Column 1	Column 2	Modifier 0=not allowed 1=allowed 9=not applicable
G0120	G0427	1	G0120	99315	1	G0120	99478	1
G0120	76000	1	G0120	99316	1	G0120	99479	1
G0120	76001	1	G0120	99318	1	G0120	99480	1
G0120	99201	1	G0120	99324	1	G0121	G0380	1
G0120	99202	1	G0120	99325	1	G0121	G0381	1
G0120	99203	1	G0120	99326	1	G0121	G0382	1
G0120	99204	1	G0120	99327	1	G0121	G0383	1
G0120	99205	1	G0120	99328	1	G0121	G0384	1
G0120	99211	1	G0120	99334	1	G0121	G0406	1
G0120	99212	1	G0120	99335	1	G0121	G0407	1
G0120	99213	1	G0120	99336	1	G0121	G0408	1
G0120	99214	1	G0120	99337	1	G0121	G0425	1
G0120	99215	1	G0120	99341	1	G0121	G0426	1
G0120	99217	1	G0120	99342	1	G0121	G0427	1
G0120	99218	1	G0120	99343	1	G0121	0213T	0
G0120	99219	1	G0120	99344	1	G0121	0216T	0
G0120	99220	1	G0120	99345	1	G0121	0228T	0
G0120	99221	1	G0120	99347	1	G0121	0230T	0
G0120	99222	1	G0120	99348	1	G0121	36000	1
G0120	99223	1	G0120	99349	1	G0121	36400	1
G0120	99231	1	G0120	99350	1	G0121	36405	1
G0120	99232	1	G0120	99354	1	G0121	36406	1
G0120	99233	1	G0120	99355	1	G0121	36410	1
G0120	99234	1	G0120	99356	1	G0121	36420	1
G0120	99235	1	G0120	99357	1	G0121	36425	1
G0120	99236	1	G0120	99360	1	G0121	36430	1
G0120	99238	1	G0120	99455	1	G0121	36440	1
G0120	99239	1	G0120	99456	1	G0121	36600	1
G0120	99281	1	G0120	99460	1	G0121	36640	1
G0120	99282	1	G0120	99461	1	G0121	43752	1
G0120	99283	1	G0120	99462	1	G0121	51701	1
G0120	99284	1	G0120	99463	1	G0121	51702	1
G0120	99285	1	G0120	99464	1	G0121	51703	1
G0120	99291	1	G0120	99465	1	G0121	62310	0
G0120	99292	1	G0120	99466	1	G0121	62311	0
G0120	99304	1	G0120	99468	1	G0121	62318	0
G0120	99305	1	G0120	99469	1	G0121	62319	0
G0120	99306	1	G0120	99471	1	G0121	64400	0
G0120	99307	1	G0120	99472	1	G0121	64402	0
G0120	99308	1	G0120	99475	1	G0121	64405	0
G0120	99309	1	G0120	99476	1	G0121	64408	0
G0120	99310	1	G0120	99477	1	G0121	64410	0

Column 1	Column 2	Modifier 0=not allowed 1=allowed 9=not applicable	Column 1	Column 2	Modifier 0=not allowed 1=allowed 9=not applicable	Column 1	Column 2	Modifier 0=not allowed 1=allowed 9=not applicable
G0121	64412	0	G0121	95813	1	G0121	99283	1
G0121	64413	0	G0121	95816	1	G0121	99284	1
G0121	64415	0	G0121	95819	1	G0121	99285	1
G0121	64416	0	G0121	95822	1	G0121	99291	1
G0121	64417	0	G0121	95829	1	G0121	99292	1
G0121	64418	0	G0121	95955	1	G0121	99304	1
G0121	64420	0	G0121	96360	1	G0121	99305	1
G0121	64421	0	G0121	96365	1	G0121	99306	1
G0121	64425	0	G0121	96372	1	G0121	99307	1
G0121	64430	0	G0121	96374	1	G0121	99308	1
G0121	64435	0	G0121	96375	1	G0121	99309	1
G0121	64445	0	G0121	96376	1	G0121	99310	1
G0121	64446	0	G0121	99148	0	G0121	99315	1
G0121	64447	0	G0121	99149	0	G0121	99316	1
G0121	64448	0	G0121	99150	0	G0121	99318	1
G0121	64449	0	G0121	99201	1	G0121	99324	1
G0121	64450	0	G0121	99202	1	G0121	99325	1
G0121	64479	0	G0121	99203	1	G0121	99326	1
G0121	64483	0	G0121	99204	1	G0121	99327	1
G0121	64490	0	G0121	99205	1	G0121	99328	1
G0121	64493	0	G0121	99211	1	G0121	99334	1
G0121	64505	0	G0121	99212	1	G0121	99335	1
G0121	64508	0	G0121	99213	1	G0121	99336	1
G0121	64510	0	G0121	99214	1	G0121	99337	1
G0121	64517	0	G0121	99215	1	G0121	99341	1
G0121	64520	0	G0121	99217	1	G0121	99342	1
G0121	64530	0	G0121	99218	1	G0121	99343	1
G0121	93000	1	G0121	99219	1	G0121	99344	1
G0121	93005	1	G0121	99220	1	G0121	99345	1
G0121	93010	1	G0121	99221	1	G0121	99347	1
G0121	93040	1	G0121	99222	1	G0121	99348	1
G0121	93041	1	G0121	99223	1	G0121	99349	1
G0121	93042	1	G0121	99231	1	G0121	99350	1
G0121	93318	1	G0121	99232	1	G0121	99354	1
G0121	94002	1	G0121	99233	1	G0121	99355	1
G0121	94200	1	G0121	99234	1	G0121	99356	1
G0121	94250	1	G0121	99235	1	G0121	99357	1
G0121	94680	1	G0121	99236	1	G0121	99360	1
G0121	94681	1	G0121	99238	1	G0121	99455	1
G0121	94690	1	G0121	99239	1	G0121	99456	1
G0121	94770	1	G0121	99281	1	G0121	99460	1
G0121	95812	1	G0121	99282	1	G0121	99461	1

Column 1	Column 2	Modifier 0=not allowed 1=allowed 9=not applicable
G0121	99462	1
G0121	99463	1
G0121	99465	1
G0121	99466	1
G0121	99468	1
G0121	99469	1
G0121	99471	1
G0121	99472	1
G0121	99475	1
G0121	99476	1
G0121	99477	1
G0121	99478	1
G0121	99479	1
G0121	99480	1
G0123	P3000	0
G0124	G0141	0
G0124	G0147	0
G0124	G0148	0
G0124	P3000	0
G0124	P3001	0
G0124	88142	0
G0124	88143	0
G0124	88147	0
G0124	88148	0
G0124	88150	0
G0124	88152	0
G0124	88153	0
G0124	88154	0
G0124	88164	0
G0124	88165	0
G0124	88166	0
G0124	88167	0
G0124	88174	0
G0124	88175	0
G0127	11040	1
G0127	11041	1
G0127	11042	1
G0127	51701	1
G0127	51702	1
G0127	51703	1
G0127	96360	1
G0127	96365	1

Column 1	Column 2	Modifier 0=not allowed 1=allowed 9=not applicable
G0127	96372	1
G0127	96374	1
G0127	96375	1
G0127	96376	1
G0127	97597	1
G0127	97598	1
G0127	97602	1
G0127	97605	1
G0127	97606	1
G0127	99148	0
G0127	99149	0
G0127	99150	0
G0129	97001	0
G0129	97002	0
G0129	97003	1
G0129	97004	1
G0129	97150	1
G0129	97530	1
G0129	97532	1
G0129	97533	1
G0129	97535	1
G0129	97537	1
G0129	97542	1
G0129	97545	1
G0129	97750	1
G0141	G0123	0
G0141	G0143	0
G0141	G0144	0
G0141	P3000	0
G0141	88142	0
G0141	88143	0
G0141	88147	0
G0141	88148	0
G0141	88150	0
G0141	88152	0
G0141	88153	0
G0141	88154	0
G0141	88164	0
G0141	88165	0
G0141	88166	0
G0141	88167	0
G0141	88174	0

Column 1	Column 2	Modifier 0=not allowed 1=allowed 9=not applicable
G0141	88175	0
G0145	G0147	0
G0145	G0148	0
G0148	G0147	0
G0151	G0281	1
G0151	G0283	1
G0151	G0329	1
G0151	97001	1
G0151	97002	1
G0151	97003	0
G0151	97004	0
G0151	97012	1
G0151	97016	1
G0151	97018	1
G0151	97022	1
G0151	97024	1
G0151	97026	1
G0151	97028	1
G0151	97032	1
G0151	97033	1
G0151	97034	1
G0151	97035	1
G0151	97036	1
G0151	97110	1
G0151	97112	1
G0151	97113	1
G0151	97116	1
G0151	97124	1
G0151	97140	1
G0151	97150	1
G0151	97530	1
G0151	97532	1
G0151	97533	1
G0151	97535	1
G0151	97537	1
G0151	97542	1
G0151	97545	1
G0151	97546	1
G0151	97750	1
G0151	97760	1
G0151	97761	1
G0151	97762	1

Column 1	Column 2	Modifier 0=not allowed 1=allowed 9=not applicable
G0152	97001	0
G0152	97002	0
G0152	97003	1
G0152	97004	1
G0152	97150	1
G0152	97530	1
G0152	97532	1
G0152	97533	1
G0152	97535	1
G0152	97542	1
G0152	97545	1
G0152	97750	1
G0153	0208T	1
G0153	0209T	1
G0153	0210T	1
G0153	0211T	1
G0153	0212T	1
G0153	92506	1
G0153	92507	1
G0153	92508	1
G0153	92526	1
G0153	92550	1
G0153	92552	1
G0153	92553	1
G0153	92555	1
G0153	92556	1
G0153	92557	1
G0153	92561	1
G0153	92562	1
G0153	92563	1
G0153	92564	1
G0153	92565	1
G0153	92567	1
G0153	92568	1
G0153	92570	1
G0153	92571	1
G0153	92572	1
G0153	92575	1
G0153	92576	1
G0153	92577	1
G0153	92579	1
G0153	92582	1

Column 1	Column 2	Modifier 0=not allowed 1=allowed 9=not applicable
G0153	92583	1
G0153	92584	1
G0153	92585	1
G0153	92587	1
G0153	92588	1
G0153	92596	1
G0153	92620	0
G0153	92621	0
G0153	92625	0
G0154	G0008	1
G0154	G0009	1
G0154	G0010	1
G0154	P9612	1
G0154	P9615	1
G0154	36000	1
G0154	36410	1
G0154	36430	1
G0154	96360	1
G0154	96365	1
G0155	97537	1
G0157	G0281	1
G0157	G0283	1
G0157	G0329	1
G0157	97001	1
G0157	97002	1
G0157	97003	0
G0157	97004	0
G0157	97012	1
G0157	97016	1
G0157	97018	1
G0157	97022	1
G0157	97024	1
G0157	97026	1
G0157	97028	1
G0157	97032	1
G0157	97033	1
G0157	97034	1
G0157	97035	1
G0157	97036	1
G0157	97110	1
G0157	97112	1
G0157	97113	1

Column 1	Column 2	Modifier 0=not allowed 1=allowed 9=not applicable
G0157	97116	1
G0157	97124	1
G0157	97140	1
G0157	97150	1
G0157	97530	1
G0157	97532	1
G0157	97533	1
G0157	97535	1
G0157	97537	1
G0157	97542	1
G0157	97545	1
G0157	97546	1
G0157	97750	1
G0157	97760	1
G0157	97761	1
G0157	97762	1
G0158	97001	0
G0158	97002	0
G0158	97003	1
G0158	97004	1
G0158	97150	1
G0158	97530	1
G0158	97532	1
G0158	97533	1
G0158	97535	1
G0158	97542	1
G0158	97545	1
G0158	97750	1
G0159	G0281	1
G0159	G0283	1
G0159	G0329	1
G0159	97001	1
G0159	97002	1
G0159	97003	0
G0159	97004	0
G0159	97012	1
G0159	97016	1
G0159	97018	1
G0159	97022	1
G0159	97024	1
G0159	97026	1
G0159	97028	1

Column 1	Column 2	Modifier 0=not allowed 1=allowed 9=not applicable
G0159	97032	1
G0159	97033	1
G0159	97034	1
G0159	97035	1
G0159	97036	1
G0159	97110	1
G0159	97112	1
G0159	97113	1
G0159	97116	1
G0159	97124	1
G0159	97140	1
G0159	97150	1
G0159	97530	1
G0159	97532	1
G0159	97533	1
G0159	97535	1
G0159	97537	1
G0159	97542	1
G0159	97545	1
G0159	97546	1
G0159	97750	1
G0159	97760	1
G0159	97761	1
G0159	97762	1
G0160	97001	0
G0160	97002	0
G0160	97003	1
G0160	97004	1
G0160	97150	1
G0160	97530	1
G0160	97532	1
G0160	97533	1
G0160	97535	1
G0160	97542	1
G0160	97545	1
G0160	97750	1
G0161	0208T	1
G0161	0209T	1
G0161	0210T	1
G0161	0211T	1
G0161	0212T	1
G0161	92506	1

Column 1	Column 2	Modifier 0=not allowed 1=allowed 9=not applicable
G0161	92507	1
G0161	92508	1
G0161	92526	1
G0161	92550	1
G0161	92552	1
G0161	92553	1
G0161	92555	1
G0161	92556	1
G0161	92557	1
G0161	92561	1
G0161	92562	1
G0161	92563	1
G0161	92564	1
G0161	92565	1
G0161	92567	1
G0161	92568	1
G0161	92570	1
G0161	92571	1
G0161	92572	1
G0161	92575	1
G0161	92576	1
G0161	92577	1
G0161	92579	1
G0161	92582	1
G0161	92583	1
G0161	92584	1
G0161	92585	1
G0161	92587	1
G0161	92588	1
G0161	92596	1
G0161	92620	0
G0161	92621	0
G0161	92625	0
G0162	G0008	1
G0162	G0009	1
G0162	G0010	1
G0162	P9612	1
G0162	P9615	1
G0162	36000	1
G0162	36410	1
G0162	36430	1
G0162	96360	1

Column 1	Column 2	Modifier 0=not allowed 1=allowed 9=not applicable
G0162	96365	1
G0163	G0008	1
G0163	G0009	1
G0163	G0010	1
G0163	P9612	1
G0163	P9615	1
G0163	36000	1
G0163	36410	1
G0163	36430	1
G0163	96360	1
G0163	96365	1
G0164	G0008	1
G0164	G0009	1
G0164	G0010	1
G0164	P9612	1
G0164	P9615	1
G0164	36000	1
G0164	36410	1
G0164	36430	1
G0164	96360	1
G0164	96365	1
G0166	0178T	1
G0166	0179T	1
G0166	0180T	1
G0166	92971	0
G0166	93000	1
G0166	93005	1
G0166	93010	1
G0166	93040	0
G0166	93041	0
G0166	93042	0
G0166	93701	0
G0166	93720	0
G0166	93721	0
G0166	93722	0
G0166	93922	1
G0166	93923	1
G0166	93924	0
G0166	93965	1
G0166	97016	0
G0166	99211	1
G0168	J0670	1

2011 PHYSICIAN COL 1/2 EDITS

Column 1	Column 2	Modifier 0=not allowed 1=allowed 9=not applicable
G0168	J2001	1
G0168	0213T	0
G0168	0216T	0
G0168	0228T	0
G0168	0230T	0
G0168	11900	1
G0168	11901	1
G0168	36000	1
G0168	36400	1
G0168	36405	1
G0168	36406	1
G0168	36410	1
G0168	36420	1
G0168	36425	1
G0168	36430	1
G0168	36440	1
G0168	36600	1
G0168	36640	1
G0168	43752	1
G0168	51701	1
G0168	51702	1
G0168	51703	1
G0168	62310	0
G0168	62311	0
G0168	62318	0
G0168	62319	0
G0168	64400	0
G0168	64402	0
G0168	64405	0
G0168	64408	0
G0168	64410	0
G0168	64412	0
G0168	64413	0
G0168	64415	0
G0168	64416	0
G0168	64417	0
G0168	64418	0
G0168	64420	0
G0168	64421	0
G0168	64425	0
G0168	64430	0
G0168	64435	0

Column 1	Column 2	Modifier 0=not allowed 1=allowed 9=not applicable
G0168	64445	0
G0168	64446	0
G0168	64447	0
G0168	64448	0
G0168	64449	0
G0168	64450	0
G0168	64479	0
G0168	64483	0
G0168	64490	0
G0168	64493	0
G0168	64505	0
G0168	64508	0
G0168	64510	0
G0168	64517	0
G0168	64520	0
G0168	64530	0
G0168	93000	1
G0168	93005	1
G0168	93010	1
G0168	93040	1
G0168	93041	1
G0168	93042	1
G0168	93318	1
G0168	94002	1
G0168	94200	1
G0168	94250	1
G0168	94680	1
G0168	94681	1
G0168	94690	1
G0168	94770	1
G0168	95812	1
G0168	95813	1
G0168	95816	1
G0168	95819	1
G0168	95822	1
G0168	95829	1
G0168	95955	1
G0168	96360	1
G0168	96365	1
G0168	96372	1
G0168	96374	1
G0168	96375	1

Column 1	Column 2	Modifier 0=not allowed 1=allowed 9=not applicable
G0168	96376	1
G0168	99148	0
G0168	99149	0
G0168	99150	0
G0173	M0064	0
G0173	11920	0
G0173	11921	0
G0173	16000	0
G0173	16020	0
G0173	16025	0
G0173	16030	0
G0173	20660	1
G0173	20661	1
G0173	20693	1
G0173	20694	1
G0173	36000	1
G0173	36410	1
G0173	36425	0
G0173	51701	0
G0173	51702	0
G0173	51703	0
G0173	61795	1
G0173	69990	0
G0173	77321	1
G0173	77326	1
G0173	77327	1
G0173	77328	1
G0173	77336	1
G0173	77418	1
G0173	77421	0
G0173	90804	0
G0173	90805	0
G0173	90806	0
G0173	90807	0
G0173	90808	0
G0173	90809	0
G0173	90810	0
G0173	90811	0
G0173	90812	0
G0173	90813	0
G0173	90814	0
G0173	90815	0

Column 1	Column 2	Modifier 0=not allowed 1=allowed 9=not applicable
G0173	90816	0
G0173	90817	0
G0173	90818	0
G0173	90819	0
G0173	90821	0
G0173	90822	0
G0173	90846	0
G0173	90847	0
G0173	90862	0
G0173	96360	0
G0173	96361	0
G0173	96365	0
G0173	96366	0
G0173	96367	0
G0173	96368	0
G0173	97802	0
G0173	97803	0
G0173	97804	0
G0173	99143	0
G0173	99144	0
G0173	99145	0
G0173	99201	0
G0173	99202	0
G0173	99203	0
G0173	99204	0
G0173	99205	0
G0173	99211	0
G0173	99212	0
G0173	99213	0
G0173	99214	0
G0173	99215	0
G0173	99217	0
G0173	99218	0
G0173	99219	0
G0173	99220	0
G0173	99221	0
G0173	99222	0
G0173	99223	0
G0173	99231	0
G0173	99232	0
G0173	99233	0
G0173	99234	0

Column 1	Column 2	Modifier 0=not allowed 1=allowed 9=not applicable
G0173	99235	0
G0173	99236	0
G0173	99238	0
G0173	99239	0
G0173	99281	0
G0173	99282	0
G0173	99283	0
G0173	99284	0
G0173	99285	0
G0173	99291	0
G0173	99292	0
G0173	99304	0
G0173	99305	0
G0173	99306	0
G0173	99307	0
G0173	99308	0
G0173	99309	0
G0173	99310	0
G0173	99315	0
G0173	99316	0
G0173	99318	0
G0173	99324	0
G0173	99325	0
G0173	99326	0
G0173	99327	0
G0173	99328	0
G0173	99334	0
G0173	99335	0
G0173	99336	0
G0173	99337	0
G0173	99341	0
G0173	99342	0
G0173	99343	0
G0173	99344	0
G0173	99345	0
G0173	99347	0
G0173	99348	0
G0173	99349	0
G0173	99350	0
G0173	99360	0
G0173	99455	0
G0173	99456	0

Column 1	Column 2	Modifier 0=not allowed 1=allowed 9=not applicable
G0173	99460	0
G0173	99461	0
G0173	99462	0
G0173	99463	0
G0173	99464	0
G0173	99465	0
G0173	99466	0
G0173	99467	0
G0173	99468	0
G0173	99469	0
G0173	99471	0
G0173	99472	0
G0173	99475	0
G0173	99476	0
G0173	99477	0
G0173	99478	0
G0173	99479	0
G0173	99480	0
G0181	G0102	1
G0181	93040	1
G0181	93041	1
G0181	93042	1
G0182	G0102	1
G0182	93040	1
G0182	93041	1
G0182	93042	1
G0186	36000	1
G0186	36410	1
G0186	67005	1
G0186	67010	1
G0186	67015	1
G0186	67145	1
G0186	67220	1
G0186	67221	1
G0186	67500	1
G0186	69990	0
G0186	96360	1
G0186	96365	1
G0202	76150	0
G0202	77057	0
G0204	G0206	0
G0204	76150	0

Column 1	Column 2	Modifier 0=not allowed 1=allowed 9=not applicable
G0204	77055	0
G0204	77056	0
G0206	76150	0
G0206	77055	0
G0168	0228T	0
G0168	0230T	0
G0237	94010	1
G0237	94060	1
G0237	94150	1
G0237	94200	1
G0237	94240	1
G0237	94250	1
G0237	94260	1
G0237	94350	1
G0237	94360	1
G0237	94370	1
G0237	94375	1
G0237	94400	1
G0237	94450	1
G0237	94620	0
G0237	94621	0
G0237	94680	1
G0237	94681	1
G0237	94690	1
G0237	94720	1
G0237	94725	1
G0237	94750	1
G0237	94760	0
G0237	94761	0
G0237	94762	1
G0237	94770	0
G0237	97001	1
G0237	97002	1
G0237	97003	1
G0237	97004	1
G0237	97110	1
G0237	97112	1
G0237	97150	1
G0237	97530	1
G0237	97750	1
G0237	97802	1
G0237	97803	1

Column 1	Column 2	Modifier 0=not allowed 1=allowed 9=not applicable
G0237	97804	1
G0238	94010	1
G0238	94060	1
G0238	94150	1
G0238	94200	1
G0238	94240	1
G0238	94250	1
G0238	94260	1
G0238	94350	1
G0238	94360	1
G0238	94370	1
G0238	94375	1
G0238	94400	1
G0238	94450	1
G0238	94620	0
G0238	94621	0
G0238	94667	0
G0238	94668	0
G0238	94680	1
G0238	94681	1
G0238	94690	1
G0238	94720	1
G0238	94725	1
G0238	94750	1
G0238	94760	0
G0238	94761	0
G0238	94762	1
G0238	94770	0
G0238	97001	1
G0238	97002	1
G0238	97003	1
G0238	97004	1
G0238	97110	1
G0238	97112	1
G0238	97150	1
G0238	97530	1
G0238	97750	1
G0238	97802	1
G0238	97803	1
G0238	97804	1
G0239	G0237	1
G0239	G0238	1

Column 1	Column 2	Modifier 0=not allowed 1=allowed 9=not applicable
G0239	94010	1
G0239	94060	1
G0239	94150	1
G0239	94200	1
G0239	94240	1
G0239	94250	1
G0239	94260	1
G0239	94350	1
G0239	94360	1
G0239	94370	1
G0239	94375	1
G0239	94400	1
G0239	94450	1
G0239	94620	0
G0239	94621	0
G0239	94667	0
G0239	94668	0
G0239	94680	1
G0239	94681	1
G0239	94690	1
G0239	94720	1
G0239	94725	1
G0239	94750	1
G0239	94760	0
G0239	94761	0
G0239	94762	1
G0239	94770	0
G0239	97001	1
G0239	97002	1
G0239	97003	1
G0239	97004	1
G0239	97110	1
G0239	97112	1
G0239	97150	1
G0239	97530	1
G0239	97750	1
G0239	97802	1
G0239	97803	1
G0239	97804	1
G0245	G0127	0
G0245	G0246	0
G0245	0183T	0

Column 1	Column 2	Modifier 0=not allowed 1=allowed 9=not applicable
G0245	11040	0
G0245	11041	0
G0245	11042	0
G0245	11043	0
G0245	11044	0
G0245	11055	0
G0245	11056	0
G0245	11057	0
G0245	11305	0
G0245	11306	0
G0245	11307	0
G0245	11308	0
G0245	11420	1
G0245	11421	1
G0245	11422	1
G0245	11423	1
G0245	11424	1
G0245	11426	1
G0245	11719	0
G0245	11720	0
G0245	11721	0
G0245	11755	0
G0245	11765	0
G0245	97597	0
G0245	97598	0
G0245	97602	0
G0245	97605	0
G0245	97606	0
G0246	G0127	0
G0246	0183T	0
G0246	11040	0
G0246	11041	0
G0246	11042	0
G0246	11043	0
G0246	11044	0
G0246	11055	0
G0246	11056	0
G0246	11057	0
G0246	11305	0
G0246	11306	0
G0246	11307	0
G0246	11308	0

Column 1	Column 2	Modifier 0=not allowed 1=allowed 9=not applicable
G0246	11420	1
G0246	11421	1
G0246	11422	1
G0246	11423	1
G0246	11424	1
G0246	11426	1
G0246	11719	0
G0246	11720	0
G0246	11721	0
G0246	11755	0
G0246	11765	0
G0246	97597	0
G0246	97598	0
G0246	97602	0
G0246	97605	0
G0246	97606	0
G0247	G0127	0
G0247	0183T	0
G0247	11040	0
G0247	11041	0
G0247	11042	0
G0247	11043	1
G0247	11044	1
G0247	11055	0
G0247	11056	0
G0247	11057	0
G0247	11305	0
G0247	11306	0
G0247	11307	0
G0247	11308	0
G0247	11420	1
G0247	11421	1
G0247	11422	1
G0247	11423	1
G0247	11424	1
G0247	11426	1
G0247	11719	0
G0247	11720	0
G0247	11721	0
G0247	11755	1
G0247	11765	1
G0247	97597	0

Column 1	Column 2	Modifier 0=not allowed 1=allowed 9=not applicable
G0247	97598	0
G0247	97602	0
G0247	97605	0
G0247	97606	0
G0251	M0064	0
G0251	0073T	0
G0251	11920	0
G0251	11921	0
G0251	16000	0
G0251	16020	0
G0251	16025	0
G0251	16030	0
G0251	20660	0
G0251	36000	1
G0251	36410	1
G0251	36425	0
G0251	51701	0
G0251	51702	0
G0251	51703	0
G0251	61795	0
G0251	69990	0
G0251	77321	1
G0251	77326	1
G0251	77327	1
G0251	77328	1
G0251	77401	0
G0251	77402	0
G0251	77403	0
G0251	77404	0
G0251	77406	0
G0251	77407	0
G0251	77408	0
G0251	77409	0
G0251	77411	0
G0251	77412	0
G0251	77413	0
G0251	77414	0
G0251	77416	0
G0251	77418	1
G0251	77421	0
G0251	77422	0
G0251	77423	0

Column 1	Column 2	Modifier 0=not allowed 1=allowed 9=not applicable
G0251	90804	0
G0251	90805	0
G0251	90806	0
G0251	90807	0
G0251	90808	0
G0251	90809	0
G0251	90810	0
G0251	90811	0
G0251	90812	0
G0251	90813	0
G0251	90814	0
G0251	90815	0
G0251	90816	0
G0251	90817	0
G0251	90818	0
G0251	90819	0
G0251	90821	0
G0251	90822	0
G0251	90846	0
G0251	90847	0
G0251	90862	0
G0251	96360	0
G0251	96361	0
G0251	96365	0
G0251	96366	0
G0251	96367	0
G0251	96368	0
G0251	97802	0
G0251	97803	0
G0251	97804	0
G0251	99143	0
G0251	99144	0
G0251	99145	0
G0251	99201	0
G0251	99202	0
G0251	99203	0
G0251	99204	0
G0251	99205	0
G0251	99211	0
G0251	99212	0
G0251	99213	0
G0251	99214	0

Column 1	Column 2	Modifier 0=not allowed 1=allowed 9=not applicable
G0251	99215	0
G0251	99217	0
G0251	99218	0
G0251	99219	0
G0251	99220	0
G0251	99221	0
G0251	99222	0
G0251	99223	0
G0251	99231	0
G0251	99232	0
G0251	99233	0
G0251	99234	0
G0251	99235	0
G0251	99236	0
G0251	99238	0
G0251	99239	0
G0251	99281	0
G0251	99282	0
G0251	99283	0
G0251	99284	0
G0251	99285	0
G0251	99291	0
G0251	99292	0
G0251	99304	0
G0251	99305	0
G0251	99306	0
G0251	99307	0
G0251	99308	0
G0251	99309	0
G0251	99310	0
G0251	99315	0
G0251	99316	0
G0251	99318	0
G0251	99324	0
G0251	99325	0
G0251	99326	0
G0251	99327	0
G0251	99328	0
G0251	99334	0
G0251	99335	0
G0251	99336	0
G0251	99337	0

Column 1	Column 2	Modifier 0=not allowed 1=allowed 9=not applicable
G0251	99341	0
G0251	99342	0
G0251	99343	0
G0251	99344	0
G0251	99345	0
G0251	99347	0
G0251	99348	0
G0251	99349	0
G0251	99350	0
G0251	99354	0
G0251	99355	0
G0251	99356	0
G0251	99357	0
G0251	99360	0
G0251	99455	0
G0251	99456	0
G0251	99460	0
G0251	99461	0
G0251	99462	0
G0251	99463	0
G0251	99464	0
G0251	99465	0
G0251	99466	0
G0251	99467	0
G0251	99468	0
G0251	99469	0
G0251	99471	0
G0251	99472	0
G0251	99475	0
G0251	99476	0
G0251	99477	0
G0251	99478	0
G0251	99479	0
G0251	99480	0
G0257	36000	1
G0257	36147	1
G0257	36410	1
G0257	36430	1
G0257	90935	1
G0257	90937	1
G0257	90945	1
G0257	90947	1

Column 1	Column 2	Modifier 0=not allowed 1=allowed 9=not applicable
G0257	90997	1
G0257	96360	1
G0257	96365	1
G0257	97802	1
G0257	97803	1
G0257	97804	1
G0259	0213T	1
G0259	0216T	1
G0259	20600	1
G0259	20605	1
G0259	20610	1
G0259	27096	0
G0259	36000	1
G0259	36410	1
G0259	37202	1
G0259	62318	1
G0259	62319	1
G0259	64415	1
G0259	64417	1
G0259	64450	1
G0259	64490	1
G0259	64493	1
G0259	69990	0
G0259	76000	1
G0259	76001	1
G0259	77002	1
G0259	96360	1
G0259	96365	1
G0259	96372	1
G0259	96374	1
G0259	96375	1
G0259	96376	1
G0260	0228T	1
G0260	0230T	1
G0260	62310	1
G0260	62311	1
G0260	62318	1
G0260	62319	1
G0260	64400	1
G0260	64402	1
G0260	64405	1
G0260	64408	1

Column 1	Column 2	Modifier 0=not allowed 1=allowed 9=not applicable
G0260	64410	1
G0260	64412	1
G0260	64413	1
G0260	64415	1
G0260	64416	1
G0260	64417	1
G0260	64418	1
G0260	64420	1
G0260	64421	1
G0260	64425	1
G0260	64430	1
G0260	64435	1
G0260	64445	1
G0260	64446	1
G0260	64447	1
G0260	64448	1
G0260	64449	1
G0260	64450	1
G0260	64479	1
G0260	64483	1
G0260	64505	1
G0260	64508	1
G0260	64510	1
G0260	64517	1
G0260	64520	1
G0260	64530	1
G0268	0213T	0
G0268	0216T	0
G0268	36000	1
G0268	36410	1
G0268	37202	1
G0268	51701	1
G0268	51702	1
G0268	51703	1
G0268	62318	0
G0268	62319	0
G0268	64415	0
G0268	64417	0
G0268	64450	0
G0268	64490	0
G0268	64493	0
G0268	69990	0

Column 1	Column 2	Modifier 0=not allowed 1=allowed 9=not applicable
G0268	92504	0
G0268	96360	1
G0268	96365	1
G0268	96372	1
G0268	96374	1
G0268	96375	1
G0268	96376	1
G0268	99148	0
G0268	99149	0
G0268	99150	0
G0270	97802	0
G0270	97803	0
G0270	97804	0
G0271	97802	0
G0271	97803	0
G0271	97804	0
G0275	36140	0
G0275	36200	0
G0275	36245	1
G0275	36246	1
G0275	36247	1
G0275	75625	0
G0275	75630	0
G0275	75722	0
G0275	75724	0
G0275	76942	1
G0275	77002	1
G0278	36140	0
G0278	36200	0
G0278	36245	1
G0278	36246	1
G0278	36247	1
G0278	75625	1
G0278	75630	0
G0278	75710	1
G0278	75716	0
G0278	76942	1
G0278	77002	1
G0281	64550	1
G0281	97002	1
G0281	97004	1
G0281	97032	1

Column 1	Column 2	Modifier 0=not allowed 1=allowed 9=not applicable
G0283	97002	1
G0283	97004	1
G0283	97032	1
G0288	76376	1
G0288	76377	1
G0290	01924	0
G0290	01925	0
G0290	01926	0
G0290	34812	1
G0290	35206	1
G0290	35226	1
G0290	36000	1
G0290	36120	1
G0290	36140	1
G0290	36200	1
G0290	36410	1
G0290	36600	1
G0290	36620	1
G0290	36625	1
G0290	37202	1
G0290	92975	1
G0290	92980	0
G0290	92982	1
G0290	92995	1
G0290	93040	1
G0290	93041	1
G0290	93042	1
G0290	96360	1
G0290	96365	1
G0291	01924	0
G0291	01925	0
G0291	01926	0
G0291	34812	1
G0291	35206	1
G0291	35226	1
G0291	36000	1
G0291	36120	1
G0291	36140	1
G0291	36200	1
G0291	36410	1
G0291	36600	1
G0291	36620	1

Column 1	Column 2	Modifier 0=not allowed 1=allowed 9=not applicable
G0291	36625	1
G0291	37202	1
G0291	92975	1
G0291	92980	0
G0291	92982	1
G0291	92995	1
G0291	93040	1
G0291	93041	1
G0291	93042	1
G0291	93555	1
G0291	93556	1
G0291	96360	1
G0291	96365	1
G0302	G0303	0
G0302	G0304	0
G0302	G0380	1
G0302	G0381	1
G0302	G0382	1
G0302	G0383	1
G0302	G0384	1
G0302	G0406	1
G0302	G0407	1
G0302	G0408	1
G0302	G0425	1
G0302	G0426	1
G0302	G0427	1
G0302	99201	1
G0302	99202	1
G0302	99203	1
G0302	99204	1
G0302	99205	1
G0302	99211	1
G0302	99212	1
G0302	99213	1
G0302	99214	1
G0302	99215	1
G0302	99217	1
G0302	99218	1
G0302	99219	1
G0302	99220	1
G0302	99221	1
G0302	99222	1

Column 1	Column 2	Modifier 0=not allowed 1=allowed 9=not applicable
G0302	99223	1
G0302	99231	1
G0302	99232	1
G0302	99233	1
G0302	99234	1
G0302	99235	1
G0302	99236	1
G0302	99238	1
G0302	99239	1
G0302	99281	1
G0302	99282	1
G0302	99283	1
G0302	99284	1
G0302	99285	1
G0302	99291	1
G0302	99304	1
G0302	99305	1
G0302	99306	1
G0302	99307	1
G0302	99308	1
G0302	99309	1
G0302	99310	1
G0302	99315	1
G0302	99316	1
G0302	99318	1
G0302	99324	1
G0302	99325	1
G0302	99326	1
G0302	99327	1
G0302	99328	1
G0302	99334	1
G0302	99335	1
G0302	99336	1
G0302	99337	1
G0302	99341	1
G0302	99342	1
G0302	99343	1
G0302	99344	1
G0302	99345	1
G0302	99347	1
G0302	99348	1
G0302	99349	1

Column 1	Column 2	Modifier 0=not allowed 1=allowed 9=not applicable
G0302	99350	1
G0302	99466	1
G0302	99468	1
G0302	99469	1
G0302	99471	1
G0302	99472	1
G0302	99475	1
G0302	99476	1
G0302	99477	1
G0302	99478	1
G0302	99479	1
G0302	99480	1
G0303	G0304	0
G0303	G0380	1
G0303	G0381	1
G0303	G0382	1
G0303	G0383	1
G0303	G0384	1
G0303	G0406	1
G0303	G0407	1
G0303	G0408	1
G0303	G0425	1
G0303	G0426	1
G0303	G0427	1
G0303	99201	1
G0303	99202	1
G0303	99203	1
G0303	99204	1
G0303	99205	1
G0303	99211	1
G0303	99212	1
G0303	99213	1
G0303	99214	1
G0303	99215	1
G0303	99217	1
G0303	99218	1
G0303	99219	1
G0303	99220	1
G0303	99221	1
G0303	99222	1
G0303	99223	1
G0303	99231	1

Column 1	Column 2	Modifier 0=not allowed 1=allowed 9=not applicable
G0303	99232	1
G0303	99233	1
G0303	99234	1
G0303	99235	1
G0303	99236	1
G0303	99238	1
G0303	99239	1
G0303	99281	1
G0303	99282	1
G0303	99283	1
G0303	99284	1
G0303	99285	1
G0303	99291	1
G0303	99304	1
G0303	99305	1
G0303	99306	1
G0303	99307	1
G0303	99308	1
G0303	99309	1
G0303	99310	1
G0303	99315	1
G0303	99316	1
G0303	99318	1
G0303	99324	1
G0303	99325	1
G0303	99326	1
G0303	99327	1
G0303	99328	1
G0303	99334	1
G0303	99335	1
G0303	99336	1
G0303	99337	1
G0303	99341	1
G0303	99342	1
G0303	99343	1
G0303	99344	1
G0303	99345	1
G0303	99347	1
G0303	99348	1
G0303	99349	1
G0303	99350	1
G0303	99466	1

Column 1	Column 2	Modifier 0=not allowed 1=allowed 9=not applicable
G0303	99468	1
G0303	99469	1
G0303	99471	1
G0303	99472	1
G0303	99475	1
G0303	99476	1
G0303	99477	1
G0303	99478	1
G0303	99479	1
G0303	99480	1
G0304	G0380	1
G0304	G0381	1
G0304	G0382	1
G0304	G0383	1
G0304	G0384	1
G0304	G0406	1
G0304	G0407	1
G0304	G0408	1
G0304	G0425	1
G0304	G0426	1
G0304	G0427	1
G0304	99201	1
G0304	99202	1
G0304	99203	1
G0304	99204	1
G0304	99205	1
G0304	99211	1
G0304	99212	1
G0304	99213	1
G0304	99214	1
G0304	99215	1
G0304	99217	1
G0304	99218	1
G0304	99219	1
G0304	99220	1
G0304	99221	1
G0304	99222	1
G0304	99223	1
G0304	99231	1
G0304	99232	1
G0304	99233	1
G0304	99234	1

Column 1	Column 2	Modifier 0=not allowed 1=allowed 9=not applicable
G0304	99235	1
G0304	99236	1
G0304	99238	1
G0304	99239	1
G0304	99281	1
G0304	99282	1
G0304	99283	1
G0304	99284	1
G0304	99285	1
G0304	99291	1
G0304	99304	1
G0304	99305	1
G0304	99306	1
G0304	99307	1
G0304	99308	1
G0304	99309	1
G0304	99310	1
G0304	99315	1
G0304	99316	1
G0304	99318	1
G0304	99324	1
G0304	99325	1
G0304	99326	1
G0304	99327	1
G0304	99328	1
G0304	99334	1
G0304	99335	1
G0304	99336	1
G0304	99337	1
G0304	99341	1
G0304	99342	1
G0304	99343	1
G0304	99344	1
G0304	99345	1
G0304	99347	1
G0304	99348	1
G0304	99349	1
G0304	99350	1
G0304	99466	1
G0304	99468	1
G0304	99469	1
G0304	99471	1

Column 1	Column 2	Modifier 0=not allowed 1=allowed 9=not applicable
G0304	99472	1
G0304	99475	1
G0304	99476	1
G0304	99477	1
G0304	99478	1
G0304	99479	1
G0304	99480	1
G0305	G0380	1
G0305	G0381	1
G0305	G0382	1
G0305	G0383	1
G0305	G0384	1
G0305	G0406	1
G0305	G0407	1
G0305	G0408	1
G0305	G0425	1
G0305	G0426	1
G0305	G0427	1
G0305	99201	1
G0305	99202	1
G0305	99203	1
G0305	99204	1
G0305	99205	1
G0305	99211	1
G0305	99212	1
G0305	99213	1
G0305	99214	1
G0305	99215	1
G0305	99217	1
G0305	99218	1
G0305	99219	1
G0305	99220	1
G0305	99221	1
G0305	99222	1
G0305	99223	1
G0305	99231	1
G0305	99232	1
G0305	99233	1
G0305	99234	1
G0305	99235	1
G0305	99236	1
G0305	99238	1

Column 1	Column 2	Modifier 0=not allowed 1=allowed 9=not applicable
G0305	99239	1
G0305	99281	1
G0305	99282	1
G0305	99283	1
G0305	99284	1
G0305	99285	1
G0305	99291	1
G0305	99304	1
G0305	99305	1
G0305	99306	1
G0305	99307	1
G0305	99308	1
G0305	99309	1
G0305	99310	1
G0305	99315	1
G0305	99316	1
G0305	99318	1
G0305	99324	1
G0305	99325	1
G0305	99326	1
G0305	99327	1
G0305	99328	1
G0305	99334	1
G0305	99335	1
G0305	99336	1
G0305	99337	1
G0305	99341	1
G0305	99342	1
G0305	99343	1
G0305	99344	1
G0305	99345	1
G0305	99347	1
G0305	99348	1
G0305	99349	1
G0305	99350	1
G0305	99466	1
G0305	99468	1
G0305	99469	1
G0305	99471	1
G0305	99472	1
G0305	99475	1
G0305	99476	1

Column 1	Column 2	Modifier 0=not allowed 1=allowed 9=not applicable
G0305	99477	1
G0305	99478	1
G0305	99479	1
G0305	99480	1
G0306	G0307	0
G0306	85004	0
G0306	85007	0
G0306	85008	0
G0306	85009	0
G0306	85013	1
G0306	85014	1
G0306	85018	1
G0306	85027	0
G0306	85032	0
G0306	85041	1
G0306	85048	1
G0306	85049	0
G0307	85004	0
G0307	85008	0
G0307	85013	1
G0307	85014	1
G0307	85018	1
G0307	85032	0
G0307	85041	1
G0307	85048	1
G0307	85049	0
G0328	82270	0
G0328	82272	1
G0329	97002	1
G0329	97004	1
G0337	G0101	0
G0337	G0102	0
G0337	G0104	0
G0337	G0105	0
G0337	G0106	0
G0337	G0117	0
G0337	G0118	0
G0337	G0120	0
G0337	G0121	0
G0337	G0245	0
G0337	G0246	0
G0337	G0248	0

Column 1	Column 2	Modifier 0=not allowed 1=allowed 9=not applicable
G0337	G0250	1
G0337	G0270	0
G0337	G0271	0
G0337	G0410	1
G0337	G0411	1
G0337	M0064	0
G0337	P3000	0
G0337	P3001	0
G0337	Q0091	0
G0337	90802	0
G0337	90804	0
G0337	90805	0
G0337	90806	0
G0337	90807	0
G0337	90808	0
G0337	90809	0
G0337	90810	0
G0337	90811	0
G0337	90812	0
G0337	90813	0
G0337	90814	0
G0337	90815	0
G0337	90816	0
G0337	90817	0
G0337	90818	0
G0337	90819	0
G0337	90821	0
G0337	90822	0
G0337	90823	0
G0337	90824	0
G0337	90826	0
G0337	90827	0
G0337	90828	0
G0337	90829	0
G0337	90845	1
G0337	90846	1
G0337	90847	1
G0337	90849	1
G0337	90853	1
G0337	90857	1
G0337	90862	0
G0337	90865	1

Column 1	Column 2	Modifier 0=not allowed 1=allowed 9=not applicable
G0337	90880	1
G0337	92002	0
G0337	92004	0
G0337	92012	0
G0337	92014	0
G0337	95831	0
G0337	95832	0
G0337	95833	0
G0337	95834	0
G0337	95851	0
G0337	95852	0
G0337	96116	1
G0337	96150	0
G0337	96151	0
G0337	96152	0
G0337	96153	0
G0337	96154	0
G0337	97802	0
G0337	97803	0
G0337	97804	0
G0339	M0064	0
G0339	11920	0
G0339	11921	0
G0339	16000	0
G0339	16020	0
G0339	16025	0
G0339	16030	0
G0339	20660	0
G0339	36000	1
G0339	36410	1
G0339	36425	0
G0339	51701	0
G0339	51702	0
G0339	51703	0
G0339	61795	0
G0339	69990	0
G0339	77321	1
G0339	77326	1
G0339	77327	1
G0339	77328	1
G0339	77336	1
G0339	77401	1

Column 1	Column 2	Modifier 0=not allowed 1=allowed 9=not applicable
G0339	77402	1
G0339	77403	1
G0339	77404	1
G0339	77406	1
G0339	77407	1
G0339	77408	1
G0339	77409	1
G0339	77411	1
G0339	77412	1
G0339	77413	1
G0339	77414	1
G0339	77416	1
G0339	77421	0
G0339	77422	1
G0339	77423	1
G0339	90804	0
G0339	90805	0
G0339	90806	0
G0339	90807	0
G0339	90808	0
G0339	90809	0
G0339	90810	0
G0339	90811	0
G0339	90812	0
G0339	90813	0
G0339	90814	0
G0339	90815	0
G0339	90816	0
G0339	90817	0
G0339	90818	0
G0339	90819	0
G0339	90821	0
G0339	90822	0
G0339	90846	0
G0339	90847	0
G0339	90862	0
G0339	96360	0
G0339	96361	0
G0339	96365	0
G0339	96366	0
G0339	96367	0
G0339	96368	0

Column 1	Column 2	Modifier 0=not allowed 1=allowed 9=not applicable
G0339	97802	0
G0339	97803	0
G0339	97804	0
G0339	99143	0
G0339	99144	0
G0339	99145	0
G0339	99201	0
G0339	99202	0
G0339	99203	0
G0339	99204	0
G0339	99205	0
G0339	99211	0
G0339	99212	0
G0339	99213	0
G0339	99214	0
G0339	99215	0
G0339	99217	0
G0339	99218	0
G0339	99219	0
G0339	99220	0
G0339	99221	0
G0339	99222	0
G0339	99223	0
G0339	99231	0
G0339	99232	0
G0339	99233	0
G0339	99234	0
G0339	99235	0
G0339	99236	0
G0339	99238	0
G0339	99239	0
G0339	99281	0
G0339	99282	0
G0339	99283	0
G0339	99284	0
G0339	99285	0
G0339	99291	0
G0339	99292	0
G0339	99304	0
G0339	99305	0
G0339	99306	0
G0339	99307	0

Column 1	Column 2	Modifier 0=not allowed 1=allowed 9=not applicable
G0339	99308	0
G0339	99309	0
G0339	99310	0
G0339	99315	0
G0339	99316	0
G0339	99318	0
G0339	99324	0
G0339	99325	0
G0339	99326	0
G0339	99327	0
G0339	99328	0
G0339	99334	0
G0339	99335	0
G0339	99336	0
G0339	99337	0
G0339	99341	0
G0339	99342	0
G0339	99343	0
G0339	99344	0
G0339	99345	0
G0339	99347	0
G0339	99348	0
G0339	99349	0
G0339	99350	0
G0339	99354	0
G0339	99355	0
G0339	99356	0
G0339	99357	0
G0339	99360	0
G0339	99455	0
G0339	99456	0
G0339	99460	0
G0339	99461	0
G0339	99462	0
G0339	99463	0
G0339	99464	0
G0339	99465	0
G0339	99466	0
G0339	99467	0
G0339	99468	0
G0339	99469	0
G0339	99471	0

Column 1	Column 2	Modifier 0=not allowed 1=allowed 9=not applicable
G0339	99472	0
G0339	99475	0
G0339	99476	0
G0339	99477	0
G0339	99478	0
G0339	99479	0
G0339	99480	0
G0340	M0064	0
G0340	11920	0
G0340	11921	0
G0340	16000	0
G0340	16020	0
G0340	16025	0
G0340	16030	0
G0340	20660	0
G0340	36000	1
G0340	36410	1
G0340	36425	0
G0340	51701	0
G0340	51702	0
G0340	51703	0
G0340	61795	0
G0340	69990	0
G0340	77321	1
G0340	77326	1
G0340	77327	1
G0340	77328	1
G0340	77401	1
G0340	77402	1
G0340	77403	1
G0340	77404	1
G0340	77406	1
G0340	77407	1
G0340	77408	1
G0340	77409	1
G0340	77411	1
G0340	77412	1
G0340	77413	1
G0340	77414	1
G0340	77416	1
G0340	77421	0
G0340	77422	1

Column 1	Column 2	Modifier 0=not allowed 1=allowed 9=not applicable
G0340	77423	1
G0340	90804	0
G0340	90805	0
G0340	90806	0
G0340	90807	0
G0340	90808	0
G0340	90809	0
G0340	90810	0
G0340	90811	0
G0340	90812	0
G0340	90813	0
G0340	90814	0
G0340	90815	0
G0340	90816	0
G0340	90817	0
G0340	90818	0
G0340	90819	0
G0340	90821	0
G0340	90822	0
G0340	90846	0
G0340	90847	0
G0340	90862	0
G0340	96360	0
G0340	96361	0
G0340	96365	0
G0340	96366	0
G0340	96367	0
G0340	96368	0
G0340	97802	0
G0340	97803	0
G0340	97804	0
G0340	99143	0
G0340	99144	0
G0340	99145	0
G0340	99201	0
G0340	99202	0
G0340	99203	0
G0340	99204	0
G0340	99205	0
G0340	99211	0
G0340	99212	0
G0340	99213	0

Column 1	Column 2	Modifier 0=not allowed 1=allowed 9=not applicable
G0340	99214	0
G0340	99215	0
G0340	99217	0
G0340	99218	0
G0340	99219	0
G0340	99220	0
G0340	99221	0
G0340	99222	0
G0340	99223	0
G0340	99231	0
G0340	99232	0
G0340	99233	0
G0340	99234	0
G0340	99235	0
G0340	99236	0
G0340	99238	0
G0340	99239	0
G0340	99281	0
G0340	99282	0
G0340	99283	0
G0340	99284	0
G0340	99285	0
G0340	99291	0
G0340	99292	0
G0340	99304	0
G0340	99305	0
G0340	99306	0
G0340	99307	0
G0340	99308	0
G0340	99309	0
G0340	99310	0
G0340	99315	0
G0340	99316	0
G0340	99318	0
G0340	99324	0
G0340	99325	0
G0340	99326	0
G0340	99327	0
G0340	99328	0
G0340	99334	0
G0340	99335	0
G0340	99336	0

Column 1	Column 2	Modifier 0=not allowed 1=allowed 9=not applicable
G0340	99337	0
G0340	99341	0
G0340	99342	0
G0340	99343	0
G0340	99344	0
G0340	99345	0
G0340	99347	0
G0340	99348	0
G0340	99349	0
G0340	99350	0
G0340	99354	0
G0340	99355	0
G0340	99356	0
G0340	99357	0
G0340	99360	0
G0340	99455	0
G0340	99456	0
G0340	99460	0
G0340	99461	0
G0340	99462	0
G0340	99463	0
G0340	99464	0
G0340	99465	0
G0340	99466	0
G0340	99467	0
G0340	99468	0
G0340	99469	0
G0340	99471	0
G0340	99472	0
G0340	99475	0
G0340	99476	0
G0340	99477	0
G0340	99478	0
G0340	99479	0
G0340	99480	0
G0341	J1644	1
G0341	0213T	0
G0341	0216T	0
G0341	0228T	0
G0341	0230T	0
G0341	36000	1
G0341	36400	1

Column 1	Column 2	Modifier 0=not allowed 1=allowed 9=not applicable
G0341	36405	1
G0341	36406	1
G0341	36410	1
G0341	36420	1
G0341	36425	1
G0341	36430	1
G0341	36440	1
G0341	36481	0
G0341	36600	1
G0341	36640	1
G0341	37202	1
G0341	43752	1
G0341	51701	1
G0341	51702	1
G0341	51703	1
G0341	62310	0
G0341	62311	0
G0341	62318	0
G0341	62319	0
G0341	64400	0
G0341	64402	0
G0341	64405	0
G0341	64408	0
G0341	64410	0
G0341	64412	0
G0341	64413	0
G0341	64415	0
G0341	64416	0
G0341	64417	0
G0341	64418	0
G0341	64420	0
G0341	64421	0
G0341	64425	0
G0341	64430	0
G0341	64435	0
G0341	64445	0
G0341	64446	0
G0341	64447	0
G0341	64448	0
G0341	64449	0
G0341	64450	0
G0341	64479	0

Column 1	Column 2	Modifier 0=not allowed 1=allowed 9=not applicable
G0341	64483	0
G0341	64490	0
G0341	64493	0
G0341	64505	0
G0341	64508	0
G0341	64510	0
G0341	64517	0
G0341	64520	0
G0341	64530	0
G0341	76000	1
G0341	76001	1
G0341	76942	1
G0341	76998	1
G0341	77002	1
G0341	93000	1
G0341	93005	1
G0341	93010	1
G0341	93040	1
G0341	93041	1
G0341	93042	1
G0341	93318	1
G0341	94002	1
G0341	94200	1
G0341	94250	1
G0341	94680	1
G0341	94681	1
G0341	94690	1
G0341	94770	1
G0341	95812	1
G0341	95813	1
G0341	95816	1
G0341	95819	1
G0341	95822	1
G0341	95829	1
G0341	95955	1
G0341	96360	1
G0341	96365	1
G0341	96372	1
G0341	96374	1
G0341	96375	1
G0341	96376	1
G0341	99148	0

Column 1	Column 2	Modifier 0=not allowed 1=allowed 9=not applicable
G0341	99149	0
G0341	99150	0
G0342	G0341	0
G0342	0213T	0
G0342	0216T	0
G0342	0228T	0
G0342	0230T	0
G0342	36000	1
G0342	36400	1
G0342	36405	1
G0342	36406	1
G0342	36410	1
G0342	36420	1
G0342	36425	1
G0342	36430	1
G0342	36440	1
G0342	36481	0
G0342	36600	1
G0342	36640	1
G0342	37202	1
G0342	43752	1
G0342	44180	0
G0342	44602	1
G0342	44603	1
G0342	44604	1
G0342	44605	1
G0342	49320	0
G0342	51701	1
G0342	51702	1
G0342	51703	1
G0342	62310	0
G0342	62311	0
G0342	62318	0
G0342	62319	0
G0342	64400	0
G0342	64402	0
G0342	64405	0
G0342	64408	0
G0342	64410	0
G0342	64412	0
G0342	64413	0
G0342	64415	0

Column 1	Column 2	Modifier 0=not allowed 1=allowed 9=not applicable
G0342	64416	0
G0342	64417	0
G0342	64418	0
G0342	64420	0
G0342	64421	0
G0342	64425	0
G0342	64430	0
G0342	64435	0
G0342	64445	0
G0342	64446	0
G0342	64447	0
G0342	64448	0
G0342	64449	0
G0342	64450	0
G0342	64479	0
G0342	64483	0
G0342	64490	0
G0342	64493	0
G0342	64505	0
G0342	64508	0
G0342	64510	0
G0342	64517	0
G0342	64520	0
G0342	64530	0
G0342	76000	1
G0342	76001	1
G0342	76942	1
G0342	76998	1
G0342	77002	1
G0342	93000	1
G0342	93005	1
G0342	93010	1
G0342	93040	1
G0342	93041	1
G0342	93042	1
G0342	93318	1
G0342	94002	1
G0342	94200	1
G0342	94250	1
G0342	94680	1
G0342	94681	1
G0342	94690	1

Column 1	Column 2	Modifier 0=not allowed 1=allowed 9=not applicable
G0342	94770	1
G0342	95812	1
G0342	95813	1
G0342	95816	1
G0342	95819	1
G0342	95822	1
G0342	95829	1
G0342	95955	1
G0342	96360	1
G0342	96365	1
G0342	96372	1
G0342	96374	1
G0342	96375	1
G0342	96376	1
G0342	99148	0
G0342	99149	0
G0342	99150	0
G0343	G0341	0
G0343	G0342	0
G0343	0213T	0
G0343	0216T	0
G0343	0228T	0
G0343	0230T	0
G0343	36000	1
G0343	36400	1
G0343	36405	1
G0343	36406	1
G0343	36410	1
G0343	36420	1
G0343	36425	1
G0343	36430	1
G0343	36440	1
G0343	36481	0
G0343	36600	1
G0343	36640	1
G0343	37202	1
G0343	43752	1
G0343	44005	0
G0343	44180	0
G0343	44602	1
G0343	44603	1
G0343	44604	1

Column 1	Column 2	Modifier 0=not allowed 1=allowed 9=not applicable
G0343	44605	1
G0343	44820	0
G0343	44850	0
G0343	44950	0
G0343	44970	0
G0343	49000	0
G0343	49002	1
G0343	49010	0
G0343	49255	0
G0343	49320	1
G0343	49570	0
G0343	51701	1
G0343	51702	1
G0343	51703	1
G0343	62310	0
G0343	62311	0
G0343	62318	0
G0343	62319	0
G0343	64400	0
G0343	64402	0
G0343	64405	0
G0343	64408	0
G0343	64410	0
G0343	64412	0
G0343	64413	0
G0343	64415	0
G0343	64416	0
G0343	64417	0
G0343	64418	0
G0343	64420	0
G0343	64421	0
G0343	64425	0
G0343	64430	0
G0343	64435	0
G0343	64445	0
G0343	64446	0
G0343	64447	0
G0343	64448	0
G0343	64449	0
G0343	64450	0
G0343	64479	0
G0343	64483	0

Column 1	Column 2	Modifier 0=not allowed 1=allowed 9=not applicable
G0343	64490	0
G0343	64493	0
G0343	64505	0
G0343	64508	0
G0343	64510	0
G0343	64517	0
G0343	64520	0
G0343	64530	0
G0343	76000	1
G0343	76001	1
G0343	76942	1
G0343	76998	1
G0343	77002	1
G0343	93000	1
G0343	93005	1
G0343	93010	1
G0343	93040	1
G0343	93041	1
G0343	93042	1
G0343	93318	1
G0343	94002	1
G0343	94200	1
G0343	94250	1
G0343	94680	1
G0343	94681	1
G0343	94690	1
G0343	94770	1
G0343	95812	1
G0343	95813	1
G0343	95816	1
G0343	95819	1
G0343	95822	1
G0343	95829	1
G0343	95955	1
G0343	96360	1
G0343	96365	1
G0343	96372	1
G0343	96374	1
G0343	96375	1
G0343	96376	1
G0343	99148	0
G0343	99149	0

Column 1	Column 2	Modifier 0=not allowed 1=allowed 9=not applicable
G0343	99150	0
G0364	01112	0
G0364	01120	0
G0364	36000	1
G0364	36410	1
G0364	80500	1
G0364	80502	1
G0365	76970	1
G0365	93922	1
G0365	93931	1
G0365	93965	1
G0380	G0102	1
G0380	G0245	1
G0380	G0246	1
G0380	G0270	1
G0380	G0271	1
G0380	M0064	1
G0380	43752	1
G0380	90862	1
G0380	90940	1
G0380	92002	1
G0380	92004	1
G0380	92012	1
G0380	92014	1
G0380	94002	1
G0380	94003	1
G0380	94004	1
G0380	94644	1
G0380	94660	1
G0380	94662	1
G0380	95831	1
G0380	95832	1
G0380	95833	1
G0380	95834	1
G0380	95851	1
G0380	95852	1
G0380	96020	1
G0380	96116	1
G0380	96150	1
G0380	96151	1
G0380	96152	1
G0380	96153	1

Column 1	Column 2	Modifier 0=not allowed 1=allowed 9=not applicable
G0380	96154	1
G0380	96401	1
G0380	96402	1
G0380	96405	1
G0380	96406	1
G0380	96409	1
G0380	96413	1
G0380	96416	1
G0380	96420	1
G0380	96422	1
G0380	96425	1
G0380	96440	1
G0380	96445	1
G0380	96450	1
G0380	96523	1
G0380	97802	1
G0380	97803	1
G0380	97804	1
G0380	99605	1
G0380	99606	1
G0381	G0102	1
G0381	G0245	1
G0381	G0246	1
G0381	G0270	1
G0381	G0271	1
G0381	M0064	1
G0381	43752	1
G0381	90862	1
G0381	90940	1
G0381	92002	1
G0381	92004	1
G0381	92012	1
G0381	92014	1
G0381	94002	1
G0381	94003	1
G0381	94004	1
G0381	94644	1
G0381	94660	1
G0381	94662	1
G0381	95831	1
G0381	95832	1
G0381	95833	1

Column 1	Column 2	Modifier 0=not allowed 1=allowed 9=not applicable
G0381	95834	1
G0381	95851	1
G0381	95852	1
G0381	96020	1
G0381	96116	1
G0381	96150	1
G0381	96151	1
G0381	96152	1
G0381	96153	1
G0381	96154	1
G0381	96401	1
G0381	96402	1
G0381	96405	1
G0381	96406	1
G0381	96409	1
G0381	96413	1
G0381	96416	1
G0381	96420	1
G0381	96422	1
G0381	96425	1
G0381	96440	1
G0381	96445	1
G0381	96450	1
G0381	96523	1
G0381	97802	1
G0381	97803	1
G0381	97804	1
G0381	99605	1
G0381	99606	1
G0382	G0102	1
G0382	G0245	1
G0382	G0246	1
G0382	G0270	1
G0382	G0271	1
G0382	M0064	1
G0382	43752	1
G0382	90862	1
G0382	90940	1
G0382	92002	1
G0382	92004	1
G0382	92012	1
G0382	92014	1

Column 1	Column 2	Modifier 0=not allowed 1=allowed 9=not applicable
G0382	94002	1
G0382	94003	1
G0382	94004	1
G0382	94644	1
G0382	94660	1
G0382	94662	1
G0382	95831	1
G0382	95832	1
G0382	95833	1
G0382	95834	1
G0382	95851	1
G0382	95852	1
G0382	96020	1
G0382	96116	1
G0382	96150	1
G0382	96151	1
G0382	96152	1
G0382	96153	1
G0382	96154	1
G0382	96401	1
G0382	96402	1
G0382	96405	1
G0382	96406	1
G0382	96409	1
G0382	96413	1
G0382	96416	1
G0382	96420	1
G0382	96422	1
G0382	96425	1
G0382	96440	1
G0382	96445	1
G0382	96450	1
G0382	96523	1
G0382	97802	1
G0382	97803	1
G0382	97804	1
G0382	99605	1
G0382	99606	1
G0383	G0102	1
G0383	G0245	1
G0383	G0246	1
G0383	G0270	1

Column 1	Column 2	Modifier 0=not allowed 1=allowed 9=not applicable	Column 1	Column 2	Modifier 0=not allowed 1=allowed 9=not applicable	Column 1	Column 2	Modifier 0=not allowed 1=allowed 9=not applicable
G0383	G0271	1	G0383	97802	1	G0384	96413	1
G0383	M0064	1	G0383	97803	1	G0384	96416	1
G0383	43752	1	G0383	97804	1	G0384	96420	1
G0383	90862	1	G0383	99605	1	G0384	96422	1
G0383	90940	1	G0383	99606	1	G0384	96425	1
G0383	92002	1	G0384	G0102	1	G0384	96440	1
G0383	92004	1	G0384	G0245	1	G0384	96445	1
G0383	92012	1	G0384	G0246	1	G0384	96450	1
G0383	92014	1	G0384	G0270	1	G0384	96523	1
G0383	94002	1	G0384	G0271	1	G0384	97802	1
G0383	94003	1	G0384	M0064	1	G0384	97803	1
G0383	94004	1	G0384	43752	1	G0384	97804	1
G0383	94644	1	G0384	90862	1	G0384	99605	1
G0383	94660	1	G0384	90940	1	G0384	99606	1
G0383	94662	1	G0384	92002	1	G0389	76998	1
G0383	95831	1	G0384	92004	1	G0398	92270	0
G0383	95832	1	G0384	92012	1	G0398	93000	1
G0383	95833	1	G0384	92014	1	G0398	93005	1
G0383	95834	1	G0384	94002	1	G0398	93010	1
G0383	95851	1	G0384	94003	1	G0398	93040	1
G0383	95852	1	G0384	94004	1	G0398	93041	1
G0383	96020	1	G0384	94644	1	G0398	93042	1
G0383	96116	1	G0384	94660	1	G0398	93224	0
G0383	96150	1	G0384	94662	1	G0398	93225	0
G0383	96151	1	G0384	95831	1	G0398	93226	0
G0383	96152	1	G0384	95832	1	G0398	93227	0
G0383	96153	1	G0384	95833	1	G0398	93230	0
G0383	96154	1	G0384	95834	1	G0398	93231	0
G0383	96401	1	G0384	95851	1	G0398	93232	0
G0383	96402	1	G0384	95852	1	G0398	93233	0
G0383	96405	1	G0384	96020	1	G0398	93235	0
G0383	96406	1	G0384	96116	1	G0398	93236	0
G0383	96409	1	G0384	96150	1	G0398	93237	0
G0383	96413	1	G0384	96151	1	G0398	94200	1
G0383	96416	1	G0384	96152	1	G0398	94360	0
G0383	96420	1	G0384	96153	1	G0398	94620	1
G0383	96422	1	G0384	96154	1	G0398	94681	0
G0383	96425	1	G0384	96401	1	G0398	94760	0
G0383	96440	1	G0384	96402	1	G0398	94761	0
G0383	96445	1	G0384	96405	1	G0398	94762	0
G0383	96450	1	G0384	96406	1	G0398	94770	1
G0383	96523	1	G0384	96409	1	G0398	95812	1

Column 1	Column 2	Modifier 0=not allowed 1=allowed 9=not applicable	Column 1	Column 2	Modifier 0=not allowed 1=allowed 9=not applicable	Column 1	Column 2	Modifier 0=not allowed 1=allowed 9=not applicable
G0398	95813	1	G0399	93236	0	G0400	93041	1
G0398	95816	1	G0399	93237	0	G0400	93042	1
G0398	95819	0	G0399	94200	1	G0400	93224	0
G0398	95822	0	G0399	94360	0	G0400	93225	0
G0398	95824	0	G0399	94620	1	G0400	93226	0
G0398	95827	0	G0399	94681	0	G0400	93227	0
G0398	95860	1	G0399	94760	0	G0400	93230	0
G0398	95861	1	G0399	94761	0	G0400	93231	0
G0398	95863	1	G0399	94762	0	G0400	93232	0
G0398	95864	1	G0399	94770	1	G0400	93233	0
G0398	95865	1	G0399	95812	1	G0400	93235	0
G0398	95866	1	G0399	95813	1	G0400	93236	0
G0398	95867	1	G0399	95816	1	G0400	93237	0
G0398	95868	1	G0399	95819	0	G0400	94200	1
G0398	95869	1	G0399	95822	0	G0400	94360	0
G0398	95870	1	G0399	95824	0	G0400	94620	1
G0398	95872	1	G0399	95827	0	G0400	94681	0
G0398	95950	1	G0399	95860	1	G0400	94760	0
G0398	95951	1	G0399	95861	1	G0400	94761	0
G0398	95953	1	G0399	95863	1	G0400	94762	0
G0398	95954	1	G0399	95864	1	G0400	94770	1
G0398	95955	1	G0399	95865	1	G0400	95812	1
G0398	95956	1	G0399	95866	1	G0400	95813	1
G0398	95957	1	G0399	95867	1	G0400	95816	1
G0398	95958	1	G0399	95868	1	G0400	95819	0
G0398	95961	1	G0399	95869	1	G0400	95822	0
G0399	92270	0	G0399	95870	1	G0400	95824	0
G0399	93000	1	G0399	95872	1	G0400	95827	0
G0399	93005	1	G0399	95950	1	G0400	95860	1
G0399	93010	1	G0399	95951	1	G0400	95861	1
G0399	93040	1	G0399	95953	1	G0400	95863	1
G0399	93041	1	G0399	95954	1	G0400	95864	1
G0399	93042	1	G0399	95955	1	G0400	95865	1
G0399	93224	0	G0399	95956	1	G0400	95866	1
G0399	93225	0	G0399	95957	1	G0400	95867	1
G0399	93226	0	G0399	95958	1	G0400	95868	1
G0399	93227	0	G0399	95961	1	G0400	95869	1
G0399	93230	0	G0400	92270	0	G0400	95870	1
G0399	93231	0	G0400	93000	1	G0400	95872	1
G0399	93232	0	G0400	93005	1	G0400	95950	1
G0399	93233	0	G0400	93010	1	G0400	95951	1
G0399	93235	0	G0400	93040	1	G0400	95953	1

Column 1	Column 2	Modifier 0=not allowed 1=allowed 9=not applicable
G0400	95954	1
G0400	95955	1
G0400	95956	1
G0400	95957	1
G0400	95958	1
G0400	95961	1
G0402	G0250	1
G0402	G0270	0
G0402	G0271	0
G0402	M0064	1
G0402	90801	1
G0402	90802	1
G0402	90804	1
G0402	90805	1
G0402	90806	1
G0402	90807	1
G0402	90808	1
G0402	90809	1
G0402	90810	1
G0402	90811	1
G0402	90812	1
G0402	90813	1
G0402	90814	1
G0402	90815	1
G0402	90816	1
G0402	90817	1
G0402	90818	1
G0402	90819	1
G0402	90821	1
G0402	90822	1
G0402	90823	1
G0402	90824	1
G0402	90826	1
G0402	90827	1
G0402	90828	1
G0402	90829	1
G0402	90845	1
G0402	90862	1
G0402	92002	1
G0402	92004	1
G0402	92012	1
G0402	92014	1

Column 1	Column 2	Modifier 0=not allowed 1=allowed 9=not applicable
G0402	93000	1
G0402	93005	1
G0402	93010	1
G0402	93012	1
G0402	93014	1
G0402	93040	1
G0402	93041	1
G0402	93042	1
G0402	95831	1
G0402	95832	1
G0402	95833	1
G0402	95834	1
G0402	95851	1
G0402	95852	1
G0402	96116	1
G0402	96150	0
G0402	96151	0
G0402	96152	0
G0402	96153	0
G0402	96154	0
G0402	97802	0
G0402	97803	0
G0402	97804	0
G0403	G0404	0
G0403	G0405	0
G0406	G0102	0
G0406	G0245	0
G0406	G0246	0
G0406	G0270	0
G0406	G0271	0
G0406	M0064	0
G0406	43752	1
G0406	80500	0
G0406	80502	0
G0406	90862	0
G0406	90940	0
G0406	92002	0
G0406	92004	0
G0406	92012	0
G0406	92014	0
G0406	92531	0
G0406	92532	0

Column 1	Column 2	Modifier 0=not allowed 1=allowed 9=not applicable
G0406	94002	0
G0406	94003	0
G0406	94004	0
G0406	94644	1
G0406	94660	0
G0406	94662	0
G0406	95831	0
G0406	95832	0
G0406	95833	0
G0406	95834	0
G0406	95851	0
G0406	95852	0
G0406	96020	1
G0406	96116	1
G0406	96150	0
G0406	96151	0
G0406	96152	0
G0406	96153	0
G0406	96154	0
G0406	96360	1
G0406	96365	1
G0406	96369	1
G0406	96372	1
G0406	96373	1
G0406	96374	1
G0406	96401	1
G0406	96402	1
G0406	96405	1
G0406	96406	1
G0406	96409	1
G0406	96413	1
G0406	96416	1
G0406	96420	1
G0406	96422	1
G0406	96425	1
G0406	96440	1
G0406	96445	1
G0406	96450	1
G0406	96523	0
G0406	97802	0
G0406	97803	0
G0406	97804	0

Column 1	Column 2	Modifier 0=not allowed 1=allowed 9=not applicable	Column 1	Column 2	Modifier 0=not allowed 1=allowed 9=not applicable	Column 1	Column 2	Modifier 0=not allowed 1=allowed 9=not applicable
G0407	G0102	0	G0407	96374	1	G0408	94662	0
G0407	G0245	0	G0407	96401	1	G0408	95831	0
G0407	G0246	0	G0407	96402	1	G0408	95832	0
G0407	G0270	0	G0407	96405	1	G0408	95833	0
G0407	G0271	0	G0407	96406	1	G0408	95834	0
G0407	G0406	0	G0407	96409	1	G0408	95851	0
G0407	M0064	0	G0407	96413	1	G0408	95852	0
G0407	43752	1	G0407	96416	1	G0408	96020	1
G0407	80500	0	G0407	96420	1	G0408	96116	1
G0407	80502	0	G0407	96422	1	G0408	96150	0
G0407	90862	0	G0407	96425	1	G0408	96151	0
G0407	90940	0	G0407	96440	1	G0408	96152	0
G0407	92002	0	G0407	96445	1	G0408	96153	0
G0407	92004	0	G0407	96450	1	G0408	96154	0
G0407	92012	0	G0407	96523	0	G0408	96360	1
G0407	92014	0	G0407	97802	0	G0408	96365	1
G0407	92531	0	G0407	97803	0	G0408	96369	1
G0407	92532	0	G0407	97804	0	G0408	96372	1
G0407	94002	0	G0408	G0102	0	G0408	96373	1
G0407	94003	0	G0408	G0245	0	G0408	96374	1
G0407	94004	0	G0408	G0246	0	G0408	96401	1
G0407	94644	1	G0408	G0270	0	G0408	96402	1
G0407	94660	0	G0408	G0271	0	G0408	96405	1
G0407	94662	0	G0408	G0406	0	G0408	96406	1
G0407	95831	0	G0408	G0407	0	G0408	96409	1
G0407	95832	0	G0408	M0064	0	G0408	96413	1
G0407	95833	0	G0408	43752	1	G0408	96416	1
G0407	95834	0	G0408	80500	0	G0408	96420	1
G0407	95851	0	G0408	80502	0	G0408	96422	1
G0407	95852	0	G0408	90862	0	G0408	96425	1
G0407	96020	1	G0408	90940	0	G0408	96440	1
G0407	96116	1	G0408	92002	0	G0408	96445	1
G0407	96150	0	G0408	92004	0	G0408	96450	1
G0407	96151	0	G0408	92012	0	G0408	96523	0
G0407	96152	0	G0408	92014	0	G0408	97802	0
G0407	96153	0	G0408	92531	0	G0408	97803	0
G0407	96154	0	G0408	92532	0	G0408	97804	0
G0407	96360	1	G0408	94002	0	G0410	G0176	1
G0407	96365	1	G0408	94003	0	G0410	G0177	1
G0407	96369	1	G0408	94004	0	G0410	G0270	0
G0407	96372	1	G0408	94644	1	G0410	G0271	0
G0407	96373	1	G0408	94660	0	G0410	G0380	1

Column 1	Column 2	Modifier 0=not allowed 1=allowed 9=not applicable
G0410	G0381	1
G0410	G0382	1
G0410	G0383	1
G0410	G0384	1
G0410	M0064	0
G0410	36640	1
G0410	90802	1
G0410	90862	0
G0410	96116	1
G0410	96150	0
G0410	96151	0
G0410	96152	0
G0410	96153	0
G0410	96154	0
G0410	97802	0
G0410	97803	0
G0410	97804	0
G0410	99201	1
G0410	99202	1
G0410	99203	1
G0410	99204	1
G0410	99205	1
G0410	99211	1
G0410	99212	1
G0410	99213	1
G0410	99214	1
G0410	99215	1
G0410	99217	1
G0410	99218	1
G0410	99219	1
G0410	99220	1
G0410	99221	1
G0410	99222	1
G0410	99223	1
G0410	99231	1
G0410	99232	1
G0410	99233	1
G0410	99234	1
G0410	99235	1
G0410	99236	1
G0410	99238	1
G0410	99239	1

Column 1	Column 2	Modifier 0=not allowed 1=allowed 9=not applicable
G0410	99281	1
G0410	99282	1
G0410	99283	1
G0410	99284	1
G0410	99285	1
G0410	99291	1
G0410	99292	1
G0410	99304	1
G0410	99305	1
G0410	99306	1
G0410	99307	1
G0410	99308	1
G0410	99309	1
G0410	99310	1
G0410	99315	1
G0410	99316	1
G0410	99318	1
G0410	99324	1
G0410	99325	1
G0410	99326	1
G0410	99327	1
G0410	99328	1
G0410	99334	1
G0410	99335	1
G0410	99336	1
G0410	99337	1
G0410	99341	1
G0410	99342	1
G0410	99343	1
G0410	99344	1
G0410	99345	1
G0410	99347	1
G0410	99348	1
G0410	99349	1
G0410	99350	1
G0410	99354	1
G0410	99355	1
G0410	99356	1
G0410	99357	1
G0410	99605	1
G0410	99606	1
G0411	G0176	1

Column 1	Column 2	Modifier 0=not allowed 1=allowed 9=not applicable
G0411	G0177	1
G0411	G0270	0
G0411	G0271	0
G0411	G0380	1
G0411	G0381	1
G0411	G0382	1
G0411	G0383	1
G0411	G0384	1
G0411	M0064	0
G0411	90802	1
G0411	90862	0
G0411	96116	1
G0411	96150	0
G0411	96151	0
G0411	96152	0
G0411	96153	0
G0411	96154	0
G0411	97802	0
G0411	97803	0
G0411	97804	0
G0411	99201	1
G0411	99202	1
G0411	99203	1
G0411	99204	1
G0411	99205	1
G0411	99211	1
G0411	99212	1
G0411	99213	1
G0411	99214	1
G0411	99215	1
G0411	99217	1
G0411	99218	1
G0411	99219	1
G0411	99220	1
G0411	99221	1
G0411	99222	1
G0411	99223	1
G0411	99231	1
G0411	99232	1
G0411	99233	1
G0411	99234	1
G0411	99235	1

Column 1	Column 2	Modifier 0=not allowed 1=allowed 9=not applicable	Column 1	Column 2	Modifier 0=not allowed 1=allowed 9=not applicable	Column 1	Column 2	Modifier 0=not allowed 1=allowed 9=not applicable
G0411	99236	1	G0411	99605	1	G0412	96374	1
G0411	99238	1	G0411	99606	1	G0412	96375	1
G0411	99239	1	G0412	0213T	1	G0412	97597	1
G0411	99281	1	G0412	0216T	1	G0412	97598	1
G0411	99282	1	G0412	20680	1	G0412	97602	1
G0411	99283	1	G0412	27275	1	G0412	97605	1
G0411	99284	1	G0412	29000	1	G0412	97606	1
G0411	99285	1	G0412	29010	1	G0412	99148	0
G0411	99291	1	G0412	29015	1	G0412	99149	0
G0411	99292	1	G0412	29020	1	G0412	99150	0
G0411	99304	0	G0412	29025	1	G0413	0213T	1
G0411	99305	0	G0412	29035	1	G0413	0216T	1
G0411	99306	0	G0412	29040	1	G0413	20650	1
G0411	99307	1	G0412	29044	1	G0413	20680	1
G0411	99308	1	G0412	29046	1	G0413	27193	1
G0411	99309	1	G0412	29049	1	G0413	27194	1
G0411	99310	1	G0412	29305	1	G0413	27275	1
G0411	99315	1	G0412	29325	1	G0413	29000	1
G0411	99316	1	G0412	29520	1	G0413	29010	1
G0411	99318	1	G0412	29700	1	G0413	29015	1
G0411	99324	1	G0412	29705	1	G0413	29020	1
G0411	99325	1	G0412	29710	1	G0413	29025	1
G0411	99326	1	G0412	29715	1	G0413	29035	1
G0411	99327	1	G0412	36000	1	G0413	29040	1
G0411	99328	1	G0412	36410	1	G0413	29044	1
G0411	99334	1	G0412	37202	1	G0413	29046	1
G0411	99335	1	G0412	51701	1	G0413	29049	1
G0411	99336	1	G0412	51702	1	G0413	29305	1
G0411	99337	1	G0412	51703	1	G0413	29325	1
G0411	99341	1	G0412	62318	1	G0413	29520	1
G0411	99342	1	G0412	62319	1	G0413	29700	1
G0411	99343	1	G0412	64415	1	G0413	29705	1
G0411	99344	1	G0412	64416	1	G0413	29710	1
G0411	99345	1	G0412	64417	1	G0413	29715	1
G0411	99347	1	G0412	64450	1	G0413	36000	1
G0411	99348	1	G0412	64490	1	G0413	36410	1
G0411	99349	1	G0412	64493	1	G0413	37202	1
G0411	99350	1	G0412	69990	0	G0413	51701	1
G0411	99354	1	G0412	73530	0	G0413	51702	1
G0411	99355	1	G0412	96360	1	G0413	51703	1
G0411	99356	1	G0412	96365	1	G0413	62318	1
G0411	99357	1	G0412	96372	1	G0413	62319	1

Column 1	Column 2	Modifier 0=not allowed 1=allowed 9=not applicable
G0413	64415	1
G0413	64416	1
G0413	64417	1
G0413	64450	1
G0413	64490	1
G0413	64493	1
G0413	69990	0
G0413	73530	0
G0413	96360	1
G0413	96365	1
G0413	96372	1
G0413	96374	1
G0413	96375	1
G0413	97597	1
G0413	97598	1
G0413	97602	1
G0413	97605	1
G0413	97606	1
G0413	99148	0
G0413	99149	0
G0413	99150	0
G0414	0213T	1
G0414	0216T	1
G0414	20650	1
G0414	20680	1
G0414	27275	1
G0414	29000	1
G0414	29010	1
G0414	29015	1
G0414	29020	1
G0414	29025	1
G0414	29035	1
G0414	29040	1
G0414	29044	1
G0414	29046	1
G0414	29049	1
G0414	29305	1
G0414	29325	1
G0414	29520	1
G0414	29700	1
G0414	29705	1
G0414	29710	1

Column 1	Column 2	Modifier 0=not allowed 1=allowed 9=not applicable
G0414	29715	1
G0414	36000	1
G0414	36410	1
G0414	37202	1
G0414	51701	1
G0414	51702	1
G0414	51703	1
G0414	62318	1
G0414	62319	1
G0414	64415	1
G0414	64416	1
G0414	64417	1
G0414	64450	1
G0414	64490	1
G0414	64493	1
G0414	69990	0
G0414	73530	0
G0414	96360	1
G0414	96365	1
G0414	96372	1
G0414	96374	1
G0414	96375	1
G0414	97597	1
G0414	97598	1
G0414	97602	1
G0414	97605	1
G0414	97606	1
G0414	99148	0
G0414	99149	0
G0414	99150	0
G0415	G0413	1
G0415	0213T	1
G0415	0216T	1
G0415	20650	1
G0415	20680	1
G0415	27275	1
G0415	29000	1
G0415	29010	1
G0415	29015	1
G0415	29020	1
G0415	29025	1
G0415	29035	1

Column 1	Column 2	Modifier 0=not allowed 1=allowed 9=not applicable
G0415	29040	1
G0415	29044	1
G0415	29046	1
G0415	29049	1
G0415	29305	1
G0415	29325	1
G0415	29520	1
G0415	29700	1
G0415	29705	1
G0415	29710	1
G0415	29715	1
G0415	36000	1
G0415	36410	1
G0415	37202	1
G0415	51701	1
G0415	51702	1
G0415	51703	1
G0415	62318	1
G0415	62319	1
G0415	64415	1
G0415	64416	1
G0415	64417	1
G0415	64450	1
G0415	64490	1
G0415	64493	1
G0415	69990	0
G0415	73530	0
G0415	96360	1
G0415	96365	1
G0415	96372	1
G0415	96374	1
G0415	96375	1
G0415	97597	1
G0415	97598	1
G0415	97602	1
G0415	97605	1
G0415	97606	1
G0415	99148	0
G0415	99149	0
G0415	99150	0
G0416	88160	1
G0416	88161	1

Column 1	Column 2	Modifier 0=not allowed 1=allowed 9=not applicable
G0416	88162	1
G0416	88302	1
G0416	88304	1
G0416	88305	1
G0416	88321	1
G0416	88323	1
G0416	88325	1
G0416	89060	1
G0417	G0416	0
G0417	88160	1
G0417	88161	1
G0417	88162	1
G0417	88302	1
G0417	88304	1
G0417	88305	1
G0417	88321	1
G0417	88323	1
G0417	88325	1
G0417	89060	1
G0418	G0416	0
G0418	G0417	0
G0418	88160	1
G0418	88161	1
G0418	88162	1
G0418	88302	1
G0418	88304	1
G0418	88305	1
G0418	88321	1
G0418	88323	1
G0418	88325	1
G0418	89060	1
G0419	G0416	0
G0419	G0417	0
G0419	G0418	0
G0419	88160	1
G0419	88161	1
G0419	88162	1
G0419	88302	1
G0419	88304	1
G0419	88305	1
G0419	88321	1
G0419	88323	1

Column 1	Column 2	Modifier 0=not allowed 1=allowed 9=not applicable
G0419	88325	1
G0419	89060	1
G0420	G0421	1
G0422	G0423	0
G0422	0178T	1
G0422	0179T	1
G0422	0180T	1
G0422	36000	1
G0422	36410	1
G0422	51701	1
G0422	51702	1
G0422	51703	1
G0422	93000	1
G0422	93005	1
G0422	93010	1
G0422	93040	1
G0422	93041	1
G0422	93042	1
G0422	93268	1
G0422	93797	0
G0422	93798	0
G0422	94760	0
G0422	94761	0
G0422	97001	1
G0422	97002	1
G0422	97003	1
G0422	97004	1
G0422	97110	1
G0422	97112	1
G0422	97116	1
G0422	97140	1
G0422	97150	1
G0422	97530	1
G0422	97750	1
G0422	97802	1
G0422	97803	1
G0422	97804	1
G0422	99148	0
G0422	99149	0
G0422	99150	0
G0423	0178T	1
G0423	0179T	1

Column 1	Column 2	Modifier 0=not allowed 1=allowed 9=not applicable
G0423	0180T	1
G0423	36000	1
G0423	36410	1
G0423	51701	1
G0423	51702	1
G0423	51703	1
G0423	93000	1
G0423	93005	1
G0423	93010	1
G0423	93040	1
G0423	93041	1
G0423	93042	1
G0423	93268	1
G0423	93797	0
G0423	93798	0
G0423	94760	0
G0423	94761	0
G0423	97001	1
G0423	97002	1
G0423	97003	1
G0423	97004	1
G0423	97110	1
G0423	97112	1
G0423	97116	1
G0423	97140	1
G0423	97150	1
G0423	97530	1
G0423	97750	1
G0423	97802	1
G0423	97803	1
G0423	97804	1
G0423	99148	0
G0423	99149	0
G0423	99150	0
G0424	G0406	1
G0424	G0407	1
G0424	G0408	1
G0424	0178T	1
G0424	0179T	1
G0424	0180T	1
G0424	36000	1
G0424	36410	1

Column 1	Column 2	Modifier 0=not allowed 1=allowed 9=not applicable	Column 1	Column 2	Modifier 0=not allowed 1=allowed 9=not applicable	Column 1	Column 2	Modifier 0=not allowed 1=allowed 9=not applicable
G0424	51701	1	G0424	97112	1	G0425	95852	0
G0424	51702	1	G0424	97150	1	G0425	96020	1
G0424	51703	1	G0424	97530	1	G0425	96116	1
G0424	93000	1	G0424	97750	1	G0425	96150	0
G0424	93005	1	G0424	97802	1	G0425	96151	0
G0424	93010	1	G0424	97803	1	G0425	96152	0
G0424	93040	1	G0424	97804	1	G0425	96153	0
G0424	93041	1	G0424	99148	0	G0425	96154	0
G0424	93042	1	G0424	99149	0	G0425	96360	1
G0424	93268	1	G0424	99150	0	G0425	96365	1
G0424	94010	1	G0425	G0102	0	G0425	96369	1
G0424	94060	1	G0425	G0245	0	G0425	96372	1
G0424	94150	1	G0425	G0246	0	G0425	96373	1
G0424	94200	1	G0425	G0270	0	G0425	96374	1
G0424	94240	1	G0425	G0271	0	G0425	96401	1
G0424	94250	1	G0425	G0406	0	G0425	96402	1
G0424	94260	1	G0425	G0407	0	G0425	96405	1
G0424	94350	1	G0425	G0408	0	G0425	96406	1
G0424	94360	1	G0425	G0424	1	G0425	96409	1
G0424	94370	1	G0425	M0064	0	G0425	96413	1
G0424	94375	1	G0425	43752	1	G0425	96416	1
G0424	94400	1	G0425	80500	0	G0425	96420	1
G0424	94450	1	G0425	80502	0	G0425	96422	1
G0424	94620	0	G0425	90862	0	G0425	96425	1
G0424	94621	0	G0425	90940	0	G0425	96440	1
G0424	94667	0	G0425	92002	0	G0425	96445	1
G0424	94668	0	G0425	92004	0	G0425	96450	1
G0424	94680	1	G0425	92012	0	G0425	96523	0
G0424	94681	1	G0425	92014	0	G0425	97802	0
G0424	94690	1	G0425	92531	0	G0425	97803	0
G0424	94720	1	G0425	92532	0	G0425	97804	0
G0424	94725	1	G0425	94002	0	G0426	G0102	0
G0424	94750	1	G0425	94003	0	G0426	G0245	0
G0424	94760	0	G0425	94004	0	G0426	G0246	0
G0424	94761	0	G0425	94644	1	G0426	G0270	0
G0424	94762	1	G0425	94660	0	G0426	G0271	0
G0424	94770	0	G0425	94662	0	G0426	G0406	0
G0424	97001	1	G0425	95831	0	G0426	G0407	0
G0424	97002	1	G0425	95832	0	G0426	G0408	0
G0424	97003	1	G0425	95833	0	G0426	G0424	1
G0424	97004	1	G0425	95834	0	G0426	G0425	0
G0424	97110	1	G0425	95851	0	G0426	M0064	0

Column 1	Column 2	Modifier 0=not allowed 1=allowed 9=not applicable
G0426	43752	1
G0426	80500	0
G0426	80502	0
G0426	90862	0
G0426	90940	0
G0426	92002	0
G0426	92004	0
G0426	92012	0
G0426	92014	0
G0426	92531	0
G0426	92532	0
G0426	94002	0
G0426	94003	0
G0426	94004	0
G0426	94644	1
G0426	94660	0
G0426	94662	0
G0426	95831	0
G0426	95832	0
G0426	95833	0
G0426	95834	0
G0426	95851	0
G0426	95852	0
G0426	96020	1
G0426	96116	1
G0426	96150	0
G0426	96151	0
G0426	96152	0
G0426	96153	0
G0426	96154	0
G0426	96360	1
G0426	96365	1
G0426	96369	1
G0426	96372	1
G0426	96373	1
G0426	96374	1
G0426	96401	1
G0426	96402	1
G0426	96405	1
G0426	96406	1
G0426	96409	1
G0426	96413	1

Column 1	Column 2	Modifier 0=not allowed 1=allowed 9=not applicable
G0426	96416	1
G0426	96420	1
G0426	96422	1
G0426	96425	1
G0426	96440	1
G0426	96445	1
G0426	96450	1
G0426	96523	0
G0426	97802	0
G0426	97803	0
G0426	97804	0
G0427	G0102	0
G0427	G0245	0
G0427	G0246	0
G0427	G0270	0
G0427	G0271	0
G0427	G0406	0
G0427	G0407	0
G0427	G0408	0
G0427	G0424	1
G0427	G0425	0
G0427	G0426	0
G0427	M0064	0
G0427	43752	1
G0427	80500	0
G0427	80502	0
G0427	90862	0
G0427	90940	0
G0427	92002	0
G0427	92004	0
G0427	92012	0
G0427	92014	0
G0427	92531	0
G0427	92532	0
G0427	94002	0
G0427	94003	0
G0427	94004	0
G0427	94644	1
G0427	94660	0
G0427	94662	0
G0427	95831	0
G0427	95832	0

Column 1	Column 2	Modifier 0=not allowed 1=allowed 9=not applicable
G0427	95833	0
G0427	95834	0
G0427	95851	0
G0427	95852	0
G0427	96020	1
G0427	96116	1
G0427	96150	0
G0427	96151	0
G0427	96152	0
G0427	96153	0
G0427	96154	0
G0427	96360	1
G0427	96365	1
G0427	96369	1
G0427	96372	1
G0427	96373	1
G0427	96374	1
G0427	96401	1
G0427	96402	1
G0427	96405	1
G0427	96406	1
G0427	96409	1
G0427	96413	1
G0427	96416	1
G0427	96420	1
G0427	96422	1
G0427	96425	1
G0427	96440	1
G0427	96445	1
G0427	96450	1
G0427	96523	0
G0427	97802	0
G0427	97803	0
G0427	97804	0
G0428	01250	0
G0428	01320	0
G0428	01400	0
G0428	0213T	0
G0428	0216T	0
G0428	0228T	0
G0428	0230T	0
G0428	20600	1

Column 1	Column 2	Modifier 0=not allowed 1=allowed 9=not applicable
G0428	20605	1
G0428	20610	1
G0428	27347	1
G0428	27570	1
G0428	29870	1
G0428	29871	1
G0428	29874	0
G0428	29875	1
G0428	29877	0
G0428	29881	1
G0428	29884	1
G0428	36000	1
G0428	36400	1
G0428	36405	1
G0428	36406	1
G0428	36410	1
G0428	36420	1
G0428	36425	1
G0428	36430	1
G0428	36440	1
G0428	36600	1
G0428	36640	1
G0428	37202	1
G0428	43752	1
G0428	51701	1
G0428	51702	1
G0428	51703	1
G0428	62310	0
G0428	62311	0
G0428	62318	0
G0428	62319	0
G0428	64400	0
G0428	64402	0
G0428	64405	0
G0428	64408	0
G0428	64410	0
G0428	64412	0
G0428	64413	0
G0428	64415	0
G0428	64416	0
G0428	64417	0
G0428	64418	0

Column 1	Column 2	Modifier 0=not allowed 1=allowed 9=not applicable
G0428	64420	0
G0428	64421	0
G0428	64425	0
G0428	64430	0
G0428	64435	0
G0428	64445	0
G0428	64446	0
G0428	64447	0
G0428	64448	0
G0428	64449	0
G0428	64450	1
G0428	64479	0
G0428	64483	0
G0428	64490	0
G0428	64493	0
G0428	64505	0
G0428	64508	0
G0428	64510	0
G0428	64517	0
G0428	64520	0
G0428	64530	0
G0428	69990	0
G0428	76000	1
G0428	76001	1
G0428	77001	1
G0428	77002	1
G0428	93000	1
G0428	93005	1
G0428	93010	1
G0428	93040	1
G0428	93041	1
G0428	93042	1
G0428	93318	1
G0428	94002	1
G0428	94200	1
G0428	94250	1
G0428	94680	1
G0428	94681	1
G0428	94690	1
G0428	94770	1
G0428	95812	1
G0428	95813	1

Column 1	Column 2	Modifier 0=not allowed 1=allowed 9=not applicable
G0428	95816	1
G0428	95819	1
G0428	95822	1
G0428	95829	1
G0428	95955	1
G0428	96360	1
G0428	96365	1
G0428	96372	1
G0428	96374	1
G0428	96375	1
G0428	96376	1
G0428	99148	0
G0428	99149	0
G0428	99150	0
G0429	J2001	1
G0429	0213T	0
G0429	0216T	0
G0429	0228T	0
G0429	0230T	0
G0429	36000	1
G0429	36400	1
G0429	36405	1
G0429	36406	1
G0429	36410	1
G0429	36420	1
G0429	36425	1
G0429	36430	1
G0429	36440	1
G0429	36600	1
G0429	36640	1
G0429	37202	1
G0429	43752	1
G0429	51701	1
G0429	51702	1
G0429	51703	1
G0429	62310	0
G0429	62311	0
G0429	62318	0
G0429	62319	0
G0429	64400	0
G0429	64402	0
G0429	64405	0

Column 1	Column 2	Modifier 0=not allowed 1=allowed 9=not applicable
G0429	64408	0
G0429	64410	0
G0429	64412	0
G0429	64413	0
G0429	64415	0
G0429	64416	0
G0429	64417	0
G0429	64418	0
G0429	64420	0
G0429	64421	0
G0429	64425	0
G0429	64430	0
G0429	64435	0
G0429	64445	0
G0429	64446	0
G0429	64447	0
G0429	64448	0
G0429	64449	0
G0429	64450	0
G0429	64479	0
G0429	64483	0
G0429	64490	0
G0429	64493	0
G0429	64505	0
G0429	64508	0
G0429	64510	0
G0429	64517	0
G0429	64520	0
G0429	64530	0
G0429	69990	0
G0429	93000	1
G0429	93005	1
G0429	93010	1
G0429	93040	1
G0429	93041	1
G0429	93042	1
G0429	93318	1
G0429	94002	1
G0429	94200	1
G0429	94250	1
G0429	94680	1
G0429	94681	1

Column 1	Column 2	Modifier
G0429	94690	1
G0429	94770	1
G0429	95812	1
G0429	95813	1
G0429	95816	1
G0429	95819	1
G0429	95822	1
G0429	95829	1
G0429	95955	1
G0429	96360	1
G0429	96365	1
G0429	96372	1
G0429	96374	1
G0429	96375	1
G0429	96376	1
G0429	99148	0
G0429	99149	0
G0429	99150	0
G0431	80500	1
G0431	80502	1
G0431	83516	1
G0431	83518	1
G0436	G0396	1
G0436	G0397	1
G0436	92531	0
G0436	92532	0
G0436	96101	1
G0436	96102	1
G0436	96103	1
G0436	96105	1
G0436	96118	1
G0436	96119	1
G0436	96120	1
G0436	96125	1
G0436	99408	0
G0436	99409	0
G0437	G0396	1
G0437	G0397	1
G0437	G0436	0
G0437	92531	0
G0437	92532	0
G0437	96101	1

Column 1	Column 2	Modifier
G0437	96102	1
G0437	96103	1
G0437	96105	1
G0437	96118	1
G0437	96119	1
G0437	96120	1
G0437	96125	1
G0437	99408	0
G0437	99409	0
G0438	G0250	1
G0438	G0270	0
G0438	G0271	0
G0438	G0439	0
G0438	M0064	1
G0438	90801	1
G0438	90802	1
G0438	90804	1
G0438	90805	1
G0438	90806	1
G0438	90807	1
G0438	90808	1
G0438	90809	1
G0438	90810	1
G0438	90811	1
G0438	90812	1
G0438	90813	1
G0438	90814	1
G0438	90815	1
G0438	90816	1
G0438	90817	1
G0438	90818	1
G0438	90819	1
G0438	90821	1
G0438	90822	1
G0438	90823	1
G0438	90824	1
G0438	90826	1
G0438	90827	1
G0438	90828	1
G0438	90829	1
G0438	90845	1
G0438	90862	1

Column 1	Column 2	Modifier 0=not allowed 1=allowed 9=not applicable
G0438	92002	1
G0438	92004	1
G0438	92012	1
G0438	92014	1
G0438	95831	1
G0438	95832	1
G0438	95833	1
G0438	95834	1
G0438	95851	1
G0438	95852	1
G0438	96116	1
G0438	96150	0
G0438	96151	0
G0438	96152	0
G0438	96153	0
G0438	96154	0
G0438	97802	0
G0438	97803	0
G0438	97804	0
G0439	G0250	1
G0439	G0270	0
G0439	G0271	0
G0439	M0064	1
G0439	90801	1
G0439	90802	1
G0439	90804	1
G0439	90805	1
G0439	90806	1
G0439	90807	1
G0439	90808	1
G0439	90809	1
G0439	90810	1
G0439	90811	1
G0439	90812	1
G0439	90813	1
G0439	90814	1
G0439	90815	1
G0439	90816	1
G0439	90817	1
G0439	90818	1
G0439	90819	1
G0439	90821	1

Column 1	Column 2	Modifier 0=not allowed 1=allowed 9=not applicable
G0439	90822	1
G0439	90823	1
G0439	90824	1
G0439	90826	1
G0439	90827	1
G0439	90828	1
G0439	90829	1
G0439	90845	1
G0439	90862	1
G0439	92002	1
G0439	92004	1
G0439	92012	1
G0439	92014	1
G0439	95831	1
G0439	95832	1
G0439	95833	1
G0439	95834	1
G0439	95851	1
G0439	95852	1
G0439	96116	1
G0439	96150	0
G0439	96151	0
G0439	96152	0
G0439	96153	0
G0439	96154	0
G0439	97802	0
G0439	97803	0
G0439	97804	0
G0440	G0168	1
G0440	J0670	1
G0440	J2001	1
G0440	01951	0
G0440	01952	0
G0440	0213T	0
G0440	0216T	0
G0440	0228T	0
G0440	0230T	0
G0440	11000	1
G0440	11042	1
G0440	12001	1
G0440	12002	1
G0440	12004	1

Column 1	Column 2	Modifier 0=not allowed 1=allowed 9=not applicable
G0440	12005	1
G0440	12006	1
G0440	12007	1
G0440	12020	1
G0440	12021	1
G0440	12031	1
G0440	12032	1
G0440	12034	1
G0440	12035	1
G0440	12036	1
G0440	12037	1
G0440	13100	1
G0440	13101	1
G0440	13120	1
G0440	13121	1
G0440	15852	1
G0440	16020	1
G0440	16025	1
G0440	16030	1
G0440	29000	1
G0440	29010	1
G0440	29015	1
G0440	29020	1
G0440	29025	1
G0440	29035	1
G0440	29040	1
G0440	29044	1
G0440	29046	1
G0440	29049	1
G0440	29055	1
G0440	29058	1
G0440	29065	1
G0440	29075	1
G0440	29085	1
G0440	29086	1
G0440	29105	1
G0440	29125	1
G0440	29126	1
G0440	29130	1
G0440	29131	1
G0440	29200	1
G0440	29240	1

Column 1	Column 2	Modifier 0=not allowed 1=allowed 9=not applicable	Column 1	Column 2	Modifier 0=not allowed 1=allowed 9=not applicable	Column 1	Column 2	Modifier 0=not allowed 1=allowed 9=not applicable
G0440	29260	1	G0440	62319	0	G0440	94200	1
G0440	29280	1	G0440	64400	0	G0440	94250	1
G0440	29305	1	G0440	64402	0	G0440	94680	1
G0440	29325	1	G0440	64405	0	G0440	94681	1
G0440	29345	1	G0440	64408	0	G0440	94690	1
G0440	29355	1	G0440	64410	0	G0440	94770	1
G0440	29358	1	G0440	64412	0	G0440	95812	1
G0440	29365	1	G0440	64413	0	G0440	95813	1
G0440	29405	1	G0440	64415	0	G0440	95816	1
G0440	29425	1	G0440	64416	0	G0440	95819	1
G0440	29435	1	G0440	64417	0	G0440	95822	1
G0440	29440	1	G0440	64418	0	G0440	95829	1
G0440	29445	1	G0440	64420	0	G0440	95955	1
G0440	29450	1	G0440	64421	0	G0440	96360	1
G0440	29505	1	G0440	64425	0	G0440	96365	1
G0440	29515	1	G0440	64430	0	G0440	96372	1
G0440	29520	1	G0440	64435	0	G0440	96374	1
G0440	29530	1	G0440	64445	0	G0440	96375	1
G0440	29540	1	G0440	64446	0	G0440	96376	1
G0440	29550	1	G0440	64447	0	G0440	97597	1
G0440	29580	1	G0440	64448	0	G0440	97598	1
G0440	29581	1	G0440	64449	0	G0440	97602	1
G0440	29590	1	G0440	64450	0	G0440	97605	1
G0440	36000	1	G0440	64479	0	G0440	97606	1
G0440	36400	1	G0440	64483	0	G0440	99148	0
G0440	36405	1	G0440	64490	0	G0440	99149	0
G0440	36406	1	G0440	64493	0	G0440	99150	0
G0440	36410	1	G0440	64505	0	G0441	J0670	1
G0440	36420	1	G0440	64508	0	G0441	J2001	1
G0440	36425	1	G0440	64510	0	G0441	36000	1
G0440	36430	1	G0440	64517	0	G0441	36400	1
G0440	36440	1	G0440	64520	0	G0441	36405	1
G0440	36600	1	G0440	64530	0	G0441	36406	1
G0440	36640	1	G0440	69990	0	G0441	36410	1
G0440	37202	1	G0440	93000	1	G0441	36420	1
G0440	43752	1	G0440	93005	1	G0441	36425	1
G0440	51701	1	G0440	93010	1	G0441	36430	1
G0440	51702	1	G0440	93040	1	G0441	36440	1
G0440	51703	1	G0440	93041	1	G0441	36600	1
G0440	62310	0	G0440	93042	1	G0441	36640	1
G0440	62311	0	G0440	93318	1	G0441	37202	1
G0440	62318	0	G0440	94002	1	G0441	43752	1

Column 1	Column 2	Modifier 0=not allowed 1=allowed 9=not applicable
G0441	62310	0
G0441	62311	0
G0441	62318	0
G0441	62319	0
G0441	64400	0
G0441	64402	0
G0441	64405	0
G0441	64408	0
G0441	64410	0
G0441	64412	0
G0441	64413	0
G0441	64415	0
G0441	64416	0
G0441	64417	0
G0441	64418	0
G0441	64420	0
G0441	64421	0
G0441	64425	0
G0441	64430	0
G0441	64435	0
G0441	64445	0
G0441	64446	0
G0441	64447	0
G0441	64448	0
G0441	64449	0
G0441	64450	0
G0441	64479	0
G0441	64483	0
G0441	64490	0
G0441	64493	0
G0441	64505	0
G0441	64508	0
G0441	64510	0
G0441	64517	0
G0441	64520	0
G0441	64530	0
G0441	93000	1
G0441	93005	1
G0441	93010	1
G0441	93040	1
G0441	93041	1
G0441	93042	1

Column 1	Column 2	Modifier 0=not allowed 1=allowed 9=not applicable
G0441	93318	1
G0441	94002	1
G0441	94200	1
G0441	94250	1
G0441	94680	1
G0441	94681	1
G0441	94690	1
G0441	94770	1
G0441	95812	1
G0441	95813	1
G0441	95816	1
G0441	95819	1
G0441	95822	1
G0441	95829	1
G0441	95955	1
G0441	96360	1
G0441	96365	1
G0441	96372	1
G0441	96374	1
G0441	96375	1
G0441	96376	1
G0441	99148	0
G0441	99149	0
G0441	99150	0
G3001	C8957	1
G3001	36000	1
G3001	36410	1
G3001	77750	0
G3001	78800	0
G3001	78801	0
G3001	78802	0
G3001	78803	0
G3001	78999	0
G3001	96360	1
G3001	96365	1
G3001	96372	1
G3001	96374	1
G3001	96375	1
G3001	96376	1
G3001	96409	1
G3001	96413	1
G3001	96416	1

Column 1	Column 2	Modifier 0=not allowed 1=allowed 9=not applicable
J1470	J1460	0
J1480	J1460	0
J1480	J1470	0
J1490	J1460	0
J1490	J1470	0
J1490	J1480	0
J1500	J1460	0
J1500	J1470	0
J1500	J1480	0
J1500	J1490	0
J1510	J1460	0
J1510	J1470	0
J1510	J1480	0
J1510	J1490	0
J1510	J1500	0
J1520	J1460	0
J1520	J1470	0
J1520	J1480	0
J1520	J1490	0
J1520	J1500	0
J1520	J1510	0
J1530	J1460	0
J1530	J1470	0
J1530	J1480	0
J1530	J1490	0
J1530	J1500	0
J1530	J1510	0
J1530	J1520	0
J1540	J1460	0
J1540	J1470	0
J1540	J1480	0
J1540	J1490	0
J1540	J1500	0
J1540	J1510	0
J1540	J1520	0
J1540	J1530	0
J1550	J1460	0
J1550	J1470	0
J1550	J1480	0
J1550	J1490	0
J1550	J1500	0
J1550	J1510	0

Column 1	Column 2	Modifier 0=not allowed 1=allowed 9=not applicable	Column 1	Column 2	Modifier 0=not allowed 1=allowed 9=not applicable	Column 1	Column 2	Modifier 0=not allowed 1=allowed 9=not applicable
J1550	J1520	0	P3000	99219	1	P3000	99344	1
J1550	J1530	0	P3000	99220	1	P3000	99345	1
J1550	J1540	0	P3000	99221	1	P3000	99347	1
J1560	J1460	0	P3000	99222	1	P3000	99348	1
J1560	J1470	0	P3000	99223	1	P3000	99349	1
J1560	J1480	0	P3000	99231	1	P3000	99350	1
J1560	J1490	0	P3000	99232	1	P3000	99354	1
J1560	J1500	0	P3000	99233	1	P3000	99355	1
J1560	J1510	0	P3000	99234	1	P3000	99356	1
J1560	J1520	0	P3000	99235	1	P3000	99357	1
J1560	J1530	0	P3000	99236	1	P3000	99360	1
J1560	J1540	0	P3000	99238	1	P3000	99455	1
J1560	J1550	0	P3000	99239	1	P3000	99456	1
J2790	90385	1	P3000	99281	1	P3000	99460	1
J2792	90385	0	P3000	99282	1	P3000	99461	1
M0064	99605	1	P3000	99283	1	P3000	99462	1
M0064	99606	1	P3000	99284	1	P3000	99463	1
P3000	G0380	1	P3000	99285	1	P3000	99464	1
P3000	G0381	1	P3000	99291	1	P3000	99465	1
P3000	G0382	1	P3000	99292	1	P3000	99466	1
P3000	G0383	1	P3000	99304	1	P3000	99468	1
P3000	G0384	1	P3000	99305	1	P3000	99469	1
P3000	G0406	1	P3000	99306	1	P3000	99471	1
P3000	G0407	1	P3000	99307	1	P3000	99472	1
P3000	G0408	1	P3000	99308	1	P3000	99475	1
P3000	G0425	1	P3000	99309	1	P3000	99476	1
P3000	G0426	1	P3000	99310	1	P3000	99477	1
P3000	G0427	1	P3000	99315	1	P3000	99478	1
P3000	88160	1	P3000	99316	1	P3000	99479	1
P3000	88161	1	P3000	99318	1	P3000	99480	1
P3000	99201	1	P3000	99324	1	P3001	G0123	0
P3000	99202	1	P3000	99325	1	P3001	G0141	0
P3000	99203	1	P3000	99326	1	P3001	G0143	0
P3000	99204	1	P3000	99327	1	P3001	G0144	0
P3000	99205	1	P3000	99328	1	P3001	G0145	0
P3000	99211	1	P3000	99334	1	P3001	G0147	0
P3000	99212	1	P3000	99335	1	P3001	G0148	0
P3000	99213	1	P3000	99336	1	P3001	G0380	1
P3000	99214	1	P3000	99337	1	P3001	G0381	1
P3000	99215	1	P3000	99341	1	P3001	G0382	1
P3000	99217	1	P3000	99342	1	P3001	G0383	1
P3000	99218	1	P3000	99343	1	P3001	G0384	1

Column 1	Column 2	Modifier 0=not allowed 1=allowed 9=not applicable	Column 1	Column 2	Modifier 0=not allowed 1=allowed 9=not applicable	Column 1	Column 2	Modifier 0=not allowed 1=allowed 9=not applicable
P3001	G0406	1	P3001	99235	1	P3001	99357	1
P3001	G0407	1	P3001	99236	1	P3001	99360	1
P3001	G0408	1	P3001	99238	1	P3001	99455	1
P3001	G0425	1	P3001	99239	1	P3001	99456	1
P3001	G0426	1	P3001	99281	1	P3001	99460	1
P3001	G0427	1	P3001	99282	1	P3001	99461	1
P3001	88141	0	P3001	99283	1	P3001	99462	1
P3001	88142	0	P3001	99284	1	P3001	99463	1
P3001	88143	0	P3001	99285	1	P3001	99464	1
P3001	88147	0	P3001	99291	1	P3001	99465	1
P3001	88148	0	P3001	99292	1	P3001	99466	1
P3001	88150	0	P3001	99304	1	P3001	99468	1
P3001	88152	0	P3001	99305	1	P3001	99469	1
P3001	88153	0	P3001	99306	1	P3001	99471	1
P3001	88154	0	P3001	99307	1	P3001	99472	1
P3001	88164	0	P3001	99308	1	P3001	99475	1
P3001	88165	0	P3001	99309	1	P3001	99476	1
P3001	88166	0	P3001	99310	1	P3001	99477	1
P3001	88167	0	P3001	99315	1	P3001	99478	1
P3001	88174	0	P3001	99316	1	P3001	99479	1
P3001	88175	0	P3001	99318	1	P3001	99480	1
P3001	99201	1	P3001	99324	1	P9017	86927	1
P3001	99202	1	P3001	99325	1	P9023	86927	1
P3001	99203	1	P3001	99326	1	P9023	86965	1
P3001	99204	1	P3001	99327	1	P9032	P9010	1
P3001	99205	1	P3001	99328	1	P9032	P9011	1
P3001	99211	1	P3001	99334	1	P9032	P9016	1
P3001	99212	1	P3001	99335	1	P9032	P9019	1
P3001	99213	1	P3001	99336	1	P9032	P9020	1
P3001	99214	1	P3001	99337	1	P9032	P9021	1
P3001	99215	1	P3001	99341	1	P9032	P9022	1
P3001	99217	1	P3001	99342	1	P9032	P9031	1
P3001	99218	1	P3001	99343	1	P9032	P9034	1
P3001	99219	1	P3001	99344	1	P9032	P9035	1
P3001	99220	1	P3001	99345	1	P9032	P9039	1
P3001	99221	1	P3001	99347	1	P9032	86945	1
P3001	99222	1	P3001	99348	1	P9033	P9010	1
P3001	99223	1	P3001	99349	1	P9033	P9011	1
P3001	99231	1	P3001	99350	1	P9033	P9016	1
P3001	99232	1	P3001	99354	1	P9033	P9019	1
P3001	99233	1	P3001	99355	1	P9033	P9020	1
P3001	99234	1	P3001	99356	1	P9033	P9021	1

Column 1	Column 2	Modifier 0=not allowed 1=allowed 9=not applicable
P9033	P9022	1
P9033	P9031	1
P9033	P9034	1
P9033	P9035	1
P9033	P9039	1
P9033	86945	1
P9036	P9010	1
P9036	P9011	1
P9036	P9016	1
P9036	P9019	1
P9036	P9020	1
P9036	P9021	1
P9036	P9022	1
P9036	P9031	1
P9036	P9034	1
P9036	P9035	1
P9036	P9039	1
P9036	86945	1
P9037	P9010	1
P9037	P9011	1
P9037	P9016	1
P9037	P9019	1
P9037	P9020	1
P9037	P9021	1
P9037	P9022	1
P9037	P9031	1
P9037	P9034	1
P9037	P9035	1
P9037	P9039	1
P9037	86945	1
P9038	P9010	1
P9038	P9011	1
P9038	P9016	1
P9038	P9019	1
P9038	P9020	1
P9038	P9021	1
P9038	P9022	1
P9038	P9031	1
P9038	P9034	1
P9038	P9035	1
P9038	P9039	1
P9038	86945	1

Column 1	Column 2	Modifier 0=not allowed 1=allowed 9=not applicable
P9039	86930	1
P9039	86931	1
P9039	86932	1
P9040	P9010	1
P9040	P9011	1
P9040	P9016	1
P9040	P9019	1
P9040	P9020	1
P9040	P9021	1
P9040	P9022	1
P9040	P9031	1
P9040	P9034	1
P9040	P9035	1
P9040	P9039	1
P9040	86945	1
P9051	86644	1
P9051	86645	1
P9053	86644	1
P9053	86645	1
P9053	86945	1
P9054	86930	1
P9054	86931	1
P9054	86932	1
P9055	86644	1
P9055	86645	1
P9056	86945	1
P9057	86930	1
P9057	86931	1
P9057	86932	1
P9057	86945	1
P9058	86644	1
P9058	86645	1
P9058	86945	1
P9059	86927	1
P9060	86927	1
Q0091	G0181	1
Q0091	G0182	1
Q0091	G0380	1
Q0091	G0381	1
Q0091	G0382	1
Q0091	G0383	1
Q0091	G0384	1

Column 1	Column 2	Modifier 0=not allowed 1=allowed 9=not applicable
Q0091	G0406	1
Q0091	G0407	1
Q0091	G0408	1
Q0091	G0425	1
Q0091	G0426	1
Q0091	G0427	1
Q0091	99201	1
Q0091	99202	1
Q0091	99203	1
Q0091	99204	1
Q0091	99205	1
Q0091	99211	1
Q0091	99212	1
Q0091	99213	1
Q0091	99214	1
Q0091	99215	1
Q0091	99217	1
Q0091	99218	1
Q0091	99219	1
Q0091	99220	1
Q0091	99221	1
Q0091	99222	1
Q0091	99223	1
Q0091	99231	1
Q0091	99232	1
Q0091	99233	1
Q0091	99234	1
Q0091	99235	1
Q0091	99236	1
Q0091	99238	1
Q0091	99239	1
Q0091	99281	1
Q0091	99282	1
Q0091	99283	1
Q0091	99284	1
Q0091	99285	1
Q0091	99291	1
Q0091	99292	1
Q0091	99304	1
Q0091	99305	1
Q0091	99306	1
Q0091	99307	1

Column 1	Column 2	Modifier 0=not allowed 1=allowed 9=not applicable
Q0091	99308	1
Q0091	99309	1
Q0091	99310	1
Q0091	99315	1
Q0091	99316	1
Q0091	99318	1
Q0091	99324	1
Q0091	99325	1
Q0091	99326	1
Q0091	99327	1
Q0091	99328	1
Q0091	99334	1
Q0091	99335	1
Q0091	99336	1
Q0091	99337	1
Q0091	99341	1
Q0091	99342	1
Q0091	99343	1
Q0091	99344	1
Q0091	99345	1
Q0091	99347	1
Q0091	99348	1
Q0091	99349	1
Q0091	99350	1
Q0091	99354	1
Q0091	99355	1
Q0091	99356	1
Q0091	99357	1
Q0091	99360	1
Q0091	99455	1
Q0091	99456	1
Q0091	99460	1
Q0091	99461	1
Q0091	99462	1
Q0091	99463	1
Q0091	99464	1
Q0091	99465	1
Q0091	99466	1
Q0091	99468	1
Q0091	99469	1
Q0091	99471	1
Q0091	99472	1

Column 1	Column 2	Modifier 0=not allowed 1=allowed 9=not applicable
Q0091	99475	1
Q0091	99476	1
Q0091	99477	1
Q0091	99478	1
Q0091	99479	1
Q0091	99480	1
Q2043	G0380	1
Q2043	G0381	1
Q2043	G0382	1
Q2043	G0383	1
Q2043	G0384	1
Q2043	0213T	0
Q2043	0216T	0
Q2043	0228T	0
Q2043	0230T	0
Q2043	36000	1
Q2043	36400	1
Q2043	36405	1
Q2043	36406	1
Q2043	36410	1
Q2043	36420	1
Q2043	36425	1
Q2043	36430	1
Q2043	36440	1
Q2043	36600	1
Q2043	36640	1
Q2043	37202	1
Q2043	38206	0
Q2043	38210	0
Q2043	38211	0
Q2043	38212	0
Q2043	38213	0
Q2043	38214	0
Q2043	38215	0
Q2043	38241	0
Q2043	43752	1
Q2043	51701	1
Q2043	51702	1
Q2043	51703	1
Q2043	62310	0
Q2043	62311	0
Q2043	62318	0

Column 1	Column 2	Modifier 0=not allowed 1=allowed 9=not applicable
Q2043	62319	0
Q2043	64400	0
Q2043	64402	0
Q2043	64405	0
Q2043	64408	0
Q2043	64410	0
Q2043	64412	0
Q2043	64413	0
Q2043	64415	0
Q2043	64416	0
Q2043	64417	0
Q2043	64418	0
Q2043	64420	0
Q2043	64421	0
Q2043	64425	0
Q2043	64430	0
Q2043	64435	0
Q2043	64445	0
Q2043	64446	0
Q2043	64447	0
Q2043	64448	0
Q2043	64449	0
Q2043	64450	0
Q2043	64479	0
Q2043	64483	0
Q2043	64490	0
Q2043	64493	0
Q2043	64505	0
Q2043	64508	0
Q2043	64510	0
Q2043	64517	0
Q2043	64520	0
Q2043	64530	0
Q2043	69990	0
Q2043	93000	1
Q2043	93005	1
Q2043	93010	1
Q2043	93040	1
Q2043	93041	1
Q2043	93042	1
Q2043	93318	1
Q2043	94002	1

Column 1	Column 2	Modifier 0=not allowed 1=allowed 9=not applicable
Q2043	94200	1
Q2043	94250	1
Q2043	94680	1
Q2043	94681	1
Q2043	94690	1
Q2043	94770	1
Q2043	95812	1
Q2043	95813	1
Q2043	95816	1
Q2043	95819	1
Q2043	95822	1
Q2043	95829	1
Q2043	95955	1
Q2043	96360	1
Q2043	96365	1
Q2043	96372	1
Q2043	96374	1
Q2043	96375	1
Q2043	96376	1
Q2043	99148	0
Q2043	99149	0
Q2043	99150	0
Q2043	99201	1
Q2043	99202	1
Q2043	99203	1
Q2043	99204	1
Q2043	99205	1
Q2043	99211	1
Q2043	99212	1
Q2043	99213	1
Q2043	99214	1

Column 1	Column 2	Modifier 0=not allowed 1=allowed 9=not applicable
Q2043	99215	1
Q2043	99217	1
Q2043	99218	1
Q2043	99219	1
Q2043	99220	1
Q2043	99224	1
Q2043	99225	1
Q2043	99226	1
Q2043	99231	1
Q2043	99232	1
Q2043	99233	1
Q2043	99234	1
Q2043	99235	1
Q2043	99236	1
Q2043	99281	1
Q2043	99282	1
Q2043	99283	1
Q2043	99284	1
Q2043	99285	1
Q2043	99291	1
Q2043	99292	1
Q2043	99304	1
Q2043	99305	1
Q2043	99306	1
Q2043	99307	1
Q2043	99308	1
Q2043	99309	1
Q2043	99310	1
Q2043	99315	1
Q2043	99316	1
Q2043	99318	1

Column 1	Column 2	Modifier 0=not allowed 1=allowed 9=not applicable
Q2043	99324	1
Q2043	99325	1
Q2043	99326	1
Q2043	99327	1
Q2043	99328	1
Q2043	99334	1
Q2043	99335	1
Q2043	99336	1
Q2043	99337	1
Q2043	99341	1
Q2043	99342	1
Q2043	99343	1
Q2043	99344	1
Q2043	99345	1
Q2043	99347	1
Q2043	99348	1
Q2043	99349	1
Q2043	99350	1
Q2043	99466	1
Q2043	99468	1
Q2043	99469	1
Q2043	99471	1
Q2043	99472	1
Q2043	99475	1
Q2043	99476	1
Q2043	99477	1
Q2043	99478	1
Q2043	99479	1
Q2043	99480	1
R0075	R0070	1

APPENDIX B

Hospital Outpatient Prospective Payment System Edits
(Effective Date: 10/01/11-12/31/11, Version: 17.3)

Appendix C contains three sets of edits that provide guidance when reporting HCPCS codes within the Hospital Outpatient Prospective Payment System (PPS).

1. Practitioner/DME Supplier **Medically Unlikely Edits** (MUE) units indicate the maximum allowable number of units of service per day, per patient. The purpose of the MUEs project is to detect and deny unlikely Medicare claims on a pre-payment basis in order to stop inappropriate payment. The MUE project is not meant to establish Medicare payment policy, but rather to improve the accuracy of the Medicare payments.

2. **Mutually Exclusive Code Edits** (MEEs) are National Correct Coding Initiative (NCCI) edits for physicians and list codes that are not reported together.

3. **Columns 1 and 2 Correct Coding Edits** are National Correct Coding Initiative (NCCI) edits for physicians and list codes that are not reported together.

2011 Hospital Outpatient Services Medically Unlikely Edits (MUE)

CODE	MUE UNIT	CODE	MUE UNIT	CODE	MUE UNIT	CODE	MUE UNIT
A4258	1	A7025	1	A9554	1	C1783	2
A4470	1	A7026	1	A9555	3	C1785	2
A4480	1	A7027	1	A9557	2	C1786	2
A4557	2	A7035	1	A9559	1	C1787	2
A4561	1	A7036	1	A9560	2	C1788	2
A4562	1	A7040	2	A9561	1	C1789	3
A4614	1	A7041	2	A9562	2	C1813	2
A4640	1	A7042	2	A9566	1	C1814	3
A4642	1	A7043	2	A9567	2	C1815	2
A4650	3	A9284	1	A9569	1	C1816	2
A4660	1	A9500	3	A9570	1	C1817	3
A4663	1	A9501	3	A9571	1	C1818	2
A5500	2	A9502	3	A9580	1	C1820	3
A5501	2	A9503	1	A9582	1	C1878	2
A5503	2	A9504	1	A9604	1	C1880	2
A5504	2	A9507	1	A9700	2	C1881	2
A5505	2	A9510	1	C1721	2	C1882	2
A5506	2	A9521	2	C1722	2	C1888	2
A5507	2	A9526	2	C1749	1	C1891	2
A6501	1	A9536	1	C1750	2	C1895	2
A6502	1	A9537	1	C1752	2	C1896	2
A6503	1	A9538	1	C1753	3	C1897	3
A6504	2	A9539	2	C1755	2	C1899	2
A6505	2	A9540	2	C1756	2	C1900	2
A6506	2	A9541	1	C1758	3	C2614	3
A6507	2	A9542	1	C1764	2	C2615	2
A6508	2	A9543	1	C1767	3	C2616	1
A6509	1	A9544	1	C1768	3	C2619	2
A6510	1	A9545	1	C1770	3	C2620	2
A6511	1	A9546	1	C1771	3	C2621	2
A6513	1	A9550	1	C1772	2	C2622	2
A6545	2	A9551	1	C1777	2	C2626	2
A7017	1	A9552	1	C1780	3	C2627	3
A7020	1	A9553	1	C1782	2	C8900	1

CODE	MUE UNIT	CODE	MUE UNIT	CODE	MUE UNIT	CODE	MUE UNIT
C8901	1	E0619	1	E1240	1	G0102	1
C8902	1	E0656	1	E1250	1	G0103	1
C8903	1	E0657	1	E1260	1	G0104	1
C8904	1	E0746	1	E1270	1	G0105	1
C8905	1	E0749	1	E1280	1	G0106	1
C8906	1	E0782	1	E1285	1	G0117	1
C8907	1	E0783	1	E1290	1	G0118	1
C8908	1	E0785	1	E1295	1	G0120	1
C8909	1	E0856	1	E1500	1	G0121	1
C8910	1	E0950	1	E1510	1	G0123	1
C8911	1	E0951	2	E1520	1	G0124	1
C8912	2	E0952	2	E1530	1	G0127	1
C8913	2	E0958	2	E1540	1	G0128	1
C8914	2	E1036	1	E1550	1	G0129	3
C8918	1	E1050	1	E1560	1	G0130	1
C8919	1	E1060	1	E1570	1	G0143	1
C8920	1	E1070	1	E1580	1	G0144	1
C8921	1	E1083	1	E1590	1	G0145	1
C8922	1	E1084	1	E1592	1	G0147	1
C8923	1	E1085	1	E1594	1	G0148	1
C8924	1	E1086	1	E1600	1	G0166	2
C8925	1	E1087	1	E1610	1	G0168	2
C8926	1	E1088	1	E1615	1	G0173	1
C8927	1	E1089	1	E1620	1	G0175	1
C8928	1	E1090	1	E1625	1	G0176	5
C8929	1	E1092	1	E1630	1	G0186	1
C8930	1	E1093	1	E1635	1	G0202	1
C8931	1	E1100	1	E1639	1	G0204	1
C8932	1	E1110	1	E1831	2	G0206	1
C8933	1	E1130	1	E1902	1	G0239	2
C8934	2	E1140	1	E2231	1	G0245	1
C8935	2	E1160	1	E2295	1	G0246	1
C8936	2	E1161	1	E2313	1	G0247	1
C8957	1	E1170	1	E2397	1	G0248	1
C9716	1	E1171	1	E2609	1	G0249	3
C9724	1	E1172	1	E2617	1	G0251	1
C9725	1	E1180	1	E2622	1	G0257	2
C9726	2	E1190	1	E2623	1	G0259	2
C9727	1	E1195	1	E2624	1	G0260	2
C9728	1	E1200	1	E2625	1	G0268	1
C9800	1	E1220	1	G0008	1	G0275	1
C9898	1	E1221	1	G0009	1	G0278	1
E0433	1	E1222	1	G0010	1	G0281	1
E0616	1	E1223	1	G0027	1	G0283	1
E0618	1	E1224	1	G0101	1	G0288	1

CODE	MUE UNIT
G0289	2
G0290	1
G0291	2
G0293	1
G0294	1
G0302	1
G0303	1
G0304	1
G0305	1
G0306	2
G0307	2
G0328	1
G0329	1
G0337	1
G0339	1
G0340	1
G0364	2
G0365	2
G0379	1
G0380	2
G0381	2
G0382	2
G0383	2
G0384	2
G0389	1
G0390	1
G0396	1
G0397	1
G0398	1
G0399	1
G0400	1
G0416	1
G0417	1
G0418	1
G0419	1
G0429	1
G0431	1
G0432	1
G0433	1
G0434	1
G0435	1
G0436	1
G0437	1
G0438	1
G0439	1

CODE	MUE UNIT
G0440	1
L0112	1
L0113	1
L0120	1
L0130	1
L0140	1
L0150	1
L0160	1
L0170	1
L0172	1
L0174	1
L0180	1
L0190	1
L0200	1
L0220	1
L0430	1
L0450	1
L0452	1
L0454	1
L0456	1
L0458	1
L0460	1
L0462	1
L0464	1
L0466	1
L0468	1
L0470	1
L0472	1
L0480	1
L0482	1
L0484	1
L0486	1
L0488	1
L0490	1
L0491	1
L0492	1
L0621	1
L0622	1
L0623	1
L0624	1
L0625	1
L0626	1
L0627	1
L0628	1
L0629	1

CODE	MUE UNIT
L0630	1
L0631	1
L0632	1
L0633	1
L0634	1
L0635	1
L0636	1
L0637	1
L0638	1
L0639	1
L0640	1
L0700	1
L0710	1
L0810	1
L0820	1
L0830	1
L0859	1
L0861	1
L0970	1
L0972	1
L0974	1
L0976	1
L0978	2
L0980	1
L1000	1
L1005	1
L1010	2
L1020	2
L1025	1
L1030	1
L1040	1
L1050	1
L1060	1
L1070	2
L1080	2
L1085	1
L1090	1
L1100	2
L1110	2
L1120	3
L1200	1
L1210	2
L1220	1
L1230	1
L1240	1

CODE	MUE UNIT
L1250	2
L1260	1
L1270	3
L1280	2
L1290	2
L1300	1
L1310	1
L1500	1
L1510	1
L1520	1
L1600	1
L1610	1
L1620	1
L1630	1
L1640	1
L1650	1
L1652	1
L1660	1
L1680	1
L1685	1
L1686	1
L1690	1
L1700	1
L1710	1
L1720	2
L1730	1
L1755	2
L1810	2
L1820	2
L1830	2
L1831	2
L1832	2
L1834	2
L1836	2
L1840	2
L1843	2
L1844	2
L1845	2
L1846	2
L1847	2
L1850	2
L1860	2
L1900	2
L1902	2
L1904	2

CODE	MUE UNIT	CODE	MUE UNIT	CODE	MUE UNIT	CODE	MUE UNIT
L1906	2	L2230	2	L2820	2	L3430	2
L1907	2	L2232	2	L2830	2	L3440	2
L1910	2	L2240	2	L3000	2	L3450	2
L1920	2	L2250	2	L3001	2	L3455	2
L1930	2	L2260	2	L3002	2	L3460	2
L1932	2	L2265	2	L3003	2	L3465	2
L1940	2	L2270	2	L3010	2	L3470	2
L1945	2	L2275	2	L3020	2	L3480	2
L1950	2	L2280	2	L3030	2	L3485	2
L1951	2	L2300	1	L3031	2	L3500	2
L1960	2	L2310	1	L3040	2	L3510	2
L1970	2	L2320	2	L3050	2	L3520	2
L1971	2	L2330	2	L3060	2	L3530	2
L1980	2	L2335	2	L3070	2	L3540	2
L1990	2	L2340	2	L3080	2	L3550	2
L2000	2	L2350	2	L3090	2	L3560	2
L2005	2	L2360	2	L3100	2	L3570	2
L2010	2	L2370	2	L3140	1	L3580	2
L2020	2	L2375	2	L3150	1	L3590	2
L2030	2	L2380	2	L3160	2	L3595	2
L2034	2	L2500	2	L3170	2	L3600	2
L2035	2	L2510	2	L3215	2	L3610	2
L2036	2	L2520	2	L3216	2	L3620	2
L2037	2	L2525	2	L3217	2	L3630	2
L2038	2	L2526	2	L3219	2	L3640	1
L2040	1	L2530	2	L3221	2	L3650	1
L2050	1	L2540	2	L3222	2	L3660	1
L2060	1	L2550	2	L3224	2	L3670	1
L2070	1	L2570	2	L3225	2	L3671	1
L2080	1	L2580	2	L3230	2	L3674	2
L2090	1	L2600	2	L3250	2	L3675	1
L2106	2	L2610	2	L3251	2	L3677	1
L2108	2	L2620	2	L3252	2	L3702	2
L2112	2	L2622	2	L3253	2	L3710	2
L2114	2	L2624	2	L3330	2	L3720	2
L2116	2	L2627	1	L3332	2	L3730	2
L2126	2	L2628	1	L3340	2	L3740	2
L2128	2	L2630	1	L3350	2	L3760	2
L2132	2	L2640	1	L3360	2	L3762	2
L2134	2	L2650	2	L3370	2	L3763	2
L2136	2	L2660	1	L3380	2	L3764	2
L2180	2	L2670	2	L3390	2	L3765	2
L2188	2	L2680	2	L3400	2	L3766	2
L2190	2	L2795	2	L3410	2	L3806	2
L2192	2	L2800	2	L3420	2	L3807	2

CODE	MUE UNIT
L3808	2
L3900	2
L3901	2
L3904	2
L3905	2
L3912	2
L3913	2
L3917	2
L3919	2
L3921	2
L3923	2
L3929	2
L3931	2
L3933	3
L3935	3
L3960	1
L3961	1
L3962	1
L3967	1
L3971	1
L3973	1
L3975	1
L3976	1
L3977	1
L3978	1
L3980	2
L3982	2
L3984	2
L4000	1
L4010	2
L4020	2
L4030	2
L4040	2
L4045	2
L4050	2
L4055	2
L4060	2
L4070	2
L4080	2
L4100	2
L4130	2
L4350	2
L4360	2
L4370	2
L4380	2

CODE	MUE UNIT
L4386	2
L4392	2
L4394	2
L4396	2
L4398	2
L4631	2
L5000	2
L5010	2
L5020	2
L5050	2
L5060	2
L5100	2
L5105	2
L5150	2
L5160	2
L5200	2
L5210	2
L5220	2
L5230	2
L5250	2
L5270	2
L5280	2
L5301	2
L5311	2
L5321	2
L5331	2
L5341	2
L5400	2
L5410	2
L5420	2
L5430	2
L5450	2
L5460	2
L5500	2
L5505	2
L5510	2
L5520	2
L5530	2
L5535	2
L5540	2
L5560	2
L5570	2
L5580	2
L5585	2
L5590	2

CODE	MUE UNIT
L5595	2
L5600	2
L5610	2
L5611	2
L5613	2
L5614	2
L5616	2
L5617	2
L5628	2
L5629	2
L5630	2
L5631	2
L5632	2
L5634	2
L5636	2
L5637	2
L5638	2
L5639	2
L5640	2
L5642	2
L5643	2
L5644	2
L5645	2
L5646	2
L5647	2
L5648	2
L5649	2
L5650	2
L5651	2
L5652	2
L5653	2
L5654	2
L5655	2
L5656	2
L5658	2
L5661	2
L5665	2
L5666	2
L5668	2
L5670	2
L5671	2
L5672	2
L5676	2
L5677	2
L5678	2

CODE	MUE UNIT
L5680	2
L5681	2
L5682	2
L5683	2
L5684	2
L5686	2
L5688	2
L5690	2
L5692	2
L5694	2
L5695	2
L5696	2
L5697	2
L5698	2
L5699	2
L5700	2
L5701	2
L5702	2
L5703	2
L5704	2
L5705	2
L5706	2
L5707	2
L5710	2
L5711	2
L5712	2
L5714	2
L5716	2
L5718	2
L5722	2
L5724	2
L5726	2
L5728	2
L5780	2
L5781	2
L5782	2
L5785	2
L5790	2
L5795	2
L5810	2
L5811	2
L5812	2
L5814	2
L5816	2
L5818	2

CODE	MUE UNIT
L5822	2
L5824	2
L5826	2
L5828	2
L5830	2
L5840	2
L5845	2
L5848	2
L5850	2
L5855	2
L5856	2
L5857	2
L5858	2
L5910	2
L5920	2
L5925	2
L5930	2
L5940	2
L5950	2
L5960	2
L5961	2
L5962	2
L5964	2
L5966	2
L5968	2
L5970	2
L5971	2
L5972	2
L5973	2
L5974	2
L5975	2
L5976	2
L5978	2
L5979	2
L5980	2
L5981	2
L5982	2
L5984	2
L5985	2
L5986	2
L5987	2
L5988	2
L5990	2
L6000	2
L6010	2

CODE	MUE UNIT
L6020	2
L6025	2
L6050	2
L6055	2
L6100	2
L6110	2
L6120	2
L6130	2
L6200	2
L6205	2
L6250	2
L6300	2
L6310	2
L6320	2
L6350	2
L6360	2
L6370	2
L6380	2
L6382	2
L6384	2
L6386	2
L6388	2
L6400	2
L6450	2
L6500	2
L6550	2
L6570	2
L6580	2
L6582	2
L6584	2
L6586	2
L6588	2
L6590	2
L6600	2
L6605	2
L6610	2
L6711	2
L6712	2
L6713	2
L6714	2
L6721	2
L6722	2
L6615	2
L6616	2
L6620	2

CODE	MUE UNIT
L6621	2
L6623	2
L6625	2
L6628	2
L6629	2
L6630	2
L6635	2
L6637	2
L6638	2
L6640	2
L6641	2
L6642	2
L6645	2
L6646	2
L6647	2
L6648	2
L6650	2
L6670	2
L6672	2
L6675	2
L6676	2
L6677	2
L6686	2
L6687	2
L6688	2
L6689	2
L6690	2
L6693	2
L6694	2
L6695	2
L6696	2
L6697	2
L6698	2
L6711	2
L6712	2
L6713	2
L6714	2
L6721	2
L6722	2
L6805	2
L6810	2
L6881	2
L6882	2
L6883	2
L6884	2

CODE	MUE UNIT
L6885	2
L6890	2
L6895	2
L6900	2
L6905	2
L6910	2
L6915	2
L6920	2
L6925	2
L6930	2
L6935	2
L6940	2
L6945	2
L6950	2
L6955	2
L6960	2
L6965	2
L6970	2
L6975	2
L7040	2
L7045	2
L7170	2
L7180	2
L7181	2
L7185	2
L7186	2
L7190	2
L7191	2
L7260	2
L7261	2
L7266	2
L7272	2
L7274	2
L7362	1
L7366	1
L7368	1
L7400	2
L7401	2
L7402	2
L7403	2
L7404	2
L7405	2
L7900	1
L8030	2
L8031	2

CODE	MUE UNIT
L8032	2
L8035	2
L8039	2
L8040	1
L8041	1
L8042	2
L8043	1
L8044	1
L8045	2
L8046	1
L8047	1
L8300	1
L8310	1
L8320	2
L8330	2
L8500	1
L8501	2
L8507	3
L8509	1
L8510	1
L8511	1
L8514	1
L8515	1
L8600	2
L8604	3
L8610	2
L8612	2
L8613	2
L8614	2
L8615	2
L8616	2
L8617	2
L8618	2
L8619	2
L8622	2
L8627	2
L8628	2
L8629	2
L8631	4
L8641	4
L8642	2
L8658	4
L8659	4
L8670	4
L8681	1

CODE	MUE UNIT
L8683	1
L8684	1
L8686	2
L8687	2
L8689	1
L8690	1
L8691	1
L8693	1
L8695	1
M0064	1
P2028	1
P2029	1
P2033	1
P2038	1
P3000	1
P3001	1
P9612	1
P9615	1
Q0035	1
Q0085	2
Q0091	1
Q0111	2
Q0112	3
Q0113	2
Q0114	1
Q0115	1
Q0478	1
Q0479	1
Q0480	1
Q0481	1
Q0482	1
Q0483	1
Q0484	1
Q0485	1
Q0486	1
Q0487	1
Q0488	1
Q0489	1
Q0490	1
Q0491	1
Q0492	1
Q0493	1
Q0494	1
Q0495	1
Q0497	2

CODE	MUE UNIT
Q0498	1
Q0499	1
Q0501	1
Q0502	1
Q0503	3
Q0504	1
Q1003	2
Q2035	1
Q2036	1
Q2037	1
Q2038	1
Q2039	1
Q2043	1
Q4001	1
Q4002	1
Q4003	2
Q4004	2
Q4025	1
Q4026	1
Q4027	1
Q4028	1
R0070	2
R0075	2
R0076	1
V2020	1
V2101	2
V2102	2
V2104	2
V2105	2
V2106	2
V2107	2
V2108	2
V2109	2
V2110	2
V2111	2
V2112	2
V2113	2
V2114	2
V2115	2
V2118	2
V2121	2
V2200	2
V2201	2
V2202	2
V2203	2

CODE	MUE UNIT
V2204	2
V2205	2
V2206	2
V2207	2
V2208	2
V2209	2
V2210	2
V2211	2
V2212	2
V2213	2
V2214	2
V2215	2
V2218	2
V2219	2
V2220	2
V2221	2
V2299	2
V2300	2
V2301	2
V2302	2
V2303	2
V2304	2
V2305	2
V2306	2
V2307	2
V2308	2
V2309	2
V2310	2
V2311	2
V2312	2
V2313	2
V2314	2
V2315	2
V2318	2
V2319	2
V2320	2
V2321	2
V2399	2
V2410	2
V2430	2
V2500	2
V2501	2
V2502	2
V2503	2
V2510	2

CODE	MUE UNIT
V2511	2
V2512	2
V2513	2
V2520	2
V2521	2
V2522	2
V2523	2
V2530	2
V2531	2

CODE	MUE UNIT
V2600	1
V2610	1
V2615	2
V2623	2
V2624	2
V2625	2
V2626	2
V2627	2

CODE	MUE UNIT
V2628	2
V2629	2
V2630	2
V2631	2
V2632	2
V2700	2
V2710	2
V2718	2

CODE	MUE UNIT
V2730	2
V2770	2
V2780	2
V2782	2
V2783	2
V2785	2
V2790	1
V2797	1

Hospital Outpatient Prospective Payment System (PPS)
Mutually Exclusive Edits (MEEs)
(Effective Date: 10/01/11-12/31/11, Version: 17.3)
Codes in Column 1 are not reported with codes in Column 2 with 0 or 9

Column 1	Column 2	Modifier 0=not allowed 1=allowed 9=not applicable	Column 1	Column 2	Modifier 0=not allowed 1=allowed 9=not applicable	Column 1	Column 2	Modifier 0=not allowed 1=allowed 9=not applicable
C8928	C8923	1	C9800	11952	1	G0104	45381	0
C8928	C8924	1	C9800	11954	1	G0104	45382	0
C8928	C8925	1	E0781	E0782	1	G0104	45383	0
C8928	C8927	0	G0101	57410	1	G0104	45384	0
C8928	C8929	1	G0103	84153	0	G0104	45385	0
C8928	93306	1	G0103	84154	1	G0104	45386	0
C8928	93307	1	G0104	G0105	0	G0104	45387	0
C8928	93308	1	G0104	G0106	1	G0104	46604	0
C8928	93312	1	G0104	G0120	1	G0104	46608	0
C8928	93313	1	G0104	G0121	0	G0104	46614	0
C8928	93314	1	G0104	45300	0	G0105	45300	0
C8928	93318	0	G0104	45303	0	G0105	45303	0
C8930	93303	1	G0104	45305	0	G0105	45305	0
C8930	93304	1	G0104	45307	0	G0105	45307	0
C8930	93313	1	G0104	45308	0	G0105	45308	0
C8930	93314	1	G0104	45309	0	G0105	45309	0
C8930	93797	1	G0104	45315	0	G0105	45315	0
C8930	93798	1	G0104	45317	0	G0105	45317	0
C8931	72159	0	G0104	45320	0	G0105	45320	0
C8932	72159	0	G0104	45321	0	G0105	45321	0
C8933	72159	0	G0104	45327	0	G0105	45327	0
C8934	73225	0	G0104	45330	0	G0105	45330	0
C8935	73225	0	G0104	45331	0	G0105	45331	0
C8936	73225	0	G0104	45332	0	G0105	45332	0
C8957	96415	0	G0104	45333	0	G0105	45333	0
C9273	36512	0	G0104	45334	0	G0105	45334	0
C9273	36513	0	G0104	45335	0	G0105	45335	0
C9273	36514	0	G0104	45337	0	G0105	45337	0
C9273	36515	0	G0104	45338	0	G0105	45338	0
C9273	36516	0	G0104	45339	0	G0105	45339	0
C9716	46750	0	G0104	45340	0	G0105	45340	0
C9716	46751	0	G0104	45341	0	G0105	45341	0
C9716	46760	0	G0104	45342	0	G0105	45342	0
C9716	46761	0	G0104	45345	0	G0105	45345	0
C9716	46762	0	G0104	45355	0	G0105	45355	0
C9800	G0429	0	G0104	45378	0	G0106	G0105	0
C9800	11950	1	G0104	45379	0	G0106	G0121	0
C9800	11951	1	G0104	45380	0	G0106	74270	1

Column 1	Column 2	Modifier 0=not allowed 1=allowed 9=not applicable	Column 1	Column 2	Modifier 0=not allowed 1=allowed 9=not applicable	Column 1	Column 2	Modifier 0=not allowed 1=allowed 9=not applicable
G0106	74280	1	G0127	99213	1	G0127	99335	1
G0120	G0105	0	G0127	99214	1	G0127	99336	1
G0120	G0106	0	G0127	99215	1	G0127	99337	1
G0120	G0121	0	G0127	99217	1	G0127	99341	1
G0120	74270	1	G0127	99218	1	G0127	99342	1
G0120	74280	1	G0127	99219	1	G0127	99343	1
G0121	G0105	0	G0127	99220	1	G0127	99344	1
G0121	45300	0	G0127	99221	1	G0127	99345	1
G0121	45303	0	G0127	99222	1	G0127	99347	1
G0121	45305	0	G0127	99223	1	G0127	99348	1
G0121	45307	0	G0127	99224	1	G0127	99349	1
G0121	45308	0	G0127	99225	1	G0127	99350	1
G0121	45309	0	G0127	99226	1	G0127	99354	1
G0121	45315	0	G0127	99231	1	G0127	99355	1
G0121	45317	0	G0127	99232	1	G0127	99356	1
G0121	45320	0	G0127	99233	1	G0127	99357	1
G0121	45321	0	G0127	99234	1	G0130	76977	0
G0121	45327	0	G0127	99235	1	G0130	77080	1
G0121	45330	0	G0127	99236	1	G0154	G0128	1
G0121	45331	0	G0127	99238	1	G0159	G0151	0
G0121	45332	0	G0127	99239	1	G0160	G0152	0
G0121	45333	0	G0127	99281	1	G0161	G0153	0
G0121	45334	0	G0127	99282	1	G0162	G0128	1
G0121	45335	0	G0127	99283	1	G0163	G0128	1
G0121	45337	0	G0127	99284	1	G0164	G0128	1
G0121	45338	0	G0127	99285	1	G0173	G0251	1
G0121	45339	0	G0127	99304	1	G0173	G0339	0
G0121	45340	0	G0127	99305	1	G0173	G0340	0
G0121	45341	0	G0127	99306	1	G0173	61304	1
G0121	45342	0	G0127	99307	1	G0173	61305	1
G0121	45345	0	G0127	99308	1	G0173	61312	1
G0121	45355	0	G0127	99309	1	G0173	61313	1
G0127	G0380	1	G0127	99310	1	G0173	61314	1
G0127	G0381	1	G0127	99315	1	G0173	61315	1
G0127	G0382	1	G0127	99316	1	G0173	61320	1
G0127	G0383	1	G0127	99318	1	G0173	61321	1
G0127	G0384	1	G0127	99324	1	G0173	61330	1
G0127	99203	1	G0127	99325	1	G0173	61332	1
G0127	99204	1	G0127	99326	1	G0173	61333	1
G0127	99205	1	G0127	99327	1	G0173	61440	1
G0127	99211	1	G0127	99328	1	G0173	61450	1
G0127	99212	1	G0127	99334	1	G0173	61458	1

Column 1	Column 2	Modifier 0=not allowed 1=allowed 9=not applicable
G0173	61460	1
G0173	61470	1
G0173	61480	1
G0173	61490	1
G0173	61500	1
G0173	61501	1
G0173	61510	1
G0173	61512	1
G0173	61514	1
G0173	61516	1
G0173	61518	1
G0173	61519	1
G0173	61520	1
G0173	61521	1
G0173	61522	1
G0173	61524	1
G0173	61526	1
G0173	61530	1
G0173	61563	1
G0173	61564	1
G0173	61720	1
G0173	61735	1
G0173	61790	1
G0173	61791	1
G0173	77371	1
G0173	77372	1
G0173	77373	1
G0173	77427	1
G0173	77431	1
G0173	77470	1
G0175	90804	1
G0175	90805	1
G0175	90806	1
G0175	90807	1
G0175	90808	1
G0175	90809	1
G0175	90810	1
G0175	90811	1
G0175	90812	1
G0175	90813	1
G0175	90814	1
G0175	90815	1

Column 1	Column 2	Modifier 0=not allowed 1=allowed 9=not applicable
G0175	90816	1
G0175	90817	1
G0175	90818	1
G0175	90819	1
G0175	90821	1
G0175	90822	1
G0175	90823	1
G0175	90824	1
G0175	90826	1
G0175	90827	1
G0175	90828	1
G0175	90829	1
G0175	90846	1
G0175	90847	1
G0179	G0180	0
G0181	G0182	1
G0186	67210	1
G0186	67228	1
G0251	G0339	0
G0251	G0340	0
G0251	20661	1
G0251	20693	1
G0251	20694	1
G0251	61304	1
G0251	61305	1
G0251	61312	1
G0251	61313	1
G0251	61314	1
G0251	61315	1
G0251	61320	1
G0251	61321	1
G0251	61330	1
G0251	61332	1
G0251	61333	1
G0251	61440	1
G0251	61450	1
G0251	61458	1
G0251	61460	1
G0251	61470	1
G0251	61480	1
G0251	61490	1
G0251	61500	1

Column 1	Column 2	Modifier 0=not allowed 1=allowed 9=not applicable
G0251	61510	1
G0251	61512	1
G0251	61514	1
G0251	61516	1
G0251	61518	1
G0251	61519	1
G0251	61520	1
G0251	61521	1
G0251	61522	1
G0251	61524	1
G0251	61530	1
G0251	61563	1
G0251	61564	1
G0251	61735	1
G0268	69210	0
G0270	G0271	0
G0281	G0283	1
G0281	G0329	0
G0328	82274	0
G0329	G0283	1
G0337	99201	1
G0337	99202	1
G0337	99203	1
G0337	99204	1
G0337	99205	1
G0337	99211	1
G0337	99212	1
G0337	99213	1
G0337	99214	1
G0337	99215	1
G0339	G0340	1
G0339	20661	1
G0339	20693	1
G0339	20694	1
G0339	61304	1
G0339	61305	1
G0339	61312	1
G0339	61313	1
G0339	61314	1
G0339	61315	1
G0339	61320	1
G0339	61321	1

Column 1	Column 2	Modifier 0=not allowed 1=allowed 9=not applicable
G0339	61330	1
G0339	61332	1
G0339	61333	1
G0339	61440	1
G0339	61450	1
G0339	61458	1
G0339	61460	1
G0339	61470	1
G0339	61480	1
G0339	61490	1
G0339	61500	1
G0339	61510	1
G0339	61512	1
G0339	61514	1
G0339	61516	1
G0339	61518	1
G0339	61519	1
G0339	61520	1
G0339	61521	1
G0339	61522	1
G0339	61524	1
G0339	61526	1
G0339	61530	1
G0339	61563	1
G0339	61564	1
G0339	61735	1
G0340	20661	1
G0340	20693	1
G0340	20694	1
G0340	61304	1
G0340	61305	1
G0340	61312	1
G0340	61313	1
G0340	61314	1
G0340	61315	1
G0340	61320	1
G0340	61321	1
G0340	61330	1
G0340	61332	1
G0340	61333	1
G0340	61440	1
G0340	61450	1

Column 1	Column 2	Modifier 0=not allowed 1=allowed 9=not applicable
G0340	61458	1
G0340	61460	1
G0340	61470	1
G0340	61480	1
G0340	61490	1
G0340	61500	1
G0340	61510	1
G0340	61512	1
G0340	61514	1
G0340	61516	1
G0340	61518	1
G0340	61519	1
G0340	61520	1
G0340	61521	1
G0340	61522	1
G0340	61524	1
G0340	61526	1
G0340	61530	1
G0340	61563	1
G0340	61564	1
G0340	61735	1
G0341	48554	0
G0342	48554	0
G0343	48554	0
G0365	76998	1
G0365	93971	1
G0380	99239	1
G0381	G0380	1
G0381	99239	1
G0382	G0380	1
G0382	G0381	1
G0382	99239	1
G0383	G0380	1
G0383	G0381	1
G0383	G0382	1
G0383	99463	1
G0384	G0380	1
G0384	G0381	1
G0384	G0382	1
G0384	G0383	1
G0384	99463	1
G0398	G0399	0

Column 1	Column 2	Modifier 0=not allowed 1=allowed 9=not applicable
G0398	G0400	0
G0399	G0400	0
G0402	G0380	1
G0402	G0381	1
G0402	G0382	1
G0402	G0383	1
G0402	G0384	1
G0402	99201	1
G0402	99202	1
G0402	99203	1
G0402	99204	1
G0402	99205	1
G0402	99211	1
G0402	99212	1
G0402	99213	1
G0402	99214	1
G0402	99215	1
G0402	99281	1
G0402	99282	1
G0402	99283	1
G0402	99284	1
G0402	99285	1
G0402	99304	1
G0402	99305	1
G0402	99306	1
G0402	99307	1
G0402	99308	1
G0402	99309	1
G0402	99310	1
G0402	99315	1
G0402	99316	1
G0402	99318	1
G0402	99324	1
G0402	99325	1
G0402	99326	1
G0402	99327	1
G0402	99328	1
G0402	99334	1
G0402	99335	1
G0402	99336	1
G0402	99337	1
G0402	99341	1

Column 1	Column 2	Modifier 0=not allowed 1=allowed 9=not applicable
G0402	99342	1
G0402	99343	1
G0402	99344	1
G0402	99345	1
G0402	99347	1
G0402	99348	1
G0402	99349	1
G0402	99350	1
G0403	93000	1
G0403	93005	1
G0403	93010	1
G0403	93040	1
G0403	93041	1
G0403	93042	1
G0404	93000	1
G0404	93005	1
G0404	93010	1
G0404	93040	1
G0404	93041	1
G0404	93042	1
G0405	93000	1
G0405	93005	1
G0405	93010	1
G0405	93040	1
G0405	93041	1
G0405	93042	1
G0409	G0155	1
G0409	G0176	1
G0409	G0177	1
G0409	90801	1
G0409	90802	1
G0409	90804	1
G0409	90805	1
G0409	90806	1
G0409	90807	1
G0409	90808	1
G0409	90809	1
G0409	90810	1
G0409	90811	1
G0409	90812	1
G0409	90813	1
G0409	90814	1

Column 1	Column 2	Modifier 0=not allowed 1=allowed 9=not applicable
G0409	90815	1
G0409	90816	1
G0409	90817	1
G0409	90818	1
G0409	90819	1
G0409	90821	1
G0409	90822	1
G0409	90823	1
G0409	90824	1
G0409	90826	1
G0409	90827	1
G0409	90828	1
G0409	90829	1
G0409	90845	1
G0409	90846	1
G0409	90847	1
G0409	90849	1
G0409	90853	1
G0409	90857	1
G0409	90862	1
G0409	90865	1
G0409	90870	1
G0409	90880	1
G0410	90804	1
G0410	90805	1
G0410	90806	1
G0410	90807	1
G0410	90808	1
G0410	90809	1
G0410	90810	1
G0410	90811	1
G0410	90812	1
G0410	90813	1
G0410	90814	1
G0410	90815	1
G0410	90870	1
G0411	90804	1
G0411	90805	1
G0411	90806	1
G0411	90807	1
G0411	90808	1
G0411	90809	1

Column 1	Column 2	Modifier 0=not allowed 1=allowed 9=not applicable
G0411	90810	1
G0411	90811	1
G0411	90812	1
G0411	90813	1
G0411	90814	1
G0411	90815	1
G0411	90870	1
G0422	93015	1
G0422	93016	0
G0422	93017	1
G0422	93018	1
G0422	93025	1
G0423	93015	1
G0423	93016	0
G0423	93017	1
G0423	93018	1
G0423	93025	1
G0424	G0237	1
G0424	G0238	1
G0424	G0239	1
G0424	G0422	1
G0424	G0423	1
G0424	93015	1
G0424	93016	0
G0424	93017	1
G0424	93018	1
G0424	93025	1
G0424	93797	1
G0424	93798	1
G0428	29882	1
G0428	29883	1
G0429	11950	1
G0429	11951	1
G0429	11952	1
G0429	11954	1
G0436	99406	0
G0436	99407	0
G0437	99406	0
G0437	99407	0
G0438	G0380	1
G0438	G0381	1
G0438	G0382	1

Column 1	Column 2	Modifier 0=not allowed 1=allowed 9=not applicable
G0438	G0383	1
G0438	G0384	1
G0438	99201	1
G0438	99202	1
G0438	99203	1
G0438	99204	1
G0438	99205	1
G0438	99211	1
G0438	99212	1
G0438	99213	1
G0438	99214	1
G0438	99215	1
G0438	99281	1
G0438	99282	1
G0438	99283	1
G0438	99284	1
G0438	99285	1
G0438	99304	1
G0438	99305	1
G0438	99306	1
G0438	99307	1
G0438	99308	1
G0438	99309	1
G0438	99310	1
G0438	99315	1
G0438	99316	1
G0438	99318	1
G0438	99324	1
G0438	99325	1
G0438	99326	1
G0438	99327	1
G0438	99328	1
G0438	99334	1
G0438	99335	1
G0438	99336	1
G0438	99337	1
G0438	99341	1
G0438	99342	1
G0438	99343	1
G0438	99344	1
G0438	99345	1
G0438	99347	1

Column 1	Column 2	Modifier 0=not allowed 1=allowed 9=not applicable
G0438	99348	1
G0438	99349	1
G0438	99350	1
G0439	G0380	1
G0439	G0381	1
G0439	G0382	1
G0439	G0383	1
G0439	G0384	1
G0439	99201	1
G0439	99202	1
G0439	99203	1
G0439	99204	1
G0439	99205	1
G0439	99211	1
G0439	99212	1
G0439	99213	1
G0439	99214	1
G0439	99215	1
G0439	99281	1
G0439	99282	1
G0439	99283	1
G0439	99284	1
G0439	99285	1
G0439	99304	1
G0439	99305	1
G0439	99306	1
G0439	99307	1
G0439	99308	1
G0439	99309	1
G0439	99310	1
G0439	99315	1
G0439	99316	1
G0439	99318	1
G0439	99324	1
G0439	99325	1
G0439	99326	1
G0439	99327	1
G0439	99328	1
G0439	99334	1
G0439	99335	1
G0439	99336	1
G0439	99337	1

Column 1	Column 2	Modifier 0=not allowed 1=allowed 9=not applicable
G0439	99341	1
G0439	99342	1
G0439	99343	1
G0439	99344	1
G0439	99345	1
G0439	99347	1
G0439	99348	1
G0439	99349	1
G0439	99350	1
G0440	15170	1
G0440	15171	1
G0440	15175	1
G0440	15176	1
G0440	15300	1
G0440	15301	1
G0440	15320	1
G0440	15321	1
G0440	15330	1
G0440	15331	1
G0440	15335	1
G0440	15336	1
G0440	15340	1
G0440	15341	1
G0440	15360	1
G0440	15361	1
G0440	15365	1
G0440	15366	1
G0441	15170	1
G0441	15171	1
G0441	15175	1
G0441	15176	1
G0441	15300	1
G0441	15301	1
G0441	15320	1
G0441	15321	1
G0441	15330	1
G0441	15331	1
G0441	15335	1
G0441	15336	1
G0441	15340	1
G0441	15341	1
G0441	15360	1

Column 1	Column 2	Modifier 0=not allowed 1=allowed 9=not applicable
G0441	15361	1
G0441	15365	1
G0441	15366	1
M0064	90862	1
P9011	P9010	1
P9011	P9021	0
P9011	P9022	0

Column 1	Column 2	Modifier 0=not allowed 1=allowed 9=not applicable
P9011	P9039	0
P9022	P9010	1
P9022	P9016	1
P9022	P9021	1
P9022	P9039	1
P9039	P9010	1
P9039	P9016	1

Column 1	Column 2	Modifier 0=not allowed 1=allowed 9=not applicable
P9039	P9021	1
P9603	P9604	1
P9612	P9615	0
Q1003	Q1004	1
Q1003	Q1005	1
Q1004	Q1005	1

Column 1/2 NCCI Edits
Hospital Outpatient Prospective Payment System (PPS)
(Effective Date: 10/01/11-12/31/11, Version: 17.2)
Codes in Column 1 are not reported with codes in Column 2 with 0 or 9

Column 1	Column 2	Modifier 0=not allowed 1=allowed 9=not applicable	Column 1	Column 2	Modifier 0=not allowed 1=allowed 9=not applicable	Column 1	Column 2	Modifier 0=not allowed 1=allowed 9=not applicable
A9500	A9512	1	C8900	96376	1	C8903	76998	1
A9501	A9512	0	C8901	36000	1	C8903	77001	1
A9502	A9512	0	C8901	36410	1	C8903	77002	1
A9503	A9512	0	C8901	76000	1	C8903	96360	1
A9504	A9512	0	C8901	76001	1	C8903	96365	1
A9510	A9512	0	C8901	76376	1	C8903	96372	1
A9521	A9512	0	C8901	76377	1	C8903	96374	1
A9536	A9512	0	C8901	76942	1	C8903	96375	1
A9537	A9512	0	C8901	76998	1	C8903	96376	1
A9538	A9512	0	C8901	77001	1	C8904	36000	1
A9539	A9512	0	C8901	77002	1	C8904	36410	1
A9540	A9512	1	C8901	96360	1	C8904	76000	1
A9541	A9512	1	C8901	96365	1	C8904	76001	1
A9550	A9512	0	C8901	96372	1	C8904	76942	1
A9551	A9512	0	C8901	96374	1	C8904	76998	1
A9557	A9512	0	C8901	96375	1	C8904	77001	1
A9560	A9512	0	C8901	96376	1	C8904	77002	1
A9561	A9512	0	C8902	36000	1	C8904	96360	1
A9562	A9512	0	C8902	36410	1	C8904	96365	1
A9566	A9512	0	C8902	76000	1	C8904	96372	1
A9567	A9512	0	C8902	76001	1	C8904	96374	1
A9568	A9512	0	C8902	76376	1	C8904	96375	1
A9569	A9512	0	C8902	76377	1	C8904	96376	1
C8900	36000	1	C8902	76942	1	C8905	36000	1
C8900	36410	1	C8902	76998	1	C8905	36410	1
C8900	76000	1	C8902	77001	1	C8905	76000	1
C8900	76001	1	C8902	77002	1	C8905	76001	1
C8900	76376	1	C8902	96360	1	C8905	76942	1
C8900	76377	1	C8902	96365	1	C8905	76998	1
C8900	76942	1	C8902	96372	1	C8905	77001	1
C8900	76998	1	C8902	96374	1	C8905	77002	1
C8900	77001	1	C8902	96375	1	C8905	96360	1
C8900	77002	1	C8902	96376	1	C8905	96365	1
C8900	96360	1	C8903	36000	1	C8905	96372	1
C8900	96365	1	C8903	36410	1	C8905	96374	1
C8900	96372	1	C8903	76000	1	C8905	96375	1
C8900	96374	1	C8903	76001	1	C8905	96376	1
C8900	96375	1	C8903	76942	1	C8906	C8903	1

Column 1	Column 2	Modifier 0=not allowed 1=allowed 9=not applicable
C8906	C8904	1
C8906	C8905	1
C8906	36000	1
C8906	36410	1
C8906	76000	1
C8906	76001	1
C8906	76942	1
C8906	76998	1
C8906	77001	1
C8906	77002	1
C8906	96360	1
C8906	96365	1
C8906	96372	1
C8906	96374	1
C8906	96375	1
C8906	96376	1
C8907	C8903	1
C8907	C8904	1
C8907	C8905	1
C8907	36000	1
C8907	36410	1
C8907	76000	1
C8907	76001	1
C8907	76942	1
C8907	76998	1
C8907	77001	1
C8907	77002	1
C8907	96360	1
C8907	96365	1
C8907	96372	1
C8907	96374	1
C8907	96375	1
C8907	96376	1
C8908	C8903	1
C8908	C8904	1
C8908	C8905	1
C8908	36000	1
C8908	36410	1
C8908	76000	1
C8908	76001	1
C8908	76942	1
C8908	76998	1

Column 1	Column 2	Modifier 0=not allowed 1=allowed 9=not applicable
C8908	77001	1
C8908	77002	1
C8908	96360	1
C8908	96365	1
C8908	96372	1
C8908	96374	1
C8908	96375	1
C8908	96376	1
C8909	36000	1
C8909	36410	1
C8909	76000	1
C8909	76001	1
C8909	76376	1
C8909	76377	1
C8909	76942	1
C8909	76998	1
C8909	77001	1
C8909	77002	1
C8909	96360	1
C8909	96365	1
C8909	96372	1
C8909	96374	1
C8909	96375	1
C8909	96376	1
C8910	36000	1
C8910	36410	1
C8910	76000	1
C8910	76001	1
C8910	76376	1
C8910	76377	1
C8910	76942	1
C8910	76998	1
C8910	77001	1
C8910	77002	1
C8910	96360	1
C8910	96365	1
C8910	96372	1
C8910	96374	1
C8910	96375	1
C8910	96376	1
C8911	36000	1
C8911	36410	1

Column 1	Column 2	Modifier 0=not allowed 1=allowed 9=not applicable
C8911	76000	1
C8911	76001	1
C8911	76376	1
C8911	76377	1
C8911	76942	1
C8911	76998	1
C8911	77001	1
C8911	77002	1
C8911	96360	1
C8911	96365	1
C8911	96372	1
C8911	96374	1
C8911	96375	1
C8911	96376	1
C8912	36000	1
C8912	36410	1
C8912	76000	1
C8912	76001	1
C8912	76376	1
C8912	76377	1
C8912	76942	1
C8912	76998	1
C8912	77001	1
C8912	77002	1
C8912	96360	1
C8912	96365	1
C8912	96372	1
C8912	96374	1
C8912	96375	1
C8912	96376	1
C8913	36000	1
C8913	36410	1
C8913	76000	1
C8913	76001	1
C8913	76376	1
C8913	76377	1
C8913	76942	1
C8913	76998	1
C8913	77001	1
C8913	77002	1
C8913	96360	1
C8913	96365	1

Column 1	Column 2	Modifier 0=not allowed 1=allowed 9=not applicable
C8913	96372	1
C8913	96374	1
C8913	96375	1
C8913	96376	1
C8914	36000	1
C8914	36410	1
C8914	76000	1
C8914	76001	1
C8914	76376	1
C8914	76377	1
C8914	76942	1
C8914	76998	1
C8914	77001	1
C8914	77002	1
C8914	96360	1
C8914	96365	1
C8914	96372	1
C8914	96374	1
C8914	96375	1
C8914	96376	1
C8918	36000	1
C8918	36410	1
C8918	76000	1
C8918	76376	1
C8918	76377	1
C8918	76942	1
C8918	76998	1
C8918	77001	1
C8918	77002	1
C8918	96372	1
C8918	96374	1
C8918	96375	1
C8918	96376	1
C8919	36000	1
C8919	36410	1
C8919	76000	1
C8919	76001	1
C8919	76376	1
C8919	76377	1
C8919	76942	1
C8919	76998	1
C8919	77001	1

Column 1	Column 2	Modifier 0=not allowed 1=allowed 9=not applicable
C8919	77002	1
C8919	96372	1
C8919	96374	1
C8919	96375	1
C8919	96376	1
C8920	36000	1
C8920	36410	1
C8920	76000	1
C8920	76001	1
C8920	76376	1
C8920	76377	1
C8920	76942	1
C8920	76998	1
C8920	77001	1
C8920	77002	1
C8920	96372	1
C8920	96374	1
C8920	96375	1
C8920	96376	1
C8921	C8922	1
C8921	36000	1
C8921	36005	1
C8921	36410	1
C8921	76998	1
C8921	93040	1
C8921	93041	1
C8921	93042	1
C8921	93303	0
C8921	93304	1
C8921	96360	1
C8921	96365	1
C8921	96372	1
C8921	96374	1
C8921	96375	1
C8921	96376	1
C8922	36000	1
C8922	36005	1
C8922	36410	1
C8922	76998	1
C8922	93040	1
C8922	93041	1
C8922	93042	1

Column 1	Column 2	Modifier 0=not allowed 1=allowed 9=not applicable
C8922	93304	1
C8922	96360	1
C8922	96365	1
C8922	96372	1
C8922	96374	1
C8922	96375	1
C8922	96376	1
C8923	C8924	1
C8923	C8929	0
C8923	36000	1
C8923	36005	1
C8923	36410	1
C8923	76998	1
C8923	93040	1
C8923	93041	1
C8923	93042	1
C8923	93306	0
C8923	93307	0
C8923	93308	1
C8923	96360	1
C8923	96365	1
C8923	96372	1
C8923	96374	1
C8923	96375	1
C8923	96376	1
C8924	36000	1
C8924	36005	1
C8924	36410	1
C8924	76998	1
C8924	93040	1
C8924	93041	1
C8924	93042	1
C8924	93308	1
C8924	96360	1
C8924	96365	1
C8924	96372	1
C8924	96374	1
C8924	96375	1
C8924	96376	1
C8925	36000	1
C8925	36005	1
C8925	36410	1

Column 1	Column 2	Modifier 0=not allowed 1=allowed 9=not applicable
C8925	76998	1
C8925	93040	1
C8925	93041	1
C8925	93042	1
C8925	93312	0
C8925	93313	0
C8925	93314	0
C8925	96360	1
C8925	96365	1
C8925	96372	1
C8925	96374	1
C8925	96375	1
C8925	96376	1
C8926	36000	1
C8926	36005	1
C8926	36410	1
C8926	76998	1
C8926	93040	1
C8926	93041	1
C8926	93042	1
C8926	93315	0
C8926	93316	0
C8926	93317	0
C8926	96360	1
C8926	96365	1
C8926	96372	1
C8926	96374	1
C8926	96375	1
C8926	96376	1
C8927	36000	1
C8927	36005	1
C8927	36410	1
C8927	76998	1
C8927	93040	1
C8927	93041	1
C8927	93042	1
C8927	93318	0
C8927	96360	1
C8927	96365	1
C8927	96372	1
C8927	96374	1
C8927	96375	1

Column 1	Column 2	Modifier 0=not allowed 1=allowed 9=not applicable
C8927	96376	1
C8928	C8930	0
C8928	36000	1
C8928	36005	1
C8928	36410	1
C8928	76998	1
C8928	93040	1
C8928	93041	1
C8928	93042	1
C8928	93350	0
C8928	93351	0
C8928	94761	0
C8928	96360	1
C8928	96365	1
C8928	96372	1
C8928	96374	1
C8928	96375	1
C8928	96376	1
C8929	C8924	1
C8929	36000	1
C8929	36005	1
C8929	36410	1
C8929	76604	1
C8929	76998	1
C8929	93040	1
C8929	93041	1
C8929	93042	1
C8929	93304	1
C8929	93307	0
C8929	93308	1
C8929	93320	0
C8929	93321	0
C8929	93325	0
C8929	96360	1
C8929	96365	1
C8929	96372	1
C8929	96374	1
C8929	96375	1
C8929	96376	1
C8930	C8929	1
C8930	36000	1
C8930	36005	1

Column 1	Column 2	Modifier 0=not allowed 1=allowed 9=not applicable
C8930	36410	1
C8930	76998	1
C8930	93000	1
C8930	93005	1
C8930	93010	1
C8930	93015	0
C8930	93016	0
C8930	93017	0
C8930	93018	0
C8930	93040	1
C8930	93041	1
C8930	93042	1
C8930	93306	1
C8930	93308	1
C8930	93350	0
C8930	93351	0
C8930	94620	1
C8930	94621	0
C8930	94760	0
C8930	94761	0
C8930	96360	1
C8930	96365	1
C8930	96372	1
C8930	96374	1
C8930	96375	1
C8930	96376	1
C8931	C8932	0
C8931	36000	1
C8931	36005	1
C8931	36410	1
C8931	72141	1
C8931	72142	1
C8931	72146	1
C8931	72147	1
C8931	72148	1
C8931	72149	1
C8931	72156	1
C8931	72157	1
C8931	72158	1
C8931	76000	1
C8931	76001	1
C8931	76376	0

Column 1	Column 2	Modifier 0=not allowed 1=allowed 9=not applicable
C8931	76377	0
C8931	76942	1
C8931	76998	1
C8931	77002	1
C8931	96360	1
C8931	96365	1
C8931	96372	1
C8931	96374	1
C8931	96375	1
C8931	96376	1
C8932	36000	1
C8932	36005	1
C8932	36410	1
C8932	72141	1
C8932	72142	1
C8932	72146	1
C8932	72147	1
C8932	72148	1
C8932	72149	1
C8932	72156	1
C8932	72157	1
C8932	72158	1
C8932	76000	1
C8932	76001	1
C8932	76376	0
C8932	76377	0
C8932	76942	1
C8932	76998	1
C8932	77002	1
C8932	96360	1
C8932	96365	1
C8932	96372	1
C8932	96374	1
C8932	96375	1
C8932	96376	1
C8933	C8931	0
C8933	C8932	0
C8933	36000	1
C8933	36005	1
C8933	36410	1
C8933	72141	1
C8933	72142	1

Column 1	Column 2	Modifier 0=not allowed 1=allowed 9=not applicable
C8933	72146	1
C8933	72147	1
C8933	72148	1
C8933	72149	1
C8933	72156	1
C8933	72157	1
C8933	72158	1
C8933	76000	1
C8933	76001	1
C8933	76376	0
C8933	76377	0
C8933	76942	1
C8933	76998	1
C8933	77002	1
C8933	96360	1
C8933	96365	1
C8933	96372	1
C8933	96374	1
C8933	96375	1
C8933	96376	1
C8934	C8935	0
C8934	36000	1
C8934	36005	1
C8934	36410	1
C8934	73218	1
C8934	73219	1
C8934	73220	1
C8934	73221	1
C8934	73222	1
C8934	73223	1
C8934	76000	1
C8934	76001	1
C8934	76376	0
C8934	76377	0
C8934	76942	1
C8934	76998	1
C8934	77002	1
C8934	96360	1
C8934	96365	1
C8934	96372	1
C8934	96374	1
C8934	96375	1

Column 1	Column 2	Modifier 0=not allowed 1=allowed 9=not applicable
C8934	96376	1
C8935	36000	1
C8935	36005	1
C8935	36410	1
C8935	73218	1
C8935	73219	1
C8935	73220	1
C8935	73221	1
C8935	73222	1
C8935	73223	1
C8935	76000	1
C8935	76001	1
C8935	76376	0
C8935	76377	0
C8935	76942	1
C8935	76998	1
C8935	77002	1
C8935	96360	1
C8935	96365	1
C8935	96372	1
C8935	96374	1
C8935	96375	1
C8935	96376	1
C8936	C8934	0
C8936	C8935	0
C8936	36000	1
C8936	36005	1
C8936	36410	1
C8936	73218	1
C8936	73219	1
C8936	73220	1
C8936	73221	1
C8936	73222	1
C8936	73223	1
C8936	76000	1
C8936	76001	1
C8936	76376	0
C8936	76377	0
C8936	76942	1
C8936	76998	1
C8936	77002	1
C8936	96360	1

Column 1	Column 2	Modifier 0=not allowed 1=allowed 9=not applicable
C8936	96365	1
C8936	96372	1
C8936	96374	1
C8936	96375	1
C8936	96376	1
C8957	36000	1
C8957	36410	1
C8957	64450	1
C8957	96360	1
C8957	96365	1
C8957	96372	1
C8957	96374	1
C8957	96521	0
C8957	96522	0
C8957	96523	0
C8957	99201	1
C8957	99202	1
C8957	99203	1
C8957	99204	1
C8957	99205	1
C8957	99211	1
C8957	99212	1
C8957	99213	1
C8957	99214	1
C8957	99215	1
C9273	G0380	1
C9273	G0381	1
C9273	G0382	1
C9273	G0383	1
C9273	G0384	1
C9273	0213T	1
C9273	0216T	1
C9273	0228T	1
C9273	0230T	1
C9273	36000	1
C9273	36400	1
C9273	36405	1
C9273	36406	1
C9273	36410	1
C9273	36420	1
C9273	36425	1
C9273	36430	1

Column 1	Column 2	Modifier 0=not allowed 1=allowed 9=not applicable
C9273	36440	1
C9273	36600	1
C9273	36640	1
C9273	37202	1
C9273	38206	0
C9273	38210	0
C9273	38211	0
C9273	38212	0
C9273	38213	0
C9273	38214	0
C9273	38215	0
C9273	38241	0
C9273	43752	1
C9273	51701	1
C9273	51702	1
C9273	51703	1
C9273	62310	1
C9273	62311	1
C9273	62318	1
C9273	62319	1
C9273	64400	1
C9273	64402	1
C9273	64405	1
C9273	64408	1
C9273	64410	1
C9273	64412	1
C9273	64413	1
C9273	64415	1
C9273	64416	1
C9273	64417	1
C9273	64418	1
C9273	64420	1
C9273	64421	1
C9273	64425	1
C9273	64430	1
C9273	64435	1
C9273	64445	1
C9273	64446	1
C9273	64447	1
C9273	64448	1
C9273	64449	1
C9273	64450	1

Column 1	Column 2	Modifier 0=not allowed 1=allowed 9=not applicable
C9273	64479	1
C9273	64483	1
C9273	64490	1
C9273	64493	1
C9273	64505	1
C9273	64508	1
C9273	64510	1
C9273	64517	1
C9273	64520	1
C9273	64530	1
C9273	69990	0
C9273	93000	1
C9273	93005	1
C9273	93010	1
C9273	93040	1
C9273	93041	1
C9273	93042	1
C9273	93318	1
C9273	94002	1
C9273	94200	1
C9273	94250	1
C9273	94680	1
C9273	94681	1
C9273	94690	1
C9273	94770	1
C9273	95812	1
C9273	95813	1
C9273	95816	1
C9273	95819	1
C9273	95822	1
C9273	95829	1
C9273	95955	1
C9273	96360	1
C9273	96365	1
C9273	96372	1
C9273	96374	1
C9273	96375	1
C9273	96376	1
C9273	99148	1
C9273	99149	1
C9273	99150	1
C9273	99201	1

Column 1	Column 2	Modifier 0=not allowed 1=allowed 9=not applicable
C9273	99202	1
C9273	99203	1
C9273	99204	1
C9273	99205	1
C9273	99211	1
C9273	99212	1
C9273	99213	1
C9273	99214	1
C9273	99215	1
C9273	99217	1
C9273	99218	1
C9273	99219	1
C9273	99220	1
C9273	99224	1
C9273	99225	1
C9273	99226	1
C9273	99231	1
C9273	99232	1
C9273	99233	1
C9273	99234	1
C9273	99235	1
C9273	99236	1
C9273	99281	1
C9273	99282	1
C9273	99283	1
C9273	99284	1
C9273	99285	1
C9273	99291	1
C9273	99292	1
C9273	99304	1
C9273	99305	1
C9273	99306	1
C9273	99307	1
C9273	99308	1
C9273	99309	1
C9273	99310	1
C9273	99315	1
C9273	99316	1
C9273	99318	1
C9273	99324	1
C9273	99325	1
C9273	99326	1

Column 1	Column 2	Modifier 0=not allowed 1=allowed 9=not applicable
C9273	99327	1
C9273	99328	1
C9273	99334	1
C9273	99335	1
C9273	99336	1
C9273	99337	1
C9273	99341	1
C9273	99342	1
C9273	99343	1
C9273	99344	1
C9273	99345	1
C9273	99347	1
C9273	99348	1
C9273	99349	1
C9273	99350	1
C9273	99466	1
C9273	99468	1
C9273	99469	1
C9273	99471	1
C9273	99472	1
C9273	99475	1
C9273	99476	1
C9273	99477	1
C9273	99478	1
C9273	99479	1
C9273	99480	1
C9716	0213T	1
C9716	0216T	1
C9716	0226T	0
C9716	36000	1
C9716	36410	1
C9716	37202	1
C9716	43752	1
C9716	45900	0
C9716	45905	0
C9716	45910	0
C9716	45915	0
C9716	45990	0
C9716	46040	0
C9716	46080	0
C9716	46220	0
C9716	46600	0

Column 1	Column 2	Modifier 0=not allowed 1=allowed 9=not applicable
C9716	46940	0
C9716	46942	0
C9716	62318	1
C9716	62319	1
C9716	64415	1
C9716	64416	1
C9716	64417	1
C9716	64450	1
C9716	64490	1
C9716	64493	1
C9716	96360	1
C9716	96365	1
C9716	96372	1
C9716	96374	1
C9716	96375	1
C9716	96376	1
C9724	0213T	1
C9724	0216T	1
C9724	31505	0
C9724	31525	0
C9724	31575	0
C9724	36000	1
C9724	36410	1
C9724	37202	1
C9724	43200	0
C9724	43201	0
C9724	43202	0
C9724	43204	0
C9724	43205	0
C9724	43215	0
C9724	43216	0
C9724	43217	0
C9724	43219	0
C9724	43220	0
C9724	43226	0
C9724	43227	0
C9724	43228	0
C9724	43231	0
C9724	43232	0
C9724	43234	0
C9724	43235	0
C9724	43255	1

Column 1	Column 2	Modifier 0=not allowed 1=allowed 9=not applicable
C9724	43752	1
C9724	43753	1
C9724	43754	0
C9724	62318	1
C9724	62319	1
C9724	64415	1
C9724	64416	1
C9724	64417	1
C9724	64450	1
C9724	64490	1
C9724	64493	1
C9724	92511	0
C9724	94760	0
C9724	94761	0
C9724	96360	1
C9724	96365	1
C9724	96372	1
C9724	96374	1
C9724	96375	1
C9724	96376	1
C9725	0213T	1
C9725	0216T	1
C9725	0226T	0
C9725	36000	1
C9725	36410	1
C9725	37202	1
C9725	43752	1
C9725	45900	0
C9725	45905	0
C9725	45910	0
C9725	45915	0
C9725	45990	0
C9725	46040	0
C9725	46080	0
C9725	46220	0
C9725	46600	0
C9725	46940	0
C9725	46942	0
C9725	62318	1
C9725	62319	1
C9725	64415	1
C9725	64416	1

Column 1	Column 2	Modifier 0=not allowed 1=allowed 9=not applicable
C9725	64417	1
C9725	64450	1
C9725	64490	1
C9725	64493	1
C9725	96360	1
C9725	96365	1
C9725	96372	1
C9725	96374	1
C9725	96375	1
C9725	96376	1
C9800	Q2026	0
C9800	Q2027	0
C9800	0213T	1
C9800	0216T	1
C9800	0228T	1
C9800	0230T	1
C9800	36000	1
C9800	36400	1
C9800	36405	1
C9800	36406	1
C9800	36410	1
C9800	36420	1
C9800	36425	1
C9800	36430	1
C9800	36440	1
C9800	36600	1
C9800	36640	1
C9800	37202	1
C9800	43752	1
C9800	51701	1
C9800	51702	1
C9800	51703	1
C9800	62310	1
C9800	62311	1
C9800	62318	1
C9800	62319	1
C9800	64400	1
C9800	64402	1
C9800	64405	1
C9800	64408	1
C9800	64410	1
C9800	64412	1

Column 1	Column 2	Modifier 0=not allowed 1=allowed 9=not applicable
C9800	64413	1
C9800	64415	1
C9800	64416	1
C9800	64417	1
C9800	64418	1
C9800	64420	1
C9800	64421	1
C9800	64425	1
C9800	64430	1
C9800	64435	1
C9800	64445	1
C9800	64446	1
C9800	64447	1
C9800	64448	1
C9800	64449	1
C9800	64450	1
C9800	64479	1
C9800	64483	1
C9800	64490	1
C9800	64493	1
C9800	64505	1
C9800	64508	1
C9800	64510	1
C9800	64517	1
C9800	64520	1
C9800	64530	1
C9800	69990	0
C9800	93000	1
C9800	93005	1
C9800	93010	1
C9800	93040	1
C9800	93041	1
C9800	93042	1
C9800	93318	1
C9800	94002	1
C9800	94200	1
C9800	94250	1
C9800	94680	1
C9800	94681	1
C9800	94690	1
C9800	94770	1
C9800	95812	1

Column 1	Column 2	Modifier 0=not allowed 1=allowed 9=not applicable	Column 1	Column 2	Modifier 0=not allowed 1=allowed 9=not applicable	Column 1	Column 2	Modifier 0=not allowed 1=allowed 9=not applicable
C9800	95813	1	G0101	99221	1	G0101	99343	1
C9800	95816	1	G0101	99222	1	G0101	99344	1
C9800	95819	1	G0101	99223	1	G0101	99345	1
C9800	95822	1	G0101	99224	1	G0101	99347	1
C9800	95829	1	G0101	99225	1	G0101	99348	1
C9800	95955	1	G0101	99226	1	G0101	99349	1
C9800	96360	1	G0101	99231	1	G0101	99350	1
C9800	96365	1	G0101	99232	1	G0101	99354	1
C9800	96372	1	G0101	99233	1	G0101	99355	1
C9800	96374	1	G0101	99234	1	G0101	99356	1
C9800	96375	1	G0101	99235	1	G0101	99357	1
C9800	96376	1	G0101	99236	1	G0101	99360	1
C9800	99148	1	G0101	99238	1	G0101	99455	1
C9800	99149	1	G0101	99239	1	G0101	99456	1
C9800	99150	1	G0101	99281	1	G0101	99460	1
G0008	99211	1	G0101	99282	1	G0101	99461	1
G0009	99211	1	G0101	99283	1	G0101	99462	1
G0010	99211	1	G0101	99284	1	G0101	99463	1
G0027	80500	1	G0101	99285	1	G0101	99464	1
G0027	80502	1	G0101	99291	1	G0101	99465	1
G0027	89321	0	G0101	99292	1	G0101	99466	1
G0101	G0181	1	G0101	99304	1	G0101	99468	1
G0101	G0182	1	G0101	99305	1	G0101	99469	1
G0101	G0380	1	G0101	99306	1	G0101	99471	1
G0101	G0381	1	G0101	99307	1	G0101	99472	1
G0101	G0382	1	G0101	99308	1	G0101	99475	1
G0101	G0383	1	G0101	99309	1	G0101	99476	1
G0101	G0384	1	G0101	99310	1	G0101	99477	1
G0101	99201	1	G0101	99315	1	G0101	99478	1
G0101	99202	1	G0101	99316	1	G0101	99479	1
G0101	99203	1	G0101	99318	1	G0101	99480	1
G0101	99204	1	G0101	99324	1	G0102	99463	1
G0101	99205	1	G0101	99325	1	G0104	G0181	1
G0101	99211	1	G0101	99326	1	G0104	G0182	1
G0101	99212	1	G0101	99327	1	G0104	G0380	1
G0101	99213	1	G0101	99328	1	G0104	G0381	1
G0101	99214	1	G0101	99334	1	G0104	G0382	1
G0101	99215	1	G0101	99335	1	G0104	G0383	1
G0101	99217	1	G0101	99336	1	G0104	G0384	1
G0101	99218	1	G0101	99337	1	G0104	0213T	1
G0101	99219	1	G0101	99341	1	G0104	0216T	1
G0101	99220	1	G0101	99342	1	G0104	0228T	1

Column 1	Column 2	Modifier 0=not allowed 1=allowed 9=not applicable	Column 1	Column 2	Modifier 0=not allowed 1=allowed 9=not applicable	Column 1	Column 2	Modifier 0=not allowed 1=allowed 9=not applicable
G0104	0230T	1	G0104	64450	1	G0104	99202	1
G0104	36000	1	G0104	64479	1	G0104	99203	1
G0104	36400	1	G0104	64483	1	G0104	99204	1
G0104	36405	1	G0104	64490	1	G0104	99205	1
G0104	36406	1	G0104	64493	1	G0104	99211	1
G0104	36410	1	G0104	64505	1	G0104	99212	1
G0104	36420	1	G0104	64508	1	G0104	99213	1
G0104	36425	1	G0104	64510	1	G0104	99214	1
G0104	36430	1	G0104	64517	1	G0104	99215	1
G0104	36440	1	G0104	64520	1	G0104	99217	1
G0104	36600	1	G0104	64530	1	G0104	99218	1
G0104	36640	1	G0104	93000	1	G0104	99219	1
G0104	37202	1	G0104	93005	1	G0104	99220	1
G0104	43752	1	G0104	93010	1	G0104	99221	1
G0104	51701	1	G0104	93040	1	G0104	99222	1
G0104	51702	1	G0104	93041	1	G0104	99223	1
G0104	51703	1	G0104	93042	1	G0104	99224	1
G0104	62310	1	G0104	93318	1	G0104	99225	1
G0104	62311	1	G0104	94002	1	G0104	99226	1
G0104	62318	1	G0104	94200	1	G0104	99231	1
G0104	62319	1	G0104	94250	1	G0104	99232	1
G0104	64400	1	G0104	94680	1	G0104	99233	1
G0104	64402	1	G0104	94681	1	G0104	99234	1
G0104	64405	1	G0104	94690	1	G0104	99235	1
G0104	64408	1	G0104	94770	1	G0104	99236	1
G0104	64410	1	G0104	95812	1	G0104	99238	1
G0104	64412	1	G0104	95813	1	G0104	99239	1
G0104	64413	1	G0104	95816	1	G0104	99281	1
G0104	64415	1	G0104	95819	1	G0104	99282	1
G0104	64416	1	G0104	95822	1	G0104	99283	1
G0104	64417	1	G0104	95829	1	G0104	99284	1
G0104	64418	1	G0104	95955	1	G0104	99285	1
G0104	64420	1	G0104	96360	1	G0104	99291	1
G0104	64421	1	G0104	96365	1	G0104	99292	1
G0104	64425	1	G0104	96372	1	G0104	99304	1
G0104	64430	1	G0104	96374	1	G0104	99305	1
G0104	64435	1	G0104	96375	1	G0104	99306	1
G0104	64445	1	G0104	96376	1	G0104	99307	1
G0104	64446	1	G0104	99148	1	G0104	99308	1
G0104	64447	1	G0104	99149	1	G0104	99309	1
G0104	64448	1	G0104	99150	1	G0104	99310	1
G0104	64449	1	G0104	99201	1	G0104	99315	1

Column 1	Column 2	Modifier 0=not allowed 1=allowed 9=not applicable
G0104	99316	1
G0104	99318	1
G0104	99324	1
G0104	99325	1
G0104	99326	1
G0104	99327	1
G0104	99328	1
G0104	99334	1
G0104	99335	1
G0104	99336	1
G0104	99337	1
G0104	99341	1
G0104	99342	1
G0104	99343	1
G0104	99344	1
G0104	99345	1
G0104	99347	1
G0104	99348	1
G0104	99349	1
G0104	99350	1
G0104	99354	1
G0104	99355	1
G0104	99356	1
G0104	99357	1
G0104	99360	1
G0104	99455	1
G0104	99456	1
G0104	99460	1
G0104	99461	1
G0104	99462	1
G0104	99463	1
G0104	99464	1
G0104	99465	1
G0104	99466	1
G0104	99468	1
G0104	99469	1
G0104	99471	1
G0104	99472	1
G0104	99475	1
G0104	99476	1
G0104	99477	1
G0104	99478	1

Column 1	Column 2	Modifier 0=not allowed 1=allowed 9=not applicable
G0104	99479	1
G0104	99480	1
G0105	G0181	1
G0105	G0182	1
G0105	G0380	1
G0105	G0381	1
G0105	G0382	1
G0105	G0383	1
G0105	G0384	1
G0105	0213T	1
G0105	0216T	1
G0105	0228T	1
G0105	0230T	1
G0105	36000	1
G0105	36400	1
G0105	36405	1
G0105	36406	1
G0105	36410	1
G0105	36420	1
G0105	36425	1
G0105	36430	1
G0105	36440	1
G0105	36600	1
G0105	36640	1
G0105	37202	1
G0105	43752	1
G0105	51701	1
G0105	51702	1
G0105	51703	1
G0105	62310	1
G0105	62311	1
G0105	62318	1
G0105	62319	1
G0105	64400	1
G0105	64402	1
G0105	64405	1
G0105	64408	1
G0105	64410	1
G0105	64412	1
G0105	64413	1
G0105	64415	1
G0105	64416	1

Column 1	Column 2	Modifier 0=not allowed 1=allowed 9=not applicable
G0105	64417	1
G0105	64418	1
G0105	64420	1
G0105	64421	1
G0105	64425	1
G0105	64430	1
G0105	64435	1
G0105	64445	1
G0105	64446	1
G0105	64447	1
G0105	64448	1
G0105	64449	1
G0105	64450	1
G0105	64479	1
G0105	64483	1
G0105	64490	1
G0105	64493	1
G0105	64505	1
G0105	64508	1
G0105	64510	1
G0105	64517	1
G0105	64520	1
G0105	64530	1
G0105	93000	1
G0105	93005	1
G0105	93010	1
G0105	93040	1
G0105	93041	1
G0105	93042	1
G0105	93318	1
G0105	94002	1
G0105	94200	1
G0105	94250	1
G0105	94680	1
G0105	94681	1
G0105	94690	1
G0105	94770	1
G0105	95812	1
G0105	95813	1
G0105	95816	1
G0105	95819	1
G0105	95822	1

Column 1	Column 2	Modifier 0=not allowed 1=allowed 9=not applicable	Column 1	Column 2	Modifier 0=not allowed 1=allowed 9=not applicable	Column 1	Column 2	Modifier 0=not allowed 1=allowed 9=not applicable
G0105	95829	1	G0105	99284	1	G0105	99463	1
G0105	95955	1	G0105	99285	1	G0105	99464	1
G0105	96360	1	G0105	99291	1	G0105	99465	1
G0105	96365	1	G0105	99292	1	G0105	99466	1
G0105	96372	1	G0105	99304	1	G0105	99468	1
G0105	96374	1	G0105	99305	1	G0105	99469	1
G0105	96375	1	G0105	99306	1	G0105	99471	1
G0105	96376	1	G0105	99307	1	G0105	99472	1
G0105	99148	1	G0105	99308	1	G0105	99475	1
G0105	99149	1	G0105	99309	1	G0105	99476	1
G0105	99150	1	G0105	99310	1	G0105	99477	1
G0105	99201	1	G0105	99315	1	G0105	99478	1
G0105	99202	1	G0105	99316	1	G0105	99479	1
G0105	99203	1	G0105	99318	1	G0105	99480	1
G0105	99204	1	G0105	99324	1	G0106	G0181	1
G0105	99205	1	G0105	99325	1	G0106	G0182	1
G0105	99211	1	G0105	99326	1	G0106	G0380	1
G0105	99212	1	G0105	99327	1	G0106	G0381	1
G0105	99213	1	G0105	99328	1	G0106	G0382	1
G0105	99214	1	G0105	99334	1	G0106	G0383	1
G0105	99215	1	G0105	99335	1	G0106	G0384	1
G0105	99217	1	G0105	99336	1	G0106	74010	1
G0105	99218	1	G0105	99337	1	G0106	76000	1
G0105	99219	1	G0105	99341	1	G0106	76001	1
G0105	99220	1	G0105	99342	1	G0106	77001	1
G0105	99221	1	G0105	99343	1	G0106	99201	1
G0105	99222	1	G0105	99344	1	G0106	99202	1
G0105	99223	1	G0105	99345	1	G0106	99203	1
G0105	99224	1	G0105	99347	1	G0106	99204	1
G0105	99225	1	G0105	99348	1	G0106	99205	1
G0105	99226	1	G0105	99349	1	G0106	99211	1
G0105	99231	1	G0105	99350	1	G0106	99212	1
G0105	99232	1	G0105	99354	1	G0106	99213	1
G0105	99233	1	G0105	99355	1	G0106	99214	1
G0105	99234	1	G0105	99356	1	G0106	99215	1
G0105	99235	1	G0105	99357	1	G0106	99217	1
G0105	99236	1	G0105	99360	1	G0106	99218	1
G0105	99238	1	G0105	99455	1	G0106	99219	1
G0105	99239	1	G0105	99456	1	G0106	99220	1
G0105	99281	1	G0105	99460	1	G0106	99221	1
G0105	99282	1	G0105	99461	1	G0106	99222	1
G0105	99283	1	G0105	99462	1	G0106	99223	1

Column 1	Column 2	Modifier 0=not allowed 1=allowed 9=not applicable
G0106	99224	1
G0106	99225	1
G0106	99226	1
G0106	99231	1
G0106	99232	1
G0106	99233	1
G0106	99234	1
G0106	99235	1
G0106	99236	1
G0106	99238	1
G0106	99239	1
G0106	99281	1
G0106	99282	1
G0106	99283	1
G0106	99284	1
G0106	99285	1
G0106	99291	1
G0106	99292	1
G0106	99304	1
G0106	99305	1
G0106	99306	1
G0106	99307	1
G0106	99308	1
G0106	99309	1
G0106	99310	1
G0106	99315	1
G0106	99316	1
G0106	99318	1
G0106	99324	1
G0106	99325	1
G0106	99326	1
G0106	99327	1
G0106	99328	1
G0106	99334	1
G0106	99335	1
G0106	99336	1
G0106	99337	1
G0106	99341	1
G0106	99342	1
G0106	99343	1
G0106	99344	1
G0106	99345	1

Column 1	Column 2	Modifier 0=not allowed 1=allowed 9=not applicable
G0106	99347	1
G0106	99348	1
G0106	99350	1
G0106	99354	1
G0106	99355	1
G0106	99356	1
G0106	99357	1
G0106	99360	1
G0106	99455	1
G0106	99456	1
G0106	99460	1
G0106	99461	1
G0106	99462	1
G0106	99463	1
G0106	99464	1
G0106	99465	1
G0106	99466	1
G0106	99468	1
G0106	99469	1
G0106	99471	1
G0106	99472	1
G0106	99475	1
G0106	99476	1
G0106	99477	1
G0106	99478	1
G0106	99479	1
G0106	99480	1
G0108	G0270	0
G0108	G0271	0
G0108	97802	0
G0108	97803	0
G0108	97804	0
G0109	G0270	0
G0109	G0271	0
G0109	97802	0
G0109	97803	0
G0109	97804	0
G0117	G0118	0
G0120	G0181	1
G0120	G0182	1
G0120	G0380	1
G0120	G0381	1

Column 1	Column 2	Modifier 0=not allowed 1=allowed 9=not applicable
G0120	G0382	1
G0120	G0383	1
G0120	G0384	1
G0120	76000	1
G0120	76001	1
G0120	77001	1
G0120	99201	1
G0120	99202	1
G0120	99203	1
G0120	99204	1
G0120	99205	1
G0120	99211	1
G0120	99212	1
G0120	99213	1
G0120	99214	1
G0120	99215	1
G0120	99217	1
G0120	99218	1
G0120	99219	1
G0120	99220	1
G0120	99221	1
G0120	99222	1
G0120	99223	1
G0120	99224	1
G0120	99225	1
G0120	99226	1
G0120	99231	1
G0120	99232	1
G0120	99233	1
G0120	99234	1
G0120	99235	1
G0120	99236	1
G0120	99238	1
G0120	99239	1
G0120	99281	1
G0120	99282	1
G0120	99283	1
G0120	99284	1
G0120	99285	1
G0120	99291	1
G0120	99292	1
G0120	99304	1

Column 1	Column 2	Modifier 0=not allowed 1=allowed 9=not applicable
G0120	99305	1
G0120	99306	1
G0120	99307	1
G0120	99308	1
G0120	99309	1
G0120	99310	1
G0120	99315	1
G0120	99316	1
G0120	99318	1
G0120	99324	1
G0120	99325	1
G0120	99326	1
G0120	99327	1
G0120	99328	1
G0120	99334	1
G0120	99335	1
G0120	99336	1
G0120	99337	1
G0120	99341	1
G0120	99342	1
G0120	99343	1
G0120	99344	1
G0120	99345	1
G0120	99347	1
G0120	99348	1
G0120	99349	1
G0120	99350	1
G0120	99354	1
G0120	99355	1
G0120	99356	1
G0120	99357	1
G0120	99360	1
G0120	99455	1
G0120	99456	1
G0120	99460	1
G0120	99461	1
G0120	99462	1
G0120	99463	1
G0120	99464	1
G0120	99465	1
G0120	99466	1
G0120	99468	1

Column 1	Column 2	Modifier 0=not allowed 1=allowed 9=not applicable
G0120	99469	1
G0120	99471	1
G0120	99472	1
G0120	99475	1
G0120	99476	1
G0120	99477	1
G0120	99478	1
G0120	99479	1
G0120	99480	1
G0121	G0380	1
G0121	G0381	1
G0121	G0382	1
G0121	G0383	1
G0121	G0384	1
G0121	0213T	1
G0121	0216T	1
G0121	0228T	1
G0121	0230T	1
G0121	36000	1
G0121	36400	1
G0121	36405	1
G0121	36406	1
G0121	36410	1
G0121	36420	1
G0121	36425	1
G0121	36430	1
G0121	36440	1
G0121	36600	1
G0121	36640	1
G0121	37202	1
G0121	43752	1
G0121	51701	1
G0121	51702	1
G0121	51703	1
G0121	62310	1
G0121	62311	1
G0121	62318	1
G0121	62319	1
G0121	64400	1
G0121	64402	1
G0121	64405	1
G0121	64408	1

Column 1	Column 2	Modifier 0=not allowed 1=allowed 9=not applicable
G0121	64410	1
G0121	64412	1
G0121	64413	1
G0121	64415	1
G0121	64416	1
G0121	64417	1
G0121	64418	1
G0121	64420	1
G0121	64421	1
G0121	64425	1
G0121	64430	1
G0121	64435	1
G0121	64445	1
G0121	64446	1
G0121	64447	1
G0121	64448	1
G0121	64449	1
G0121	64450	1
G0121	64479	1
G0121	64483	1
G0121	64490	1
G0121	64493	1
G0121	64505	1
G0121	64508	1
G0121	64510	1
G0121	64517	1
G0121	64520	1
G0121	64530	1
G0121	93000	1
G0121	93005	1
G0121	93010	1
G0121	93040	1
G0121	93041	1
G0121	93042	1
G0121	93318	1
G0121	94002	1
G0121	94200	1
G0121	94250	1
G0121	94680	1
G0121	94681	1
G0121	94690	1
G0121	94770	1

Column 1	Column 2	Modifier 0=not allowed 1=allowed 9=not applicable	Column 1	Column 2	Modifier 0=not allowed 1=allowed 9=not applicable	Column 1	Column 2	Modifier 0=not allowed 1=allowed 9=not applicable
G0121	95812	1	G0121	99238	1	G0121	99455	1
G0121	95813	1	G0121	99239	1	G0121	99456	1
G0121	95816	1	G0121	99281	1	G0121	99460	1
G0121	95819	1	G0121	99282	1	G0121	99461	1
G0121	95822	1	G0121	99283	1	G0121	99462	1
G0121	95829	1	G0121	99284	1	G0121	99463	1
G0121	95955	1	G0121	99285	1	G0121	99465	1
G0121	96360	1	G0121	99291	1	G0121	99466	1
G0121	96365	1	G0121	99292	1	G0121	99468	1
G0121	96372	1	G0121	99304	1	G0121	99469	1
G0121	96374	1	G0121	99305	1	G0121	99471	1
G0121	96375	1	G0121	99306	1	G0121	99472	1
G0121	96376	1	G0121	99307	1	G0121	99475	1
G0121	99148	1	G0121	99308	1	G0121	99476	1
G0121	99149	1	G0121	99309	1	G0121	99477	1
G0121	99150	1	G0121	99310	1	G0121	99478	1
G0121	99201	1	G0121	99315	1	G0121	99479	1
G0121	99202	1	G0121	99316	1	G0121	99480	1
G0121	99203	1	G0121	99318	1	G0123	P3000	0
G0121	99204	1	G0121	99324	1	G0124	G0141	0
G0121	99205	1	G0121	99325	1	G0124	G0147	0
G0121	99211	1	G0121	99326	1	G0124	G0148	0
G0121	99212	1	G0121	99327	1	G0124	P3000	0
G0121	99213	1	G0121	99328	1	G0124	P3001	0
G0121	99214	1	G0121	99334	1	G0124	88142	0
G0121	99215	1	G0121	99335	1	G0124	88143	0
G0121	99217	1	G0121	99336	1	G0124	88147	0
G0121	99218	1	G0121	99337	1	G0124	88148	0
G0121	99219	1	G0121	99341	1	G0124	88150	0
G0121	99220	1	G0121	99342	1	G0124	88152	0
G0121	99221	1	G0121	99343	1	G0124	88153	0
G0121	99222	1	G0121	99344	1	G0124	88154	0
G0121	99223	1	G0121	99345	1	G0124	88164	0
G0121	99224	1	G0121	99347	1	G0124	88165	0
G0121	99225	1	G0121	99348	1	G0124	88166	0
G0121	99226	1	G0121	99349	1	G0124	88167	0
G0121	99231	1	G0121	99350	1	G0124	88174	0
G0121	99232	1	G0121	99354	1	G0124	88175	0
G0121	99233	1	G0121	99355	1	G0127	11042	1
G0121	99234	1	G0121	99356	1	G0127	36000	1
G0121	99235	1	G0121	99357	1	G0127	36400	1
G0121	99236	1	G0121	99360	1	G0127	36405	1

Column 1	Column 2	Modifier 0=not allowed 1=allowed 9=not applicable
G0127	36406	1
G0127	36410	1
G0127	36420	1
G0127	36425	1
G0127	36430	1
G0127	36440	1
G0127	36600	1
G0127	36640	1
G0127	37202	1
G0127	43752	1
G0127	51701	1
G0127	51702	1
G0127	51703	1
G0127	62310	1
G0127	62311	1
G0127	62318	1
G0127	62319	1
G0127	64400	1
G0127	64402	1
G0127	64405	1
G0127	64408	1
G0127	64410	1
G0127	64412	1
G0127	64413	1
G0127	64415	1
G0127	64416	1
G0127	64417	1
G0127	64418	1
G0127	64420	1
G0127	64421	1
G0127	64425	1
G0127	64430	1
G0127	64435	1
G0127	64445	1
G0127	64446	1
G0127	64447	1
G0127	64448	1
G0127	64449	1
G0127	64450	1
G0127	64479	1
G0127	64483	1
G0127	64490	1

Column 1	Column 2	Modifier 0=not allowed 1=allowed 9=not applicable
G0127	64493	1
G0127	64505	1
G0127	64508	1
G0127	64510	1
G0127	64517	1
G0127	64520	1
G0127	64530	1
G0127	93000	1
G0127	93005	1
G0127	93010	1
G0127	93040	1
G0127	93041	1
G0127	93042	1
G0127	93318	1
G0127	94002	1
G0127	94200	1
G0127	94250	1
G0127	94680	1
G0127	94681	1
G0127	94690	1
G0127	94770	1
G0127	95812	1
G0127	95813	1
G0127	95816	1
G0127	95819	1
G0127	95822	1
G0127	95829	1
G0127	95955	1
G0127	96360	1
G0127	96365	1
G0127	96372	1
G0127	96374	1
G0127	96375	1
G0127	96376	1
G0127	97597	1
G0127	97598	1
G0127	97602	1
G0127	97605	1
G0127	97606	1
G0127	99148	1
G0127	99149	1
G0127	99150	1

Column 1	Column 2	Modifier 0=not allowed 1=allowed 9=not applicable
G0129	97001	0
G0129	97002	0
G0129	97003	1
G0129	97004	1
G0129	97150	1
G0129	97530	1
G0129	97532	1
G0129	97533	1
G0129	97535	1
G0129	97537	1
G0129	97542	1
G0129	97545	1
G0129	97750	1
G0141	G0123	0
G0141	G0143	0
G0141	G0144	0
G0141	P3000	0
G0141	88142	0
G0141	88143	0
G0141	88147	0
G0141	88148	0
G0141	88150	0
G0141	88152	0
G0141	88153	0
G0141	88154	0
G0141	88164	0
G0141	88165	0
G0141	88166	0
G0141	88167	0
G0141	88174	0
G0141	88175	0
G0145	G0147	0
G0145	G0148	0
G0148	G0147	0
G0151	G0281	1
G0151	G0283	1
G0151	G0329	1
G0151	97001	1
G0151	97002	1
G0151	97003	0
G0151	97004	0
G0151	97012	1

Column 1	Column 2	Modifier 0=not allowed 1=allowed 9=not applicable
G0151	97016	1
G0151	97018	1
G0151	97022	1
G0151	97024	1
G0151	97026	1
G0151	97028	1
G0151	97032	1
G0151	97033	1
G0151	97034	1
G0151	97035	1
G0151	97036	1
G0151	97110	1
G0151	97112	1
G0151	97113	1
G0151	97116	1
G0151	97124	1
G0151	97140	1
G0151	97150	1
G0151	97530	1
G0151	97532	1
G0151	97533	1
G0151	97535	1
G0151	97537	1
G0151	97542	1
G0151	97545	1
G0151	97546	1
G0151	97750	1
G0151	97760	1
G0151	97761	1
G0151	97762	1
G0152	97001	0
G0152	97002	0
G0152	97003	1
G0152	97004	1
G0152	97150	1
G0152	97530	1
G0152	97532	1
G0152	97533	1
G0152	97535	1
G0152	97542	1
G0152	97545	1
G0152	97750	1

Column 1	Column 2	Modifier 0=not allowed 1=allowed 9=not applicable
G0153	0208T	1
G0153	0209T	1
G0153	0210T	1
G0153	0211T	1
G0153	0212T	1
G0153	92506	1
G0153	92507	1
G0153	92508	1
G0153	92526	1
G0153	92550	1
G0153	92552	1
G0153	92553	1
G0153	92555	1
G0153	92556	1
G0153	92557	1
G0153	92561	1
G0153	92562	1
G0153	92563	1
G0153	92564	1
G0153	92565	1
G0153	92567	1
G0153	92568	1
G0153	92570	1
G0153	92571	1
G0153	92572	1
G0153	92575	1
G0153	92576	1
G0153	92577	1
G0153	92579	1
G0153	92582	1
G0153	92583	1
G0153	92584	1
G0153	92585	1
G0153	92587	1
G0153	92588	1
G0153	92596	1
G0153	92620	0
G0153	92621	0
G0153	92625	0
G0154	G0008	1
G0154	G0009	1
G0154	G0010	1

Column 1	Column 2	Modifier 0=not allowed 1=allowed 9=not applicable
G0154	P9612	1
G0154	P9615	1
G0154	36000	1
G0154	36410	1
G0154	36430	1
G0154	96360	1
G0154	96365	1
G0155	97537	1
G0157	G0281	1
G0157	G0283	1
G0157	G0329	1
G0157	97001	1
G0157	97002	1
G0157	97003	0
G0157	97004	0
G0157	97012	1
G0157	97016	1
G0157	97018	1
G0157	97022	1
G0157	97024	1
G0157	97026	1
G0157	97028	1
G0157	97032	1
G0157	97033	1
G0157	97034	1
G0157	97035	1
G0157	97036	1
G0157	97110	1
G0157	97112	1
G0157	97113	1
G0157	97116	1
G0157	97124	1
G0157	97140	1
G0157	97150	1
G0157	97530	1
G0157	97532	1
G0157	97533	1
G0157	97535	1
G0157	97537	1
G0157	97542	1
G0157	97545	1
G0157	97546	1

Column 1	Column 2	Modifier 0=not allowed 1=allowed 9=not applicable
G0157	97750	1
G0157	97760	1
G0157	97761	1
G0157	97762	1
G0158	97001	0
G0158	97002	0
G0158	97003	1
G0158	97004	1
G0158	97150	1
G0158	97530	1
G0158	97532	1
G0158	97533	1
G0158	97535	1
G0158	97542	1
G0158	97545	1
G0158	97750	1
G0159	G0157	0
G0159	G0281	1
G0159	G0283	1
G0159	G0329	1
G0159	97001	1
G0159	97002	1
G0159	97003	0
G0159	97004	0
G0159	97012	1
G0159	97016	1
G0159	97018	1
G0159	97022	1
G0159	97024	1
G0159	97026	1
G0159	97028	1
G0159	97032	1
G0159	97033	1
G0159	97034	1
G0159	97035	1
G0159	97036	1
G0159	97110	1
G0159	97112	1
G0159	97113	1
G0159	97116	1
G0159	97124	1
G0159	97140	1

Column 1	Column 2	Modifier 0=not allowed 1=allowed 9=not applicable
G0159	97150	1
G0159	97530	1
G0159	97532	1
G0159	97533	1
G0159	97535	1
G0159	97537	1
G0159	97542	1
G0159	97545	1
G0159	97546	1
G0159	97750	1
G0159	97760	1
G0159	97761	1
G0159	97762	1
G0160	G0158	0
G0160	97001	0
G0160	97002	0
G0160	97003	1
G0160	97004	1
G0160	97150	1
G0160	97530	1
G0160	97532	1
G0160	97533	1
G0160	97535	1
G0160	97542	1
G0160	97545	1
G0160	97750	1
G0161	0208T	1
G0161	0209T	1
G0161	0210T	1
G0161	0211T	1
G0161	0212T	1
G0161	92506	1
G0161	92507	1
G0161	92508	1
G0161	92526	1
G0161	92550	1
G0161	92552	1
G0161	92553	1
G0161	92555	1
G0161	92556	1
G0161	92557	1
G0161	92561	1

Column 1	Column 2	Modifier 0=not allowed 1=allowed 9=not applicable
G0161	92562	1
G0161	92563	1
G0161	92564	1
G0161	92565	1
G0161	92567	1
G0161	92568	1
G0161	92570	1
G0161	92571	1
G0161	92572	1
G0161	92575	1
G0161	92576	1
G0161	92577	1
G0161	92579	1
G0161	92582	1
G0161	92583	1
G0161	92584	1
G0161	92585	1
G0161	92587	1
G0161	92588	1
G0161	92596	1
G0161	92620	0
G0161	92621	0
G0161	92625	0
G0162	G0008	1
G0162	G0009	1
G0162	G0010	1
G0162	P9612	1
G0162	P9615	1
G0162	36000	1
G0162	36410	1
G0162	36430	1
G0162	96360	1
G0162	96365	1
G0163	G0008	1
G0163	G0009	1
G0163	G0010	1
G0163	P9612	1
G0163	P9615	1
G0163	36000	1
G0163	36410	1
G0163	36430	1
G0163	96360	1

Column 1	Column 2	Modifier 0=not allowed 1=allowed 9=not applicable
G0163	96365	1
G0164	G0008	1
G0164	G0009	1
G0164	G0010	1
G0164	P9612	1
G0164	P9615	1
G0164	36000	1
G0164	36410	1
G0164	36430	1
G0164	96360	1
G0164	96365	1
G0166	0178T	1
G0166	0179T	1
G0166	0180T	1
G0166	92971	0
G0166	93000	1
G0166	93005	1
G0166	93010	1
G0166	93040	0
G0166	93041	0
G0166	93042	0
G0166	93701	0
G0166	93720	0
G0166	93721	0
G0166	93722	0
G0166	93922	1
G0166	93923	1
G0166	93924	0
G0166	93965	1
G0166	97016	0
G0166	99211	1
G0168	0213T	1
G0168	0216T	1
G0168	0228T	1
G0168	0230T	1
G0168	11900	1
G0168	11901	1
G0168	36000	1
G0168	36400	1
G0168	36405	1
G0168	36406	1
G0168	36410	1

Column 1	Column 2	Modifier 0=not allowed 1=allowed 9=not applicable
G0168	36420	1
G0168	36425	1
G0168	36430	1
G0168	36440	1
G0168	36600	1
G0168	36640	1
G0168	37202	1
G0168	43752	1
G0168	51701	1
G0168	51702	1
G0168	51703	1
G0168	62310	1
G0168	62311	1
G0168	62318	1
G0168	62319	1
G0168	64400	1
G0168	64402	1
G0168	64405	1
G0168	64408	1
G0168	64410	1
G0168	64412	1
G0168	64413	1
G0168	64415	1
G0168	64416	1
G0168	64417	1
G0168	64418	1
G0168	64420	1
G0168	64421	1
G0168	64425	1
G0168	64430	1
G0168	64435	1
G0168	64445	1
G0168	64446	1
G0168	64447	1
G0168	64448	1
G0168	64449	1
G0168	64450	1
G0168	64479	1
G0168	64483	1
G0168	64490	1
G0168	64493	1
G0168	64505	1

Column 1	Column 2	Modifier 0=not allowed 1=allowed 9=not applicable
G0168	64508	1
G0168	64510	1
G0168	64517	1
G0168	64520	1
G0168	64530	1
G0168	93000	1
G0168	93005	1
G0168	93010	1
G0168	93040	1
G0168	93041	1
G0168	93042	1
G0168	93318	1
G0168	94002	1
G0168	94200	1
G0168	94250	1
G0168	94680	1
G0168	94681	1
G0168	94690	1
G0168	94770	1
G0168	95812	1
G0168	95813	1
G0168	95816	1
G0168	95819	1
G0168	95822	1
G0168	95829	1
G0168	95955	1
G0168	96360	1
G0168	96365	1
G0168	96372	1
G0168	96374	1
G0168	96375	1
G0168	96376	1
G0168	99148	1
G0168	99149	1
G0168	99150	1
G0173	11920	1
G0173	11921	1
G0173	16000	1
G0173	16020	1
G0173	16025	1
G0173	16030	1
G0173	20660	1

Column 1	Column 2	Modifier 0=not allowed 1=allowed 9=not applicable
G0173	20661	1
G0173	20693	1
G0173	20694	1
G0173	36000	1
G0173	36410	1
G0173	36425	1
G0173	51701	1
G0173	51702	1
G0173	51703	1
G0173	61781	1
G0173	61782	1
G0173	61783	1
G0173	69990	0
G0173	77321	1
G0173	77326	1
G0173	77327	1
G0173	77328	1
G0173	77336	1
G0173	77418	1
G0173	77421	0
G0173	97802	1
G0173	97803	1
G0173	97804	1
G0173	99143	1
G0173	99144	1
G0173	99145	1
G0177	G0151	1
G0177	G0152	1
G0177	G0153	1
G0177	G0154	1
G0177	G0155	1
G0177	G0156	1
G0177	G0270	1
G0177	G0271	1
G0177	92065	1
G0177	97112	1
G0177	97116	1
G0177	97530	1
G0177	97532	1
G0177	97533	1
G0177	97535	1
G0177	97537	1

Column 1	Column 2	Modifier 0=not allowed 1=allowed 9=not applicable
G0177	97542	1
G0177	97545	1
G0177	97802	0
G0177	97803	0
G0177	97804	0
G0181	G0102	1
G0181	93040	1
G0181	93041	1
G0181	93042	1
G0182	G0102	1
G0182	93040	1
G0182	93041	1
G0182	93042	1
G0186	36000	1
G0186	36410	1
G0186	67005	1
G0186	67010	1
G0186	67015	1
G0186	67145	1
G0186	67220	1
G0186	67221	1
G0186	67500	1
G0186	69990	0
G0186	96360	1
G0186	96365	1
G0202	77057	0
G0204	G0206	0
G0204	77055	0
G0204	77056	0
G0206	77055	0
G0237	94010	1
G0237	94060	1
G0237	94150	1
G0237	94200	1
G0237	94240	1
G0237	94250	1
G0237	94260	1
G0237	94350	1
G0237	94360	1
G0237	94370	1
G0237	94375	1
G0237	94400	1

Column 1	Column 2	Modifier 0=not allowed 1=allowed 9=not applicable
G0237	94450	1
G0237	94620	0
G0237	94621	0
G0237	94680	1
G0237	94681	1
G0237	94690	1
G0237	94720	1
G0237	94725	1
G0237	94750	1
G0237	94760	0
G0237	94761	0
G0237	94762	1
G0237	94770	0
G0237	97001	1
G0237	97002	1
G0237	97003	1
G0237	97004	1
G0237	97110	1
G0237	97112	1
G0237	97150	1
G0237	97530	1
G0237	97750	1
G0237	97802	1
G0237	97803	1
G0237	97804	1
G0238	94010	1
G0238	94060	1
G0238	94150	1
G0238	94200	1
G0238	94240	1
G0238	94250	1
G0238	94260	1
G0238	94350	1
G0238	94360	1
G0238	94370	1
G0238	94375	1
G0238	94400	1
G0238	94450	1
G0238	94620	0
G0238	94621	0
G0238	94667	1
G0238	94668	1

Column 1	Column 2	Modifier 0=not allowed 1=allowed 9=not applicable
G0238	94680	1
G0238	94681	1
G0238	94690	1
G0238	94720	1
G0238	94725	1
G0238	94750	1
G0238	94760	0
G0238	94761	0
G0238	94762	1
G0238	94770	0
G0238	97001	1
G0238	97002	1
G0238	97003	1
G0238	97004	1
G0238	97110	1
G0238	97112	1
G0238	97150	1
G0238	97530	1
G0238	97750	1
G0238	97802	1
G0238	97803	1
G0238	97804	1
G0239	G0237	1
G0239	G0238	1
G0239	94010	1
G0239	94060	1
G0239	94150	1
G0239	94200	1
G0239	94240	1
G0239	94250	1
G0239	94260	1
G0239	94350	1
G0239	94360	1
G0239	94370	1
G0239	94375	1
G0239	94400	1
G0239	94450	1
G0239	94620	0
G0239	94621	0
G0239	94667	1
G0239	94668	1
G0239	94680	1

Column 1	Column 2	Modifier 0=not allowed 1=allowed 9=not applicable
G0239	94681	1
G0239	94690	1
G0239	94720	1
G0239	94725	1
G0239	94750	1
G0239	94760	0
G0239	94761	0
G0239	94762	1
G0239	94770	0
G0239	97001	1
G0239	97002	1
G0239	97003	1
G0239	97004	1
G0239	97110	1
G0239	97112	1
G0239	97150	1
G0239	97530	1
G0239	97750	1
G0239	97802	1
G0239	97803	1
G0239	97804	1
G0245	G0127	0
G0245	G0246	0
G0245	0183T	0
G0245	11042	0
G0245	11043	0
G0245	11044	0
G0245	11055	0
G0245	11056	0
G0245	11057	0
G0245	11305	0
G0245	11306	0
G0245	11307	0
G0245	11308	0
G0245	11420	1
G0245	11421	1
G0245	11422	1
G0245	11423	1
G0245	11424	1
G0245	11426	1
G0245	11719	0
G0245	11720	0

Column 1	Column 2	Modifier 0=not allowed 1=allowed 9=not applicable
G0245	11721	0
G0245	11755	0
G0245	11765	0
G0245	97597	1
G0245	97598	1
G0245	97602	1
G0245	97605	1
G0245	97606	1
G0246	G0127	0
G0246	0183T	0
G0246	11042	0
G0246	11043	0
G0246	11044	0
G0246	11055	0
G0246	11056	0
G0246	11057	0
G0246	11305	0
G0246	11306	0
G0246	11307	0
G0246	11308	0
G0246	11420	1
G0246	11421	1
G0246	11422	1
G0246	11423	1
G0246	11424	1
G0246	11426	1
G0246	11719	0
G0246	11720	0
G0246	11721	0
G0246	11755	0
G0246	11765	0
G0246	97597	1
G0246	97598	1
G0246	97602	1
G0246	97605	1
G0246	97606	1
G0247	G0127	0
G0247	0183T	0
G0247	11042	0
G0247	11043	1
G0247	11044	1
G0247	11055	0

Column 1	Column 2	Modifier 0=not allowed 1=allowed 9=not applicable
G0247	11056	0
G0247	11057	0
G0247	11305	0
G0247	11306	0
G0247	11307	0
G0247	11308	0
G0247	11420	1
G0247	11421	1
G0247	11422	1
G0247	11423	1
G0247	11424	1
G0247	11426	1
G0247	11719	0
G0247	11720	0
G0247	11721	0
G0247	11755	1
G0247	11765	1
G0247	97597	1
G0247	97598	1
G0247	97602	1
G0247	97605	1
G0247	97606	1
G0251	0073T	0
G0251	11920	1
G0251	11921	1
G0251	16000	1
G0251	16020	1
G0251	16025	1
G0251	16030	1
G0251	20660	0
G0251	36000	1
G0251	36410	1
G0251	36425	1
G0251	51701	1
G0251	51702	1
G0251	51703	1
G0251	61781	0
G0251	61782	0
G0251	61783	0
G0251	69990	0
G0251	77321	1
G0251	77326	1

Column 1	Column 2	Modifier 0=not allowed 1=allowed 9=not applicable
G0251	77327	1
G0251	77328	1
G0251	77401	0
G0251	77402	0
G0251	77403	0
G0251	77404	0
G0251	77406	0
G0251	77407	0
G0251	77408	0
G0251	77409	0
G0251	77411	0
G0251	77412	0
G0251	77413	0
G0251	77414	0
G0251	77416	0
G0251	77418	1
G0251	77421	0
G0251	77422	0
G0251	77423	0
G0251	97802	1
G0251	97803	1
G0251	97804	1
G0251	99143	1
G0251	99144	1
G0251	99145	1
G0257	36000	1
G0257	36147	1
G0257	36410	1
G0257	36430	1
G0257	90935	1
G0257	90937	1
G0257	90945	1
G0257	90947	1
G0257	90997	1
G0257	96360	1
G0257	96365	1
G0257	96372	1
G0257	96374	1
G0257	96375	1
G0257	96376	1
G0257	97802	1
G0257	97803	1

Column 1	Column 2	Modifier 0=not allowed 1=allowed 9=not applicable
G0257	97804	1
G0259	0213T	1
G0259	0216T	1
G0259	20600	1
G0259	20605	1
G0259	20610	1
G0259	27096	0
G0259	36000	1
G0259	36410	1
G0259	37202	1
G0259	62318	1
G0259	62319	1
G0259	64415	1
G0259	64417	1
G0259	64450	1
G0259	64490	1
G0259	64493	1
G0259	69990	0
G0259	76000	1
G0259	76001	1
G0259	77001	1
G0259	77002	1
G0259	77003	1
G0259	96360	1
G0259	96365	1
G0259	96372	1
G0259	96374	1
G0259	96375	1
G0259	96376	1
G0260	0213T	1
G0260	0216T	1
G0260	0228T	1
G0260	0230T	1
G0260	62310	1
G0260	62311	1
G0260	62318	1
G0260	62319	1
G0260	64400	1
G0260	64402	1
G0260	64405	1
G0260	64408	1
G0260	64410	1

Column 1	Column 2	Modifier 0=not allowed 1=allowed 9=not applicable
G0260	64412	1
G0260	64413	1
G0260	64415	1
G0260	64416	1
G0260	64417	1
G0260	64418	1
G0260	64420	1
G0260	64421	1
G0260	64425	1
G0260	64430	1
G0260	64435	1
G0260	64445	1
G0260	64446	1
G0260	64447	1
G0260	64448	1
G0260	64449	1
G0260	64450	1
G0260	64479	1
G0260	64483	1
G0260	64490	1
G0260	64493	1
G0260	64505	1
G0260	64508	1
G0260	64510	1
G0260	64517	1
G0260	64520	1
G0260	64530	1
G0268	0213T	1
G0268	0216T	1
G0268	36000	1
G0268	36400	1
G0268	36405	1
G0268	36406	1
G0268	36410	1
G0268	36420	1
G0268	36425	1
G0268	36430	1
G0268	36440	1
G0268	36600	1
G0268	36640	1
G0268	37202	1
G0268	43752	1

Column 1	Column 2	Modifier 0=not allowed 1=allowed 9=not applicable
G0268	51701	1
G0268	51702	1
G0268	51703	1
G0268	62310	1
G0268	62311	1
G0268	62318	1
G0268	62319	1
G0268	64400	1
G0268	64402	1
G0268	64405	1
G0268	64408	1
G0268	64410	1
G0268	64412	1
G0268	64413	1
G0268	64415	1
G0268	64416	1
G0268	64417	1
G0268	64418	1
G0268	64420	1
G0268	64421	1
G0268	64425	1
G0268	64430	1
G0268	64435	1
G0268	64445	1
G0268	64446	1
G0268	64447	1
G0268	64448	1
G0268	64449	1
G0268	64450	1
G0268	64490	1
G0268	64493	1
G0268	64505	1
G0268	64508	1
G0268	64510	1
G0268	64517	1
G0268	64520	1
G0268	64530	1
G0268	69990	0
G0268	92504	0
G0268	93000	1
G0268	93005	1
G0268	93010	1

Column 1	Column 2	Modifier 0=not allowed 1=allowed 9=not applicable
G0268	93040	1
G0268	93041	1
G0268	93042	1
G0268	93318	1
G0268	94002	1
G0268	94200	1
G0268	94250	1
G0268	94680	1
G0268	94681	1
G0268	94690	1
G0268	94770	1
G0268	95812	1
G0268	95813	1
G0268	95816	1
G0268	95819	1
G0268	95822	1
G0268	95829	1
G0268	95955	1
G0268	96360	1
G0268	96365	1
G0268	96372	1
G0268	96374	1
G0268	96375	1
G0268	96376	1
G0268	99148	1
G0268	99149	1
G0268	99150	1
G0270	97802	0
G0270	97803	0
G0270	97804	0
G0271	97802	0
G0271	97803	0
G0271	97804	0
G0275	36140	0
G0275	36200	0
G0275	36245	1
G0275	36246	1
G0275	36247	1
G0275	75625	0
G0275	75630	0
G0275	75722	0
G0275	75724	0

Column 1	Column 2	Modifier 0=not allowed 1=allowed 9=not applicable
G0275	76000	1
G0275	76001	1
G0275	76942	1
G0275	77001	1
G0275	77002	1
G0278	36140	0
G0278	36200	0
G0278	36245	1
G0278	36246	1
G0278	36247	1
G0278	75625	1
G0278	75630	0
G0278	75710	1
G0278	75716	0
G0278	76000	1
G0278	76001	1
G0278	76942	1
G0278	77001	1
G0278	77002	1
G0281	64550	1
G0281	97002	1
G0281	97004	1
G0281	97032	1
G0283	97002	1
G0283	97004	1
G0283	97032	1
G0288	76376	1
G0288	76377	1
G0290	34812	1
G0290	35206	1
G0290	35226	1
G0290	36000	1
G0290	36120	1
G0290	36140	1
G0290	36200	1
G0290	36410	1
G0290	36600	1
G0290	36620	1
G0290	36625	1
G0290	37202	1
G0290	92975	1
G0290	92980	0

Column 1	Column 2	Modifier 0=not allowed 1=allowed 9=not applicable
G0290	92982	1
G0290	92995	1
G0290	93040	1
G0290	93041	1
G0290	93042	1
G0290	96360	1
G0290	96365	1
G0291	34812	1
G0291	35206	1
G0291	35226	1
G0291	36000	1
G0291	36120	1
G0291	36140	1
G0291	36200	1
G0291	36410	1
G0291	36600	1
G0291	36620	1
G0291	36625	1
G0291	37202	1
G0291	92975	1
G0291	92980	0
G0291	92982	1
G0291	92995	1
G0291	93040	1
G0291	93041	1
G0291	93042	1
G0291	93555	1
G0291	93556	1
G0291	96360	1
G0291	96365	1
G0302	G0303	0
G0302	G0304	0
G0302	G0380	1
G0302	G0381	1
G0302	G0382	1
G0302	G0383	1
G0302	G0384	1
G0302	99201	1
G0302	99202	1
G0302	99203	1
G0302	99204	1
G0302	99205	1

Column 1	Column 2	Modifier 0=not allowed 1=allowed 9=not applicable
G0302	99211	1
G0302	99212	1
G0302	99213	1
G0302	99214	1
G0302	99215	1
G0302	99217	1
G0302	99218	1
G0302	99219	1
G0302	99220	1
G0302	99221	1
G0302	99222	1
G0302	99223	1
G0302	99224	1
G0302	99225	1
G0302	99226	1
G0302	99231	1
G0302	99232	1
G0302	99233	1
G0302	99234	1
G0302	99235	1
G0302	99236	1
G0302	99238	1
G0302	99239	1
G0302	99281	1
G0302	99282	1
G0302	99283	1
G0302	99284	1
G0302	99285	1
G0302	99291	1
G0302	99304	1
G0302	99305	1
G0302	99306	1
G0302	99307	1
G0302	99308	1
G0302	99309	1
G0302	99310	1
G0302	99315	1
G0302	99316	1
G0302	99318	1
G0302	99324	1
G0302	99325	1
G0302	99326	1

Column 1	Column 2	Modifier 0=not allowed 1=allowed 9=not applicable
G0302	99327	1
G0302	99328	1
G0302	99334	1
G0302	99335	1
G0302	99336	1
G0302	99337	1
G0302	99341	1
G0302	99342	1
G0302	99343	1
G0302	99344	1
G0302	99345	1
G0302	99347	1
G0302	99348	1
G0302	99349	1
G0302	99350	1
G0302	99466	1
G0302	99468	1
G0302	99469	1
G0302	99471	1
G0302	99472	1
G0302	99475	1
G0302	99476	1
G0302	99477	1
G0302	99478	1
G0302	99479	1
G0302	99480	1
G0303	G0304	0
G0303	G0380	1
G0303	G0381	1
G0303	G0382	1
G0303	G0383	1
G0303	G0384	1
G0303	99201	1
G0303	99202	1
G0303	99203	1
G0303	99204	1
G0303	99205	1
G0303	99211	1
G0303	99212	1
G0303	99213	1
G0303	99214	1
G0303	99215	1

Column 1	Column 2	Modifier 0=not allowed 1=allowed 9=not applicable
G0303	99217	1
G0303	99218	1
G0303	99219	1
G0303	99220	1
G0303	99221	1
G0303	99222	1
G0303	99223	1
G0303	99224	1
G0303	99225	1
G0303	99226	1
G0303	99231	1
G0303	99232	1
G0303	99233	1
G0303	99234	1
G0303	99235	1
G0303	99236	1
G0303	99238	1
G0303	99239	1
G0303	99281	1
G0303	99282	1
G0303	99283	1
G0303	99284	1
G0303	99285	1
G0303	99291	1
G0303	99304	1
G0303	99305	1
G0303	99306	1
G0303	99307	1
G0303	99308	1
G0303	99309	1
G0303	99310	1
G0303	99315	1
G0303	99316	1
G0303	99318	1
G0303	99324	1
G0303	99325	1
G0303	99326	1
G0303	99327	1
G0303	99328	1
G0303	99334	1
G0303	99335	1
G0303	99336	1

Column 1	Column 2	Modifier 0=not allowed 1=allowed 9=not applicable
G0303	99337	1
G0303	99341	1
G0303	99342	1
G0303	99343	1
G0303	99344	1
G0303	99345	1
G0303	99347	1
G0303	99348	1
G0303	99349	1
G0303	99350	1
G0303	99466	1
G0303	99468	1
G0303	99469	1
G0303	99471	1
G0303	99472	1
G0303	99475	1
G0303	99476	1
G0303	99477	1
G0303	99478	1
G0303	99479	1
G0303	99480	1
G0304	G0380	1
G0304	G0381	1
G0304	G0382	1
G0304	G0383	1
G0304	G0384	1
G0304	99201	1
G0304	99202	1
G0304	99203	1
G0304	99204	1
G0304	99205	1
G0304	99211	1
G0304	99212	1
G0304	99213	1
G0304	99214	1
G0304	99215	1
G0304	99217	1
G0304	99218	1
G0304	99219	1
G0304	99220	1
G0304	99221	1
G0304	99222	1

Column 1	Column 2	Modifier 0=not allowed 1=allowed 9=not applicable
G0304	99223	1
G0304	99224	1
G0304	99225	1
G0304	99226	1
G0304	99231	1
G0304	99232	1
G0304	99233	1
G0304	99234	1
G0304	99235	1
G0304	99236	1
G0304	99238	1
G0304	99239	1
G0304	99281	1
G0304	99282	1
G0304	99283	1
G0304	99284	1
G0304	99285	1
G0304	99291	1
G0304	99304	1
G0304	99305	1
G0304	99306	1
G0304	99307	1
G0304	99308	1
G0304	99309	1
G0304	99310	1
G0304	99315	1
G0304	99316	1
G0304	99318	1
G0304	99324	1
G0304	99325	1
G0304	99326	1
G0304	99327	1
G0304	99328	1
G0304	99334	1
G0304	99335	1
G0304	99336	1
G0304	99337	1
G0304	99341	1
G0304	99342	1
G0304	99343	1
G0304	99344	1
G0304	99345	1

Column 1	Column 2	Modifier 0=not allowed 1=allowed 9=not applicable
G0304	99347	1
G0304	99348	1
G0304	99349	1
G0304	99350	1
G0304	99466	1
G0304	99468	1
G0304	99469	1
G0304	99471	1
G0304	99472	1
G0304	99475	1
G0304	99476	1
G0304	99477	1
G0304	99478	1
G0304	99479	1
G0304	99480	1
G0305	G0380	1
G0305	G0381	1
G0305	G0382	1
G0305	G0383	1
G0305	G0384	1
G0305	99201	1
G0305	99202	1
G0305	99203	1
G0305	99204	1
G0305	99205	1
G0305	99211	1
G0305	99212	1
G0305	99213	1
G0305	99214	1
G0305	99215	1
G0305	99217	1
G0305	99218	1
G0305	99219	1
G0305	99220	1
G0305	99221	1
G0305	99222	1
G0305	99223	1
G0305	99224	1
G0305	99225	1
G0305	99226	1
G0305	99231	1
G0305	99232	1

Column 1	Column 2	Modifier 0=not allowed 1=allowed 9=not applicable
G0305	99233	1
G0305	99234	1
G0305	99235	1
G0305	99236	1
G0305	99238	1
G0305	99239	1
G0305	99281	1
G0305	99282	1
G0305	99283	1
G0305	99284	1
G0305	99285	1
G0305	99291	1
G0305	99304	1
G0305	99305	1
G0305	99306	1
G0305	99307	1
G0305	99308	1
G0305	99309	1
G0305	99310	1
G0305	99315	1
G0305	99316	1
G0305	99318	1
G0305	99324	1
G0305	99325	1
G0305	99326	1
G0305	99327	1
G0305	99328	1
G0305	99334	1
G0305	99335	1
G0305	99336	1
G0305	99337	1
G0305	99341	1
G0305	99342	1
G0305	99343	1
G0305	99344	1
G0305	99345	1
G0305	99347	1
G0305	99348	1
G0305	99349	1
G0305	99350	1
G0305	99466	1
G0305	99468	1

Column 1	Column 2	Modifier 0=not allowed 1=allowed 9=not applicable
G0305	99469	1
G0305	99471	1
G0305	99472	1
G0305	99475	1
G0305	99476	1
G0305	99477	1
G0305	99478	1
G0305	99479	1
G0305	99480	1
G0306	G0307	0
G0306	85004	0
G0306	85007	0
G0306	85008	0
G0306	85009	0
G0306	85013	1
G0306	85014	1
G0306	85018	1
G0306	85027	0
G0306	85032	0
G0306	85041	1
G0306	85048	1
G0306	85049	0
G0307	85004	0
G0307	85008	0
G0307	85013	1
G0307	85014	1
G0307	85018	1
G0307	85032	0
G0307	85041	1
G0307	85048	1
G0307	85049	0
G0328	82270	0
G0328	82272	1
G0329	97002	1
G0329	97004	1
G0337	G0101	0
G0337	G0102	0
G0337	G0104	0
G0337	G0105	0
G0337	G0106	0
G0337	G0117	0
G0337	G0118	0

Column 1	Column 2	Modifier 0=not allowed 1=allowed 9=not applicable
G0337	G0120	0
G0337	G0121	0
G0337	G0245	0
G0337	G0246	0
G0337	G0248	0
G0337	G0250	1
G0337	G0270	0
G0337	G0271	0
G0337	G0410	1
G0337	G0411	1
G0337	M0064	1
G0337	P3000	0
G0337	P3001	0
G0337	Q0091	0
G0337	90802	0
G0337	90804	1
G0337	90805	1
G0337	90806	1
G0337	90807	1
G0337	90808	1
G0337	90809	1
G0337	90810	1
G0337	90811	1
G0337	90812	1
G0337	90813	1
G0337	90814	1
G0337	90815	1
G0337	90816	1
G0337	90817	1
G0337	90818	1
G0337	90819	1
G0337	90821	1
G0337	90822	1
G0337	90823	1
G0337	90824	1
G0337	90826	1
G0337	90827	1
G0337	90828	1
G0337	90829	1
G0337	90845	1
G0337	90846	1
G0337	90847	1

Column 1	Column 2	Modifier 0=not allowed 1=allowed 9=not applicable
G0337	90849	1
G0337	90853	1
G0337	90857	1
G0337	90862	1
G0337	90865	1
G0337	90880	1
G0337	92002	1
G0337	92004	1
G0337	92012	1
G0337	92014	1
G0337	95831	0
G0337	95832	0
G0337	95833	0
G0337	95834	0
G0337	95851	0
G0337	95852	0
G0337	96116	1
G0337	96150	0
G0337	96151	0
G0337	96152	0
G0337	96153	0
G0337	96154	0
G0337	97802	0
G0337	97803	0
G0337	97804	0
G0339	11920	1
G0339	11921	1
G0339	16000	1
G0339	16020	1
G0339	16025	1
G0339	16030	1
G0339	20660	0
G0339	36000	1
G0339	36410	1
G0339	36425	1
G0339	51701	1
G0339	51702	1
G0339	51703	1
G0339	61781	0
G0339	61782	0
G0339	61783	0
G0339	69990	0

Column 1	Column 2	Modifier 0=not allowed 1=allowed 9=not applicable	Column 1	Column 2	Modifier 0=not allowed 1=allowed 9=not applicable	Column 1	Column 2	Modifier 0=not allowed 1=allowed 9=not applicable
G0339	77321	1	G0340	61783	0	G0341	36600	1
G0339	77326	1	G0340	69990	0	G0341	36640	1
G0339	77327	1	G0340	77321	1	G0341	37202	1
G0339	77328	1	G0340	77326	1	G0341	43752	1
G0339	77336	1	G0340	77327	1	G0341	51701	1
G0339	77401	1	G0340	77328	1	G0341	51702	1
G0339	77402	1	G0340	77401	1	G0341	51703	1
G0339	77403	1	G0340	77402	1	G0341	62310	1
G0339	77404	1	G0340	77403	1	G0341	62311	1
G0339	77406	1	G0340	77404	1	G0341	62318	1
G0339	77407	1	G0340	77406	1	G0341	62319	1
G0339	77408	1	G0340	77407	1	G0341	64400	1
G0339	77409	1	G0340	77408	1	G0341	64402	1
G0339	77411	1	G0340	77409	1	G0341	64405	1
G0339	77412	1	G0340	77411	1	G0341	64408	1
G0339	77413	1	G0340	77412	1	G0341	64410	1
G0339	77414	1	G0340	77413	1	G0341	64412	1
G0339	77416	1	G0340	77414	1	G0341	64413	1
G0339	77421	0	G0340	77416	1	G0341	64415	1
G0339	77422	1	G0340	77421	0	G0341	64416	1
G0339	77423	1	G0340	77422	1	G0341	64417	1
G0339	97802	1	G0340	77423	1	G0341	64418	1
G0339	97803	1	G0340	97802	1	G0341	64420	1
G0339	97804	1	G0340	97803	1	G0341	64421	1
G0339	99143	1	G0340	97804	1	G0341	64425	1
G0339	99144	1	G0340	99143	1	G0341	64430	1
G0339	99145	1	G0340	99144	1	G0341	64435	1
G0340	11920	1	G0340	99145	1	G0341	64445	1
G0340	11921	1	G0341	0213T	1	G0341	64446	1
G0340	16000	1	G0341	0216T	1	G0341	64447	1
G0340	16020	1	G0341	0228T	1	G0341	64448	1
G0340	16025	1	G0341	0230T	1	G0341	64449	1
G0340	16030	1	G0341	36000	1	G0341	64450	1
G0340	20660	0	G0341	36400	1	G0341	64479	1
G0340	36000	1	G0341	36405	1	G0341	64483	1
G0340	36410	1	G0341	36406	1	G0341	64490	1
G0340	36425	1	G0341	36410	1	G0341	64493	1
G0340	51701	1	G0341	36420	1	G0341	64505	1
G0340	51702	1	G0341	36425	1	G0341	64508	1
G0340	51703	1	G0341	36430	1	G0341	64510	1
G0340	61781	0	G0341	36440	1	G0341	64517	1
G0340	61782	0	G0341	36481	0	G0341	64520	1

Column 1	Column 2	Modifier 0=not allowed 1=allowed 9=not applicable	Column 1	Column 2	Modifier 0=not allowed 1=allowed 9=not applicable	Column 1	Column 2	Modifier 0=not allowed 1=allowed 9=not applicable
G0341	64530	1	G0342	36000	1	G0342	64435	1
G0341	76000	1	G0342	36400	1	G0342	64445	1
G0341	76001	1	G0342	36405	1	G0342	64446	1
G0341	76942	1	G0342	36406	1	G0342	64447	1
G0341	76998	1	G0342	36410	1	G0342	64448	1
G0341	77001	1	G0342	36420	1	G0342	64449	1
G0341	77002	1	G0342	36425	1	G0342	64450	1
G0341	93000	1	G0342	36430	1	G0342	64479	1
G0341	93005	1	G0342	36440	1	G0342	64483	1
G0341	93010	1	G0342	36481	0	G0342	64490	1
G0341	93040	1	G0342	36600	1	G0342	64493	1
G0341	93041	1	G0342	36640	1	G0342	64505	1
G0341	93042	1	G0342	37202	1	G0342	64508	1
G0341	93318	1	G0342	43752	1	G0342	64510	1
G0341	94002	1	G0342	44180	0	G0342	64517	1
G0341	94200	1	G0342	44602	1	G0342	64520	1
G0341	94250	1	G0342	44603	1	G0342	64530	1
G0341	94680	1	G0342	44604	1	G0342	76000	1
G0341	94681	1	G0342	44605	1	G0342	76001	1
G0341	94690	1	G0342	49320	0	G0342	76942	1
G0341	94770	1	G0342	51701	1	G0342	76998	1
G0341	95812	1	G0342	51702	1	G0342	77001	1
G0341	95813	1	G0342	51703	1	G0342	77002	1
G0341	95816	1	G0342	62310	1	G0342	93000	1
G0341	95819	1	G0342	62311	1	G0342	93005	1
G0341	95822	1	G0342	62318	1	G0342	93010	1
G0341	95829	1	G0342	62319	1	G0342	93040	1
G0341	95955	1	G0342	64400	1	G0342	93041	1
G0341	96360	1	G0342	64402	1	G0342	93042	1
G0341	96365	1	G0342	64405	1	G0342	93318	1
G0341	96372	1	G0342	64408	1	G0342	94002	1
G0341	96374	1	G0342	64410	1	G0342	94200	1
G0341	96375	1	G0342	64412	1	G0342	94250	1
G0341	96376	1	G0342	64413	1	G0342	94680	1
G0341	99148	1	G0342	64415	1	G0342	94681	1
G0341	99149	1	G0342	64416	1	G0342	94690	1
G0341	99150	1	G0342	64417	1	G0342	94770	1
G0342	G0341	0	G0342	64418	1	G0342	95812	1
G0342	0213T	1	G0342	64420	1	G0342	95813	1
G0342	0216T	1	G0342	64421	1	G0342	95816	1
G0342	0228T	1	G0342	64425	1	G0342	95819	1
G0342	0230T	1	G0342	64430	1	G0342	95822	1

Column 1	Column 2	Modifier 0=not allowed 1=allowed 9=not applicable
G0342	95829	1
G0342	95955	1
G0342	96360	1
G0342	96365	1
G0342	96372	1
G0342	96374	1
G0342	96375	1
G0342	96376	1
G0342	99148	1
G0342	99149	1
G0342	99150	1
G0343	G0341	0
G0343	G0342	0
G0343	0213T	1
G0343	0216T	1
G0343	0228T	1
G0343	0230T	1
G0343	36000	1
G0343	36400	1
G0343	36405	1
G0343	36406	1
G0343	36410	1
G0343	36420	1
G0343	36425	1
G0343	36430	1
G0343	36440	1
G0343	36481	0
G0343	36600	1
G0343	36640	1
G0343	37202	1
G0343	43752	1
G0343	44005	0
G0343	44180	0
G0343	44602	1
G0343	44603	1
G0343	44604	1
G0343	44605	1
G0343	44820	0
G0343	44850	0
G0343	44950	0
G0343	49000	0
G0343	49002	1

Column 1	Column 2	Modifier 0=not allowed 1=allowed 9=not applicable
G0343	49010	0
G0343	49255	0
G0343	49320	1
G0343	49570	0
G0343	51701	1
G0343	51702	1
G0343	51703	1
G0343	62310	1
G0343	62311	1
G0343	62318	1
G0343	62319	1
G0343	64400	1
G0343	64402	1
G0343	64405	1
G0343	64408	1
G0343	64410	1
G0343	64412	1
G0343	64413	1
G0343	64415	1
G0343	64416	1
G0343	64417	1
G0343	64418	1
G0343	64420	1
G0343	64421	1
G0343	64425	1
G0343	64430	1
G0343	64435	1
G0343	64445	1
G0343	64446	1
G0343	64447	1
G0343	64448	1
G0343	64449	1
G0343	64450	1
G0343	64479	1
G0343	64483	1
G0343	64490	1
G0343	64493	1
G0343	64505	1
G0343	64508	1
G0343	64510	1
G0343	64517	1
G0343	64520	1

Column 1	Column 2	Modifier 0=not allowed 1=allowed 9=not applicable
G0343	64530	1
G0343	76000	1
G0343	76001	1
G0343	76942	1
G0343	76998	1
G0343	77001	1
G0343	77002	1
G0343	93000	1
G0343	93005	1
G0343	93010	1
G0343	93040	1
G0343	93041	1
G0343	93042	1
G0343	93318	1
G0343	94002	1
G0343	94200	1
G0343	94250	1
G0343	94680	1
G0343	94681	1
G0343	94690	1
G0343	94770	1
G0343	95812	1
G0343	95813	1
G0343	95816	1
G0343	95819	1
G0343	95822	1
G0343	95829	1
G0343	95955	1
G0343	96360	1
G0343	96365	1
G0343	96372	1
G0343	96374	1
G0343	96375	1
G0343	96376	1
G0343	99148	1
G0343	99149	1
G0343	99150	1
G0364	36000	1
G0364	36410	1
G0364	80500	1
G0364	80502	1
G0365	76970	1

Column 1	Column 2	Modifier 0=not allowed 1=allowed 9=not applicable	Column 1	Column 2	Modifier 0=not allowed 1=allowed 9=not applicable	Column 1	Column 2	Modifier 0=not allowed 1=allowed 9=not applicable
G0365	93922	1	G0380	96420	1	G0381	96153	1
G0365	93931	1	G0380	96422	1	G0381	96154	1
G0365	93965	1	G0380	96425	1	G0381	96401	1
G0380	G0102	1	G0380	96440	1	G0381	96402	1
G0380	G0245	1	G0380	96446	1	G0381	96405	1
G0380	G0246	1	G0380	96450	1	G0381	96406	1
G0380	G0270	1	G0380	96523	1	G0381	96409	1
G0380	G0271	1	G0380	97802	1	G0381	96413	1
G0380	M0064	1	G0380	97803	1	G0381	96416	1
G0380	43752	1	G0380	97804	1	G0381	96420	1
G0380	90862	1	G0380	99605	1	G0381	96422	1
G0380	90940	1	G0380	99606	1	G0381	96425	1
G0380	92002	1	G0381	G0102	1	G0381	96440	1
G0380	92004	1	G0381	G0245	1	G0381	96446	1
G0380	92012	1	G0381	G0246	1	G0381	96450	1
G0380	92014	1	G0381	G0270	1	G0381	96523	1
G0380	94002	1	G0381	G0271	1	G0381	97802	1
G0380	94003	1	G0381	M0064	1	G0381	97803	1
G0380	94004	1	G0381	43752	1	G0381	97804	1
G0380	94644	1	G0381	90862	1	G0381	99605	1
G0380	94660	1	G0381	90940	1	G0381	99606	1
G0380	94662	1	G0381	92002	1	G0382	G0102	1
G0380	95831	1	G0381	92004	1	G0382	G0245	1
G0380	95832	1	G0381	92012	1	G0382	G0246	1
G0380	95833	1	G0381	92014	1	G0382	G0270	1
G0380	95834	1	G0381	94002	1	G0382	G0271	1
G0380	95851	1	G0381	94003	1	G0382	M0064	1
G0380	95852	1	G0381	94004	1	G0382	43752	1
G0380	96020	1	G0381	94644	1	G0382	90862	1
G0380	96116	1	G0381	94660	1	G0382	90940	1
G0380	96150	1	G0381	94662	1	G0382	92002	1
G0380	96151	1	G0381	95831	1	G0382	92004	1
G0380	96152	1	G0381	95832	1	G0382	92012	1
G0380	96153	1	G0381	95833	1	G0382	92014	1
G0380	96154	1	G0381	95834	1	G0382	94002	1
G0380	96401	1	G0381	95851	1	G0382	94003	1
G0380	96402	1	G0381	95852	1	G0382	94004	1
G0380	96405	1	G0381	96020	1	G0382	94644	1
G0380	96406	1	G0381	96116	1	G0382	94660	1
G0380	96409	1	G0381	96150	1	G0382	94662	1
G0380	96413	1	G0381	96151	1	G0382	95831	1
G0380	96416	1	G0381	96152	1	G0382	95832	1

Column 1	Column 2	Modifier 0=not allowed 1=allowed 9=not applicable
G0382	95833	1
G0382	95834	1
G0382	95851	1
G0382	95852	1
G0382	96020	1
G0382	96116	1
G0382	96150	1
G0382	96151	1
G0382	96152	1
G0382	96153	1
G0382	96154	1
G0382	96401	1
G0382	96402	1
G0382	96405	1
G0382	96406	1
G0382	96409	1
G0382	96413	1
G0382	96416	1
G0382	96420	1
G0382	96422	1
G0382	96425	1
G0382	96440	1
G0382	96446	1
G0382	96450	1
G0382	96523	1
G0382	97802	1
G0382	97803	1
G0382	97804	1
G0382	99605	1
G0382	99606	1
G0383	G0102	1
G0383	G0245	1
G0383	G0246	1
G0383	G0270	1
G0383	G0271	1
G0383	M0064	1
G0383	43752	1
G0383	90862	1
G0383	90940	1
G0383	92002	1
G0383	92004	1
G0383	92012	1

Column 1	Column 2	Modifier 0=not allowed 1=allowed 9=not applicable
G0383	92014	1
G0383	94002	1
G0383	94003	1
G0383	94004	1
G0383	94644	1
G0383	94660	1
G0383	94662	1
G0383	95831	1
G0383	95832	1
G0383	95833	1
G0383	95834	1
G0383	95851	1
G0383	95852	1
G0383	96020	1
G0383	96116	1
G0383	96150	1
G0383	96151	1
G0383	96152	1
G0383	96153	1
G0383	96154	1
G0383	96401	1
G0383	96402	1
G0383	96405	1
G0383	96406	1
G0383	96409	1
G0383	96413	1
G0383	96416	1
G0383	96420	1
G0383	96422	1
G0383	96425	1
G0383	96440	1
G0383	96446	1
G0383	96450	1
G0383	96523	1
G0383	97802	1
G0383	97803	1
G0383	97804	1
G0383	99605	1
G0383	99606	1
G0384	G0102	1
G0384	G0245	1
G0384	G0246	1

Column 1	Column 2	Modifier 0=not allowed 1=allowed 9=not applicable
G0384	G0270	1
G0384	G0271	1
G0384	M0064	1
G0384	43752	1
G0384	90862	1
G0384	90940	1
G0384	92002	1
G0384	92004	1
G0384	92012	1
G0384	92014	1
G0384	94002	1
G0384	94003	1
G0384	94004	1
G0384	94644	1
G0384	94660	1
G0384	94662	1
G0384	95831	1
G0384	95832	1
G0384	95833	1
G0384	95834	1
G0384	95851	1
G0384	95852	1
G0384	96020	1
G0384	96116	1
G0384	96150	1
G0384	96151	1
G0384	96152	1
G0384	96153	1
G0384	96154	1
G0384	96401	1
G0384	96402	1
G0384	96405	1
G0384	96406	1
G0384	96409	1
G0384	96413	1
G0384	96416	1
G0384	96420	1
G0384	96422	1
G0384	96425	1
G0384	96440	1
G0384	96445	1
G0384	96446	1

Column 1	Column 2	Modifier 0=not allowed 1=allowed 9=not applicable
G0384	96523	1
G0384	97802	1
G0384	97803	1
G0384	97804	1
G0384	99605	1
G0384	99606	1
G0389	76998	1
G0396	99408	0
G0396	99409	0
G0397	G0396	0
G0397	99408	0
G0397	99409	0
G0398	92270	1
G0398	93000	1
G0398	93005	1
G0398	93010	1
G0398	93040	1
G0398	93041	1
G0398	93042	1
G0398	93224	1
G0398	93225	1
G0398	93226	1
G0398	93227	1
G0398	93230	1
G0398	94200	1
G0398	94360	0
G0398	94620	1
G0398	94681	0
G0398	94760	1
G0398	94761	1
G0398	94762	1
G0398	94770	1
G0398	95812	1
G0398	95813	1
G0398	95816	1
G0398	95819	1
G0398	95822	1
G0398	95824	1
G0398	95827	1
G0398	95860	1
G0398	95861	1
G0398	95863	1

Column 1	Column 2	Modifier 0=not allowed 1=allowed 9=not applicable
G0398	95864	1
G0398	95865	1
G0398	95866	1
G0398	95867	1
G0398	95868	1
G0398	95869	1
G0398	95870	1
G0398	95872	1
G0398	95950	1
G0398	95951	1
G0398	95953	1
G0398	95954	1
G0398	95955	1
G0398	95956	1
G0398	95957	1
G0398	95958	1
G0398	95961	1
G0399	92270	1
G0399	93000	1
G0399	93005	1
G0399	93010	1
G0399	93040	1
G0399	93041	1
G0399	93042	1
G0399	93224	1
G0399	93225	1
G0399	93226	1
G0399	93227	1
G0399	93230	1
G0399	94200	1
G0399	94360	0
G0399	94620	1
G0399	94681	0
G0399	94760	1
G0399	94761	1
G0399	94762	1
G0399	94770	1
G0399	95812	1
G0399	95813	1
G0399	95816	1
G0399	95819	1
G0399	95822	1

Column 1	Column 2	Modifier 0=not allowed 1=allowed 9=not applicable
G0399	95824	1
G0399	95827	1
G0399	95860	1
G0399	95861	1
G0399	95863	1
G0399	95864	1
G0399	95865	1
G0399	95866	1
G0399	95867	1
G0399	95868	1
G0399	95869	1
G0399	95870	1
G0399	95872	1
G0399	95950	1
G0399	95951	1
G0399	95953	1
G0399	95954	1
G0399	95955	1
G0399	95956	1
G0399	95957	1
G0399	95958	1
G0399	95961	1
G0400	92270	1
G0400	93000	1
G0400	93005	1
G0400	93010	1
G0400	93040	1
G0400	93041	1
G0400	93042	1
G0400	93224	1
G0400	93225	1
G0400	93226	1
G0400	93227	1
G0400	94200	1
G0400	94360	0
G0400	94620	1
G0400	94681	0
G0400	94760	1
G0400	94761	1
G0400	94762	1
G0400	94770	1
G0400	95812	1

Column 1	Column 2	Modifier 0=not allowed 1=allowed 9=not applicable
G0400	95813	1
G0400	95816	1
G0400	95819	1
G0400	95822	1
G0400	95824	1
G0400	95827	1
G0400	95860	1
G0400	95861	1
G0400	95863	1
G0400	95864	1
G0400	95865	1
G0400	95866	1
G0400	95867	1
G0400	95868	1
G0400	95869	1
G0400	95870	1
G0400	95872	1
G0400	95950	1
G0400	95951	1
G0400	95953	1
G0400	95954	1
G0400	95955	1
G0400	95956	1
G0400	95957	1
G0400	95958	1
G0400	95961	1
G0402	G0102	0
G0402	G0250	1
G0402	G0270	0
G0402	G0271	0
G0402	M0064	1
G0402	90801	1
G0402	90802	1
G0402	90804	1
G0402	90805	1
G0402	90806	1
G0402	90807	1
G0402	90808	1
G0402	90809	1
G0402	90810	1
G0402	90811	1
G0402	90812	1

Column 1	Column 2	Modifier 0=not allowed 1=allowed 9=not applicable
G0402	90813	1
G0402	90814	1
G0402	90815	1
G0402	90816	1
G0402	90817	1
G0402	90818	1
G0402	90819	1
G0402	90821	1
G0402	90822	1
G0402	90823	1
G0402	90824	1
G0402	90826	1
G0402	90827	1
G0402	90828	1
G0402	90829	1
G0402	90845	1
G0402	90862	1
G0402	92002	1
G0402	92004	1
G0402	92012	1
G0402	92014	1
G0402	93000	1
G0402	93005	1
G0402	93010	1
G0402	93040	1
G0402	93041	1
G0402	93042	1
G0402	95831	1
G0402	95832	1
G0402	95833	1
G0402	95834	1
G0402	95851	1
G0402	95852	1
G0402	96116	1
G0402	96150	0
G0402	96151	0
G0402	96152	0
G0402	96153	0
G0402	96154	0
G0402	97802	0
G0402	97803	0
G0402	97804	0

Column 1	Column 2	Modifier 0=not allowed 1=allowed 9=not applicable
G0403	G0404	0
G0403	G0405	0
G0410	G0270	1
G0410	G0271	1
G0410	G0380	1
G0410	G0381	1
G0410	G0382	1
G0410	G0383	1
G0410	G0384	1
G0410	M0064	1
G0410	36640	1
G0410	90862	1
G0410	96150	1
G0410	96151	1
G0410	96152	1
G0410	96153	1
G0410	96154	1
G0410	97802	1
G0410	97803	1
G0410	97804	1
G0410	99201	1
G0410	99202	1
G0410	99203	1
G0410	99204	1
G0410	99205	1
G0410	99211	1
G0410	99212	1
G0410	99213	1
G0410	99214	1
G0410	99215	1
G0410	99217	1
G0410	99218	1
G0410	99219	1
G0410	99220	1
G0410	99221	1
G0410	99222	1
G0410	99223	1
G0410	99224	1
G0410	99225	1
G0410	99226	1
G0410	99231	1
G0410	99232	1

Column 1	Column 2	Modifier 0=not allowed 1=allowed 9=not applicable	Column 1	Column 2	Modifier 0=not allowed 1=allowed 9=not applicable	Column 1	Column 2	Modifier 0=not allowed 1=allowed 9=not applicable
G0410	99233	1	G0410	99355	1	G0411	99231	1
G0410	99234	1	G0410	99356	1	G0411	99232	1
G0410	99235	1	G0410	99357	1	G0411	99233	1
G0410	99236	1	G0410	99605	1	G0411	99234	1
G0410	99238	1	G0410	99606	1	G0411	99235	1
G0410	99239	1	G0411	G0270	1	G0411	99236	1
G0410	99281	1	G0411	G0271	1	G0411	99238	1
G0410	99282	1	G0411	G0380	1	G0411	99239	1
G0410	99283	1	G0411	G0381	1	G0411	99281	1
G0410	99284	1	G0411	G0382	1	G0411	99282	1
G0410	99285	1	G0411	G0383	1	G0411	99283	1
G0410	99291	1	G0411	G0384	1	G0411	99284	1
G0410	99292	1	G0411	M0064	1	G0411	99285	1
G0410	99304	1	G0411	90862	1	G0411	99291	1
G0410	99305	1	G0411	96150	1	G0411	99292	1
G0410	99306	1	G0411	96151	1	G0411	99304	1
G0410	99307	1	G0411	96152	1	G0411	99305	1
G0410	99308	1	G0411	96153	1	G0411	99306	1
G0410	99309	1	G0411	96154	1	G0411	99307	1
G0410	99310	1	G0411	97802	1	G0411	99308	1
G0410	99315	1	G0411	97803	1	G0411	99309	1
G0410	99316	1	G0411	97804	1	G0411	99310	1
G0410	99318	1	G0411	99201	1	G0411	99315	1
G0410	99324	1	G0411	99202	1	G0411	99316	1
G0410	99325	1	G0411	99203	1	G0411	99318	1
G0410	99326	1	G0411	99204	1	G0411	99324	1
G0410	99327	1	G0411	99205	1	G0411	99325	1
G0410	99328	1	G0411	99211	1	G0411	99326	1
G0410	99334	1	G0411	99212	1	G0411	99327	1
G0410	99335	1	G0411	99213	1	G0411	99328	1
G0410	99336	1	G0411	99214	1	G0411	99334	1
G0410	99337	1	G0411	99215	1	G0411	99335	1
G0410	99341	1	G0411	99217	1	G0411	99336	1
G0410	99342	1	G0411	99218	1	G0411	99337	1
G0410	99343	1	G0411	99219	1	G0411	99341	1
G0410	99344	1	G0411	99220	1	G0411	99342	1
G0410	99345	1	G0411	99221	1	G0411	99343	1
G0410	99347	1	G0411	99222	1	G0411	99344	1
G0410	99348	1	G0411	99223	1	G0411	99345	1
G0410	99349	1	G0411	99224	1	G0411	99347	1
G0410	99350	1	G0411	99225	1	G0411	99348	1
G0410	99354	1	G0411	99226	1	G0411	99349	1

Column 1	Column 2	Modifier 0=not allowed 1=allowed 9=not applicable
G0411	99350	1
G0411	99354	1
G0411	99355	1
G0411	99356	1
G0411	99357	1
G0411	99605	1
G0411	99606	1
G0412	0213T	1
G0412	0216T	1
G0412	20680	1
G0412	27275	1
G0412	29000	1
G0412	29010	1
G0412	29015	1
G0412	29020	1
G0412	29025	1
G0412	29035	1
G0412	29040	1
G0412	29044	1
G0412	29046	1
G0412	29049	1
G0412	29305	1
G0412	29325	1
G0412	29520	1
G0412	29700	1
G0412	29705	1
G0412	29710	1
G0412	29715	1
G0412	36000	1
G0412	36400	1
G0412	36405	1
G0412	36406	1
G0412	36410	1
G0412	36420	1
G0412	36425	1
G0412	36430	1
G0412	36440	1
G0412	36600	1
G0412	36640	1
G0412	37202	1
G0412	43752	1
G0412	51701	1

Column 1	Column 2	Modifier 0=not allowed 1=allowed 9=not applicable
G0412	51702	1
G0412	51703	1
G0412	62318	1
G0412	62319	1
G0412	64400	1
G0412	64402	1
G0412	64405	1
G0412	64408	1
G0412	64410	1
G0412	64412	1
G0412	64413	1
G0412	64415	1
G0412	64416	1
G0412	64417	1
G0412	64418	1
G0412	64420	1
G0412	64421	1
G0412	64425	1
G0412	64430	1
G0412	64435	1
G0412	64445	1
G0412	64446	1
G0412	64447	1
G0412	64448	1
G0412	64449	1
G0412	64450	1
G0412	64479	1
G0412	64483	1
G0412	64490	1
G0412	64493	1
G0412	64505	1
G0412	64508	1
G0412	64510	1
G0412	64517	1
G0412	64520	1
G0412	64530	1
G0412	69990	0
G0412	73530	0
G0412	93000	1
G0412	93005	1
G0412	93010	1
G0412	93040	1

Column 1	Column 2	Modifier 0=not allowed 1=allowed 9=not applicable
G0412	93041	1
G0412	93042	1
G0412	93318	1
G0412	94002	1
G0412	94200	1
G0412	94250	1
G0412	94680	1
G0412	94681	1
G0412	94690	1
G0412	94770	1
G0412	95812	1
G0412	95813	1
G0412	95816	1
G0412	95819	1
G0412	95822	1
G0412	95829	1
G0412	95955	1
G0412	96360	1
G0412	96365	1
G0412	96372	1
G0412	96374	1
G0412	96375	1
G0412	96376	1
G0412	97597	1
G0412	97598	1
G0412	97602	1
G0412	97605	1
G0412	97606	1
G0412	99148	1
G0412	99149	1
G0412	99150	1
G0413	0213T	1
G0413	0216T	1
G0413	20650	1
G0413	20680	1
G0413	27193	1
G0413	27194	1
G0413	27275	1
G0413	29000	1
G0413	29010	1
G0413	29015	1
G0413	29020	1

Column 1	Column 2	Modifier 0=not allowed 1=allowed 9=not applicable
G0413	29025	1
G0413	29035	1
G0413	29040	1
G0413	29044	1
G0413	29046	1
G0413	29049	1
G0413	29305	1
G0413	29325	1
G0413	29520	1
G0413	29700	1
G0413	29705	1
G0413	29710	1
G0413	29715	1
G0413	36000	1
G0413	36400	1
G0413	36405	1
G0413	36406	1
G0413	36410	1
G0413	36420	1
G0413	36425	1
G0413	36430	1
G0413	36440	1
G0413	36600	1
G0413	36640	1
G0413	37202	1
G0413	43752	1
G0413	51701	1
G0413	51702	1
G0413	51703	1
G0413	62310	1
G0413	62311	1
G0413	62318	1
G0413	62319	1
G0413	64400	1
G0413	64402	1
G0413	64405	1
G0413	64408	1
G0413	64410	1
G0413	64412	1
G0413	64413	1
G0413	64415	1
G0413	64416	1

Column 1	Column 2	Modifier 0=not allowed 1=allowed 9=not applicable
G0413	64417	1
G0413	64418	1
G0413	64420	1
G0413	64421	1
G0413	64425	1
G0413	64430	1
G0413	64435	1
G0413	64445	1
G0413	64446	1
G0413	64447	1
G0413	64448	1
G0413	64449	1
G0413	64450	1
G0413	64479	1
G0413	64483	1
G0413	64490	1
G0413	64493	1
G0413	64505	1
G0413	64508	1
G0413	64510	1
G0413	64517	1
G0413	64520	1
G0413	64530	1
G0413	69990	0
G0413	73530	0
G0413	93000	1
G0413	93005	1
G0413	93010	1
G0413	93040	1
G0413	93041	1
G0413	93042	1
G0413	93318	1
G0413	94002	1
G0413	94200	1
G0413	94250	1
G0413	94680	1
G0413	94681	1
G0413	94690	1
G0413	94770	1
G0413	95812	1
G0413	95813	1
G0413	95816	1

Column 1	Column 2	Modifier 0=not allowed 1=allowed 9=not applicable
G0413	95819	1
G0413	95822	1
G0413	95829	1
G0413	95955	1
G0413	96360	1
G0413	96365	1
G0413	96372	1
G0413	96374	1
G0413	96375	1
G0413	96376	1
G0413	97597	1
G0413	97598	1
G0413	97602	1
G0413	97605	1
G0413	97606	1
G0413	99148	1
G0413	99149	1
G0413	99150	1
G0414	0213T	1
G0414	0216T	1
G0414	20650	1
G0414	20680	1
G0414	27275	1
G0414	29000	1
G0414	29010	1
G0414	29015	1
G0414	29020	1
G0414	29025	1
G0414	29035	1
G0414	29040	1
G0414	29044	1
G0414	29046	1
G0414	29049	1
G0414	29305	1
G0414	29325	1
G0414	29520	1
G0414	29700	1
G0414	29705	1
G0414	29710	1
G0414	29715	1
G0414	36000	1
G0414	36400	1

Column 1	Column 2	Modifier 0=not allowed 1=allowed 9=not applicable
G0414	36405	1
G0414	36406	1
G0414	36410	1
G0414	36420	1
G0414	36425	1
G0414	36430	1
G0414	36440	1
G0414	36600	1
G0414	36640	1
G0414	37202	1
G0414	43752	1
G0414	51701	1
G0414	51702	1
G0414	51703	1
G0414	62310	1
G0414	62311	1
G0414	62318	1
G0414	62319	1
G0414	64400	1
G0414	64402	1
G0414	64405	1
G0414	64408	1
G0414	64410	1
G0414	64412	1
G0414	64413	1
G0414	64415	1
G0414	64416	1
G0414	64417	1
G0414	64418	1
G0414	64420	1
G0414	64421	1
G0414	64425	1
G0414	64430	1
G0414	64435	1
G0414	64445	1
G0414	64446	1
G0414	64447	1
G0414	64448	1
G0414	64449	1
G0414	64450	1
G0414	64479	1
G0414	64483	1

Column 1	Column 2	Modifier
G0414	64490	1
G0414	64493	1
G0414	64505	1
G0414	64508	1
G0414	64510	1
G0414	64517	1
G0414	64520	1
G0414	64530	1
G0414	69990	0
G0414	73530	0
G0414	93000	1
G0414	93005	1
G0414	93010	1
G0414	93040	1
G0414	93041	1
G0414	93042	1
G0414	93318	1
G0414	94002	1
G0414	94200	1
G0414	94250	1
G0414	94680	1
G0414	94681	1
G0414	94690	1
G0414	94770	1
G0414	95812	1
G0414	95813	1
G0414	95816	1
G0414	95819	1
G0414	95822	1
G0414	95829	1
G0414	95955	1
G0414	96360	1
G0414	96365	1
G0414	96372	1
G0414	96374	1
G0414	96375	1
G0414	96376	1
G0414	97597	1
G0414	97598	1
G0414	97602	1
G0414	97605	1
G0414	97606	1

Column 1	Column 2	Modifier
G0414	99148	1
G0414	99149	1
G0414	99150	1
G0415	G0413	1
G0415	0213T	1
G0415	0216T	1
G0415	20650	1
G0415	20680	1
G0415	27275	1
G0415	29000	1
G0415	29010	1
G0415	29015	1
G0415	29020	1
G0415	29025	1
G0415	29035	1
G0415	29040	1
G0415	29044	1
G0415	29046	1
G0415	29049	1
G0415	29305	1
G0415	29325	1
G0415	29520	1
G0415	29700	1
G0415	29705	1
G0415	29710	1
G0415	29715	1
G0415	36000	1
G0415	36400	1
G0415	36405	1
G0415	36406	1
G0415	36410	1
G0415	36420	1
G0415	36425	1
G0415	36430	1
G0415	36440	1
G0415	36600	1
G0415	36640	1
G0415	37202	1
G0415	43752	1
G0415	51701	1
G0415	51702	1
G0415	51703	1

Column 1	Column 2	Modifier 0=not allowed 1=allowed 9=not applicable
G0415	62310	1
G0415	62311	1
G0415	62318	1
G0415	62319	1
G0415	64400	1
G0415	64402	1
G0415	64405	1
G0415	64408	1
G0415	64410	1
G0415	64412	1
G0415	64413	1
G0415	64415	1
G0415	64416	1
G0415	64417	1
G0415	64418	1
G0415	64420	1
G0415	64421	1
G0415	64425	1
G0415	64430	1
G0415	64435	1
G0415	64445	1
G0415	64446	1
G0415	64447	1
G0415	64448	1
G0415	64449	1
G0415	64450	1
G0415	64479	1
G0415	64483	1
G0415	64490	1
G0415	64493	1
G0415	64505	1
G0415	64508	1
G0415	64510	1
G0415	64517	1
G0415	64520	1
G0415	64530	1
G0415	69990	0
G0415	73530	0
G0415	93000	1
G0415	93005	1
G0415	93010	1
G0415	93040	1

Column 1	Column 2	Modifier 0=not allowed 1=allowed 9=not applicable
G0415	93041	1
G0415	93042	1
G0415	93318	1
G0415	94002	1
G0415	94200	1
G0415	94250	1
G0415	94680	1
G0415	94681	1
G0415	94690	1
G0415	94770	1
G0415	95812	1
G0415	95813	1
G0415	95816	1
G0415	95819	1
G0415	95822	1
G0415	95829	1
G0415	95955	1
G0415	96360	1
G0415	96365	1
G0415	96372	1
G0415	96374	1
G0415	96375	1
G0415	96376	1
G0415	97597	1
G0415	97598	1
G0415	97602	1
G0415	97605	1
G0415	97606	1
G0415	99148	1
G0415	99149	1
G0415	99150	1
G0416	88160	1
G0416	88161	1
G0416	88162	1
G0416	88302	1
G0416	88304	1
G0416	88305	1
G0416	88321	1
G0416	88323	1
G0416	88325	1
G0416	89060	1
G0417	G0416	0

Column 1	Column 2	Modifier 0=not allowed 1=allowed 9=not applicable
G0417	88160	1
G0417	88161	1
G0417	88162	1
G0417	88302	1
G0417	88304	1
G0417	88305	1
G0417	88321	1
G0417	88323	1
G0417	88325	1
G0417	89060	1
G0418	G0416	0
G0418	G0417	0
G0418	88160	1
G0418	88161	1
G0418	88162	1
G0418	88302	1
G0418	88304	1
G0418	88305	1
G0418	88321	1
G0418	88323	1
G0418	88325	1
G0418	89060	1
G0419	G0416	0
G0419	G0417	0
G0419	G0418	0
G0419	88160	1
G0419	88161	1
G0419	88162	1
G0419	88302	1
G0419	88304	1
G0419	88305	1
G0419	88321	1
G0419	88323	1
G0419	88325	1
G0419	89060	1
G0420	G0421	1
G0422	G0423	0
G0422	0178T	1
G0422	0179T	1
G0422	0180T	1
G0422	36000	1
G0422	36410	1

Column 1	Column 2	Modifier 0=not allowed 1=allowed 9=not applicable
G0422	51701	1
G0422	51702	1
G0422	51703	1
G0422	93000	1
G0422	93005	1
G0422	93010	1
G0422	93040	1
G0422	93041	1
G0422	93042	1
G0422	93268	1
G0422	93797	0
G0422	93798	0
G0422	94760	0
G0422	94761	0
G0422	97001	1
G0422	97002	1
G0422	97003	1
G0422	97004	1
G0422	97110	1
G0422	97112	1
G0422	97116	1
G0422	97140	1
G0422	97150	1
G0422	97530	1
G0422	97750	1
G0422	97802	1
G0422	97803	1
G0422	97804	1
G0422	99148	1
G0422	99149	1
G0422	99150	1
G0423	0178T	1
G0423	0179T	1
G0423	0180T	1
G0423	36000	1
G0423	36410	1
G0423	51701	1
G0423	51702	1
G0423	51703	1
G0423	93000	1
G0423	93005	1
G0423	93010	1

Column 1	Column 2	Modifier 0=not allowed 1=allowed 9=not applicable
G0423	93040	1
G0423	93041	1
G0423	93042	1
G0423	93268	1
G0423	93797	0
G0423	93798	0
G0423	94760	0
G0423	94761	0
G0423	97001	1
G0423	97002	1
G0423	97003	1
G0423	97004	1
G0423	97110	1
G0423	97112	1
G0423	97116	1
G0423	97140	1
G0423	97150	1
G0423	97530	1
G0423	97750	1
G0423	97802	1
G0423	97803	1
G0423	97804	1
G0423	99148	1
G0423	99149	1
G0423	99150	1
G0424	0178T	1
G0424	0179T	1
G0424	0180T	1
G0424	36000	1
G0424	36410	1
G0424	51701	1
G0424	51702	1
G0424	51703	1
G0424	93000	1
G0424	93005	1
G0424	93010	1
G0424	93040	1
G0424	93041	1
G0424	93042	1
G0424	93268	1
G0424	94010	1
G0424	94060	1

Column 1	Column 2	Modifier 0=not allowed 1=allowed 9=not applicable
G0424	94150	1
G0424	94200	1
G0424	94240	1
G0424	94250	1
G0424	94260	1
G0424	94350	1
G0424	94360	1
G0424	94370	1
G0424	94375	1
G0424	94400	1
G0424	94450	1
G0424	94620	0
G0424	94621	0
G0424	94667	1
G0424	94668	1
G0424	94680	1
G0424	94681	1
G0424	94690	1
G0424	94720	1
G0424	94725	1
G0424	94750	1
G0424	94760	0
G0424	94761	0
G0424	94762	1
G0424	94770	1
G0424	97001	1
G0424	97002	1
G0424	97003	1
G0424	97004	1
G0424	97110	1
G0424	97112	1
G0424	97150	1
G0424	97530	1
G0424	97750	1
G0424	97802	1
G0424	97803	1
G0424	97804	1
G0424	99148	1
G0424	99149	1
G0424	99150	1
G0428	0213T	1
G0428	0216T	1

Column 1	Column 2	Modifier 0=not allowed 1=allowed 9=not applicable
G0428	0228T	1
G0428	0230T	1
G0428	20600	1
G0428	20605	1
G0428	20610	1
G0428	27347	1
G0428	27570	1
G0428	29870	1
G0428	29871	1
G0428	29874	0
G0428	29875	1
G0428	29877	0
G0428	29881	1
G0428	29884	1
G0428	36000	1
G0428	36400	1
G0428	36405	1
G0428	36406	1
G0428	36410	1
G0428	36420	1
G0428	36425	1
G0428	36430	1
G0428	36440	1
G0428	36600	1
G0428	36640	1
G0428	37202	1
G0428	43752	1
G0428	51701	1
G0428	51702	1
G0428	51703	1
G0428	62310	1
G0428	62311	1
G0428	62318	1
G0428	62319	1
G0428	64400	1
G0428	64402	1
G0428	64405	1
G0428	64408	1
G0428	64410	1
G0428	64412	1
G0428	64413	1
G0428	64415	1

Column 1	Column 2	Modifier 0=not allowed 1=allowed 9=not applicable
G0428	64416	1
G0428	64417	1
G0428	64418	1
G0428	64420	1
G0428	64421	1
G0428	64425	1
G0428	64430	1
G0428	64435	1
G0428	64445	1
G0428	64446	1
G0428	64447	1
G0428	64448	1
G0428	64449	1
G0428	64450	1
G0428	64479	1
G0428	64483	1
G0428	64490	1
G0428	64493	1
G0428	64505	1
G0428	64508	1
G0428	64510	1
G0428	64517	1
G0428	64520	1
G0428	64530	1
G0428	69990	0
G0428	76000	1
G0428	76001	1
G0428	77001	1
G0428	77002	1
G0428	93000	1
G0428	93005	1
G0428	93010	1
G0428	93040	1
G0428	93041	1
G0428	93042	1
G0428	93318	1
G0428	94002	1
G0428	94200	1
G0428	94250	1
G0428	94680	1
G0428	94681	1
G0428	94690	1

Column 1	Column 2	Modifier 0=not allowed 1=allowed 9=not applicable
G0428	94770	1
G0428	95812	1
G0428	95813	1
G0428	95816	1
G0428	95819	1
G0428	95822	1
G0428	95829	1
G0428	95955	1
G0428	96360	1
G0428	96365	1
G0428	96372	1
G0428	96374	1
G0428	96375	1
G0428	96376	1
G0428	99148	1
G0428	99149	1
G0428	99150	1
G0429	0213T	1
G0429	0216T	1
G0429	0228T	1
G0429	0230T	1
G0429	36000	1
G0429	36400	1
G0429	36405	1
G0429	36406	1
G0429	36410	1
G0429	36420	1
G0429	36425	1
G0429	36430	1
G0429	36440	1
G0429	36600	1
G0429	36640	1
G0429	37202	1
G0429	43752	1
G0429	51701	1
G0429	51702	1
G0429	51703	1
G0429	62310	1
G0429	62311	1
G0429	62318	1
G0429	62319	1
G0429	64400	1

Column 1	Column 2	Modifier 0=not allowed 1=allowed 9=not applicable	Column 1	Column 2	Modifier 0=not allowed 1=allowed 9=not applicable	Column 1	Column 2	Modifier 0=not allowed 1=allowed 9=not applicable
G0429	64402	1	G0429	94680	1	G0437	92532	1
G0429	64405	1	G0429	94681	1	G0437	96101	1
G0429	64408	1	G0429	94690	1	G0437	96102	1
G0429	64410	1	G0429	94770	1	G0437	96103	1
G0429	64412	1	G0429	95812	1	G0437	96105	1
G0429	64413	1	G0429	95813	1	G0437	96118	1
G0429	64415	1	G0429	95816	1	G0437	96119	1
G0429	64416	1	G0429	95819	1	G0437	96120	1
G0429	64417	1	G0429	95822	1	G0437	96125	1
G0429	64418	1	G0429	95829	1	G0437	99408	1
G0429	64420	1	G0429	95955	1	G0437	99409	1
G0429	64421	1	G0429	96360	1	G0438	G0102	0
G0429	64425	1	G0429	96365	1	G0438	G0250	1
G0429	64430	1	G0429	96372	1	G0438	G0270	0
G0429	64435	1	G0429	96374	1	G0438	G0271	0
G0429	64445	1	G0429	96375	1	G0438	G0439	0
G0429	64446	1	G0429	96376	1	G0438	M0064	1
G0429	64447	1	G0429	99148	1	G0438	90801	1
G0429	64448	1	G0429	99149	1	G0438	90802	1
G0429	64449	1	G0429	99150	1	G0438	90804	1
G0429	64450	1	G0431	80500	1	G0438	90805	1
G0429	64479	1	G0431	80502	1	G0438	90806	1
G0429	64483	1	G0431	83516	1	G0438	90807	1
G0429	64490	1	G0431	83518	1	G0438	90808	1
G0429	64493	1	G0436	G0396	1	G0438	90809	1
G0429	64505	1	G0436	G0397	1	G0438	90810	1
G0429	64508	1	G0436	92531	1	G0438	90811	1
G0429	64510	1	G0436	92532	1	G0438	90812	1
G0429	64517	1	G0436	96101	1	G0438	90813	1
G0429	64520	1	G0436	96102	1	G0438	90814	1
G0429	64530	1	G0436	96103	1	G0438	90815	1
G0429	69990	0	G0436	96105	1	G0438	90816	1
G0429	93000	1	G0436	96118	1	G0438	90817	1
G0429	93005	1	G0436	96119	1	G0438	90818	1
G0429	93010	1	G0436	96120	1	G0438	90819	1
G0429	93040	1	G0436	96125	1	G0438	90821	1
G0429	93041	1	G0436	99408	1	G0438	90822	1
G0429	93042	1	G0436	99409	1	G0438	90823	1
G0429	93318	1	G0437	G0396	1	G0438	90824	1
G0429	94002	1	G0437	G0397	1	G0438	90826	1
G0429	94200	1	G0437	G0436	0	G0438	90827	1
G0429	94250	1	G0437	92531	1	G0438	90828	1

Column 1	Column 2	Modifier 0=not allowed 1=allowed 9=not applicable
G0438	90829	1
G0438	90845	1
G0438	90862	1
G0438	92002	1
G0438	92004	1
G0438	92012	1
G0438	92014	1
G0438	93000	1
G0438	93005	1
G0438	93010	1
G0438	93040	1
G0438	93041	1
G0438	93042	1
G0438	95831	1
G0438	95832	1
G0438	95833	1
G0438	95834	1
G0438	95851	1
G0438	95852	1
G0438	96116	1
G0438	96150	0
G0438	96151	0
G0438	96152	0
G0438	96153	0
G0438	96154	0
G0438	97802	0
G0438	97803	0
G0438	97804	0
G0439	G0102	0
G0439	G0250	1
G0439	G0270	0
G0439	G0271	0
G0439	M0064	1
G0439	90801	1
G0439	90802	1
G0439	90804	1
G0439	90805	1
G0439	90806	1
G0439	90807	1
G0439	90808	1
G0439	90809	1
G0439	90810	1

Column 1	Column 2	Modifier 0=not allowed 1=allowed 9=not applicable
G0439	90811	1
G0439	90812	1
G0439	90813	1
G0439	90814	1
G0439	90815	1
G0439	90816	1
G0439	90817	1
G0439	90818	1
G0439	90819	1
G0439	90821	1
G0439	90822	1
G0439	90823	1
G0439	90824	1
G0439	90826	1
G0439	90827	1
G0439	90828	1
G0439	90829	1
G0439	90845	1
G0439	90862	1
G0439	92002	1
G0439	92004	1
G0439	92012	1
G0439	92014	1
G0439	93000	1
G0439	93005	1
G0439	93010	1
G0439	93040	1
G0439	93041	1
G0439	93042	1
G0439	95831	1
G0439	95832	1
G0439	95833	1
G0439	95834	1
G0439	95851	1
G0439	95852	1
G0439	96116	1
G0439	96150	0
G0439	96151	0
G0439	96152	0
G0439	96153	0
G0439	96154	0
G0439	97802	0

Column 1	Column 2	Modifier 0=not allowed 1=allowed 9=not applicable
G0439	97803	0
G0439	97804	0
G0440	G0168	1
G0440	0213T	1
G0440	0216T	1
G0440	0228T	1
G0440	0230T	1
G0440	11000	1
G0440	11042	1
G0440	12001	1
G0440	12002	1
G0440	12004	1
G0440	12005	1
G0440	12006	1
G0440	12007	1
G0440	12020	1
G0440	12021	1
G0440	12031	1
G0440	12032	1
G0440	12034	1
G0440	12035	1
G0440	12036	1
G0440	12037	1
G0440	13100	1
G0440	13101	1
G0440	13120	1
G0440	13121	1
G0440	15852	1
G0440	16020	1
G0440	16025	1
G0440	16030	1
G0440	29000	1
G0440	29010	1
G0440	29015	1
G0440	29020	1
G0440	29025	1
G0440	29035	1
G0440	29040	1
G0440	29044	1
G0440	29046	1
G0440	29049	1
G0440	29055	1

Column 1	Column 2	Modifier 0=not allowed 1=allowed 9=not applicable	Column 1	Column 2	Modifier 0=not allowed 1=allowed 9=not applicable	Column 1	Column 2	Modifier 0=not allowed 1=allowed 9=not applicable
G0440	29058	1	G0440	36430	1	G0440	64517	1
G0440	29065	1	G0440	36440	1	G0440	64520	1
G0440	29075	1	G0440	36600	1	G0440	64530	1
G0440	29085	1	G0440	36640	1	G0440	69990	0
G0440	29086	1	G0440	37202	1	G0440	93000	1
G0440	29105	1	G0440	43752	1	G0440	93005	1
G0440	29125	1	G0440	51701	1	G0440	93010	1
G0440	29126	1	G0440	51702	1	G0440	93040	1
G0440	29130	1	G0440	51703	1	G0440	93041	1
G0440	29131	1	G0440	62310	1	G0440	93042	1
G0440	29200	1	G0440	62311	1	G0440	93318	1
G0440	29240	1	G0440	62318	1	G0440	94002	1
G0440	29260	1	G0440	62319	1	G0440	94200	1
G0440	29280	1	G0440	64400	1	G0440	94250	1
G0440	29305	1	G0440	64402	1	G0440	94680	1
G0440	29325	1	G0440	64405	1	G0440	94681	1
G0440	29345	1	G0440	64408	1	G0440	94690	1
G0440	29355	1	G0440	64410	1	G0440	94770	1
G0440	29358	1	G0440	64412	1	G0440	95812	1
G0440	29365	1	G0440	64413	1	G0440	95813	1
G0440	29405	1	G0440	64415	1	G0440	95816	1
G0440	29425	1	G0440	64416	1	G0440	95819	1
G0440	29435	1	G0440	64417	1	G0440	95822	1
G0440	29440	1	G0440	64418	1	G0440	95829	1
G0440	29445	1	G0440	64420	1	G0440	95955	1
G0440	29450	1	G0440	64421	1	G0440	96360	1
G0440	29505	1	G0440	64425	1	G0440	96365	1
G0440	29515	1	G0440	64430	1	G0440	96372	1
G0440	29520	1	G0440	64435	1	G0440	96374	1
G0440	29530	1	G0440	64445	1	G0440	96375	1
G0440	29540	1	G0440	64446	1	G0440	96376	1
G0440	29550	1	G0440	64447	1	G0440	97597	1
G0440	29580	1	G0440	64448	1	G0440	97598	1
G0440	29581	1	G0440	64449	1	G0440	97602	1
G0440	29590	1	G0440	64450	1	G0440	97605	1
G0440	36000	1	G0440	64479	1	G0440	97606	1
G0440	36400	1	G0440	64483	1	G0440	99148	1
G0440	36405	1	G0440	64490	1	G0440	99149	1
G0440	36406	1	G0440	64493	1	G0440	99150	1
G0440	36410	1	G0440	64505	1	G0441	36000	1
G0440	36420	1	G0440	64508	1	G0441	36400	1
G0440	36425	1	G0440	64510	1	G0441	36405	1

Column 1	Column 2	Modifier 0=not allowed 1=allowed 9=not applicable
G0441	36406	1
G0441	36410	1
G0441	36420	1
G0441	36425	1
G0441	36430	1
G0441	36440	1
G0441	36600	1
G0441	36640	1
G0441	37202	1
G0441	43752	1
G0441	62310	1
G0441	62311	1
G0441	62318	1
G0441	62319	1
G0441	64400	1
G0441	64402	1
G0441	64405	1
G0441	64408	1
G0441	64410	1
G0441	64412	1
G0441	64413	1
G0441	64415	1
G0441	64416	1
G0441	64417	1
G0441	64418	1
G0441	64420	1
G0441	64421	1
G0441	64425	1
G0441	64430	1
G0441	64435	1
G0441	64445	1
G0441	64446	1
G0441	64447	1
G0441	64448	1
G0441	64449	1
G0441	64450	1
G0441	64479	1
G0441	64483	1
G0441	64490	1
G0441	64493	1
G0441	64505	1
G0441	64508	1

Column 1	Column 2	Modifier 0=not allowed 1=allowed 9=not applicable
G0441	64510	1
G0441	64517	1
G0441	64520	1
G0441	64530	1
G0441	93000	1
G0441	93005	1
G0441	93010	1
G0441	93040	1
G0441	93041	1
G0441	93042	1
G0441	93318	1
G0441	94002	1
G0441	94200	1
G0441	94250	1
G0441	94680	1
G0441	94681	1
G0441	94690	1
G0441	94770	1
G0441	95812	1
G0441	95813	1
G0441	95816	1
G0441	95819	1
G0441	95822	1
G0441	95829	1
G0441	95955	1
G0441	96360	1
G0441	96365	1
G0441	96372	1
G0441	96374	1
G0441	96375	1
G0441	96376	1
G0441	99148	1
G0441	99149	1
G0441	99150	1
G3001	C8957	1
G3001	36000	1
G3001	36410	1
G3001	77750	0
G3001	78800	0
G3001	78801	0
G3001	78802	0
G3001	78803	0

Column 1	Column 2	Modifier 0=not allowed 1=allowed 9=not applicable
G3001	78999	0
G3001	96360	1
G3001	96365	1
G3001	96372	1
G3001	96374	1
G3001	96375	1
G3001	96376	1
G3001	96409	1
G3001	96413	1
G3001	96416	1
M0064	99605	1
M0064	99606	1
P3000	G0380	1
P3000	G0381	1
P3000	G0382	1
P3000	G0383	1
P3000	G0384	1
P3000	88160	1
P3000	88161	1
P3000	99201	1
P3000	99202	1
P3000	99203	1
P3000	99204	1
P3000	99205	1
P3000	99211	1
P3000	99212	1
P3000	99213	1
P3000	99214	1
P3000	99215	1
P3000	99217	1
P3000	99218	1
P3000	99219	1
P3000	99220	1
P3000	99221	1
P3000	99222	1
P3000	99223	1
P3000	99224	1
P3000	99225	1
P3000	99226	1
P3000	99231	1
P3000	99232	1
P3000	99233	1

Column 1	Column 2	Modifier 0=not allowed 1=allowed 9=not applicable
P3000	99234	1
P3000	99235	1
P3000	99236	1
P3000	99238	1
P3000	99239	1
P3000	99281	1
P3000	99282	1
P3000	99283	1
P3000	99284	1
P3000	99285	1
P3000	99291	1
P3000	99292	1
P3000	99304	1
P3000	99305	1
P3000	99306	1
P3000	99307	1
P3000	99308	1
P3000	99309	1
P3000	99310	1
P3000	99315	1
P3000	99316	1
P3000	99318	1
P3000	99324	1
P3000	99325	1
P3000	99326	1
P3000	99327	1
P3000	99328	1
P3000	99334	1
P3000	99335	1
P3000	99336	1
P3000	99337	1
P3000	99341	1
P3000	99342	1
P3000	99343	1
P3000	99344	1
P3000	99345	1
P3000	99347	1
P3000	99348	1
P3000	99349	1
P3000	99350	1
P3000	99354	1
P3000	99355	1

Column 1	Column 2	Modifier 0=not allowed 1=allowed 9=not applicable
P3000	99356	1
P3000	99357	1
P3000	99360	1
P3000	99455	1
P3000	99456	1
P3000	99460	1
P3000	99461	1
P3000	99462	1
P3000	99463	1
P3000	99464	1
P3000	99465	1
P3000	99466	1
P3000	99468	1
P3000	99469	1
P3000	99471	1
P3000	99472	1
P3000	99475	1
P3000	99476	1
P3000	99477	1
P3000	99478	1
P3000	99479	1
P3000	99480	1
P3001	G0123	0
P3001	G0141	0
P3001	G0143	0
P3001	G0144	0
P3001	G0145	0
P3001	G0147	0
P3001	G0148	0
P3001	G0380	1
P3001	G0381	1
P3001	G0382	1
P3001	G0383	1
P3001	G0384	1
P3001	88141	0
P3001	88142	0
P3001	88143	0
P3001	88147	0
P3001	88148	0
P3001	88150	0
P3001	88152	0
P3001	88153	0

Column 1	Column 2	Modifier 0=not allowed 1=allowed 9=not applicable
P3001	88154	0
P3001	88164	0
P3001	88165	0
P3001	88166	0
P3001	88167	0
P3001	88174	0
P3001	88175	0
P3001	99201	1
P3001	99202	1
P3001	99203	1
P3001	99204	1
P3001	99205	1
P3001	99211	1
P3001	99212	1
P3001	99213	1
P3001	99214	1
P3001	99215	1
P3001	99217	1
P3001	99218	1
P3001	99219	1
P3001	99220	1
P3001	99221	1
P3001	99222	1
P3001	99223	1
P3001	99224	1
P3001	99225	1
P3001	99226	1
P3001	99231	1
P3001	99232	1
P3001	99233	1
P3001	99234	1
P3001	99235	1
P3001	99236	1
P3001	99238	1
P3001	99239	1
P3001	99281	1
P3001	99282	1
P3001	99283	1
P3001	99284	1
P3001	99285	1
P3001	99291	1
P3001	99292	1

Column 1	Column 2	Modifier 0=not allowed 1=allowed 9=not applicable	Column 1	Column 2	Modifier 0=not allowed 1=allowed 9=not applicable	Column 1	Column 2	Modifier 0=not allowed 1=allowed 9=not applicable
P3001	99304	1	P3001	99468	1	P9036	P9039	1
P3001	99305	1	P3001	99469	1	P9037	P9010	1
P3001	99306	1	P3001	99471	1	P9037	P9011	1
P3001	99307	1	P3001	99472	1	P9037	P9016	1
P3001	99308	1	P3001	99475	1	P9037	P9019	1
P3001	99309	1	P3001	99476	1	P9037	P9020	1
P3001	99310	1	P3001	99477	1	P9037	P9021	1
P3001	99315	1	P3001	99478	1	P9037	P9022	1
P3001	99316	1	P3001	99479	1	P9037	P9031	1
P3001	99318	1	P3001	99480	1	P9037	P9034	1
P3001	99324	1	P9032	P9010	1	P9037	P9035	1
P3001	99325	1	P9032	P9011	1	P9037	P9039	1
P3001	99326	1	P9032	P9016	1	P9038	P9010	1
P3001	99327	1	P9032	P9019	1	P9038	P9011	1
P3001	99328	1	P9032	P9020	1	P9038	P9016	1
P3001	99334	1	P9032	P9021	1	P9038	P9019	1
P3001	99335	1	P9032	P9022	1	P9038	P9020	1
P3001	99336	1	P9032	P9031	1	P9038	P9021	1
P3001	99337	1	P9032	P9034	1	P9038	P9022	1
P3001	99341	1	P9032	P9035	1	P9038	P9031	1
P3001	99342	1	P9032	P9039	1	P9038	P9034	1
P3001	99343	1	P9033	P9010	1	P9038	P9035	1
P3001	99344	1	P9033	P9011	1	P9038	P9039	1
P3001	99345	1	P9033	P9016	1	P9040	P9010	1
P3001	99347	1	P9033	P9019	1	P9040	P9011	1
P3001	99348	1	P9033	P9020	1	P9040	P9016	1
P3001	99349	1	P9033	P9021	1	P9040	P9019	1
P3001	99350	1	P9033	P9022	1	P9040	P9020	1
P3001	99354	1	P9033	P9031	1	P9040	P9021	1
P3001	99355	1	P9033	P9034	1	P9040	P9022	1
P3001	99356	1	P9033	P9035	1	P9040	P9031	1
P3001	99357	1	P9033	P9039	1	P9040	P9034	1
P3001	99360	1	P9036	P9010	1	P9040	P9035	1
P3001	99455	1	P9036	P9011	1	P9040	P9039	1
P3001	99456	1	P9036	P9016	1	Q0091	G0181	1
P3001	99460	1	P9036	P9019	1	Q0091	G0182	1
P3001	99461	1	P9036	P9020	1	Q0091	G0380	1
P3001	99462	1	P9036	P9021	1	Q0091	G0381	1
P3001	99463	1	P9036	P9022	1	Q0091	G0382	1
P3001	99464	1	P9036	P9031	1	Q0091	G0383	1
P3001	99465	1	P9036	P9034	1	Q0091	G0384	1
P3001	99466	1	P9036	P9035	1	Q0091	99201	1

Column 1	Column 2	Modifier 0=not allowed 1=allowed 9=not applicable
Q0091	99202	1
Q0091	99203	1
Q0091	99204	1
Q0091	99205	1
Q0091	99211	1
Q0091	99212	1
Q0091	99213	1
Q0091	99214	1
Q0091	99215	1
Q0091	99217	1
Q0091	99218	1
Q0091	99219	1
Q0091	99220	1
Q0091	99221	1
Q0091	99222	1
Q0091	99223	1
Q0091	99224	1
Q0091	99225	1
Q0091	99226	1
Q0091	99231	1
Q0091	99232	1
Q0091	99233	1
Q0091	99234	1
Q0091	99235	1
Q0091	99236	1
Q0091	99238	1
Q0091	99239	1
Q0091	99281	1
Q0091	99282	1

Column 1	Column 2	Modifier 0=not allowed 1=allowed 9=not applicable
Q0091	99283	1
Q0091	99284	1
Q0091	99285	1
Q0091	99291	1
Q0091	99292	1
Q0091	99304	1
Q0091	99305	1
Q0091	99306	1
Q0091	99307	1
Q0091	99308	1
Q0091	99309	1
Q0091	99310	1
Q0091	99315	1
Q0091	99316	1
Q0091	99318	1
Q0091	99324	1
Q0091	99325	1
Q0091	99326	1
Q0091	99327	1
Q0091	99328	1
Q0091	99334	1
Q0091	99335	1
Q0091	99336	1
Q0091	99337	1
Q0091	99341	1
Q0091	99342	1
Q0091	99343	1
Q0091	99344	1
Q0091	99345	1

Column 1	Column 2	Modifier 0=not allowed 1=allowed 9=not applicable
Q0091	99347	1
Q0091	99348	1
Q0091	99349	1
Q0091	99350	1
Q0091	99354	1
Q0091	99355	1
Q0091	99356	1
Q0091	99357	1
Q0091	99360	1
Q0091	99455	1
Q0091	99456	1
Q0091	99460	1
Q0091	99461	1
Q0091	99462	1
Q0091	99463	1
Q0091	99464	1
Q0091	99465	1
Q0091	99466	1
Q0091	99468	1
Q0091	99469	1
Q0091	99471	1
Q0091	99472	1
Q0091	99475	1
Q0091	99476	1
Q0091	99477	1
Q0091	99478	1
Q0091	99479	1
Q0091	99480	1
R0075	R0070	1

APPENDIX C

GENERAL CORRECT CODING POLICIES FOR NATIONAL CORRECT CODING INITIATIVE POLICY MANUAL FOR MEDICARE SERVICES

Current Procedural Terminology © 2009 American Medical Association. All Rights Reserved.

Current Procedural Terminology (CPT) is copyright 2009 American Medical Association. All Rights Reserved. No fee schedules, basic units, relative values, or related listings are included in CPT. The AMA assumes no liability for the data contained herein. Applicable FARS/DFARS restrictions apply to government use.

CPT® is a trademark of the American Medical Association.

Chapter I

Version 16.3

GENERAL CORRECT CODING POLICIES

A. Introduction

Healthcare providers utilize HCPCS/CPT codes to report medical services performed on patients to Medicare Carriers (A/B MACs processing practitioner service claims) and Fiscal Intermediaries (FIs). HCPCS (Healthcare Common Procedure Coding System) consists of Level I CPT (Current Procedural Terminology) codes and Level II codes. CPT codes are defined in the American Medical Association's (AMA) *CPT Manual* which is updated and published annually. HCPCS Level II codes are defined by the Centers for Medicare and Medicaid Services (CMS) and are updated throughout the year as necessary. Changes in CPT codes are approved by the AMA CPT Editorial Panel which meets three times per year.

CPT and HCPCS Level II codes define medical and surgical procedures performed on patients. Some procedure codes are very specific defining a single service (e.g., CPT code 93000 (electrocardiogram)) while other codes define procedures consisting of many services (e.g., CPT code 58263 (vaginal hysterectomy with removal of tube(s) and ovary(s) and repair of enterocele)). Because many procedures can be performed by different approaches, different methods, or in combination with other procedures, there are often multiple HCPCS/CPT codes defining similar or related procedures.

CPT and HCPCS Level II code descriptors usually do not define all services included in a procedure. There are often services inherent in a procedure or group of procedures. For example, anesthesia services include certain preparation and monitoring services.

The CMS developed the NCCI to prevent inappropriate payment of services that should not be reported together. There are two NCCI edit tables: "Column One/Column Two Correct Coding Edit Table" and "Mutually Exclusive Edit Table." Each edit table contains edits which are pairs of HCPCS/CPT codes that in general should not be reported together. Each edit has a column one and column two HCPCS/CPT code. If a provider reports the two codes of an edit pair, the column two code is denied, and the column one code is eligible for payment. However, if it is clinically appropriate to utilize an NCCI-associated modifier, both the column one and column two codes are eligible for payment. (NCCI-associated modifiers and their appropriate use are discussed elsewhere in this chapter.) All edits are included in the "Column One/Column Two Correct Coding Edit Table" except those that are based on the "mutually exclusive" (Chapter I, Section P) and "gender-specific" (Chapter I, Section Q) criteria in which case the edits are included in the "Mutually Exclusive Edit Table."

When the NCCI was first established and during its early years, the "Column One/Column Two Correct Coding Edit Table" was termed the "Comprehensive/Component Edit Table." This latter terminology was a misnomer. Although the column two code is often a component of a more comprehensive column one code, this relationship is not true for many edits. In the latter type of edit the code pair edit simply represents two codes that should not be reported together. For example, a provider should not report a vaginal hysterectomy code and total abdominal hysterectomy code together.

In this Manual many policies are described utilizing the term "physician." Unless indicated differently the usage of this term does not restrict the policies to physicians only but applies to all practitioners, hospitals, providers, or suppliers eligible to bill the relevant HCPCS/CPT codes pursuant to applicable portions of the Social Security Act (SSA) of 1965, the Code of Federal Regulations (CFR), and Medicare rules. In some sections of this Manual, the term "physician" would not include some of these entities because specific rules do not apply to them. For example, Anesthesia Rules and Global Surgery Rules do not apply to hospitals.

In 2010 the *CPT Manual* modified the numbering of codes so that the sequence of codes as they appear in the *CPT Manual* does not necessarily correspond to a sequential numbering of codes. In the *National Correct Coding Initiative Policy Manual for Medicare Services*, use of a numerical range of codes reflects all codes that numerically fall within the range regardless of their sequential order in the *CPT Manual*.

This chapter addresses general coding principles, issues, and policies. Many of these principles, issues, and policies are addressed further in subsequent chapters dealing with specific groups of HCPCS/CPT codes. In this chapter examples are often utilized to clarify principles, issues, or policies. The examples do not represent the only codes to which the principles, issues, or policies apply.

B. Coding Based on Standards of Medical/Surgical Practice

Most HCPCS/CPT code defined procedures include services that are integral to them. Some of these integral services have specific CPT codes for reporting the service when not performed as an integral part of another procedure. (For example, CPT code 36000 (introduction of needle or intracatheter into a vein) is integral to all nuclear medicine procedures requiring injection of a radiopharmaceutical into a vein. CPT code 36000 is not separately reportable with these types of nuclear medicine procedures. However, CPT code 36000 may be reported alone if the only service provided is the introduction of a needle into a vein. Other integral services do not have specific CPT codes. (For example, wound irrigation is integral to the treatment of all wounds and does not have a HCPCS/CPT code.) Services integral to HCPCS/CPT code defined procedures are included in those procedures based on the standards of medical/surgical practice. It is inappropriate to separately report services that are integral to another procedure with that procedure.

Many NCCI edits are based on the standards of medical/surgical practice. Services that are integral to another service are component parts of the more comprehensive service. When integral component services have their own HCPCS/CPT codes, NCCI edits place the comprehensive service in column one and the component service in column two. Since a component service integral to a comprehensive service is not separately reportable, the column two code is not separately reportable with the column one code.

Some services are integral to large numbers of procedures. Other services are integral to a more limited number of procedures. Examples of services integral to a large number of procedures include:

- Cleansing, shaving and prepping of skin
- Draping and positioning of patient
- Insertion of intravenous access for medication administration
- Insertion of urinary catheter
- Sedative administration by the physician performing a procedure (see Chapter II, Anesthesia Services)
- Local, topical or regional anesthesia administered by the physician performing the procedure
- Surgical approach including identification of anatomical landmarks, incision, evaluation of the surgical field, debridement of traumatized tissue, lysis of adhesions, and isolation of structures limiting access to the surgical field such as bone, blood vessels, nerve, and muscles including stimulation for identification or monitoring
- Surgical cultures
- Wound irrigation
- Insertion and removal of drains, suction devices, and pumps into same site
- Surgical closure and dressings
- Application, management, and removal of postoperative dressings and analgesic devices (peri-incisional)
- TENS unit
- Institution of Patient Controlled Anesthesia
- Preoperative, intraoperative and postoperative documentation, including photographs, drawings, dictation, or transcription as necessary to document the services provided
- Surgical supplies, except for specific situations where CMS policy permits separate payment

Although other chapters in this Manual further address issues related to the standards of medical/surgical practice for the procedures covered by that chapter, it is not possible because of space limitations to discuss all NCCI edits based on the principle of the standards of medical/surgical practice. However, there are several general principles that can be applied to the edits as follows:

1. The component service is an accepted standard of care when performing the comprehensive service.
2. The component service is usually necessary to complete the comprehensive service.
3. The component service is not a separately distinguishable procedure when performed with the comprehensive service.

Specific examples of services that are not separately reportable because they are components of more comprehensive services follow:

Medical:

1. Since interpretation of cardiac rhythm is an integral component of the interpretation of an electrocardiogram, a rhythm strip is not separately reportable.
2. Since determination of ankle/brachial indices requires both upper and lower extremity doppler studies, an upper extremity doppler study is not separately reportable.
3. Since a cardiac stress test includes multiple electrocardiograms, an electrocardiogram is not separately reportable.

Surgical:

1. Since a myringotomy requires access to the tympanic membrane through the external auditory canal, removal of impacted cerumen from the external auditory canal is not separately reportable.
2. A "scout" bronchoscopy to assess the surgical field, anatomic landmarks, extent of disease, etc., is not separately reportable with an open pulmonary procedure such as a pulmonary lobectomy. By contrast, an initial diagnostic bronchoscopy is separately reportable. If the diagnostic bronchoscopy is performed at the same patient encounter as the open pulmonary procedure and does not duplicate an earlier diagnostic bronchoscopy by the same or another physician, the diagnostic bronchoscopy may be reported with modifier –58 to indicate a staged procedure. A cursory examination of the upper airway during a bronchoscopy with the bronchoscope should not be reported separately as a laryngoscopy. However, separate endoscopies of anatomically distinct areas with different endoscopes may be reported separately (e.g., thoracoscopy and mediastinoscopy).
3. Since a colectomy requires exposure of the colon, the laparotomy and adhesiolysis to expose the colon are not separately reportable.

C. Medical/Surgical Package

Most medical and surgical procedures include pre-procedure, intra-procedure, and post-procedure work. When multiple procedures are performed at the same patient encounter, there is often overlap of the pre-procedure and post-procedure work. Payment methodologies for surgical procedures account for the overlap of the pre-procedure and post-procedure work.

The component elements of the pre-procedure and post-procedure work for each procedure are included component services of that procedure as a standard of medical/surgical practice. Some general guidelines follow:

1. Many invasive procedures require vascular and/or airway access. The work associated with obtaining the required access is included in the pre-procedure or intra-procedure work. The work associated with returning a patient to the appropriate post-procedure state is included in the post-procedure work.

Airway access is necessary for general anesthesia and is not separately reportable. There is no CPT code for elective endotracheal intubation. CPT code 31500 describes an emergency endotracheal intubation and should not be reported for elective endotracheal intubation. Visualization of the airway is a component part of an endotracheal intubation, and CPT codes describing procedures that visualize the airway (e.g., nasal endoscopy, laryngoscopy, bronchoscopy) should not be reported with an endotracheal intubation. These CPT codes describe diagnostic and therapeutic endoscopies, and it is a misuse of these codes to report visualization of the airway for endotracheal intubation.

Intravenous access (e.g., CPT codes 36000, 36400, 36410) is not separately reportable when performed with many types of procedures (e.g., surgical procedures, anesthesia procedures, radiological procedures requiring intravenous contrast, nuclear medicine procedures requiring intravenous radiopharmaceutical).

After vascular access is achieved, the access must be maintained by a slow infusion (e.g., saline) or injection of heparin or saline into a "lock". Since these services are necessary for maintenance of the vascular access, they are not separately reportable with the vascular access CPT codes or procedures requiring vascular access as a standard of medical/surgical practice. CPT code 37201 (Transcatheter therapy, infusion for thrombolysis other than coronary) should not be reported for use of an anticoagulant to maintain vascular access.

The global surgical package includes the administration of fluids and drugs during the operative procedure. CPT codes 96360-96376 should not be reported separately. Under OPPS, the administration of fluids and drugs during or for an operative procedure are included services and are not separately reportable (e.g., CPT codes 96360-96376).

When a procedure requires more invasive vascular access services (e.g., central venous access, pulmonary artery access), the more invasive vascular service is separately reportable if it is not typical of the procedure and the work of the more invasive vascular service has not been included in the valuation of the procedure.

Insertion of a central venous access device (e.g., central venous catheter, pulmonary artery catheter) requires passage of a catheter through central venous vessels and, in the case of a pulmonary artery catheter, through the right atrium and ventricle. These services often require the use of fluoroscopic guidance. Separate reporting of CPT codes for right heart catheterization, selective venous catheterization, or pulmonary artery catheterization is not appropriate when reporting a CPT code for insertion of a central venous access device. Since CPT code 77001 describes fluoroscopic guidance for central venous access device procedures, CPT codes for more general fluoroscopy (e.g., 76000, 76001, 77002) should not be reported separately.

2. Medicare Anesthesia Rules prevent separate payment for anesthesia services by the same physician performing a surgical or medical procedure. The physician performing a surgical or medical procedure should not report CPT codes 96360-96376 for the administration of anesthetic agents during the procedure. If it is medically reasonable and necessary that a separate provider (anesthesia practitioner) perform anesthesia services (e.g., monitored anesthesia care) for a surgical or medical procedure, a separate anesthesia service may be reported by the second provider.

Under OPPS, anesthesia for a surgical procedure is an included service and is not separately reportable. For example, a provider should not report CPT codes 96360-96376 for anesthesia services.

When anesthesia services are not separately reportable, physicians and facilities should not unbundle components of anesthesia and report them in lieu of an anesthesia code.

3. Many procedures require cardiopulmonary monitoring either by the physician performing the procedure or an anesthesia practitioner. Since these services are integral to the procedure, they are not separately reportable. Examples of these services include cardiac monitoring, pulse oximetry, and ventilation management (e.g., 93000-93010, 93040-93042, 94760, 94761, 94770).
4. A biopsy performed at the time of another more extensive procedure (e.g., excision, destruction, removal) is separately reportable under specific circumstances.

If the biopsy is performed on a separate lesion, it is separately reportable. This situation may be reported with anatomic modifiers or modifier -59.

If the biopsy is performed on the same lesion on which a more extensive procedure is performed, it is separately reportable only if the biopsy is utilized for immediate pathologic diagnosis prior to the more extensive procedure, and the decision to proceed with the more extensive procedure is based on the diagnosis established by the pathologic examination. The biopsy is not separately reportable if the pathologic examination at the time of surgery is for the purpose of assessing margins of resection or verifying resectability. When separately reportable modifier -58 may be reported to indicate that the biopsy and the more extensive procedure were planned or staged procedures.

If a biopsy is performed and submitted for pathologic evaluation that will be completed after the more extensive procedure is performed, the biopsy is not separately reportable with the more extensive procedure.

If a single lesion is biopsied multiple times, only one biopsy code may be reported with a single unit of service. If multiple lesions are non-endoscopically biopsied, a biopsy code may be reported for each lesion appending a modifier indicating that each biopsy was performed on a separate lesion. For endoscopic biopsies, multiple biopsies of a single or multiple lesions are reported with one unit of service of the biopsy code. If it is medically reasonable and necessary to submit multiple biopsies of the same or different lesions for separate pathologic examination, the medical record must identify the precise location and separate nature of each biopsy.

5. Exposure and exploration of the surgical field is integral to an operative procedure and is not separately reportable. For example, an exploratory laparotomy (CPT code 49000) is not separately reportable with an intra-abdominal procedure. If exploration of the surgical field results in additional procedures other than the primary procedure, the additional procedures may generally be reported separately. However, a procedure designated by the CPT code descriptor as a "separate procedure" is not separately reportable if performed in a region anatomically related to the other procedure(s) through the same skin incision, orifice, or surgical approach.

6. If a definitive surgical procedure requires access through diseased tissue (e.g., necrotic skin, abscess, hematoma, seroma), a separate service for this access (e.g., debridement, incision and drainage) is not separately reportable. For example, debridement of skin to repair a fracture is not separately reportable.

7. If removal, destruction, or other form of elimination of a lesion requires coincidental elimination of other pathology, only the primary procedure may be reported. For example, if an area of pilonidal disease contains an abscess, incision and drainage of the abscess during the procedure to excise the area of pilonidal disease is not separately reportable.

8. An excision and removal (–ectomy) includes the incision and opening (–otomy) of the organ. A HCPCS/CPT code for an –otomy procedure should not be reported with an –ectomy code for the same organ.

9. Multiple approaches to the same procedure are mutually exclusive of one another and should not be reported separately.

For example, both a vaginal hysterectomy and abdominal hysterectomy should not be reported separately.

10. If a procedure utilizing one approach fails and is converted to a procedure utilizing a different approach, only the completed procedure may be reported. For example, if a laparoscopic hysterectomy is converted to an open hysterectomy, only the open hysterectomy procedure code may be reported.

11. If a laparoscopic procedure fails and is converted to an open procedure, the physician should not report a diagnostic laparoscopy in lieu of the failed laparoscopic procedure. For example, if a laparoscopic cholecystectomy is converted to an open cholecystectomy, the physician should not report the failed laparoscopic cholecystectomy nor a diagnostic laparoscopy.

12. If a diagnostic endoscopy is the basis for and precedes an open procedure, the diagnostic endoscopy is separately reportable with modifier -58. However, the medical record must document the medical reasonableness and necessity for the diagnostic endoscopy. A scout endoscopy to assess anatomic landmarks and extent of disease is not separately reportable with an open procedure. When an endoscopic procedure fails and is converted to another surgical procedure, only the completed surgical procedure may be reported. The endoscopic procedure is not separately reportable with the completed surgical procedure.

13. Treatment of complications of primary surgical procedures is separately reportable with some limitations. The global surgical package for an operative procedure includes all intra-operative services that are normally a usual and necessary part of the procedure. Additionally the global surgical package includes all medical and surgical services required of the surgeon during the postoperative period of the surgery to treat complications that do not require return to the operating room. Thus, treatment of a complication of a primary surgical procedure is not separately reportable (1) if it represents usual and necessary care in the operating room during the procedure or (2) if it occurs postoperatively and does not require return to the operating room. For example, control of hemorrhage is a usual and necessary component of a surgical procedure in the operating room and is not separately reportable. Control of postoperative hemorrhage is also not separately reportable unless the patient must be returned to the operating room for treatment. In the latter case, the control of hemorrhage may be separately reportable with modifier -78.

D. Evaluation and Management (E&M) Services

Medicare Global Surgery Rules define the rules for reporting evaluation and management (E&M) services with procedures covered by these rules. This section summarizes some of the rules.

All procedures on the Medicare Physician Fee Schedule are assigned a Global period of 000, 010, 090, XXX, YYY, or ZZZ. The global concept does not apply to XXX procedures. The global period for YYY procedures is defined by the Carrier (A/B MAC processing practitioner service claims). All procedures with a global period of ZZZ are related to another procedure, and the applicable global period for the ZZZ code is determined by the related procedure.

Since NCCI edits are applied to same day services by the same provider to the same beneficiary, certain Global Surgery Rules are applicable to NCCI. An E&M service is separately reportable on the same date of service as a procedure with a global period of 000, 010, or 090 under limited circumstances.

If a procedure has a global period of 090 days, it is defined as a major surgical procedure. If an E&M is performed on the same date of service as a major surgical procedure for the purpose of deciding whether to perform this surgical procedure, the E&M service is separately reportable with modifier –57. Other E&M services on the same date of service as a major surgical procedure are included in the global payment for the procedure and are not separately reportable. NCCI does not contain edits based on this rule because Medicare Carriers (A/B MACs processing practitioner service claims) have separate edits.

If a procedure has a global period of 000 or 010 days, it is defined as a minor surgical procedure. The decision to perform a minor surgical procedure is included in the payment for the minor surgical procedure and should not be reported separately as an E&M service. However, a significant and separately identifiable E&M service unrelated to the decision to perform the minor surgical procedure is separately reportable with modifier -25. The E&M service and minor surgical procedure do not require different diagnoses. If a minor surgical procedure is performed on a new patient, the same rules for reporting E&M services apply. The fact that the patient is "new" to the provider is not sufficient alone to justify reporting an E&M service on the same date of service as a minor surgical procedure. NCCI does contain some edits based on these principles, but the Medicare Carriers (A/B MACs processing practitioner service claims) have separate edits. Neither the NCCI nor Carriers (A/B MACs processing practitioner service claims) have all possible edits based on these principles.

Example: If a physician determines that a new patient with head trauma requires sutures, confirms the allergy and immunization status, obtains informed consent, and performs the repair, an E&M service is not separately reportable. However, if the physician also performs a medically reasonable and necessary full neurological examination, an E&M service may be separately reportable.

Procedures with a global surgery indicator of "XXX" are not covered by these rules. Many of these "XXX" procedures are performed by physicians and have inherent pre-procedure, intra-procedure, and post-procedure work usually performed each time the procedure is completed. This work should never be reported as a separate E&M code. Other "XXX" procedures are not usually performed by a physician and have no physician work relative value units associated with them. A physician should never report a separate E&M code with these procedures for the supervision of others performing the procedure or for the interpretation of the procedure. With most "XXX" procedures, the physician may, however, perform a significant and separately identifiable E&M service on the same date of service which may be reported by appending modifier -25 to the E&M code. This E&M service may be related to the same diagnosis necessitating performance of the "XXX" procedure but cannot include any work inherent in the "XXX" procedure, supervision of others performing the "XXX" procedure, or time for interpreting the result of the "XXX" procedure. Appending modifier -25 to a significant, separately identifiable E&M service when performed on the same date of service as an "XXX" procedure is correct coding.

E. Modifiers and Modifier Indicators

1. The AMA *CPT Manual* and CMS define modifiers that may be appended to HCPCS/CPT codes to provide additional information about the services rendered. Modifiers consist of two alphanumeric characters.

Modifiers may be appended to HCPCS/CPT codes only if the clinical circumstances justify the use of the modifier. A modifier should not be appended to a HCPCS/CPT code solely to bypass an NCCI edit if the clinical circumstances do not justify its use. If the Medicare program imposes restrictions on the use of a modifier, the modifier may only be used to bypass an NCCI edit if the Medicare restrictions are fulfilled.

Modifiers that may be used under appropriate clinical circumstances to bypass an NCCI edit include:

Anatomic modifiers: E1-E4, FA, F1-F9, TA, T1-T9, LT, RT, LC, LD, RC
Global surgery modifiers: -25, -58, -78, -79
Other modifiers: -27, -59, -91

It is very important that NCCI-associated modifiers only be used when appropriate. In general these circumstances relate to separate patient encounters, separate anatomic sites or separate specimens. (See subsequent discussion of modifiers in this section.) Most edits involving paired organs or structures (e.g., eyes, ears, extremities, lungs, kidneys) have modifier indicators of "1" because the two codes of the code pair edit may be reported if performed on the contralateral organs or structures. Most of these code pairs should not be reported with NCCI-associated modifiers when performed on the ipsilateral organ or structure unless there is a specific coding rationale to bypass the edit. The existence of the NCCI edit indicates that the two codes generally cannot be reported together unless the two corresponding procedures are performed at two separate patient encounters or two separate anatomic locations. However, if the two corresponding procedures are performed at the same patient encounter and in contiguous structures, NCCI-associated modifiers generally should not be utilized.

The appropriate use of most of these modifiers is straight-forward. However, further explanation is provided about modifiers -25, -58, and -59. Although modifier -22 is not a modifier that bypasses an NCCI edit, its use is occasionally relevant to an NCCI edit and is discussed below.

a) **Modifier -22:** Modifier -22 is defined by the *CPT Manual* as an "Increased Procedural Services." This modifier should not be reported routinely but only when the service(s) performed is(are) substantially more extensive than the usual service(s) included in the procedure described by the HCPCS/CPT code reported.

Occasionally a provider may perform two procedures that should not be reported together based on an NCCI edit. If the edit allows use of NCCI-associated modifiers to bypass it and the clinical circumstances justify use of one of these modifiers, both services may be reported with the NCCI-associated modifier. However, if the NCCI edit does not allow use of NCCI-associated modifiers to bypass it and the procedure qualifies as an unusual procedural service, the physician may report the column one HCPCS/CPT code of the NCCI edit with modifier -22. The Carrier (A/B MAC processing practitioner service claims) may then evaluate the unusual procedural service to determine whether additional payment is justified.

For example, CMS limits payment for CPT code 69990 (microsurgical techniques, requiring use of operating microscope . . .) to procedures listed in the Internet-Only Manual (IOM) (*Claims Processing Manual,* Pub. 100-4, 12-§20.4.5). If a physician reports CPT code 69990 with two other CPT codes and one of the codes is not on this list, an NCCI edit with the code not on the list will prevent payment for CPT code 69990. Claims processing systems do not determine which procedure is linked with CPT code 69990. In situations such as this, the physician may submit his claim to the local carrier (A/B MAC processing practitioner service claims) for readjudication appending modifier 22 to the CPT code. Although the carrier (A/B MAC processing practitioner service claims) cannot override an NCCI edit that does not allow use of NCCI-associated modifiers, the carrier (A/B MAC processing practitioner service claims) has discretion to adjust payment to include use of the operating microscope based on modifier 22.

b) **Modifier -25:** The *CPT Manual* defines modifier -25 as a "significant, separately identifiable evaluation and management service by the same physician on the same day of the procedure or other service." Modifier -25 may be appended to an evaluation and management (E&M) CPT code to indicate that the E&M service is significant and separately identifiable from other services reported on the same date of service. The E&M service may be related to the same or different diagnosis as the other procedure(s).

Modifier -25 may be appended to E&M services reported with minor surgical procedures (global period of 000 or 010 days) or procedures not covered by global surgery rules (global indicator of XXX). Since minor surgical procedures and XXX procedures include pre-procedure, intra-procedure, and post-procedure work inherent in the procedure, the provider should not report an E&M service for this work. Furthermore, Medicare Global Surgery rules prevent the reporting of a separate E&M service for the work associated with the decision to perform a minor surgical procedure whether the patient is a new or established patient.

c) **Modifier -58:** Modifier -58 is defined by the *CPT Manual* as a "staged or related procedure or service by the same physician during the postoperative period." It may be used to indicate that a procedure was followed by a second procedure during the post-operative period of the first procedure. This situation may occur because the second procedure was planned prospectively, was more extensive than the first procedure, or was therapy after a diagnostic surgical service. Use of modifier -58 will bypass NCCI edits that allow use of NCCI-associated modifiers.

If a diagnostic endoscopic procedure results in the decision to perform an open procedure, both procedures may be reported with modifier -58 appended to the HCPCS/CPT code for the open procedure. However, if the endoscopic procedure preceding an open procedure is a "scout" procedure to assess anatomic landmarks and/or extent of disease, it is not separately reportable.

Diagnostic endoscopy is never separately reportable with another endoscopic procedure of the same organ(s) when performed at the same patient encounter. Similarly, diagnostic laparoscopy is never separately reportable with a surgical laparoscopic procedure of the same body cavity when performed at the same patient encounter.

If a planned laparoscopic procedure fails and is converted to an open procedure, only the open procedure may be reported. The failed laparoscopic procedure is not separately reportable. The NCCI contains many, but not all, edits bundling laparoscopic procedures into open procedures. Since the number of possible code combinations bundling a laparoscopic procedure into an open procedure is much greater than the number of such edits in NCCI, the principle stated in this paragraph is applicable regardless of whether the selected code pair combination is included in the NCCI tables. A provider should not select laparoscopic and open HCPCS/CPT codes to report because the combination is not included in the NCCI tables.

d) **Modifier -59:** Modifier -59 is an important NCCI-associated modifier that is often used incorrectly. For the NCCI its primary purpose is to indicate that two or more procedures are performed at different anatomic sites or different patient encounters. It should only be used if no other modifier more appropriately describes the relationships of the two or more procedure codes. The *CPT Manual* defines modifier -59 as follows:

Modifier -59: Distinct Procedural Service: Under certain circumstances, the physician may need to indicate that a procedure or service was distinct or independent from other services performed on the same day. Modifier -59 is used to identify procedures/services that are not normally reported together, but are appropriate under the circumstances. This may represent a different session or patient encounter, different procedure or surgery, different site or organ system, separate incision/excision, separate lesion, or separate injury (or area of injury in extensive injuries) not ordinarily encountered or performed on the same day by the same physician. However, when another already established modifier is appropriate, it should be used rather than modifier -59. Only if no more descriptive modifier is available, and the use of modifier -59 best explains the circumstances, should modifier -59 be used.

NCCI edits define when two procedure HCPCS/CPT codes may not be reported together except under special circumstances. If an edit allows use of NCCI-associated modifiers, the two procedure codes may be reported together if the two procedures are performed at different anatomic sites or different patient encounters. Carrier (A/B MAC processing practitioner service claims) processing systems utilize NCCI-associated modifiers to allow payment of both codes of an edit. Modifier -59 and other NCCI-associated modifiers should NOT be used to bypass an NCCI edit unless the proper criteria for use of the modifier are met. Documentation in the medical record must satisfy the criteria required by any NCCI-associated modifier used.

Some examples of the appropriate use of modifier -59 are contained in the individual chapter policies.

One of the common misuses of modifier -59 is related to the portion of the definition of modifier -59 allowing its use to describe "different procedure or surgery." The code descriptors of the two codes of a code pair edit consisting of two surgical procedures or two diagnostic procedures usually represent different procedures or surgeries. The edit indicates that the two procedures/surgeries cannot be reported together if performed at the same anatomic site and same patient encounter. The provider cannot use modifier -59 for such an edit based on the two codes being different procedures/surgeries. However, if the two procedures/surgeries are performed at separate anatomic sites or at separate patient encounters on the same date of service, modifier -59 may be appended to indicate that they are different procedures/surgeries on that date of service.

An exception to this general principle about misuse of modifier -59 applies to some code pair edits consisting of a surgical procedure and a diagnostic procedure. If the diagnostic procedure precedes the surgical procedure and is the basis on which the decision to perform the surgical procedure is made, the two procedures may be reported with modifier -59 appended to the column two HCPCS/CPT code under appropriate circumstances. However, if the diagnostic procedure is an inherent component of the surgical procedure, it cannot be reported separately. If the diagnostic procedure follows the surgical procedure at the same patient encounter, modifier -59 may be utilized if appropriate.

Use of modifier -59 to indicate different procedures/surgeries does not require a different diagnosis for each HCPCS/CPT coded procedure/surgery. Additionally, different diagnoses are not adequate criteria for use of modifier -59. The HCPCS/CPT codes remain bundled unless the procedures/surgeries are performed at different anatomic sites or separate patient encounters.

From an NCCI perspective, the definition of different anatomic sites includes different organs or different lesions in the same organ. However, it does not include treatment of contiguous structures of the same organ. For example, treatment of the nail, nail bed, and adjacent soft tissue constitutes treatment of a single anatomic site. Treatment of posterior segment structures in the ipsilateral eye constitutes treatment of a single anatomic site. Arthroscopic treatment of a shoulder injury in adjoining areas of the ipsilateral shoulder constitutes treatment of a single anatomic site.

Example: The column one/column two code edit with column one CPT code 38221 (bone marrow biopsy) and column two CPT code 38220 (bone marrow, aspiration only) includes two distinct procedures when performed at separate anatomic sites or separate patient encounters. In these circumstances, it would be acceptable to use modifier -59. However, if both 38221 and 38220 are performed through the same skin incision at the same patient encounter which is the usual practice, modifier -59 should NOT be used. Although CMS does not allow separate payment for CPT code 38220 with CPT code 38221 when bone marrow aspiration and biopsy are performed through the same skin incision at a single patient encounter, CMS does allow separate payment for HCPCS level II code G0364 (bone marrow aspiration performed with bone marrow biopsy through same incision on the same date of service) with CPT code 38221 under these circumstances.

2. Each NCCI edit has an assigned modifier indicator. A modifier indicator of "0" indicates that NCCI-associated modifiers cannot be used to bypass the edit. A modifier indicator of "1" indicates that NCCI-associated modifiers may be used to bypass an edit under appropriate circumstances. A modifier indicator of "9" indicates that the edit has been deleted, and the modifier indicator is not relevant.
3. Modifiers -76 ("repeat procedure or service by same physician") and -77 ("repeat procedure by another physician") are not NCCI-associated modifiers. Use of either of these modifiers does not bypass an NCCI edit.

F. Standard Preparation/Monitoring Services for Anesthesia

With few exceptions anesthesia HCPCS/CPT codes do not specify the mode of anesthesia for a particular procedure. Regardless of the mode of anesthesia, preparation and monitoring services are not separately reportable with anesthesia service HCPCS/CPT codes when performed in association with the anesthesia service. However, if the provider of the anesthesia service performs one or more of these services prior to and unrelated to the anticipated anesthesia service or after the patient is released from the anesthesia practitioner's postoperative care, the service may be separately reportable with modifier -59.

G. Anesthesia Service Included in the Surgical Procedure

Under the CMS Anesthesia Rules, with limited exceptions, Medicare does not allow separate payment for anesthesia services performed by the physician who also furnishes the medical or surgical service. In this case, payment for the anesthesia service is included in the payment for the medical or surgical procedure. For example, separate payment is not allowed for the physician's performance of local, regional, or most other anesthesia including nerve blocks if the physician also performs the medical or surgical procedure. However, Medicare allows separate reporting for moderate conscious sedation services (CPT codes 99143-99145) when provided by same physician performing a medical or surgical procedure except for those procedures listed in Appendix G of the *CPT Manual*.

CPT codes describing anesthesia services (00100-01999) or services that are bundled into anesthesia should not be reported in addition to the surgical or medical procedure requiring the anesthesia services if performed by the same physician. Examples of improperly reported services that are bundled into the anesthesia service when anesthesia is provided by the physician performing the medical or surgical procedure include introduction of needle or intracatheter into a vein (CPT code 36000), venipuncture (CPT code 36410), intravenous infusion/injection (CPT codes 96360-96368, 96374-96376) or cardiac assessment (e.g., CPT codes 93000-93010, 93040-93042). However, if these services are not related to the delivery of an anesthetic agent, or are not an inherent component of the procedure or global service, they may be reported separately.

H. HCPCS/CPT Procedure Code Definition

The HCPCS/CPT code descriptors of two codes are often the basis of an NCCI edit. If two HCPCS/CPT codes describe redundant services, they should not be reported separately. Several general principles follow:

1. A family of CPT codes may include a CPT code followed by one or more indented CPT codes. The first CPT code descriptor includes a semicolon. The portion of the descriptor of the first code in the family preceding the semicolon is a common part of the descriptor for each subsequent code of the family. For example,

   CPT code 70120 Radiologic examination, mastoids; less than three views per side
   CPT code 70130 Complete, minimum of three views per side

The portion of the descriptor preceding the semicolon ("Radiologic examination, mastoids") is common to both CPT codes 70120 and 70130. The difference between the two codes is the portion of the descriptors following the semicolon. Often as in this case, two codes from a family may not be reported separately. A physician cannot report CPT codes 70120 and 70130 for a procedure performed on ipsilateral mastoids at the same patient encounter. It is important to recognize, however, that there are numerous circumstances when it may be appropriate to report more than one code from a family of codes. For example, CPT codes 70120 and 70130 may be reported separately if the two procedures are performed on contralateral mastoids or at two separate patient encounters on the same date of service.

2. If a HCPCS/CPT code is reported, it includes all components of the procedure defined by the descriptor. For example, CPT code 58291 includes a vaginal hysterectomy with "removal of tube(s) and/or ovary(s)." A physician cannot report a salpingo-oophorectomy (CPT code 58720) separately with CPT code 58291.

3. CPT code descriptors often define correct coding relationships where two codes may not be reported separately with one another at the same anatomic site and/or same patient encounter. A few examples follow:
   a. A "partial" procedure is not separately reportable with a "complete" procedure.
   b. A "partial" procedure is not separately reportable with a "total" procedure.
   c. A "unilateral" procedure is not separately reportable with a "bilateral" procedure.
   d. A "single" procedure is not separately reportable with a "multiple" procedure.
   e. A "with" procedure is not separately reportable with a "without" procedure.
   f. An "initial" procedure is not separately reportable with a "subsequent" procedure.

I. *CPT Manual* and CMS Coding Manual Instructions

CMS often publishes coding instructions in its rules, manuals, and notices. Physicians must utilize these instructions when reporting services rendered to Medicare patients.

The *CPT Manual* also includes coding instructions which may be found in the "Introduction", individual chapters, and appendices. In individual chapters the instructions may appear at the beginning of a chapter, at the beginning of a subsection of the chapter, or after specific CPT codes. Physicians should follow *CPT Manual* instructions unless CMS has provided different coding or reporting instructions.

The American Medical Association publishes *CPT Assistant* which contains coding guidelines. CMS does not review nor approve the information in this publication. In the development of NCCI edits, CMS occasionally disagrees with the information in this publication. If a physician utilizes information from *CPT Assistant* to report services rendered to Medicare patients, it is possible that Medicare Carriers (A/B MACs processing practitioner service claims) and Fiscal Intermediaries may utilize different criteria to process claims.

J. CPT "Separate Procedure" Definition

If a CPT code descriptor includes the term "separate procedure", the CPT code may not be reported separately with a related procedure. CMS interprets this designation to prohibit the separate reporting of a "separate procedure" when performed with another procedure in an anatomically related region often through the same skin incision, orifice, or surgical approach.

A CPT code with the "separate procedure" designation may be reported with another procedure if it is performed at a separate patient encounter on the same date of service or at the same patient encounter in an anatomically unrelated area often through a separate skin incision, orifice, or surgical approach. Modifier -59 or a more specific modifier (e.g., anatomic modifier) may be appended to the "separate procedure" CPT code to indicate that it qualifies as a separately reportable service.

K. Family of Codes

The *CPT Manual* often contains a group of codes that describe related procedures that may be performed in various combinations. Some codes describe limited component services, and other codes describe various combinations of component services. Physicians must utilize several principles in selecting the correct code to report:

1. A HCPCS/CPT code may be reported if and only if all services described by the code are performed.
2. The HCPCS/CPT code describing the services performed should be reported. A physician should not report multiple codes corresponding to component services if a single comprehensive code describes the services performed. There are limited exceptions to this rule which are specifically identified in this Manual.
3. HCPCS/CPT code(s) corresponding to component service(s) of other more comprehensive HCPCS/CPT code(s) should not be reported separately with the more comprehensive HCPCS/CPT code(s) that include the component service(s).
4. If the HCPCS/CPT codes do not correctly describe the procedure(s) performed, the physician should report a "not otherwise specified" CPT code rather than a HCPCS/CPT code that most closely describes the procedure(s) performed.

L. More Extensive Procedure

The *CPT Manual* often describes groups of similar codes differing in the complexity of the service. Unless services are performed at separate patient encounters or at separate anatomic sites, the less complex service is included in the more complex service and is not separately reportable. Several examples of this principle follow:

1. If two procedures only differ in that one is described as a "simple" procedure and the other as a "complex" procedure, the "simple" procedure is included in the "complex" procedure and is not separately reportable unless the two procedures are performed at separate patient encounters or at separate anatomic sites.
2. If two procedures only differ in that one is described as a "simple" procedure and the other as a "complicated" procedure, the "simple" procedure is included in the "complicated" procedure and is not separately reportable unless the two procedures are performed at separate patient encounters or at separate anatomic sites.

3. If two procedures only differ in that one is described as a "limited" procedure and the other as a "complete" procedure, the "limited" procedure is included in the "complete" procedure and is not separately reportable unless the two procedures are performed at separate patient encounters or at separate anatomic sites.

4. If two procedures only differ in that one is described as an "intermediate" procedure and the other as a "comprehensive" procedure, the "intermediate" procedure is included in the "comprehensive" procedure and is not separately reportable unless the two procedures are performed at separate patient encounters or at separate anatomic sites.

5. If two procedures only differ in that one is described as a "superficial" procedure and the other as a "deep" procedure, the "superficial" procedure is included in the "deep" procedure and is not separately reportable unless the two procedures are performed at separate patient encounters or at separate anatomic sites.

6. If two procedures only differ in that one is described as an "incomplete" procedure and the other as a "complete" procedure, the "incomplete" procedure is included in the "complete" procedure and is not separately reportable unless the two procedures are performed at separate patient encounters or at separate anatomic sites.

7. If two procedures only differ in that one is described as an "external" procedure and the other as an "internal" procedure, the "external" procedure is included in the "internal" procedure and is not separately reportable unless the two procedures are performed at separate patient encounters or at separate anatomic sites.

M. Sequential Procedure

Some surgical procedures may be performed by different surgical approaches. If an initial surgical approach to a procedure fails and a second surgical approach is utilized at the same patient encounter, only the HCPCS/CPT code corresponding to the second surgical approach may be reported. If there are different HCPCS/CPT codes for the two different surgical approaches, the two procedures are considered "sequential", and only the HCPCS/CPT code corresponding to the second surgical approach may be reported. For example, a physician may begin a cholecystectomy procedure utilizing a laparoscopic approach and have to convert the procedure to an open abdominal approach. Only the CPT code for the open cholecystectomy may be reported. The CPT code for the failed laparoscopic cholecystectomy is not separately reportable.

N. Laboratory Panel

The *CPT Manual* defines organ and disease specific panels of laboratory tests. If a laboratory performs all tests included in one of these panels, the laboratory may report the CPT code for the panel or the CPT codes for the individual tests. If the laboratory repeats one of these component tests as a medically reasonable and necessary service on the same date of service, the CPT code corresponding to the repeat laboratory test may be reported with modifier -91 appended.

O. Misuse of Column Two Code with Column One Code

CMS manuals and instructions often describe groups of HCPCS/CPT codes that should not be reported together for the Medicare program. Edits based on these instructions are often included as misuse of column two code with column one code.

A HCPCS/CPT code descriptor does not include exhaustive information about the code. Physicians who are not familiar with a HCPCS/CPT code may incorrectly report the code in a context different than intended. The NCCI has identified HCPCS/CPT codes that are incorrectly reported with other HCPCS/CPT codes as a result of the misuse of the column two code with the column one code. If these edits allow use of NCCI-associated modifiers (modifier indicator of "1"), there are limited circumstances when the column two code may be reported on the same date of service as the column one code. Two examples follow:

1. Three or more HCPCS/CPT codes may be reported on the same date of service. Although the column two code is misused if reported as a service associated with the column one code, the column two code may be appropriately reported with a third HCPCS/CPT code reported on the same date of service. For example, CMS limits separate payment for use

of the operating microscope for microsurgical techniques (CPT code 69990) to a group of procedures listed in the online *Claims Processing Manual* (Chapter 12, Section 20.4.5 (Allowable Adjustments)). The NCCI has edits with column one codes of surgical procedures not listed in this section of the manual and column two CPT code of 69990. Some of these edits allow use of NCCI-associated modifiers because the two services listed in the edit may be performed at the same patient encounter as a third procedure for which CPT code 69990 is separately reportable.

2. There may be limited circumstances when the column two code is separately reportable with the column one code. For example, the NCCI has an edit with column one CPT code of 80061 (lipid profile) and column two CPT code of 83721 (LDL cholesterol by direct measurement). If the triglyceride level is less than 400 mg/dl, the LDL is a calculated value utilizing the results from the lipid profile for the calculation, and CPT code 83721 is not separately reportable. However, if the triglyceride level is greater than 400 mg/dl, the LDL may be measured directly and may be separately reportable with CPT code 83721 utilizing an NCCI-associated modifier to bypass the edit.

P. Mutually Exclusive Procedures

Many procedure codes cannot be reported together because they are mutually exclusive of each other. Mutually exclusive procedures cannot reasonably be performed at the same anatomic site or same patient encounter. An example of a mutually exclusive situation is the repair of an organ that can be performed by two different methods. Only one method can be chosen to repair the organ. A second example is a service that can be reported as an "initial" service or a "subsequent" service. With the exception of drug administration services, the initial service and subsequent service cannot be reported at the same patient encounter.

Pairs of HCPCS/CPT codes that are mutually exclusive of one another based either on the HCPCS/CPT code descriptors or the medical impossibility/improbability that the two procedures could be performed at the same patient encounter are identified as code pair edits in the Mutually Exclusive edit table.

Many edits in the Mutually Exclusive edit table allow the use of NCCI-associated modifiers. For example, the two procedures of a code pair edit may be performed at different anatomic sites (e.g., contralateral eyes) or separate patient encounters on the same date of service.

Q. Gender-Specific Procedures (formerly Designation of Sex)

The descriptor of some HCPCS/CPT codes includes a gender-specific restriction on the use of the code. HCPCS/CPT codes specific for one gender should not be reported with HCPCS/CPT codes for the opposite gender. For example, CPT code 53210 describes a total urethrectomy including cystostomy in a female, and CPT code 53215 describes the same procedure in a male. Since the patient cannot have both the male and female procedures performed, the two CPT codes cannot be reported together. Edits based on this principle are included in the Mutually Exclusive edit table since the two procedures of a code pair edit cannot be performed on the same patient.

R. Add-on Codes

Some codes in the *CPT Manual* are identified as "add-on" codes which describe a service that can only be reported in addition to a primary procedure. *CPT Manual* instructions specify the primary procedure code(s) for some add-on codes. For other add-on codes, the primary procedure code(s) is(are) not specified. When the *CPT Manual* identifies specific primary codes, the add-on code should not be reported as a supplemental service for other HCPCS/CPT codes not listed as a primary code.

Add-on codes permit the reporting of significant supplemental services commonly performed in addition to the primary procedure. By contrast, incidental services that are necessary to accomplish the primary procedure (e.g., lysis of adhesions in the course of an open cholecystectomy) are not separately reportable with an add-on code. Similarly, complications inherent in an invasive procedure occurring during the procedure are not separately reportable. For example, control of bleeding during an invasive procedure is considered part of the procedure and is not separately reportable.

In general, NCCI does not include edits with most add-on codes because edits related to the primary procedure(s) are adequate to prevent inappropriate payment for an add-on coded procedure. (i.e., if an edit prevents payment of the primary procedure code, the add-on code should not be paid.) However, NCCI does include edits for some add-on codes when coding edits related to the primary procedures must be supplemented. Examples include edits with add-on codes 69990 (microsurgical techniques requiring use of operating microscope) and 95920 (intraoperative neurophysiology testing).

HCPCS/CPT codes that are not designated as add-on codes should not be misused as an add-on code to report a supplemental service. A HCPCS/CPT code may be reported if and only if all services described by the CPT code are performed. A HCPCS/CPT code should not be reported with another service because a portion of the service described by the HCPCS/CPT code was performed with the other procedure. For example: If an ejection fraction is estimated from an echocardiogram study, it would be inappropriate to additionally report CPT code 78472 (cardiac blood pool imaging with ejection fraction) with the echocardiography (CPT code 93307). Although the procedure described by CPT code 78472 includes an ejection fraction, it is measured by gated equilibrium with a radionuclide which is not utilized in echocardiography.

S. Excluded Service

The NCCI does not address issues related to HCPCS/CPT codes describing services that are excluded from Medicare coverage or are not otherwise recognized for payment under the Medicare program.

T. Unlisted Procedure Codes

The *CPT Manual* includes codes to identify services or procedures not described by other HCPCS/CPT codes. These unlisted procedure codes are identified as XXX99 or XXXX9 codes and are located at the end of each section or subsection of the manual. If a physician provides a service that is not accurately described by other HCPCS/CPT codes, the service should be reported utilizing an unlisted procedure code. A physician should not report a CPT code for a specific procedure if it does not accurately describe the service performed. It is inappropriate to report the best fit HCPCS/CPT code unless it accurately describes the service performed, and all components of the HCPCS/CPT code were performed. Since unlisted procedure codes may be reported for a very diverse group of services, the NCCI generally does not include edits with these codes.

U. Modified, Deleted, and Added Code Pairs/Edits

Correct coding (column one/column two) and mutually exclusive edits are adopted after due consideration of Medicare policies including the principles described in the *National Correct Coding Initiative Policy Manual for Medicare Services*, HCPCS and *CPT Manual* code descriptors, *CPT Manual* coding guidelines, coding guidelines of national societies, standards of medical and surgical practice, current coding practice, and provider billing patterns. Since the NCCI is developed by CMS for the Medicare program, the most important consideration is CMS policy.

Prior to initial implementation of the NCCI in 1996, the proposed edits were evaluated by Medicare Part B Carrier Medical Directors, representatives of the American Medical Association's CPT Advisory Committee, and representatives of other national medical and surgical societies.

The NCCI undergoes continuous refinement with revised edit tables published quarterly. There is a process to address annual changes (additions, deletions, and modifications) of HCPCS/CPT codes and *CPT Manual* coding guidelines. Other sources of refinement are initiatives by the CMS central office and comments from the CMS regional offices, AMA, national medical, surgical, and other healthcare societies/organizations, Medicare contractor medical directors, providers, consultants, other third party payors, and other interested parties. Prior to implementing new edits, CMS generally provides a review and comment period to representative national organizations that may be impacted by the edits. However, there are situations when CMS thinks that it is prudent to implement edits prior to completion of the review and comment period. CMS Central Office evaluates the input from all sources and decides which edits are modified, deleted, or added each quarter.

V. Medically Unlikely Edits (MUEs)

To lower the Medicare Fee-For-Service Paid Claims Error Rate, CMS has established units of service edits referred to as Medically Unlikely Edit(s) (MUEs).

An MUE for a HCPCS/CPT code is the maximum number of units of service (UOS) under most circumstances allowable by the same provider for the same beneficiary on the same date of service. The ideal MUE value for a HCPCS/CPT code is the unit of service that allows the vast majority of appropriately coded claims to pass the MUE.

All practitioner claims submitted to Carriers (A/B MACs processing practitioner service claims), outpatient facilities services claims (Type of Bill 13X, 14X, 85X) submitted to Fiscal Intermediaries (A/B MACs processing facility claims), and supplier claims submitted to Durable Medical Equipment (DME) MACs are tested against MUEs. Each line of a claim is adjudicated separately against the MUE value for the HCPCS/CPT code reported on that line. If the unit of service on that line exceeds the MUE value, the entire line is denied.

Medicare Administrative Contractors (MACs) process claims previously submitted to Carriers and Fiscal Intermediaries (A/B MACs). MACs apply MUEs to the same types of claims.

If appropriate use of CPT modifiers (e.g., -59, -76, -77, -91, anatomic) causes the same HCPCS/CPT code to appear on separate lines of a claim, each line is separately adjudicated against the MUE value for that HCPCS/CPT code. Claims processing contractors have rules limiting use of these modifiers with some HCPCS/CPT codes.

UOS denied based on an MUE may be appealed.

The MUE value for each HCPCS/CPT code is based on one or more of the following considerations:

(1) Anatomic considerations may limit units of service based on anatomic structures. For example, the MUE value for an appendectomy is one since there is only one appendix.
(2) CPT code descriptors/CPT coding instructions in the *CPT Manual* may limit units of service. For example, a procedure described as the "initial 30 minutes" would have an MUE value of 1 because of the use of the term "initial".
(3) Edits based on established CMS policies may limit units of service. For example, the bilateral surgery indicator on the Medicare Physician Fee Schedule Database (MPFSDB) may limit reporting of bilateral procedures.
(4) The nature of an analyte may limit units of service and is in general determined by one of three considerations:
   a) The nature of the specimen may limit the units of service as for a test requiring a 24 hour urine specimen.
   b) The nature of the test may limit the units of service as for a test that requires 24 hours to perform.
   c) The physiology, pathophysiology, or clinical application of the analyte is such that a maximum unit of service for a single date of service can be determined. For example, the MUE for RBC folic acid level is one since the test would only be necessary once on a single date of service.
(5) The nature of a procedure/service may limit units of service and is in general determined by the amount of time required to perform a procedure/service (e.g., overnight sleep studies) or clinical application of a procedure/service (e.g., motion analysis tests).
(6) The nature of equipment may limit units of service and is in general determined by the number of items of equipment that would be utilized (e.g., cochlear implant or wheelchair).
(7) Clinical judgment considerations are based on input from numerous physicians and certified coders.
(8) Submitted claims data (100%) from a six month period is utilized.

HCPCS J code and drug related C and Q code MUEs are based on prescribing information and 100% claims data for a six month period of time. Utilizing the prescribing information the highest total daily dose for each drug was determined. This dose and its corresponding units of service were evaluated against paid and submitted claims data. Some of the guiding principles utilized in developing these edits are as follows:

(1) If the prescribing information defined a maximum daily dose, this value was used to determine the MUE value. For some drugs there is an absolute maximum daily dose. For others there is a maximum "recommended" or "usual" dose. In the latter of the two cases, the daily dose calculation was evaluated against claims data.

(2) If the maximum daily dose calculation is based on actual body weight, a dose based on a weight range of 110-150 kg was evaluated against the claims data. If the maximum daily dose calculation is based on ideal body weight, a dose based on a weight range of 90-110 kg was evaluated against claims data. If the maximum daily dose calculation is based on body surface area (BSA), a dose based on a BSA range of 2.4-3.0 square meters was evaluated against claims data.

(3) For "as needed" (PRN) drugs and drugs where maximum daily dose is based on patient response, prescribing information and claims data were utilized to establish MUE values.

(4) Published off label usage of a drug was considered for the maximum daily dose calculation.

The first MUEs were implemented January 1, 2007. Additional MUEs are added on a quarterly basis on the same schedule as NCCI updates. Prior to implementation proposed MUEs are sent to numerous national healthcare organizations for a sixty day review and comment period.

Some A/B MACs allow providers to report repetitive services performed over a range of dates on a single line of a claim with multiple units of service. If a provider reports services in this fashion, the provider should report the "from date" and "to date" on the claim line. Contractors are instructed to divide the units of service reported on the claim line by the number of days in the date span and round to the nearest whole number. This number is compared to the MUE value for the code on the claim line.

Suppliers billing services to the DME MACs typically report some HCPCS codes for supply items for a period exceeding a single day. The DME MACs have billing rules for these codes. For some codes the DME MACs require that the "from date" and "to date" be reported. The MUEs for these codes are based on the maximum number of units of service that may be reported for a single date of service. For other codes the DME MACs permit multiple days' supply items to be reported on a single claim line where the "from date" and "to date" are the same. The DME MACs have rules allowing supply items for a maximum number of days to be reported at one time for each of these types of codes. The MUE values for these codes are based on the maximum number of days that may be reported at one time. As with all MUEs, the MUE value does not represent a utilization guideline. Suppliers should not assume that they may report units of service up to the MUE value on each date of service. Suppliers may only report supply items that are medically reasonable and necessary.

A denial of services due to an MUE is a coding denial, not a medical necessity denial. A provider/supplier may not issue an Advanced Beneficiary Notice of Noncoverage (ABN) in connection with services denied due to an MUE and cannot bill the beneficiary for units of service denied based on an MUE.

Most MUE values are set so that a provider or supplier would only very occasionally have a claim line denied. If a provider encounters a code with frequent denials due to the MUE, or frequent use of a CPT modifier to bypass the MUE, the provider or supplier should consider the following: (1) Is the HCPCS/CPT code being used correctly? (2) Is the unit of service being counted correctly? (3) Are all reported services medically reasonable and necessary? and (4) Why does the provider's or supplier's practice differ from national patterns? A provider or supplier may choose to discuss these questions with the local Medicare contractor or a national healthcare organization whose members frequently perform the procedure.

Most MUE values are published on the CMS MUE webpage (http://www.cms.hhs.gov/ NationalCorrectCodInitEd/08_MUE.asp#TopOfPage). However, some MUE values are not published and are confidential. These values should not be published in oral or written form by any party that acquires one or more of them.

MUEs are not utilization edits. Although the MUE value for some codes may represent the commonly reported units of service (e.g., MUE of "1" for appendectomy), the usual units of service for many HCPCS/CPT codes is less than the MUE value. Claims reporting units of service less than the MUE value may be subject to review by claims processing contractors, Program Safeguard Contractors (PSCs), Zoned Program Integrity Contractors (ZPICs), Recovery Audit Contractors (RACs), and Department of Justice (DOJ).

Since MUEs are coding edits rather than medical necessity edits, claims processing contractors may have units of service edits that are more restrictive than MUEs. In such cases, the more restrictive claims processing contractor edit would be applied to the claim. Similarly, if the MUE is more restrictive than a claims processing contractor edit, the more restrictive MUE would apply.

A provider, supplier, healthcare organization, or other interested party may request reconsideration of an MUE value for a HCPCS/CPT code. A written request proposing an alternative MUE with rationale may be sent to:

> National Correct Coding Initiative
> Correct Coding Solutions, LLC
> P.O. Box 907
> Carmel, IN 46082-0907
> Fax: 317-571-1745

FIGURE CREDITS

1. From Little J et al: *Dental management of the medically compromised patient,* ed 7, St. Louis, 2008, Mosby. *(Courtesy Medtronic, Minneapolis)*
2. From Roberts J, Hedges J: *Clinical procedures in emergency medicine,* ed 4, Philadelphia, 2004, Saunders.
3. Modified from Grosfeld J et al: *Pediatric surgery,* ed 6, Philadelphia, 2006, Mosby.
4. Modified from Hsu J, Michael J, Fisk J: *AAOS atlas of orthoses and assistive devices,* ed 4, Philadelphia, 2008, Mosby.
5. From Dionne R, Phero J, Becker D: *Management of pain and anxiety in the dental office,* ed 1, St. Louis, 2002, Saunders.
6. Modified from Roberts J, Hedges J: *Clinical procedures in emergency medicine,* ed 4, St. Louis, 2004, Saunders.
7. From Auerbach P: *Wilderness medicine,* ed 5, Philadelphia, 2007, Mosby. (Courtesy Black Diamond Equipment, Ltd.)
8. Modified from Abeloff M et al: *Clinical oncology,* ed 3, Philadelphia, 2004, Churchill Livingstone.
9. *(Original to book).*
10. Modified from Duthie E, Katz P, Malone M: *Practice of geriatrics,* ed 4, Philadelphia, 2007, Saunders.
11. Modified from Roberts J, Hedges J: *Clinical procedures in emergency medicine,* ed 4, St. Louis, 2004, Saunders.
12. From Albert R, Spiro S, Jett J: *Clinical respiratory medicine,* ed 2, Philadelphia, 2004, Mosby.
13. From Young A, Proctor D: *Kinn's the medical assistant,* ed 9, St. Louis, 2003, Saunders.
14. From Bonewit-West K: *Clinical procedures for medical assistants,* ed 5, Philadelphia, 2000, WB Saunders.
15. From Young A, Proctor D: *Kinn's the medical assistant,* ed 9, St. Louis, 2003, Saunders.
16. From Roberts J, Hedges J: *Clinical procedures in emergency medicine,* ed 4, St. Louis, 2004, Saunders.
17. From Yeo: *Shackelford's surgery of the alimentary tract,* ed 6, Philadelphia, 2007, Saunders.
18. Redrawn from Bragg D, Rubin P, Hricak H: *Oncologic imaging,* ed 2, 2002, Saunders.
19. From Lewis S, Bain B, Bates I: *Dacie and Lewis practical haematology,* ed 10, Philadelphia, 2006, Churchill Livingstone.
20. From Rutherford: *Vascular surgery,* ed 6, Philadelphia, 2005, Saunders.
21. From Roberts J, Hedges J: *Clinical procedures in emergency medicine,* ed 4, St. Louis, 2004, Saunders. *(Courtesy Atrium Medical Corp., Hudson, NH 03051)*
22. **A** From Auerbach P: *Wilderness medicine,* ed 5, Philadelphia, 2007, Mosby. **B** Modified from Hsu J, Michael J, Fisk J: *AAOS atlas of orthoses and assistive devices,* ed 4, Philadelphia, 2008, Mosby.
23. Modified from Lusardi M, Nielsen C: *Orthotics and prosthetics in rehabilitation,* ed 2, St. Louis, 2006, Butterworth-Heinemann.
24. Modified from Lusardi M, Nielsen C: *Orthotics and prosthetics in rehabilitation,* ed 2, St. Louis, 2006, Butterworth-Heinemann.
25. Modified from Lusardi M, Nielsen C: *Orthotics and prosthetics in rehabilitation,* ed 2, St. Louis, 2006, Butterworth-Heinemann.
26. From Buck C: *The next step, advanced medical coding 2009 edition,* St. Louis, 2008, Saunders.
27. From Lusardi M, Nielsen C: *Orthotics and prosthetics in rehabilitation,* ed 2, St. Louis, 2006, Butterworth-Heinemann.
28. From Hsu J, Michael J, Fisk J: *AAOS atlas of orthoses and assistive devices,* ed 4, Philadelphia, 2008, Mosby.
29. Modified from Hsu J, Michael J, Fisk J: *AAOS atlas of orthoses and assistive devices,* ed 4, Philadelphia, 2008, Mosby.
30. Modified from Hsu J, Michael J, Fisk J: *AAOS atlas of orthoses and assistive devices,* ed 4, Philadelphia, 2008, Mosby.
31. From Hsu J, Michael J, Fisk J: *AAOS atlas of orthoses and assistive devices,* ed 4, Philadelphia, 2008, Mosby.
32. From Lusardi M, Nielsen C: *Orthotics and prosthetics in rehabilitation,* ed 2, St. Louis, 2006, Butterworth-Heinemann.
33. From Lusardi M, Nielsen C: *Orthotics and prosthetics in rehabilitation,* ed 2, St. Louis, 2006, Butterworth-Heinemann.

34. Modified from Lusardi M, Nielsen C: *Orthotics and prosthetics in rehabilitation,* ed 2, St. Louis, 2006, Butterworth-Heinemann.

35. From Hsu J, Michael J, Fisk J: *AAOS atlas of orthoses and assistive devices,* ed 4, Philadelphia, 2008, Mosby.

36. *(Original to book.)*

37. From Lusardi M, Nielsen C: *Orthotics and prosthetics in rehabilitation,* ed 2, St. Louis, 2006, Butterworth-Heinemann.

38. Modified from Hsu J, Michael J, Fisk J: *AAOS atlas of orthoses and assistive devices,* ed 4, Philadelphia, 2008, Mosby.

39. From Canale S: *Campbell's operative orthopaedics,* ed 10, St. Louis, 2003, Mosby.

40. Modified from Canale S: *Campbell's operative orthopaedics,* ed 10, St. Louis, 2003, Mosby.

41. From Lusardi M, Nielsen C: *Orthotics and prosthetics in rehabilitation,* ed 2, St. Louis, 2006, Butterworth-Heinemann.

42. From Lusardi M, Nielsen C: *Orthotics and prosthetics in rehabilitation,* ed 2, St. Louis, 2006, Butterworth-Heinemann.

43. Modified from Lusardi M, Nielsen C: *Orthotics and prosthetics in rehabilitation,* ed 2, St. Louis, 2006, Butterworth-Heinemann.

44. From Lusardi M, Nielsen C: *Orthotics and prosthetics in rehabilitation,* ed 2, St. Louis, 2006, Butterworth-Heinemann. *(Courtesy Michael Curtain)*

45. Modified from Lusardi M, Nielsen C: *Orthotics and prosthetics in rehabilitation,* ed 2, St. Louis, 2006, Butterworth-Heinemann.

46. Modified from Bland K, Copeland E: *The breast: comprehensive management of benign and malignant disorders,* ed 3, St. Louis, 2004, Saunders.

47. From Cummings C et al: *Cummings otolaryngology: head and neck surgery,* ed 4, Philadelphia, 2005, Mosby.

48. Modified from Cummings C et al: *Cummings otolaryngology: head and neck surgery,* ed 4, Philadelphia, 2005, Mosby.

49. From Weinzweig J: *Plastic surgery secrets,* ed 1, Philadelphia, 1999, Hanley & Belfus, p 543.

50. Modified from Mann D: *Heart failure: a companion to Braunwald's heart disease,* ed 1, Philadelphia, 2004, Saunders.

51. Modified from Roberts J, Hedges J: *Clinical procedures in emergency medicine,* ed 4, Philadelphia, 2004, Saunders.

52. From Yanoff M, Duker J: *Ophthalmology,* ed 2, St. Louis, 2004, Mosby.

53. From Feldman M, Friedman L, Brandt L: *Sleisenger and Fordtran's gastrointestinal and liver disease,* ed 8, Philadelphia, 2006, Saunders.

54. From Katz V et al: *Comprehensive gynecology,* ed 5, Philadelphia, 2007, Mosby.

55. From Young A, Proctor D: *Kinn's the medical assistant,* ed 10, St. Louis, 2007, Saunders.

56. Modified from National Kidney and Urologic Diseases Information Clearinghouse: (http://kidney.niddk.nih.gov/kudiseases/pubs/stonesadults/index.htm)

57. From Yanoff M, Duker J: *Ophthalmology,* ed 2, St. Louis, 2004, Mosby.